To Howard,

This is nothing compared to what you should do for neurosurgery, but look over & critique

Let's go!

Jeff M.

New York

Oct 23, 2006

Laparoscopic Colorectal Surgery

Second Edition

Laparoscopic Colorectal Surgery

Second Edition

Jeffrey W. Milsom, MD
Chief, Section of Colon and Rectal Surgery, Professor of Surgery, Department of Surgery, Weill Medical College of Cornell University, New York Presbyterian Hospital, New York, New York

Bartholomäus Böhm, MD
Chief of Surgery, HELIOS Klinifum Erfurt, Klinik für Allgemeain-und Viszeralchirurgie, Erfurt, Germany

Kiyokazu Nakajima, MD, PhD
Assistant Professor, Department of Surgery, Osaka University Graduate School of Medicine, Osaka, Japan; Department of Surgery, Osaka Rosai Hospital, Osaka, Japan

Editors

With 306 Illustrations, 8 in Full Color

Illustrations by Yuko Tonohira

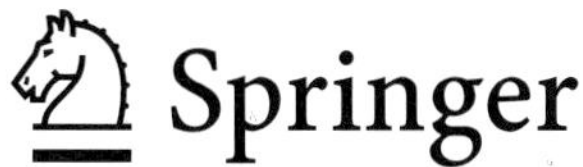

Jeffrey W. Milsom, MD
Chief, Section of Colon and Rectal Surgery
Professor of Surgery
Department of Surgery
Weill Medical College of Cornell University
New York Presbyterian Hospital
New York, NY
USA

Bartholomäus Böhm, MD
Chief of Surgery
HELIOS Klinifum Erfurt
Klinik für Allgemeain-und Viszeralchirurgie
Erfurt, Germany

Kiyokazu Nakajima, MD, PhD
Assistant Professor
Department of Surgery
Osaka University Graduate School of Medicine
Osaka, Japan
and
Department of Surgery
Osaka Rosai Hospital
Osaka, Japan

Library of Congress Control Number: 2005930723

ISBN-10: 0-387-28254-8
ISBN-13: 978-0387-28254-1

Printed on acid-free paper.

Printed in the United States of America. (BS/MVY)

9 8 7 6 5 4 3 2 1

springer.com

Preface to the Second Edition

Tempus fugit! The year 1990 was the first year for reports of laparoscopic methods to treat colonic diseases. It has been a full decade since the first edition of this book, *Laparoscopic Colorectal Surgery,* was published (1996). It was not apparent in the mid-1990s whether this specialized field would become accepted in major departments of surgery, but now it is one of the most rapidly growing areas of laparoscopic surgery. Surgeons experienced in these techniques are being aggressively recruited by medical centers around the world, and most patients are now querying their surgeons about "laparoscopic colon surgery."

Laparoscopic colorectal surgery was initially one of the slowest areas of development in minimally invasive surgery because it is often complex, multi-quadrant, and frequently involves the treatment of a malignancy. Any one of these reasons were sufficient to give great consideration to the use of a new technique, hence the careful evaluation of laparoscopic colorectal surgery has been a *modus operandi* for surgeons around the world.

This second edition of *Laparoscopic Colorectal Surgery* differs from the first in several important aspects. The first edition was wholly written by Jeffrey Milsom and Bartholomäus Böhm. The second edition now calls on a new coeditor, Kiyokazu Nakajima, a talented surgeon from Osaka University in Japan. This means that the book has major representation in thought and content from three major regions of the world: Asia (Dr. Nakajima, Japan), Europe (Dr. Böhm, Germany), and North America (Dr. Milsom, United States).

We now have authors who have written many of the most important sections of the book and are experienced surgeons, actively performing laparoscopic colorectal procedures: from Asia (Drs. Riichiro Nezu, Junji Okuda, Masahiko Watanabe, and Yoshifumi Inoue), Europe (Drs. Joel LeRoy, Hermann Kessler, Wolfgang Schwenk, Michael Seifert, Steffen Minner), and the United States (Drs. Toyooki Sonoda, Peter Marcello, Richard L. Whelan, Martin Weiser, Sang Lee, and Alessandro Fichera). Again, our intent was to create a diverse, world-wide approach to this continuously evolving field. At the end of each their chapters, we (JM, BB, KN) have added personal comments relating to the chapter.

Thirdly, our new artist, Yuko Tonohira, has added appreciable value to the book in many ways. Ms. Tonohira is a recent art major graduate from Parsons School of Design in New York City. She adds geographic depth to the book as well, since she grew up in Hokkaido, Japan. In addition to her artistic talent, she spent countless hours in the operating rooms, anatomical laboratories, and alongside the authors, learning laparoscopic colorectal surgery firsthand. Her skills and dedication have resulted in a fantastic and uniform presentation for the book, since all illustrations are her work.

The contents of the book have also changed appreciably since the first edition. All chapters have been rewritten. We have shortened some of the basic discussions about such topics as electrosurgery and optics, and have inserted a new chapter on laparoscopic colorectal anatomy (Chapter 7), expanded the number of procedures chapters (including "hand-assisted" chapters). Significantly, we have *added a whole section* on the evidence base in colorectal surgery (Chapter 11).

All in all, we believe that this book should permit the reader an opportunity to quickly grasp most of the important concepts of the field of laparoscopic colorectal surgery. Each of the procedures in Chapters 8, 9, and 10 are set up to be independent of each other, so the busy surgeon may look at the particular operation she/he is about to perform and grasp the "essentials".

We do not believe laparoscopic colorectal surgery will replace open surgery for all indications, but increasingly over the next decade, laparoscopic methods will improve and become important means to treat colorectal diseases requiring surgery. We no longer fear its use in malignancies, when done by experienced surgeons under the right circumstances, and its use in other indications will certainly continue to grow. Likewise, the technologies used in this field will also develop and greatly improve our capabilities.

As in the first edition of this book, our intent is to expose new information and methods to improve the outcomes of our patients following major colorectal surgery. We do not feel our text demonstrates the only approaches to the laparoscopic treatments of colon and rectal disease. Finally, we sincerely hope that the material presented here will fuel discussions in the surgical community, leading to further improvements in the care of patients around the world.

Jeffrey W. Milsom, MD
Bartholomäus Böhm, MD
Kiyokazu Nakajima, MD, PhD

Preface to the First Edition

Inspired by the potential of laparoscopic surgery to bring substantial advantages to patients requiring colorectal surgery, we began to apply laparoscopic techniques to colorectal surgery in late 1991. Now, several years later, this field is still in its early phases of development. Whereas laparoscopic techniques for biliary surgery quickly evolved, such techniques for effective and efficient colorectal surgery have developed slowly. Quantifying the value of laparoscopy in this field also has been difficult. Nonetheless, the possible advantages of removing a section of the intestine with safe anastomosis, all done through small "keyhole" incisions, is so tantalizing that we have continued to focus most of our research in this direction. Our philosophy has been that questions about laparoscopic colorectal surgery must be assessed in a methodical and stepwise manner. After such surgery is demonstrated to be feasible and beneficial in the short term, we plan to delve into studies assessing the underlying mechanisms of these benefits, as well as the long-term benefits.

Using animals initially in 1991, we attempted to establish basic techniques for intestinal resection and anastomosis because, at the time, the literature contained few useful descriptions. We encountered significant challenges, even in animal models in which the mesentery is thin and the bowel is relatively mobile. Early successes in the animal models led us to attempt some simple procedures for benign diseases in humans. This transition was challenging and stimulated us to pursue further training in animals and fresh human cadaver models. Many challenges presented the opportunity to pursue true gastrointestinal surgical research. We toiled over the design of techniques, procedures, and new instruments that might permit more effective laparoscopic colorectal surgery. We especially wanted to define standard techniques for curative surgery in colorectal cancer, seeking to resect along the same anatomic boundaries as in conventional surgery.

Throughout this book, we emphasize a team approach to laparoscopic surgery. Our belief in such an approach evolved naturally from many hours of working together – in the animal laboratory; operating theaters; and sitting across from each other at a table with pens, papers, and books scattered in front of us. We believe the discipline of laparoscopic colorectal surgery currently to be too intricate and complex to be taken up by the solitary surgeon performing an occasional laparoscopic intestinal operation with personnel not trained specifically in these techniques.

Laparoscopic colorectal surgery will not be an overnight revolution, as occurred with laparoscopic cholecystectomy. The techniques and teamwork that we have struggled to develop are just beginning to reap rewards – only now are laparoscopic procedures often performed in the same time as conventional procedures, with less blood loss and surgical trauma. However, only concerted, sustained efforts already begun in the surgical research laboratories of medical centers and instrument manufacturers along with adherence to the highest professional and patient care goals, will make laparoscopic techniques a genuine and substantial advance in colorectal surgery.

We eagerly present of laparoscopic colorectal surgery – equipment, instrumentation, methods of dissection and suturing, and our ideas concerning education in the field. The book details a personal approach to the surgical treatment of colorectal disease. We do not believe that our approach is the only way to achieve the goals of laparoscopic colorectal surgery and we sincerely hope our text will fuel discussion in the surgical community that will produce further advances.

Jeffrey W. Milsom, MD
Bartholomäus Böhm, MD

Acknowledgments

We wish to acknowledge that many individuals and corporations donated time and expertise in the construction of this second edition.

From the corporate world, Olympus was our staunchest supporter, giving time and energy to the project over several years. In particular we owe much to the talented engineer Mr. Hiroyuko Mino of Olympus Surgical America. His expertise is definitely appreciated for much of the technical aspects of the book. From Tyco (United States Surgical), Stryker, and Applied Medical we also owe much to the understanding and promotion of this book.

In the construct of the manuscript, Koiana Trencheva RN helped us in many tangible and intangible ways, including in the organization of the nascent research and publication efforts of our Section of Colon & Rectal Surgery section at Weill Medical College, Cornell University in New York.

Our new artist, Yuko Tonohira, shares in the direct production of the book, but she also helped in multiple aspects beyond the art work, and for this we are truly grateful.

Our editor at Springer, Beth Campbell, patiently encouraged us throughout the writing of this second edition, and she also supported us in many intangible ways. We owe her many thanks as well.

There are others who should be mentioned . . . to JI, JN, and also to PS, PK, and Dr. SA, you have helped us in many, many ways in making this book a reality, and Dr. Milsom in particular thanks you.

Finally, we again appreciate how such an endeavor, on top of our clinical and administrative responsibilities, has deprived our families of valuable time together. Thus our deepest gratitude goes to our wives Susan, Anke, and Ayako, and our children Alexandra, Geoffrey, Annika, and Stephanie, and Dr. Nakajima's parents Naomi (father) and Haruko. Without their support, it would not have been worthwhile to pursue the second edition.

Jeffrey W. Milsom, MD
Bartholomäus Böhm, MD
Kiyokazu Nakajima, MD, PhD

Contents

Contributors

Bartholomäus Böhm, MD, Chief of Surgery, HELIOS Klinifum Erfurt, Klinik für Allgemeain-und Viszeralchirurgie, Erfurt, Germany

Joseph Carter, MD, Assistant professor, New York University Medical Center, New York, NY, USA

Panchali Dhar, MD, Assistant Professor of Anesthesiology, Weill Medical College of Cornell University, New York, NY, USA

Alessandro Fichera, MD, FACS, FASCRS, Assistant Professor, Department of Surgery, University of Chicago, Chicago, IL, USA

Margaret Henri, MD, Staff Surgeon, Hôpital Maisonneuve-Rosemont; Clinical Professor, Department of Surgery, Universite de Montréal , Montréal, Canada

Yoshifumi Inoue, MD, Department of Surgery, Kawasaki Hospital, Kobe, Japan

Hermann Kessler, MD, PhD, Assistant Professor, University of Erlangen, Erlangen, Germany

Sang Lee, MD, Assistant Professor of Surgery, Section of Colon and Rectal Surgery, Department of Surgery, Weill Medical College of Cornell University, New York, NY, USA

Joel Leroy, MD, FRCS (London), Chief of Laparoscopic Colorectal Unit in the Department of General, Digestive and Endocrine Surgery of Professor Jacques Marescaux, Hopitaux Universitaires de Strasbourg; Co-director IRCAD/EITS (European Institute of TeleSurgery), Strasbourg Cedex, France

Peter W. Marcello, MD, Staff Surgeon, Department of Colon and Rectal Surgery, Lahey Clinic, Burlington, MA, USA

Jacques Marescaux, MD, FRCS, FACS, Chairman of the Department of General, Digestive and Endocrine Surgery of Professor Jacques Marescaux, Hopitaux Universitaires de Strasbourg; Chairman, IRCAD/EITS (European Institute of TeleSurgery), Strasbourg Cedex, France

Jeffrey W. Milsom, MD, Chief, Section of Colon and Rectal Surgery, Professor of Surgery, Department of Surgery, Weill Medical College of Cornell University, New York Presbyterian Hospital, New York, NY USA

Steffen Minner, MD, HELIOS Klinifum Erfurt, Klinik für Allgemeain-und Viszeralchirurgie, Erfurt, Germany

Kiyokazu Nakajima, MD, PhD, Assistant Professor, Department of Surgery, Osaka University Graduate School of Medicine, Osaka, Japan; Department of Surgery, Osaka Rosai Hospital, Osaka, Japan

Riichiro Nezu, MD, PhD, Department of Surgery, Osaka Rosai Hospital, Osaka, Japan

Junji Okuda, MD, Associate Professor and Chief Staff, Department of General and Gastroenterological Surgery, Osaka Medical College, Osaka, Japan

Francesco Rubino, MD, Assistant Professor, Universita Catholica of Roma, Policlinico Gemelli, IRCAD/EITS (European Institute of Tele-Surgery), Strasbourg Cedex, France

Wolfgang Schwenk, MD, Professor of Surgery, Department of General, Visceral, Vascular and Thoracic Surgery, Charité University of Medicine Berlin Campus Mitte, Berlin, Germany

Michael Seifert, MD, HELIOS Klinifum Erfurt, Klinik für Allgemeain-und Viszeralchirurgie, Erfurt, Germany

Toyooki Sonoda, MD, Assistant Professor of Surgery, Section of Colon and Rectal Surgery, Department of Surgery, Weill Medical college of Cornell University, New York, NY, USA

Nobuhiko Tanigawa, MD, Professor and Chairman, Department of General and Gastroenterological Surgery, Osaka Medical College, Osaka, Japan

Masahiko Watanabe, MD, FACS, Professor and Chairman, Department of Surgery, Kitasato University School of Medicine, Sagamihara, Japan

Martin R. Weiser, MD, Assistant Attending Surgeon, Memorial Sloan-Kettering Cancer Center, New York, NY, USA

Richard L. Whelan, MD, Associate Professor of Surgery, Chief, Section of Colon and Rectal Surgery Presbyterian Hospital Columbia University New York, NY, USA

James Yoo, MD, Section of Colon and Rectal Surgery, Department of Surgery, Weill Medical College of Cornell University, New York, NY, USA

Chapter 1

History of Laparoscopic Surgery

Kiyokazu Nakajima, Jeffrey W. Milsom, and Bartholomäus Böhm

Although laparoscopic surgery has transformed surgery only in the past two decades, its evolution is only the natural byproduct of the medical doctor's curiosity to directly visualize and treat surgical diseases. The earliest known attempts to look inside the living human body date from 460 to 375 BC, from the Kos school of medicine led by Hippocrates in Greece.[1,2] They described a rectal examination using a speculum remarkably similar to the instruments we use today. Similar specula were discovered in the ruins of Pompeii (70 AD) that were used to examine the vagina, the cervix, and the rectum, and obtain an inside view of the nose and ear.[1] The Babylonian Talmud written in 500 AD described a lead siphon, named "Siphophert," with a mouthpiece, which was bent inward and held a mechul (wooden drain).[1,3] The apparatus was introduced into the vagina and was used to differentiate between vaginal and uterine bleeding. During these early years ambient light was used.

The term "endoscopein" is attributed to Avicenna (Ibn Sina, 980–1037 AD) of Persia, although an Arabian physician, Albulassim (912–1013 AD), who placed a mirror in front of the exposed vagina, was the first to use reflected light as a source of illumination for an endoscopic examination. Giulio Caesare Aranzi in Venice (1530–1589) developed the first endoscopic light in 1587. He used the Benedictine monk Don Panuce's principle of the "camera obscura" for medical purposes – the rays of the sun coming through a hole in the window shutter were concentrated by a glass jar filled with marbles and then projected into the nostrils.[3]

In 1806, Bozzini looked inside the bladder using a man-made light source with an apparatus called the "Lichtleiter" (Table 1.1).[4] Bozzini envisioned and clearly described in his writings that endoscopy could someday be used as a diagnostic tool for the urethra, bladder, rectum, vagina, cervix, and pharynx as well as a surgical tool for endoscopic polypectomy or removal of bladderstones. He also surmised that endoscopy would augment understanding of the physiology and pathology of an organ if it could be visualized in vivo. His "Lichtleiter" used a candle as a light source and consisted of a light container,

Table 1.1. Chronology of important events in surgery

1806	Bozzini	"Lichtleiter" of Bozzini
1879	Nitze	Nitze cystoscope
1901	Kelling	Experimental laparoscopy in canine
1911	Jacobaeus	Laparoscopy in humans
1920	Orndoff	Sharp pyramidal trocar
1924	Zollikofer	Carbon dioxide pneumoperitoneum
1929	Kalk	Oblique scope and dual puncture technique
1938	Veress	Insufflation needle
1953	Hopkins	Rod-lens system
1967	Semm	Automatic insufflator
1985	Mühe	Laparoscopic cholecystectomy in humans
1986	Berci	Computer chip TV camera
1987	Mouret	Videolaparoscopic cholecystectomy
1991	Jacobs	Laparoscopic colectomy

mirrors, and tubes through which the light passed. As well as describing the "Lichtleiter" (Figure 1.1) in detail, he explained the difficulties of reflecting light through tubes, a problem that remained unsolved for another century.

Almost 50 years later, Desormeaux presented an improved endoscope to the Academy of Medicine of Paris. In 1853, he reported the use of a kerosene lamp as an external light source, equipped with a chimney vent and a concentrating mirror (Figure 1.2). "Endoscopy," a term coined by Desormeaux, remained crude for most of the 19th century because internal visualization remained relatively poor, and management of a light source dependent on combustion of fossil or

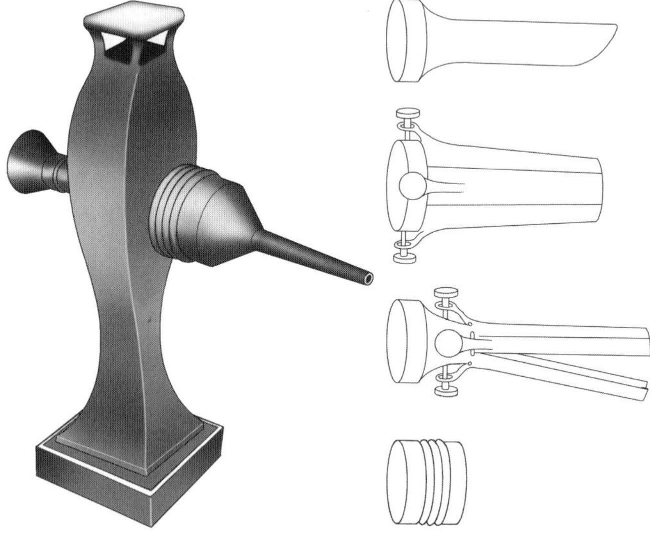

Figure 1.1. "Lichtleiter" of Bozzini (1806) with various attachments for different body orifices.

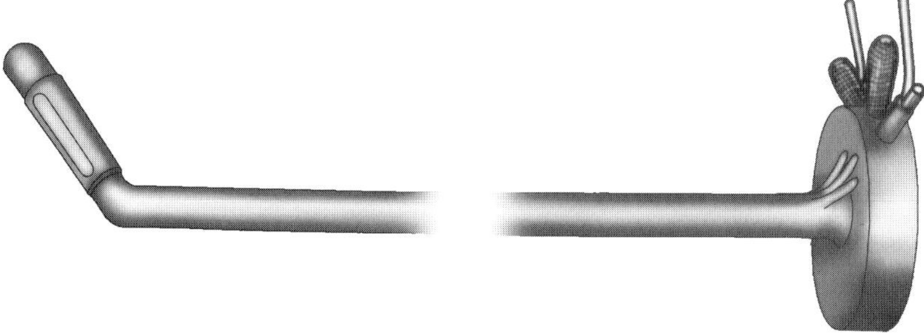

Figure 1.2. Desormeaux cystoscope (1853).

animal fuel was difficult. Nevertheless, Desormeaux described and conducted numerous investigations of the urethra and bladder.[5]

In 1867, the first internal light source was described by Bruck, a German dentist.[6] He examined the mouth using illumination provided by a loop of platinum wire connected to an electrical current. Because the wire generated intense heat, the loop was cumbersome and dangerous to use; consequently, Bruck's platinum loop never attained widespread popularity.

For most of the 19th century, cystoscopy was limited because endoscopes illuminated the interior of the bladder poorly, and they showed only a small part of the visualized object. In 1887, Nitze developed a cystoscope that dramatically overcame these major limitations.[7] To increase the intensity and extent of illumination, he placed a platinum wire powered by electricity at the tip of the cystoscope and cooled it by using a continuous stream of water through the cystoscope. Placing the light source at the tip not only increased the intensity of the light, but also was advantageous in that the light was directly coupled with the cystoscope, making the procedure much easier to perform because the light source moved with the cystoscope. Although having the light source at the tip of the endoscope widened the illuminated area, visualization was still limited until Nitze added a prismatic lens system to his cystoscope. With his newly designed instrument, which had a diameter of only 5 mm, he was able to adequately visualize an area the size of the human palm. Nitze also incorporated additional channels in his operating cystoscope through which ureteral probes could be passed. Together with Joseph Leiter, an instrument maker, they produced a commercial cystoscope that revolutionized cystoscopy and became the forerunner of modern cystoscopes and other endoscopes, including laparoscopes.

Subsequent to the invention of the incandescent lamp by Thomas Edison in 1880, Nitze and Leiter replaced the platinum wire with a light bulb in 1887 (Figure 1.3). Brenner further improved the cystoscope in 1889, building a small channel through the cystoscope for passing fluid into the bladder and for introducing ureteral catheters.

Boisseau de Rocher made the next important step in the development of modern endoscopes in 1889. He separated the ocular part of

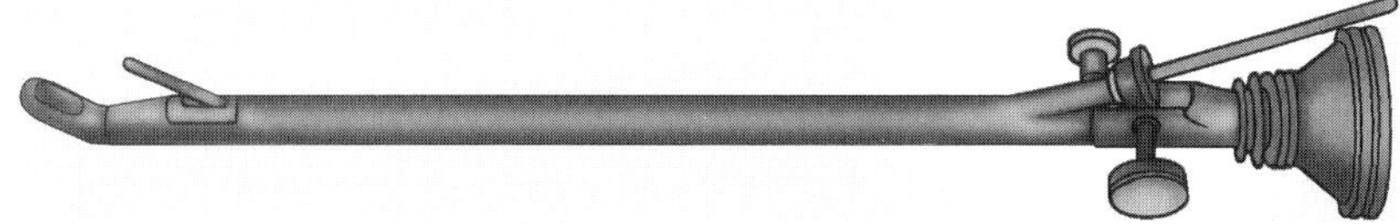

Figure 1.3. Nitze cystoscope (1887).

the cystoscope from the lamp-carrying beak by using a sheath through which multiple different telescopes could be introduced. This change allowed greater latitude of observation and manipulation through the cystoscope.

In 1902, the first actual laparoscopy, or endoscopic visualization of the peritoneal cavity, was reported by George Kelling, a surgeon from Dresden, Germany.[8] At the meeting of the German Biological and Medical Society in Hamburg in September 1901, he showed that laparoscopy could be performed in a canine model. He inserted a Nitze cystoscope into the peritoneal cavity of a living anesthetized dog and examined the viscera. The abdomen was insufflated with air filtered through a sterile cotton swab. He named the procedure "Kölioskopie." In the same year, a Russian gynecologist named Dimitri Ott independently described a technique for directly viewing the abdominal cavity in humans without an endoscope. He inspected the abdominal cavity with the help of a head mirror and a speculum introduced through a small anterior abdominal wall incision.

The first major series of laparoscopies in humans is attributed to H.C. Jacobeus. In 1910, Jacobeus reported 17 cases in which laparoscopy was accomplished using a Nitze cystoscope with "cold burning" lamps and a cannula with a valve system.[9] He also performed 20 examinations in human cadavers in which he evaluated the risk of injury to intraperitoneal structures. He achieved his first clinical experiences in patients with ascites because puncture of the abdominal cavity appeared to be easy and without risk of inadvertent injury to intraperitoneal viscera. By 1911, he had described 80 laparoscopies, with only one reported complication – a hemorrhage into the peritoneal cavity from a trocar incision.[10] With laparoscopy, he was able to recognize different kinds of liver diseases (cirrhosis, metastatic tumors, tuberculosis, and syphilis), gastric cancer, and "chronic" peritonitis.

In 1911, Bernheim, of the Johns Hopkins Medical School, reported on "organoscopy" using an ordinary proctoscope or cystoscope, with illumination from an electric headlight.[11] He made an incision in the epigastrium, inserted the scope, and inspected the viscera. He was probably the first surgeon to perform a type of laparoscopic-assisted operation: after finding nothing on "organoscopy," Bernheim drew "a part of the stomach out through the wound, made an incision in its anterior wall, and inserted the cystoscope directly into its cavity."

Roccavilla modified the method of illumination in 1914. He designed an instrument that permitted the source of light to remain outside the abdomen by reflecting the light through a trocar into the field of vision.[12]

To facilitate trocar insertion, Orndoff,[13] in 1920, used and described the pyramidal trocar point currently still in use. He reported diagnostic laparoscopies in 42 cases and described tuberculous peritonitis, extra-uterine pregnancy, salpingitis, and ovarian tumors. He was the first to stress that laparoscopy is a useful tool in diagnosing suspected post-operative hemorrhage in the peritoneal cavity.

The first automatic spring-loaded needle for initiating pneumoperitoneum was developed by Goetze in 1918.[14] He did not design the needle for laparoscopic visualization of the abdominal cavity but rather for insufflation of oxygen into the peritoneal cavity and to improve conventional plain abdominal X-ray techniques. By studying the heart rate and body temperature in 90 outpatients undergoing oxygen insufflation of the peritoneal cavity, he proved that an artificial pneumoperitoneum was not harmful or dangerous. He also defined the following contraindications for pneumoperitoneum: cardiac and pulmonary diseases, "meteorism," septic process in the peritoneal cavity, and extensive adhesions.

In 1924, W.E. Stone[15] wrote about "peritoneoscopy" in a canine model. He inserted a nasopharyngoscope through an incision in the abdominal wall and successfully completed diagnostic laparoscopies in 14 dogs. He preferred to use air insufflation instead of carbon dioxide because air insufflation did not require any special instruments. He also developed a rubber trocar gasket.

Otto Steiner,[16] unaware of the experiences of other researchers, also described in 1924 his technique of "abdominoscopy" using a cystoscope, trocar, and oxygen to insufflate the abdomen. In the same year, Zollikofer[17] first described the use of carbon dioxide gas to induce pneumoperitoneum. It quickly became the most popular distending gas because of its noncombustible properties as well as its rapid absorption after a procedure.

In 1925, Short[18] summarized the advantages of laparoscopy: "1.) It can be done without discomfort; 2.) the incision is so small that it is only necessary to keep the patient in bed for a day or two; 3.) very few special instruments are needed; 4.) it can be done at the patient's own house; and 5.) it is available when it would be dangerous to perform laparotomy."

Almost a quarter century after Kelling's initial report, an excellent review of previous experiences about "endoscopy of the abdomen" was given by Nadeau and Kampmeier[19] who also described their technique in detail as performed in three patients. They said the "appliances necessary for the performance of abdominoscopy are relatively few . . . a trocar and cannula, a cystoscope, . . . a no. 18 spinal puncture needle, a hypodermic syringe and needle, a small scalpel, and a small foot pump, rubber tubing, and connections for inflating the abdomen."

A number of important reports establishing laparoscopy as a valuable diagnostic tool were published by the German hepatologist Kalk,[20] who introduced a 45° lens system, and was the first to advocate the dual-trocar technique. This latter innovation led the way to the concept of operative laparoscopy. Kalk performed 100 laparoscopies in 4 years without any major complications and was able to diagnose various liver and gallbladder diseases, and stomach, pancreas, and renal cancer with his technique. His efforts proved that intraabdominal manipulation using laparoscopic techniques could be safely performed. He published 21 papers between 1929 and 1959 that established the use of laparoscopy to study and make accurate pathologic diagnoses of internal organs. Many authorities consider him to be the "father of modern laparoscopy."

One of the earliest reports of a therapeutic laparoscopy was in 1933, when Fervers[21] described laparoscopic lysis of adhesions. In his report, he also described the use of ureteral catheters passed through his endoscope to palpate the gallbladder for stones. In addition, while using "cold cautery" electrosurgery and insufflating the abdomen with oxygen, he described an explosion inside the peritoneal cavity with multiple audible "detonations" and "flames" visible through the abdominal wall. Laparoscopic inspection of the peritoneal cavity showed only minor injuries of the peritoneum, and the patient recovered fully after several days of observation without any additional treatment. Fervers thereafter wisely argued against use of oxygen in establishing pneumoperitoneum.

In 1937, Ruddock,[22] an internist from Los Angeles, California, reported 500 cases in which diagnostic laparoscopy was performed over a period of 4 years. He firmly established diagnostic laparoscopy as a safe procedure with very low morbidity. Injury of the intestine (stomach, small bowel, and colon) occurred in only eight patients (1.6%) in his series, and only one mortality occurred in a patient who died of hemorrhage after laparoscopic biopsy of the liver. Examinations were unsuccessful in only three patients (0.6%). He also described a biopsy forceps with electrosurgical capability to perform coagulation and tissue biopsy simultaneously. The tip of the biopsy forceps was designed so that it formed a cup containing the tissue when closed. In addition, Ruddock's patients did not experience postoperative intestinal paralysis after laparoscopy. After laparoscopy, his patients were permitted to resume eating meals without interruption. Since Ruddock's time, laparoscopy has remained the method of choice in diagnosing cases of undetermined ascites and tuberculous peritonitis, in assessing the operability of certain intraabdominal lesions, and whenever there is a question of intraabdominal metastases.

Until the 1930s, pneumoperitoneum was accomplished with a Goetze-style spring-loaded needle. In 1938, Veress[23] developed a modified spring-loaded needle to safely introduce air into the thoracic cavity. This needle, which now bears his name, is now commonly used to create pneumoperitoneum and remains almost unchanged since its invention.

A new era of endoscopy began in 1952 when Fourestier et al.[24] developed and described the "cold-light" fiberglass source that provided, at a low temperature, intense light through a quartz rod from the proximal to the distal end of the telescope. The physicist Hopkins introduced rod-shaped lenses as light transmitters with air lenses between the glass elements to further increase illumination. This design dramatically improved the resolution and contrast of the telescope in 1953.[25] Most currently used laparoscopes are designed according to the principles of the Hopkins lens system.

In the 1960s, the German gynecologist Semm,[26] one of the most innovative and productive researchers and clinicians in the field of laparoscopy, contributed several important innovations in laparoscopy: a controlled, automatic carbon dioxide insufflator, an irrigation system, the Roeder loop applicator, hook scissors, a tissue morcellator, and the pelvitrainer teaching model.

Up until the late 1970s, laparoscopic techniques were almost solely in the repertoire of gynecologists and internists. Surgeons of this era equated surgical prowess with large incisions (big surgeons: big incisions), and ignored these procedures largely. Until the early 1980s, laparoscopic visualization of the peritoneal cavity was restricted to the surgeon who held the scope. The introduction of elaborate "teaching scopes" that were connected to and branched away from the main endoscope enabled the assistant to view what the surgeon was seeing. Unfortunately, these scopes were cumbersome and ineffective when the surgeon and assistant had to coordinate actions. Thus, complex therapeutic operations were not possible using these scopes and, as a result, laparoscopy was unpopular and rarely used in general surgery during the 1970s and 1980s. The development of the computer-chip television camera allowed everyone in the operating room simultaneously to view the image generated by the laparoscope. Surgeons thereafter accelerated the technical advances of safe and improved therapeutic laparoscopy and introduced therapeutic laparoscopic procedures into the field of general surgery.

The first incidental laparoscopic appendectomy is credited to Semm in 1981[27] and the first laparoscopic cholecystectomy in humans to Mühe in 1985.[28] In March 1987, Philippe Mouret, in Lyon, France, removed a diseased gallbladder from a patient during a gynecologic laparoscopic procedure.[29] He clearly exposed the porta hepatis by forceful cephalad retraction of the gallbladder fundus, using a laparoscopic video camera. Shock and disbelief were the initial reactions when the report of the procedure was first presented at major national meetings in the United States in April 1989 (Society of American Gastrointestinal Endoscopic Surgeons, Louisville, Kentucky) and in May 1989 (American Society for Gastrointestinal Endoscopy, Washington DC). The following year, the largest lecture hall at the meeting of the American College of Surgeons in San Francisco was so full that surgeons were crowding in the entryways, craning their necks to get a view of the video presentations.

The advent of laparoscopic cholecystectomy was the single most important stimulus to the expansion of operative laparoscopy in surgery. Within a short time, various operative procedures have been performed laparoscopically including esophagectomy, selective or truncal vagotomy, abdominal cardiomyotomy, total or partial fundoplication, partial gastrectomy, gastrojejunostomy, splenectomy, adrenalectomy, choledocholithotomy, resection of liver metastases, and inguinal herniorrhaphy.[30]

The earliest report of laparoscopic colon resections was in 1991, wherein Moises Jacobs et al.[31] from Florida described their initial experience of "laparoscopic-assisted" colon resection in 20 patients. In the last 10 years, thousands of colorectal resections have been performed all over the world. Some very skillful surgeons have consistently introduced new surgical techniques with excellent outcomes and thus motivated other surgeons to apply these techniques to their patients. Every part of the large intestine colon has now been resected using laparoscopic methods. This chapter serves only as a prelude to the developments in laparoscopic colorectal surgery that are highlighted in the remainder of this book.

References

1. Gordon AG, Magos AL. The development of laparoscopic surgery. Baillieres Clin Obstet Gynaecol 1989;3:429–449.
2. Rosin D. History. In: Rosin D, ed. Minimal Access Medicine and Surgery. Oxford: Radcliffe Medical Press; 1993.
3. Semm K. The history of endoscopy. In: Vitale GC, Sanfilippo JS, Perissat J, eds. Laparoscopic Surgery: An Atlas for General Surgeons. Philadelphia: JB Lippincott; 1995.
4. Bozzini P. Lichtleiter, eine Erfindung zur Anschauung innerer Theile und Krankheiten. J Prakt Arzneikunde 1806;24:107–113.
5. Desormeaux AJ. Endoscope and its application to the diagnosis and treatment of affections of the genitourinary passage. Chicago Med J 1867.
6. Gunning JE. The history of laparoscopy. J Reprod Med 1974;12:222–225.
7. Nitze M. Beobachtungs- und Untersuchungsmethode für Harnröhre, Harnblase und Rektum. Wiener Mediz Wochenschr. 1879;29:651–652.
8. Kelling G. Ueber Oesophagoskopie, Gastroskopie und Kölioskopie. Münch Med Wochenschr 1902;49:21–24.
9. Jacobeus HC. Ueber die Möglichkeit die Zystoskopie bei Untersuchung seröser Höhlungen anzuwenden. Münch Med Wochenschr 1910;57: 2090–2092.
10. Kurze Uebersichtüber meine Erfahrungen mit der Laparo-thoraskopie. Münch Med Wochenschr 1911;58:2017–2019.
11. Bernheim BM. Organoscopy: cystoscopy of the abdominal cavity. Ann Surg 1911;53:764–767.
12. Roccavilla A. L'endoscopia delle grandi cavita sierose mediante un nuovo apparecchio ad illuminazione dirtta (laparo-toracoscopia diretta). La Riforma Medica 1914;30:991–995.
13. Orndorff BH. The peritoneoscope in diagnosis of diseases of the abdomen. J Radiol 1920;1:307–325.
14. Goetze O. Die Röntgendiagnostik bei gasgefüllter Bauchhöhle. Eine neue Methode. Münch Med Wochenschr 1918;65:1275–1280.
15. Stone WE. Intra-abdominal examination by the aid of the peritoneoscope. J Kan Med Soc. 1924;24:63–66.
16. Steiner OP. Abdominoscopy. Surg Gynecol Obstet 1924;38:266–269.
17. Zollikofer R. Zur Laparoskopie. Schweiz Med Wochenschr 1924;5: 264–265.
18. Short AR. The uses of coelioscopy. Br Med J 1925;3:254–255.
19. Nadeau OE, Kampmeier OF. Endoscopy of the abdomen: abdominoscopy. Surg Gynecol Obstet 1925;41:259–271.

20. Kalk H. Erfahrungen mit der Laparoskopie (Zugleich mit Beschreibung eines neuen Instrumentes). Zeitschr Klin Med 1929;111:303–348.
21. Fervers C. Die Laparoskopie mit dem Cystoskop. Mediz Klinik 1933;31:1042–1045.
22. Ruddock JC. Peritoneoscopy. Surg Gynecol Obstet 1937;65:623–639.
23. Veress J. Neues Instrument zur Ausführung von Brust- oder Bauchpunktionen und Pneumothoraxbehandlung. Deutsch Med Wochenschr 1938;40:1480–1481.
24. Fourestier M, Gladu A, Vulmiere J. Perfectionnements a l'endoscopie medicale. Realisation bronchoscopique. La Presse Medicale 1952;60:1292–1293.
25. Gow JG, Hopkins HH, Wallace DM, et al. The modern urological endoscope. In: Hopkins HH, ed. Handbook of Urological Endoscopy. Edinburgh: Churchill Livingstone; 1978.
26. Semm K. Operative Manual for Endoscopic Abdominal Surgery. Chicago: Thieme; 1987.
27. Semm K. Endoscopic appendectomy. Endoscopy 1983;15:59–64.
28. Mühe B. The first laparoscopic cholecystectomy. Langenbecks Arch Chir 1986;369:804.
29. Vitale GC, Cuschieri A, Perissat J. Guidelines for the future. In: Vitale GC, Sanfilippo JS, Perissat J, eds. Laparoscopic Surgery: An Atlas for General Surgeons. Philadelphia: JB Lippincott; 1995.
30. Lau WY, Leow CK, Li AK. History of endoscopic and laparoscopic surgery. World J Surg 1997;21:444–453.
31. Jacobs M, Verdeja JC, Goldstein HS. Minimally invasive colon resection (laparoscopic colectomy). Surg Laparosc Endosc 1991;1:144–150.

Chapter 2

Equipment and Instrumentation

Kiyokazu Nakajima, Jeffrey W. Milsom, and Bartholomäus Böhm

Equipment

Since the introduction of the first-generation videolaparoscope in 1986,[1] many technological improvements have followed. The main components of the laparoscopic surgical system, however, have remained the same: 1) an image processing system (a laparoscope coupled to a video camera, a light source, and a monitoring device), 2) a gas insufflator, and 3) a specialized set of instruments designed for the surgical procedures. All laparoscopic team members should have a basic working knowledge of the functions of these equipments and their various parts, to guarantee the most efficient and safe outcomes.

As for image processing, recording, and documentation, we are now in a transitional period from analog to digital systems.[2,3] Although this "digital revolution" may not affect the entire laparoscopic system immediately, we should prepare ourselves for the future changes. This chapter outlines the currently available laparoscopic equipment and discusses what kind of equipment is advisable for colorectal practice.

Laparoscopes

The majority of currently available rigid laparoscopes are derived from the Hopkins-type rod-shaped lens system developed in 1952.[4] This lens system, which is contained in the core of the laparoscope, focuses and transmits the light from the abdomen to the camera. Modern versions consist of rod-shaped lenses, air-filled spaces between the lenses, and additional lenses that compensate for peripheral distortion. Optical fibers at the periphery of the scope transmit light from the light source into the abdomen. Alternatively, the rod lens relay system can be eliminated by incorporating miniaturized charge-coupled devices mounted distally on the top of the scope.

Currently, various kinds of laparoscopes are available with different diameters and viewing angles (Figure 2.1). We generally recommend using a standard 10-mm laparoscope for routine colorectal procedures,

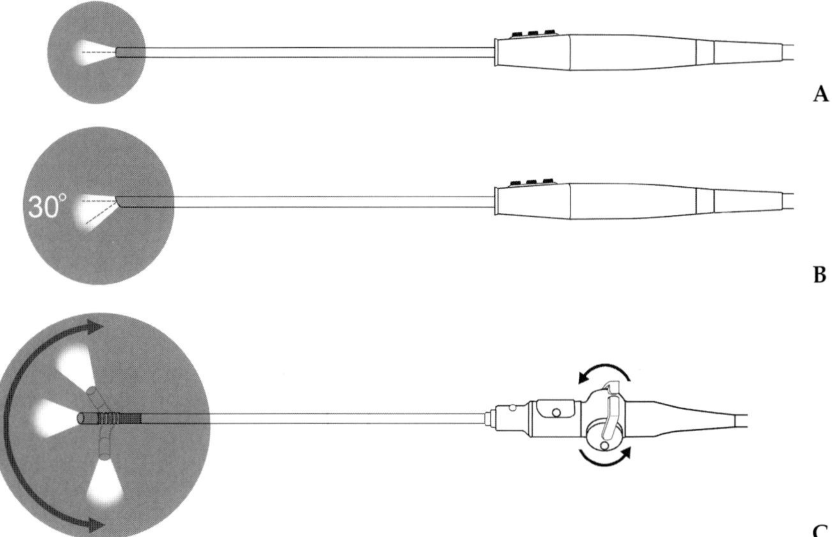

Figure 2.1. Visual field of the laparoscope depending on the viewing angle: **A** 0°, **B** 30°, **C** laparoscope with a flexible tip.

because its wide overview images are optimal for multiquadrant colorectal procedures. Miniature laparoscopes (less than 5 mm in diameter), if combined with a powerful light source and high-quality video camera, may have a certain role in selected procedures, such as biopsy, lysis of adhesion, and stoma creation. As for viewing angles, a straight-viewing (0°) laparoscope allows more intuitive perspective than an oblique-viewing laparoscope.[5] We believe, however, that colorectal laparoscopic surgeons should familiarize themselves with the oblique-viewing (i.e., 30°) laparoscope, because of its greater flexibility in viewing fixed and deeper structures that may be blind to 0° laparoscopes (e.g., the splenic flexure or deep pelvic structures).

Some surgeons have advocated theoretical advantages of the three-dimensional (3-D) viewing system in laparoscopic surgery.[6] Currently, various types of 3-D laparoscopy have become available. In general, 3-D laparoscopes provide a separate image to each eye through a variety of display mechanisms, thereby creating the perception of a stereoscopic image with true depth cues. These images may be viewed on a video monitor with specially shuttered glasses, or through a head-mounted display. The binocular information provided by such 3-D viewing systems could potentially increase the precision of laparoscopic task performance while decreasing performance time. Previous studies have shown that a 3-D system can enhance performance of surgeons in laboratory settings; however, its role in laparoscopic surgery has yet to be demonstrated. Future improvements in resolution, illumination, and ease of use, is required to widely spread this technology, and there will be an expanding role for 3-D imaging in the future.

Cameras

With the most widely used laparoscopic video systems, a video camera (so-called "camera head") is connected to the eyepiece of a traditional rod-lens laparoscope (Figure 2.2). The basis of the video camera is the 1/3–1/2 or 2/3-inch solid-state charge-coupled device (CCD), in which the imaging chip is composed of a thin, flat silicon wafer.[7] The CCD matrix comprises a rectangular grid of horizontal and vertical rows of minute image sensors called "pixels." The resolution of the CCD is determined by the number of pixels its surface can accommodate. "Single-chip" cameras use a color mosaic on a single CCD chip with 400,000 to 440,000 pixels, to detail the red, green, and blue (RGB) component of the image. However, "three-chip (3-CCD)" cameras use prisms that split the image into three paths that then pass through RGB filters into three separate CCD chips, providing a red, green, or blue signal, respectively. The resolving power of 3-CCD cameras becomes greater compared with single-chip cameras, because one CCD chip is used for each primary color, whereas only one CCD chip is used for all colors in single-chip cameras.

The information sent from CCD chips is then processed by a camera control unit (CCU) for transmission to the monitor (Figure 2.3). The majority of current CCUs have several different types of analog outputs: composite, Y/C (or S), and RGB signals. RGB signals provide the best image available with today's technology.[2] Latest model of CCU has a digital output and can be connected to a digital flat-screen display without any degradation of image quality during data transmission (as described later in this chapter).

One of the emerging technologies is the "chip-on-a-stick" videolaparoscope.[7] This system has a single 3 × 4 mm CCD chip mounted at the distal end of the laparoscope directly behind the objective lens system (Figure 2.4). With this technology (so called "direct" videoendoscopy), the conventional rod-lens system is no longer necessary, and the image-quality degradation caused by the traditional optical relay system is virtually eliminated. Although it is still technically challenging to

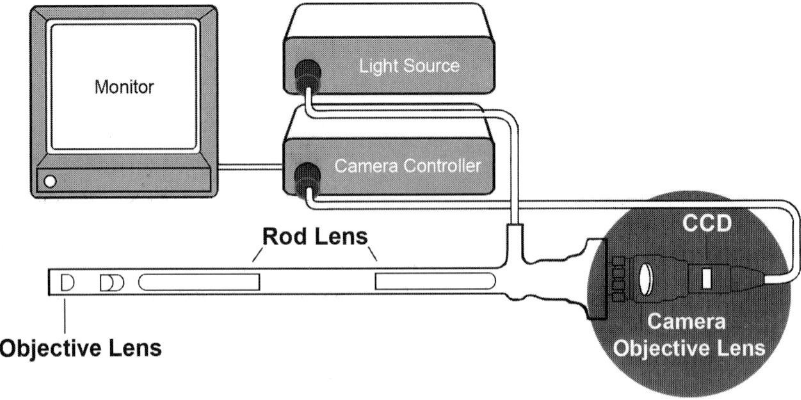

Figure 2.2. Camera head connected to conventional rod-lens laparoscope.

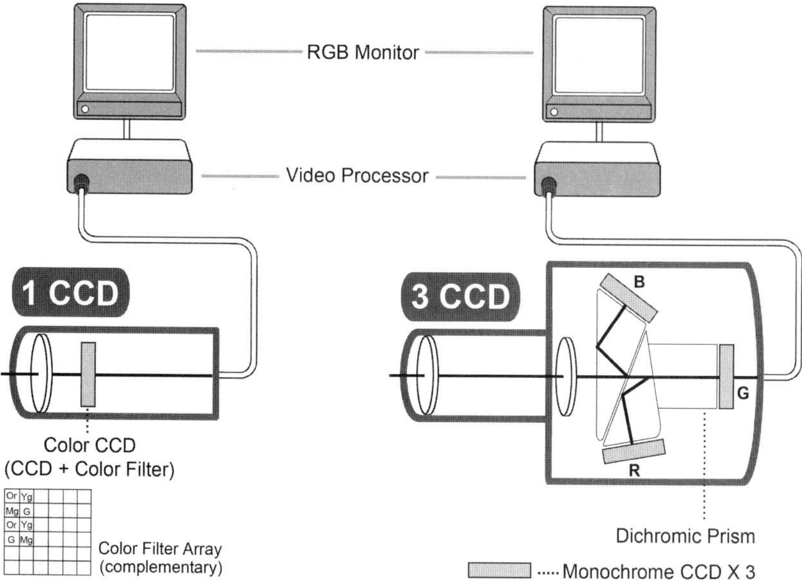

Figure 2.3. CCD, video processor, and monitor.

mount 3 CCD chips or a high-performance single CCD chip in the restricted space of the distal tip, the image quality is at least as good as "indirect" videoendoscopy. With this "chip-on-a-stick" technology, it has become possible to make the distal portion of the laparoscope either rigid or flexible. Several products have been put on the market, and our current preference is a videolaparoscope with this technology (EndoEye®; Olympus, Tokyo, Japan). One major need is to produce a laparoscope that eliminates manual lens cleaning.

Light Sources

Currently, the high-intensity xenon light source (300 W) is most widely used for advanced laparoscopic procedures, because it provides supe-

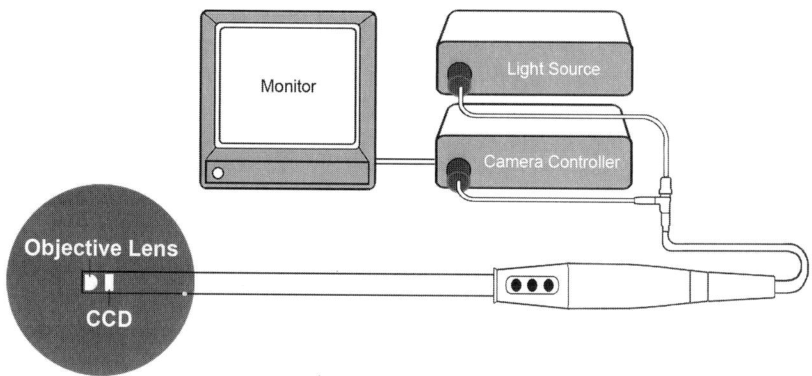

Figure 2.4. A chip-on-a-stick videolaparoscope (Endoalpha™, Olympus, Tokyo, Japan).

rior illumination compared with older halogen light sources.[8] Its performance, however, is not fully appreciated if the bulb and/or light guide (light transmission cable) has been deteriorated. The light bulb should be inspected and changed at regular intervals. The surgical team should recognize that the light guide contains bundles of fragile fiberglass cables. If damaged, it may seriously limit the quantity of light transmitted.

Monitors

The resolution of the monitor screen on which the image is displayed is determined by the number of lines exhibited.[9] With regular single-chip cameras, the resolution of a standard analog cathode ray tube (CRT) video screen ranges between 450 and 600 horizontal lines. Three-chip cameras provide an enhanced video image with 700 horizontal lines of resolution. However, the measured resolution in the monitor screen may be only marginally improved over that of a single-chip camera.[7] To fully appreciate the high-quality images of three-chip cameras, a monitor with higher resolution is required.

The digital flat-screen display (liquid crystal display: LCD) is still in a relatively early stage of development. The flat LCD screens are lighter in weight than CRT screens, therefore can be placed more easily in an optimal position for the operating surgeon to manipulate and observe in one axis. The resolution varies according to the pixel number and the size of the screen. The signal input is digital, therefore images can be displayed on the screen without any degradation in quality. Although this technology seems promising, the actual image on the digital screen has not surpassed the "analog" image generated by good laparoscope with three-chip video camera and recent CRT monitor in an RGB formation.[2] With future technological improvements, we believe the use of digital LCD screens will become mainstream in surgical laparoscopy.

Another promising technology is a head-mounted display. Early head-mounted displays suffered from low resolution and were bulky and uncomfortable to wear. However, more recent designs offer higher resolution, lighter weight, and a cordless design. The surgeon can stand in a comfortable operating position with an unobstructed view of both the operative field and the video image.[10] If head-mounted displays are used exclusively, the need for monitor booms can be eliminated, and the operating environment can be further simplified.

Recording Devices

Photodocumentation is becoming an important byproduct of laparoscopic surgery. With recent digital technological evolution, it has become easy and practical to capture still images digitally from any laparoscopic procedures. Images can be printed out in theater, but can be also transferred by a variety of storage systems to a computer and recorded in various digital formats (Figure 2.5). Those images, once stored electrically, can be easily transferred to an electric patient record (database) and utilized for various purposes.

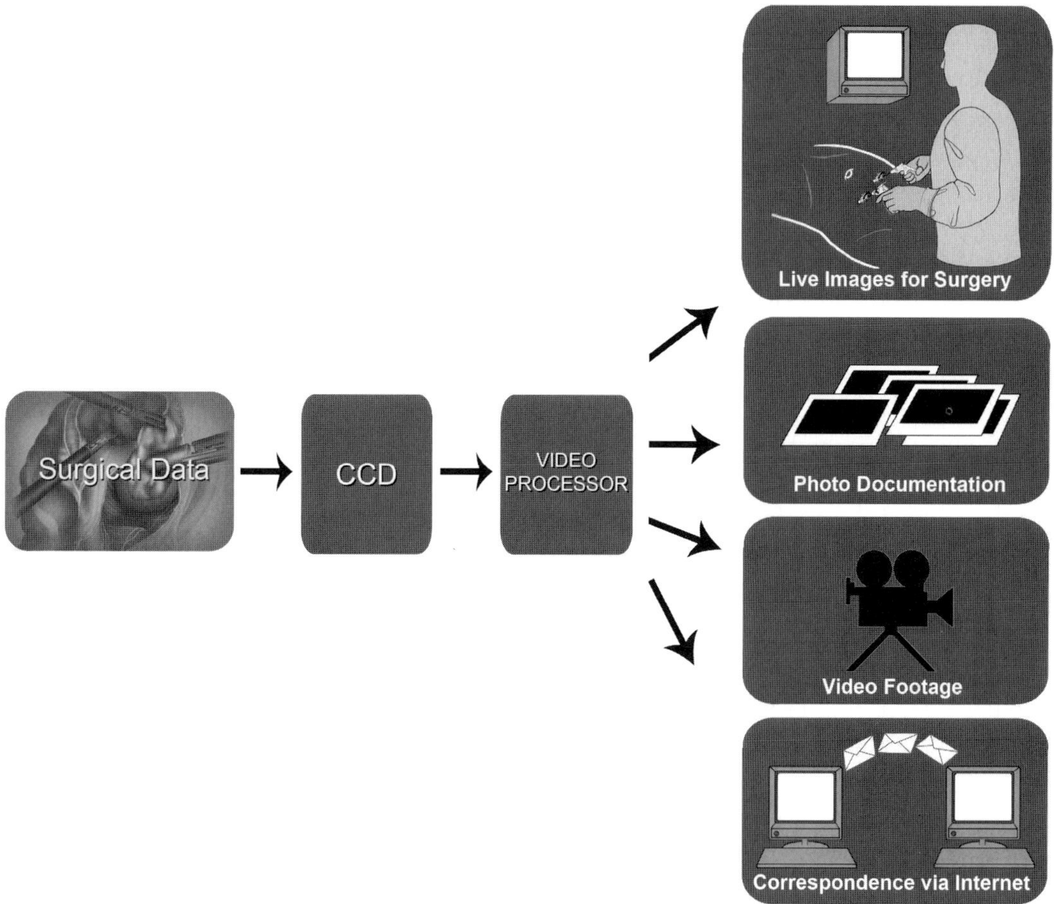

Figure 2.5. Images stored in various digital formats.

Video footage of a laparoscopic procedure is currently recorded more often in either VHS or s-VHS formats and digitized later; however, it can be also recorded directly in a digital format. Current versions of videoendoscopes used for laparoscopic procedures have an analog capture chip, and the analog signal is immediately digitized for viewing on a monitor or for recording. This will change, and chips will record the data as digital data from the start in the near future.[3]

Insufflators

An electrically controlled insufflator is often used to establish/maintain carbon dioxide (CO_2) pneumoperitoneum. The system usually has a continuously adjustable pressure selector, a digital intraabdominal pressure display, and digital delivered-flow and volume-of-gas-consumed displays. They automatically control the intraabdominal pressure by an "on-and-off" mechanism that is regulated by computer chips. For colorectal use, high-flow insufflation capability (more than 6 L/min) is desirable.

Figure 2.6 shows one of the most advanced surgical insufflators recently developed by Olympus. This system requires no second hose to monitor intraabdominal pressure, because the pressure can be monitored intermittently with the main insufflating hose. One special feature of this system is the automatic smoke/plume evacuation function that is activated when the electrosurgical device is used. The system detects and evacuates smoke/plume automatically, thus the procedure is not interrupted by poor visualization.

Previous studies have demonstrated that pneumoperitoneum using dry CO_2 gas potentially causes hypothermia.[11] Several commercial insufflators thus provide built-in heating/humidifying function. External heated humidifiers are also available in the market.

Irrigation and Suction Devices

Effective irrigation/suction system is essential for any laparoscopic procedure. Although assembling an irrigation/suction system from common operating room supplies is possible,[12] we do not believe such a system can be usefully employed under certain difficult situations occasionally encountered during laparoscopic colorectal surgery. We recommend using an electrically driven high-flow irrigator with its probe connected to a regular adjustable suction system (Figure 2.7). Even in cases of unforeseen bleeding or spillage of intestinal contents,

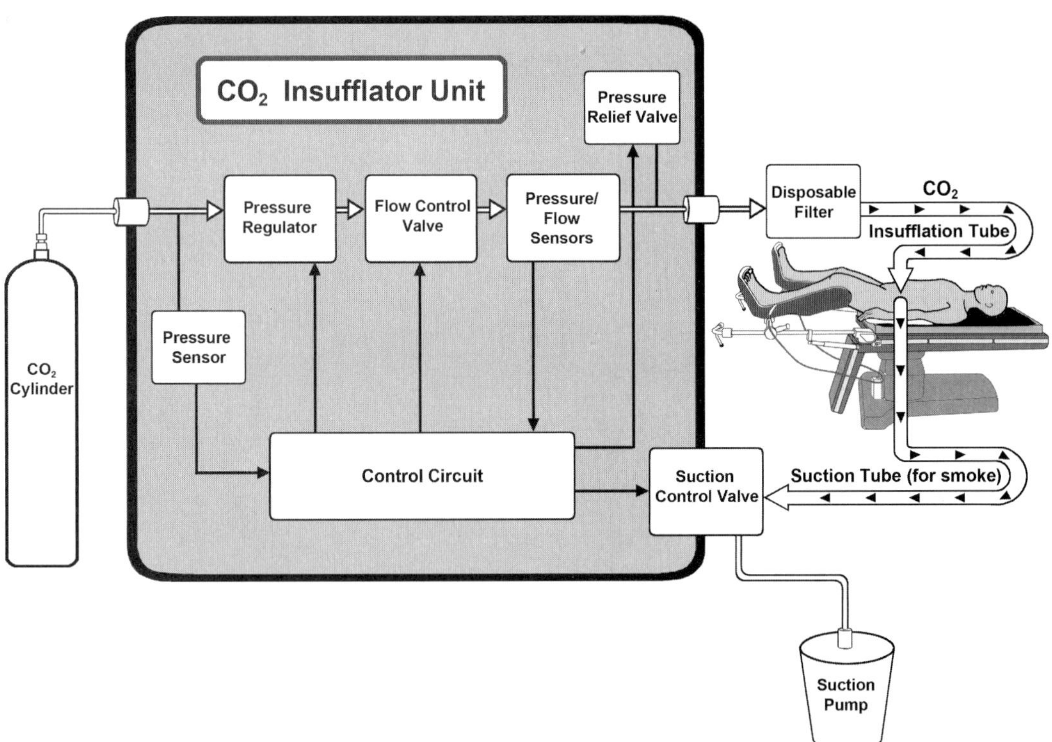

Figure 2.6. A CO_2 insufflator with automatic evacuation system (Olympus, Tokyo, Japan).

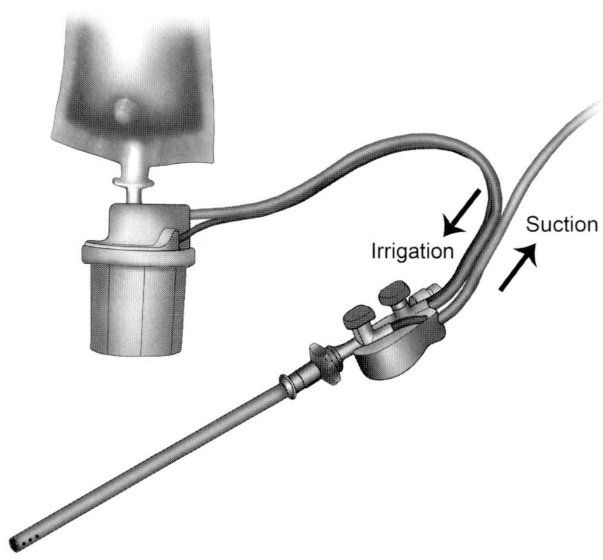

Figure 2.7. StrykeFlow™ (Stryker Endoscopy, San Jose, CA).

this device works reliably and satisfactorily both to rapidly irrigate and to effectively evacuate fluid or other material, and a variety of cannula sizes (5–10 mm) may be chosen.

A cheaper alternative is a 2- to 5-L plastic bag with saline solution on which constant pressure is applied.

Laparoscope Warmers

The view through the laparoscope may not only be impaired by blood or smoke on the lens, but also by fog. To prevent fogging after intraperitoneal insertion, the laparoscope should be adequately warmed (37° to 40°C) before intraperitoneal insertion. Although a warm saline bath can be used to keep laparoscopes warm until needed, specially designed warmers for laparoscopes are more suitable for routine use.

Special antifogging solution can be also effective to prevent fogging. Several types of products are commercially available. To achieve the best results, combined use of warmers and antifogging solution is recommended.

Instrumentation

The choice of appropriate instrumentation is a major key to success in any laparoscopic procedures. This chapter serves as a practical guide for readers to help understand which instruments are fundamental for laparoscopic colorectal surgery. All team members should aspire to constantly update themselves with recent technological developments, because new laparoscopic instruments will continue to become available as technology develops.

Miniaturization in instrumentation is one major trend in current minimally invasive surgery. Down-sized trocars with miniature instruments less than 3 mm in diameter have been put on the market, and certain procedures such as diagnostic laparoscopy, gallbladder removal, and adhesiolysis have become technically feasible. In colorectal practice, however, we believe that regular-sized instruments (10/12 mm or 5 mm in diameter) can provide maximal surgical flexibility, safety, and reliability. This chapter therefore does not include discussion of miniaturized instruments, and we have found that 5- to 10-mm instruments are still likely to be the most useful for colorectal procedures of the near future.

Insufflation Needles

The Veress needle, modified little since its invention by Janos Veress in 1938,[13] continues to be the standard instrument used for creation of pneumoperitoneum by a closed method.[8] Needles are commercially available in various lengths, all with an outside diameter of 1.8 mm. With its safety mechanism with blunt-tipped, spring-loaded inner stylet, the needle has remained the safest instrument for establishing pneumoperitoneum at laparoscopic surgery, when using an appropriate percutaneous puncture technique.

Trocars

Trocars are available in a wide array of types and sizes, and in disposable and nondisposable varieties (Figure 2.8). Although individual surgeons may have preferences, our current preference is the practical combination of disposable and reusable trocars. Recent disposable trocars no longer have sharp conical or pyramidal tips, but slim blunt tips that require less force to penetrate through the abdominal wall. Because they minimize the abdominal wall (muscles) trauma at insertion, good stabilization can be anticipated during instrument with-

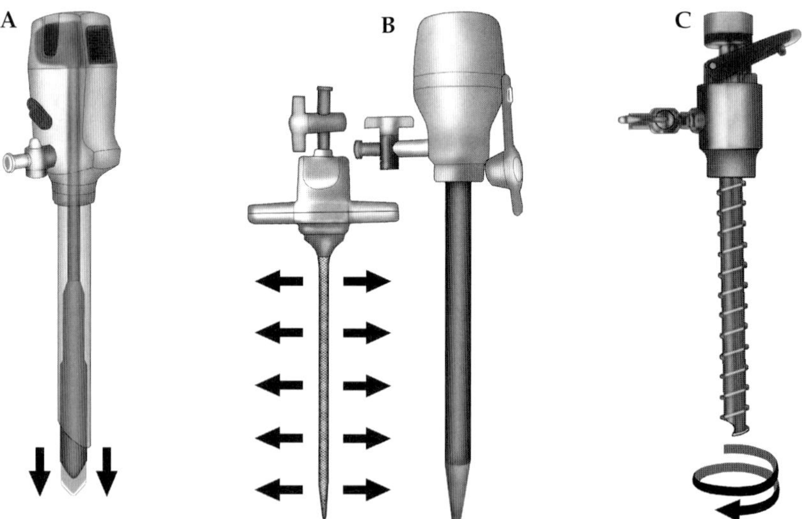

Figure 2.8. Different types of abdominal wall cannulas/trocars: **A** Endopath™ bladeless (Ethicon, Sommerville, NJ), **B** VersaStep™ (USSC, Norwalk, CT), and **C** EndoTIP™ (Storz, Tuttlingen, Germany).

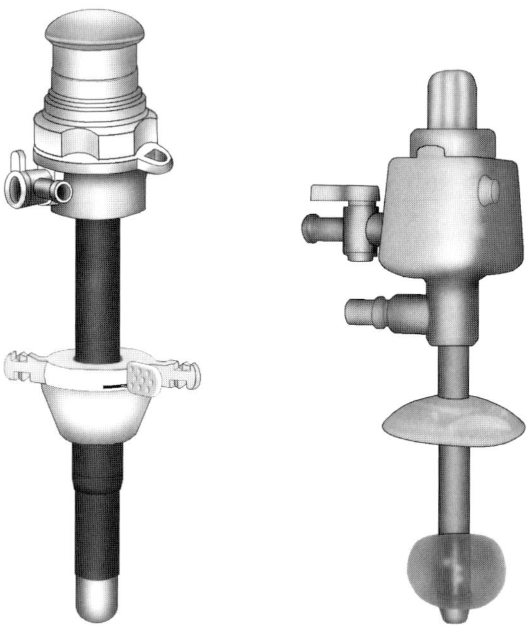

Figure 2.9. Hasson cannula (Ethicon, Sommerville, NJ) and Balloon cannula (Origin; USSC, Norwalk, CT).

drawal and manipulation, when an appropriate length of incision is made. As for reusable trocars, we no longer use classical bladed-trocars as well. Our current choice is screw-in type metal trocars (EndoTIP™; Karl-Storz, Tuttlingen, Germany), which provide safe and easy insertion with good stabilization. In general, reusable trocars are more cost-effective compared with disposable ones; however, care must be taken to keep the stylettes or screws sharp, because they tend to dull with repeated use.

An "open" technique (insertion of the initial cannula through a small laparotomy) is routinely used by some surgeons, because they believe that it is safer than "blind" Veress needle puncture. Even Veress needle users occasionally use the open technique when intraabdominal adhesions are strongly suspected. Because the open method may potentially cause continuous gas leaks around the cannula, a specially designed Hasson-type cannula with peritoneal/fascial sutures is used (Figure 2.9). Trocars with inner balloon/outer disc stabilizers may provide better fixation onto the abdominal wall, making gas leaks and sheath slippage minimal during procedures.

For the initial introduction of the cannula, the optical access trocar (e.g., Optiview™ of Ethicon, Visiport™ of USSC) is another choice. It is a blunt trocar, which is guided through the abdominal wall with the camera (laparoscope) inside and controlled by the monitor. Some surgeons prefer this device, advocating that it can combine the advantages of a safe (open method) and a fast (closed method) penetration of the abdominal cavity.[14]

In our opinion, an optimal trocar design for advanced laparoscopic surgery should meet the following conditions:

- Good fixation to the abdominal wall, both superficially and deeply, so that the cannula remains in place during instrument exchange and manipulation.
- The cannula should form an airtight seal with the abdominal wall.
- A universal seal mechanism should be present in the instrument channel, so that instruments with different diameters can be inserted and withdrawn without friction and without a converter or an adapter.

Hand-Access Devices for Colorectal Hand-Assisted Laparoscopic Surgery

Hand-assisted laparoscopic surgery (HALS) is a new development that allows a surgeon to easily insert a hand into the abdominal cavity during laparoscopic surgery. A specially designed hand-access device is necessary to maintain pneumoperitoneum and facilitate the hand insertion/withdrawal and manipulation during HALS. Because the intracorporeal manipulation is more extensive and multiquadrant in colorectal procedures compared with other general surgical procedures, the device should be durable and flexible so that a wide range of movement of the surgeon's hand causes neither gas leakage nor device malfunction. Among several commercially available products, our current preference is the GelPort™ (Applied Medical, Rancho Santa Margarita, CA; Figure 2.10).[15] The precise role of hand-access devices will be described in the specific procedure chapters.

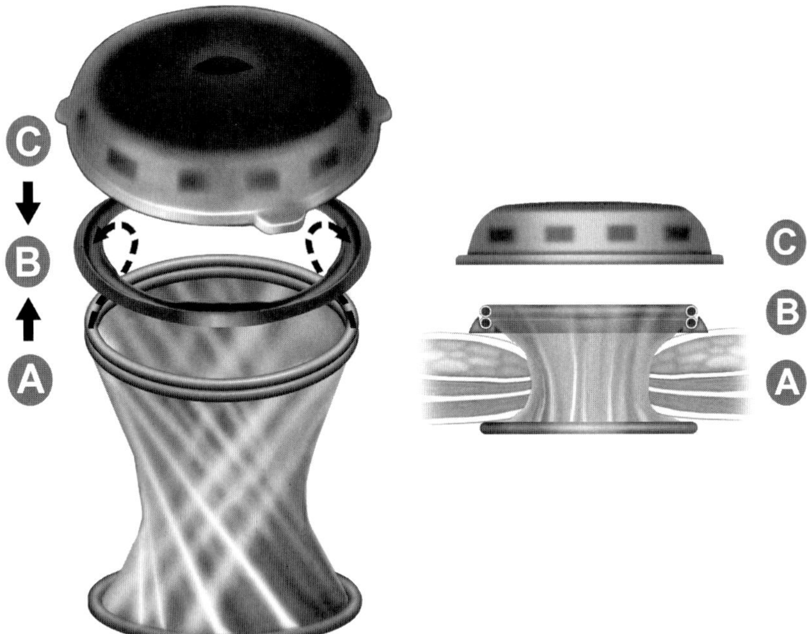

Figure 2.10. Gelport™ hand-access device (Applied Medical, Rancho Santa Margarita, CA).

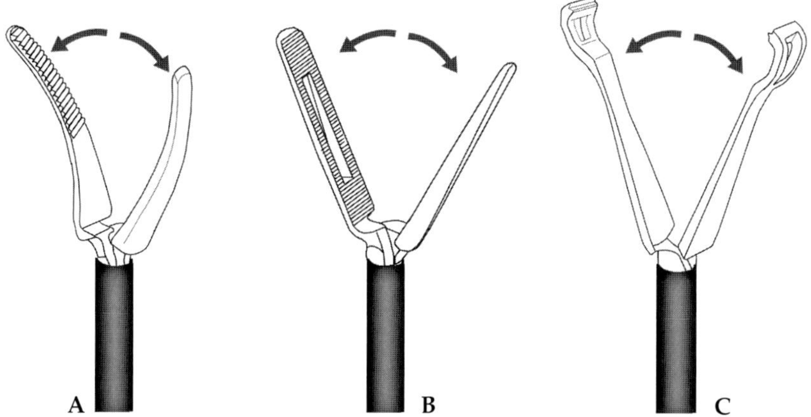

Figure 2.11. Various types of laparoscopic graspers: **A** Maryland dissector, **B** Bowel grasper, and **C** Babcock type grasper.

Grasping Instruments

Laparoscopic graspers are designed to hold the tissue firmly without exerting excessive pressure. The shaft on most of these instruments is 5 mm in diameter, 31 cm long, and isolated by a thin layer of plastic (Teflon or polyvinylchloride) that electrically insulates the instrument. The grasping blades are blunt and are about 2 cm long with a maximum jaw span of about 2 cm. Although the quantity of tissue that can be held with these graspers is limited, we use this type of grasper for almost all purposes during laparoscopic colorectal surgery (Figure 2.11). The surface area of the blades is large enough to safely hold a sufficient amount of tissue, whether it is mesentery, greater omentum, or intestine. To maintain a relatively safe grip, the inner side of the blade is serrated; the serrations are fairly atraumatic, so that the intestine can gently be grasped with this instrument. The grasper usually has a holding mechanism that is easily activated and released with a trigger.

Special dissecting instruments are useful for laparoscopic colorectal surgery. Their tips are usually more pointed than that of laparoscopic graspers, but still blunt. The blades are about 2 cm long, and are curved similar to a small curved hemostat and thus facilitate blunt dissection. Similar to the laparoscopic grasper, the shaft is 5 mm in diameter, 31 cm long, and electrically insulated. The dissector can act as a forceps during delicate dissection and can also be used for electrosurgery. Both the grasper and dissector have a dial on the handle that allows the tip to be easily rotated on its longitudinal axis. For additional maneuverability, an articulated tip is also available; a second dial moves it.

The third type of grasping instrument is an Allis-like clamp. The opposing surfaces of the blades are smaller than those of the normal grasper so that the tissue can be held more precisely. The smaller surface area and shape of the blades is very useful in certain special situations, especially in grasping bleeding vessels or the center-rod of a circular stapling instrument.

Scissors

Scissors are among the most important instruments in advanced laparoscopic surgery. Because they are used for both sharp and blunt dissection, they should have very sharp blades and a blunt tip. We do not use microscissors with small blades or the hooked scissors frequently used in gallbladder or gynecologic laparoscopic surgery because the wide dissection of mesentery and lateral and dorsal attachments of the colon can be more quickly performed with normal curved laparoscopic scissors.

The scissor shaft is 5 mm in diameter, 31 cm long, and is well insulated so that electrical current can safely be applied. The curved blades are 16 mm long with a maximum jaw span of 8 mm. The shaft can easily be rotated in its longitudinal axis by using a dial on the handle. We use the scissors for sharp and blunt dissection and for tissue desiccation, which should always be performed with closed blades. Sometimes, arcing will occur during tissue desiccation, and the extremely hot arcs may result in dulling the scissors. If the surgeon wants to desiccate the tissue while cutting, bipolar scissors should be used that combine bipolar desiccation with mechanical cutting. Because the cutting blade is ceramic in these scissors, it will neither melt nor become dull.

Retractors

Optimal exposure of the operative site is the key to success in any laparoscopic surgery. In colorectal surgery, most of this attention is directed to the small intestines, because they normally spill into all quadrants of the abdomen. Retracting instruments are mandatory if the procedure is to be successfully performed in obese patients or those with a distended intestine. The truly effective, safe, and reliable laparoscopic bowel retractors are, however, not in our hands yet.

Laparoscopic retractors often used in general laparoscopic surgery are not effective or even dangerous for colorectal practice: For instance, we do not recommend using a one-finger or a fan retractor to retract bowel loops. These designs may be useful to retract the liver or other more fixed organs, but they are not designed to retract the bowel effectively. Fan retractors also have the disadvantage that an intestinal loop may become trapped between the fingers of the retractor, exposing the loop to potential injury.

Eventually, displacement of the small bowel loops is performed most effectively using grasping devices and by gravity. Before starting the procedure, the small intestinal loops are positioned to one side of the abdomen by changing the patient's position and with gentle laparoscopic manipulation. If the small intestines still migrate into the operative field after the above technique, use of atraumatic a pad-type retractor (Endo Paddle™ Retract, USSC, Norwalk, CT; Figure 2.12) can be considered.[16]

Even after intracorporeal mobilization/transaction, the freed segment of the colon itself can also obstruct the remainder of the procedure. Safe and effective retraction of the transected colon can be achieved by an endoscopic snare device (Endo Catch™ II, USSC) with its plastic bag

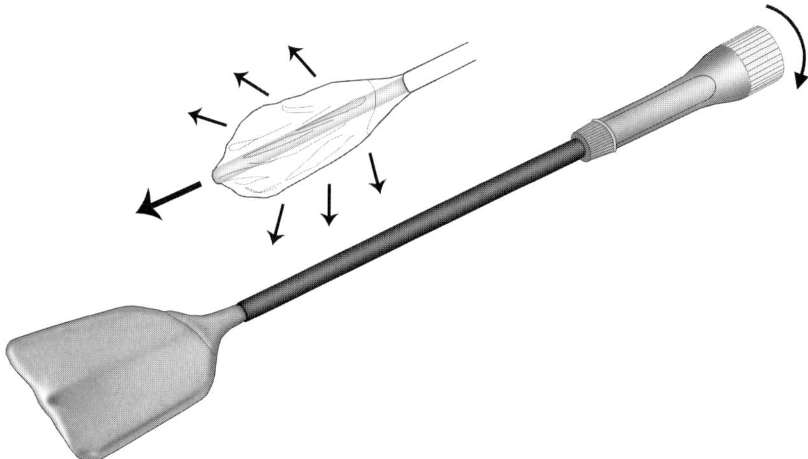

Figure 2.12. Endo Paddle™ Retract (USSC, Norwalk, CT).

removed. The snare, which is passed into the abdominal cavity inside a 10-mm-diameter tube, can be opened to a maximum diameter of about 6.5 cm and then completely or partially closed by retraction into the tube. Because the snare consists of a band of spring metal with blunt edges, it is not likely to injure the bowel if used properly. After the colon has been divided, the sling is slid over the end of the colon, and is used to retract it. Thus, not only does this sling work as a safe retractor, but it can also allow rotation of the intestine in the longitudinal axis of the instrument and facilitate dorsolateral dissection of the colon on the right or left side. The snare theoretically can be applied without transecting the intestine. One side of the loop can be detached, passed around the intestine, and then reattached. The sling may also be used to occlude the rectum before rectal washout, which is usually performed before rectal transection during rectal cancer surgery.

Despite several useful retracting techniques mentioned above, if the intestine is distended, if the patient is overly obese, or if space in the peritoneal cavity is limited in some other way, it can be difficult or sometimes impossible to expose the operative field sufficiently in laparoscopic colorectal surgery. If necessary exposure cannot be achieved, prompt conversion to HALS or open surgery should be considered.

Specimen Bags

A specimen bag is very useful for laparoscopic resections for colorectal malignancy to isolate the resected specimen from the peritoneal cavity. This may reduce the possibility of seeding tumor cells into the peritoneal cavity and abdominal wall. In general, a bag has to be inserted into the peritoneal cavity in a compressed manner and then opened. The bulky specimen may then be placed in the bag, and the bag completely closed before bringing it through the abdominal wall.

The ideal endoscopic bag for delivering the intraabdominal specimens should have the following properties:

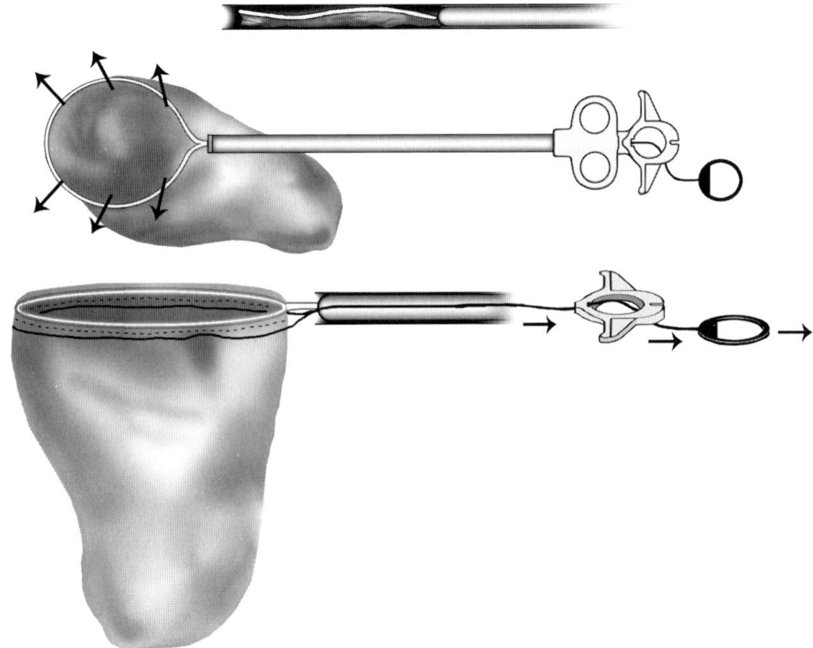

Figure 2.13. Endo Catch™ II (USSC, Norwalk, CT).

- It should be fluid-impermeable and be strong enough so that it cannot be damaged inside the abdominal cavity or when being removed.
- It should fit through a cannula 15 mm or smaller.
- It should open easily.
- It should be large enough so the entire intestinal specimen, including mesentery, can easily be placed in it in one piece.
- It should have a mechanism to quickly close the bag to prevent spills.

Our current choice is the specially designed commercially available bag, which allows excellent control of the mouth of the bag and a good drawstring mechanism (Endo Catch™ II, USSC; Figure 2.13). Using a plunger-type mechanism, the bag is expelled from the shaft once the tip of the instrument is inside the peritoneal cavity. It is initially attached to a metal hoop that holds the mouth of the bag open. Once the specimen is placed inside the bag, the drawstring is tightened, the bag is torn away from the metal hoop, and the hoop and neck of the bag are drawn up inside the metal shaft of the instrument. The cannula incision is then enlarged and the neck of the bag, including the purse string, is delivered to the anterior abdominal wall.

Clips

Clip appliers were developed to facilitate ligation of small ductal structures approximately 3 to 8 mm in diameter. The most common disposable clip appliers contain up to 20 clips and are available in 5- and 10-mm-diameter instruments. They are manufactured from a variety of materials, including absorbable polyglycolic acid and polydioxane, stainless steel, and most often, titanium. Clips are practical and effective if an electric vessel sealing device is not available, because clips require less time to apply than sutures and knots in laparoscopic surgery. In truth, the role of clips in our practice is greatly diminished, and we rarely use them. Nonetheless, they should be kept available.

Pretied Suture Loops

The pretied suture loop with slip knot (Endo Loop™, USSC) is a unique instrument that is used exclusively in laparoscopic surgery (Figure 2.14). The loops are used to obtain primary hemostasis when the vessel or vascular pedicle is divided and grasped. The loops are useful to secure unexpected bleeding after transection, where electrosurgical methods or clips are difficult to apply. After the bleeder is identified and secured with an atraumatic grasper, a second grasper is introduced from the other port and passed through the loop. The first grasper is then gently released, and the second grasper grasps the bleeding point. The loop is snugged down over the shaft of the instrument, securing the bleeder.

Another usage of this device is to secure the stump in laparoscopic appendectomy. After securing the stump, the device can be used as an effective retracting tool unless its string is cut. Various suture materials are available. We generally use a synthetic absorbable material such as

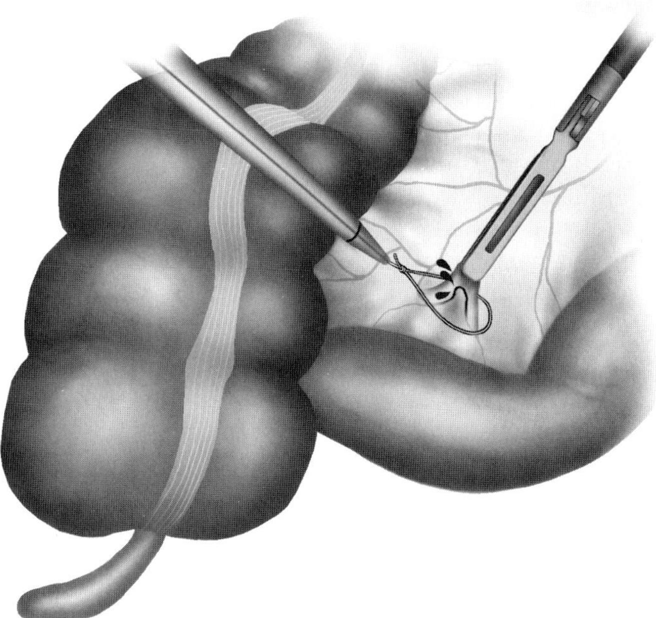

Figure 2.14. Hemostasis of a bleeding from a small mesenteric vessel using the Endo Loop™ (USSC, Norwalk, CT).

Vicryl™ (Ethicon, Somerville, NJ), or Polysorb™ (USSC), or PDS-II™ (Ethicon).

Staplers

A linear anastomotic stapler (e.g., Endo GIA™, USSC) is one of the most frequently used disposable instruments in colorectal laparoscopy. The working end of Endo GIA™ consists of two jaws, one that accommodates the staple cartridge and one that is the anvil. Several jaw lengths are available: 30, 45, and 60 mm. In the cartridge are two rows of triple-staggered staples, eight in each row; the two rows are separated by a single groove through which a small sharp knife blade advances when the stapler is fired (Figure 2.15). The staples are made of 0.21-mm titanium wire, have a backspan length of 3 mm, and a leg length of 2.0, 2.5, 3.5, and 4.8 mm, for vascular, regular, and thick bowel tissue, respectively. For safe stapling, it is critical to select adequate set of staples (cartridge) for specific organs. To staple and divide the bowel, the bowel is slid between the jaws (cartridge and anvil) and the instrument is closed and activated. Activation drives both rows of triple-staggered staples through the tissue and drives the knife to divide the intestine. The knife stops one-and-a-half staples short of the end of the staple line. Thus, both ends of intestine are divided and closed in an everted mucosa-to-mucosa manner with a triple row of staples on each side.

Although the conventional GIA™ instruments contain only two rows of double staples, we believe that the third row added to the Endo staplers probably increases their safety, which is especially important in laparoscopic surgery because the minimal access to the peritoneal cavity does not readily allow defective or bleeding intestinal anastomoses to be repaired.

Recently, articulating (roticulating) stapling devices (Endo GIA™ Roticulator, USSC) have become available. With a roticulating function, the usability of staplers has been much improved in certain laparoscopic procedures such as splenectomy and gastrectomy. However, in rectal procedures, it is still technically challenging to place staplers in the optimal direction deep inside the pelvis to transect the distal rectum. Further improvement in instrumentation is necessary to make distal rectal stapling easy and reliable.

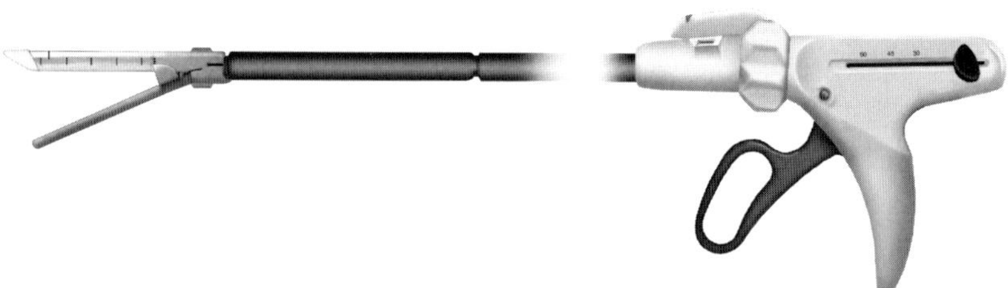

Figure 2.15. Endo GIA™ Universal stapler (USSC, Norwalk, CT).

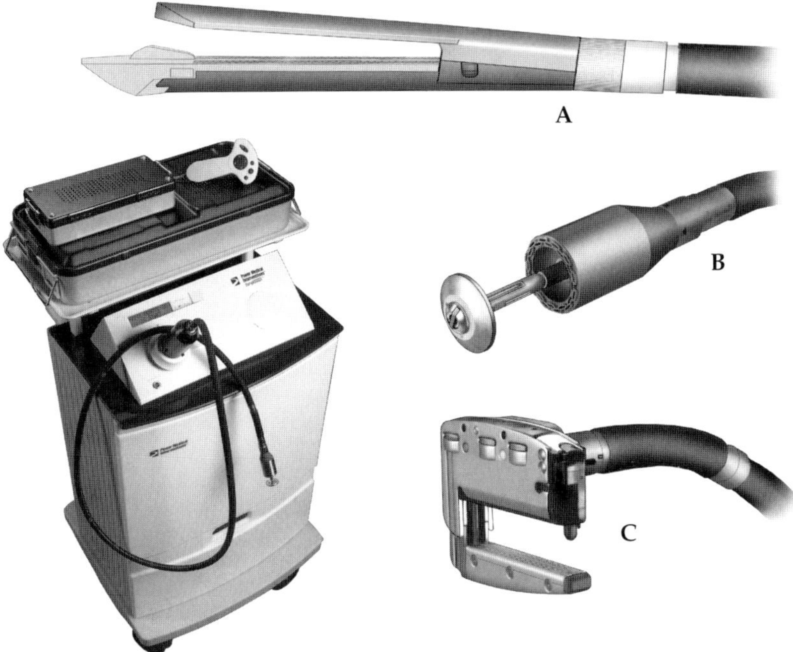

Figure 2.16. SurgASSIST™ computerized gastrointestinal stapling devices (Power Medical Interventions, New Hope, PA) **A** Straight linear cutter (SLC) 55 and 75 mm, **B** Circular stapler (CS) 25, 29, and 33 mm, **C** Right-angled linear cutter (RALC) 45 mm, which places four rows of stapler, cutting between the second and third rows.

A significant change in the means whereby staples are delivered in intestinal tissues is being developed by a new company, Power Medical Inc. (New Hope, PA). Using a 170-cm-long computer-driven cable, which attaches to a wide variety of stapling cartridges, this equipment permits the surgeon to pass certain linear staples through laparoscopic ports (straight linear cutter, SLC™ 55 and 75 mm) and angle the stapler tip over a wide range of angles (up-down and right-left). The staplers may be fired using push-button technology with a hand-held remote controller. In addition to the SLC™ stapler, there is a right-angled linear cutting device (RALC™ 45 mm) that fires four rows of staples, cutting automatically between the second and third rows. There is also a circular stapler technology, similar in some ways to the commercially available models in sizes 25, 29, and 33 mm. Advantages of this circular stapler are that it can be fired using a remote device, and also it can be passed transanally high into the large intestine, so that theoretically even right-sided end-to-end anastomoses could be made (Figure 2.16).

Trocar Wound Closure Devices

Closing small fascial defects left by trocars can be a difficult, time-consuming, and occasionally hazardous task especially in obese patients with thick abdominal walls. Inadequate closure of those wounds can lead to significant morbidities such as evisceration, incisional hernia,

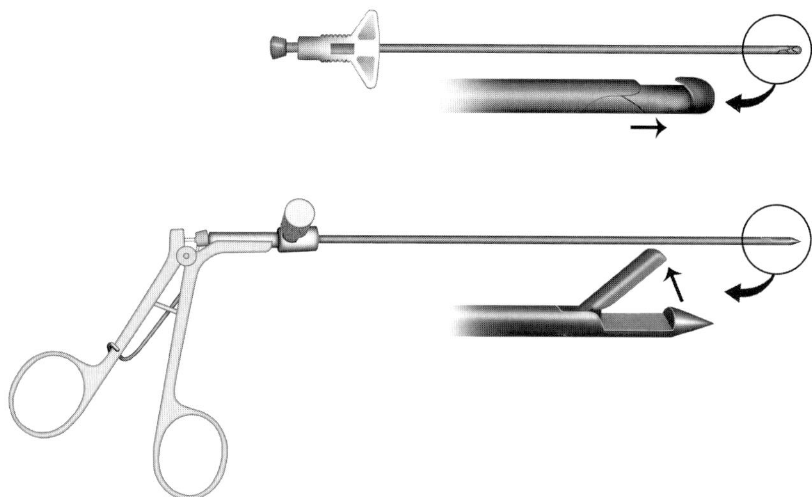

Figure 2.17. Endo Close™ (USSC, Norwalk, CT) and Suture Passer (Storz, Tuttlingen, Germany) abdominal well closure devices.

and at worst, incarcerated (Richter) hernia.[17,18] Trocar wound closure devices are commercially available in both disposable and reusable fashion (Figure 2.17). We routinely place through-and-through sutures at 10/12 mm trocar sites using Suture Passer™ (Karl-Storz). Although details of our technique are to be described later, one key is to place these sutures before trocar removal.

Fundamental Equipment and Instruments

The following list summarizes the fundamental instrumentation necessary to initiate laparoscopic colorectal surgery:

1. Image processing system
   - Laparoscopes (10 mm 0°, 30°; 5 mm 0°, 30°)
   - Laparoscopic camera – single- or three-chip camera
   - Monitors (2) – standard analog cathode ray tube or digital flat-screen
2. Gas insufflation
   - High-flow CO_2 insufflator (>6 L/min) with digital intraabdominal pressure, volume, and gas display
   - CO_2 reservoir as a tank or a connection to a "wall" reservoir
3. Instruments
   - Standard surgical instruments to incise the skin, establish trocar sites and minilaparotomy, and perform emergent laparotomy, if needed
   - Laparoscopic 5-mm bowel graspers (two per case)
   - Laparoscopic 5-mm dissector
   - Laparoscopic 5-mm scissor
   - Laparoscopic 5-mm needle holder
   - Suction/irrigation cannulae (5 and 10 mm)

References

1. Berci G, Brooks PG, Paz-Partlow M. TV laparoscopy. A new dimension in visualization and documentation of pelvic pathology. J Reprod Med 1986;31:585–588.
2. Berci G, Schwaitzberg SD. The importance of understanding the basics of imaging in the era of high-tech endoscopy. Part II. Logic, reality, and utopia. Surg Endosc 2002;16:1518–1522.
3. Birkett DH. The digital surgeon. Surg Endosc 2001;15:1059–1060.
4. Gow JG, Hopkins HH, Wallace DM, et al. The modern urological endoscope. In: Hopkins HH, ed. Handbook of Urological Endoscopy. Edingburgh: Churchill Livingstone; 1978.
5. Sanfilippo JS. Instrumentation and knot-tying. In: Vitale GC, Sanfilippo JS, Perissat J, eds. Laparoscopic Surgery: An Atlas for General Surgeons. Philadelphia: JB Lippincott; 1995.
6. Herron DM, Lantis JC, Maykel J, et al. The 3-D monitor and head-mounted display. A quantitative evaluation of advanced laparoscopic viewing technologies. Surg Endosc 1999;13:751–755.
7. Berber E, Siperstein AE. Understanding and optimizing laparoscopic videosystems. Surg Endosc 2001;15:781–787.
8. Duppler DW. Laparoscopic instrumentation, videoimaging, and equipment disinfection and sterilization. Surg Clin North Am 1992;72: 1021–1031.
9. Margulies DR, Shabot MM. Fiberoptic imaging and measurement. In: Hunter JG, Sackier JM, eds. Minimally Invasive Surgery. New York: McGraw Hill; 1993.
10. Herron DM, Gagner M, Kenyon TL, et al. The minimally invasive surgical suite enters the 21st century. A discussion of critical design elements. Surg Endosc 2001;15:415–422.
11. Ott DE. Laparoscopic hypothermia. J Laparoendosc Surg 1991;1:127–131.
12. Marshburn PB, Hulka JF. A simple irrigator-aspirator cannula for laparoscopy: the Stewart system. Obstet Gynecol 1990;75:458–460.
13. Veress J. Neues Instrument zur Ausführung von Brust- oder Bauchpunktionen und Pneumothoraxbehandlung. Deutsch Med Wochenschr 1938; 40:1480–1481.
14. String A, Berber E, Foroutani A, et al. Use of the optical access trocar for safe and rapid entry in various laparoscopic procedures. Surg Endosc 2001;15:570–573.
15. Nakajima K, Lee SW, Cocilovo C, et al. Hand-assisted laparoscopic colorectal surgery using Gelport: initial experience with a new hand access device. Surg Endosc 2004;18:102–105.
16. Milsom JW, Okuda J, Kim Seon-Hahn, et al. Atraumatic and expeditious laparoscopic bowel handling using a new endoscopic device. Dis Colon Rectum 1997;40:1394–1395.
17. Bhoyrul S, Payne J, Steffes B, et al. A randomized prospective study of radially expanding trocars in laparoscopic surgery. J Gastrointest Surg 2000;4:392–397.
18. Liu CD, McFadden DW. Laparoscopic port sites do not require fascial closure when nonbladed trocars are used. Am Surg 2000;66:853–854.

Chapter 3

Surgical Energy Sources

Bartholomäus Böhm, Jeffrey W. Milsom, and Kiyokazu Nakajima

In laparoscopic surgery, abdominal tissues are dissected using a combination of cutting and coagulation, often with specialized electrosurgical instruments or ultrasonic devices. Precise dissection with minimal bleeding is especially important in laparoscopic surgery. Even minor oozing compromises the laparoscopic view and clearing blood from the field of vision with suction and irrigation may be tedious. Therefore, dissection must be performed with tools that optimize precise tissue cutting and coagulation.

Although many different coagulation and dissection devices are available, they all divide and coagulate tissue by converting various types of energy into heat. Therefore, the effect on tissue is thermal and depends on exposure time and the amount of energy applied to the tissue. Before embarking on a specific discussion of each instrument used to cut or coagulate tissue, reviewing some basic concepts about thermal alteration of tissue is worthwhile.

Tissue reaction to thermal injury depends primarily on the temperature used (Figure 3.1). An increase in tissue temperature up to 60°C results in almost indiscernible changes to the naked eye. Coagulation begins at temperatures above 60°C; it is characterized by shrinkage and blanching caused by the denaturation of proteins, particularly collagen.[1,2] When the tissue temperature reaches 100°C, the cell water boils, water is converted to steam, and the cell wall ruptures. When the water has evaporated and heat is still applied, the tissue temperature increases rapidly until it reaches 200°–300°C. At this point, the tissue carbonizes and begins to vaporize and smoke. At temperatures more than 500°C, tissue burns and evaporates.[1–3]

The effect of heat on tissue depends not only on the absolute amount of heat applied to tissue but also on the exposure time to heat. If heat is applied over a very short time (less than 1–2 seconds), the effect is localized because the heat is not conducted to surrounding tissues; even when the heat is great enough to vaporize the tissue, the vaporization is localized. If, however, the same amount of heat is applied for a longer period (greater than 2 seconds), the heat is conducted to the

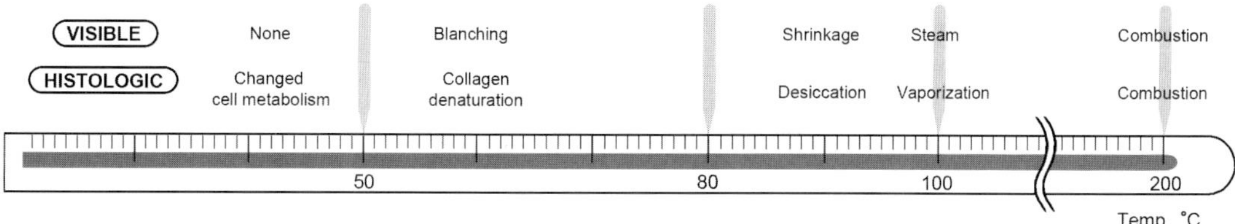

Figure 3.1. Visible and histologic alterations of tissues as related to tissue temperature.

surrounding tissue, thus increasing thermal necrosis and broadening the vaporization area.

Cutting quality and coagulation quality are inversely related, regardless of the dissection device used (Figure 3.2). Good cutting quality depends on rapid local vaporization of tissue with minimal lateral heat damage. No coagulation will occur because the lateral heat damage is not wide enough to seal the blood vessels. In contrast, the quality of coagulation depends on the width of lateral heat damage: the wider the lateral heat damage, the better the hemostasis. Because as cutting quality improves, the coagulation quality worsens, simultaneously combining excellent cutting qualities with excellent hemostasis is impossible.

Electrosurgery

Electrosurgery is universally accepted as an important tool in open surgery. Although we do not intend to describe the principles of electrosurgery in detail, some basic principles should be discussed to understand the relationship between different operating modes of the electrosurgical unit. For example, tissue heating during the desiccation is a function of the amount of current flowing through a given cross-sectional area of tissue. The electrons collide with the tissue molecules, and the current is transformed into heat energy.

The relation between current density and tissue heating must be understood particularly in monopolar surgery because if the applied current passes on its way to the dispersive electrode through a part of the body with a small conducting area, tissue may be heated far from

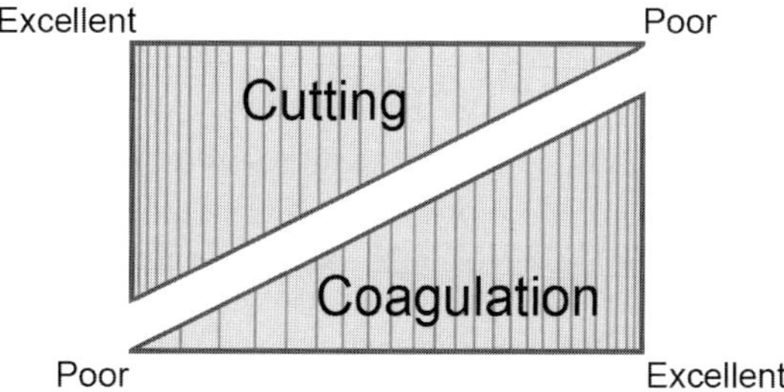

Figure 3.2. Inverse relationship between cutting and coagulation qualities of electrosurgery.

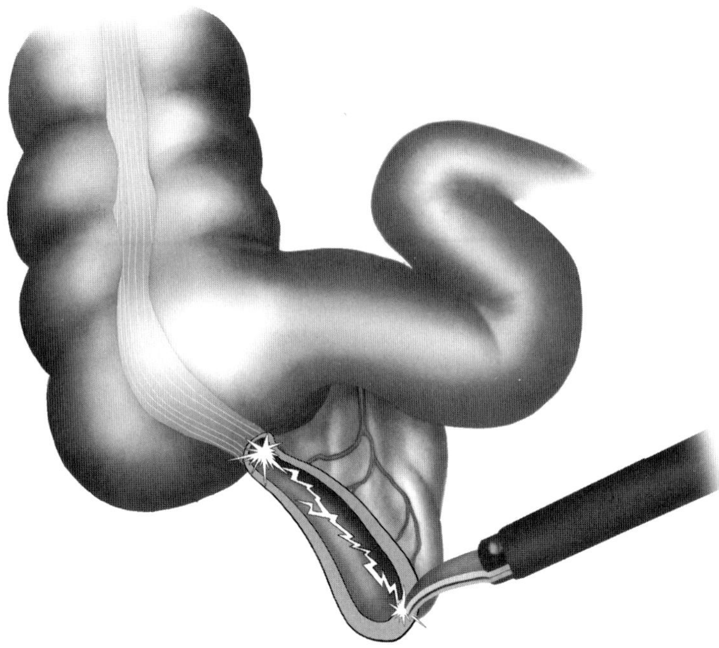

Figure 3.3. Monopolar electrosurgery, when applied to duct-like structures, may transmit a strong current through the duct-like structure, leading to damage of closely approximate tissue.

the point where the current is applied. Therefore, duct-like structures with a small area of conduction are at risk for inadvertent coagulation (Figure 3.3). Understanding the relationship between current density and heat production also is essential to understanding why smaller active electrodes have a localized effect on tissue. Because the current density of a small active electrode is greater than a larger (dispersive) electrode with the same power, a local temperature increase occurs immediately below the active electrode. The current density decreases rapidly as it radiates outward from the electrode; consequently, as the distance from the electrode increases, the temperature also rapidly decreases.

The shape and size of the active electrode influences current density at the tip – arcs ignite more readily from a sharp edge than from a rounded surface. Thus, a cutting waveform applied to tissue with the broad side of a standard blade electrode effectively desiccates, whereas its sharp edge will cut cleanly with the same power and mode.

The electrolyte content of tissue is responsible for tissue resistance, which is between 30 (blood) to 1000 (bone) ohm/cm.[4–6] Because blood has low resistance, well vascularized structures and blood vessels are major pathways for electrical current to travel through the body to the dispersive electrode. The tissue resistance increases as tissue desiccation increases, from 200–400 to 1000–3000 ohm/cm. If tissue is desiccated or carbonized, it is seldom possible to affect more tissue in that area without increasing the power or removing the eschar.

Electrosurgical Generators

In the last century, electrosurgical generators were developed that use the effect of an electrical current through tissue. The generators produce a high-frequency (HF) current (300–500 kHz).

The electrical output configuration of the electrosurgical unit is usually radiofrequency (RF) isolated. There is no direct connection between the output transformer and the power ground line, so the current seeks different return ground. This configuration is chosen to prevent tissue damage in case of a nonfunctional return electrode. RF isolation best protects the patient from burns that occur at locations other than the burn site because the electrical impedance of the return path via ground is intentionally made as high as possible.

The surgeon should always keep in mind that complete RF isolation is not possible. Any conductive object, including components and wiring inside the electrosurgical unit and even the surgeon, can act as a capacitor. Thus, some measurable RF leakage will always be grounded via the patient. However, RF leakage in electrosurgical units labeled as "RF isolated" must be within established standards. Even within these limits, small burns (an area of less than 1 mm^2) at other contact sites may occur.

Although the solid-state generators produce a standard waveform with a well-defined narrow-bandwidth, the creation of arcs during cutting or fulguration adds considerable signal energy at high and low frequencies that may interfere with other devices in the operating room. The low-frequency arc and high-intensity HF signals can interfere with pacemaker functions and stimulate tissue (muscle and nerve) to duplicate physiologic signals – for example, electrocardiogram signals.

Living tissue consists of different intra- and intercellular salt solutions separated by biologic membranes. Living cells thus represent a series of electrolytic conductors so that direct or alternating current alters the membrane permeability, resulting in muscle or nerve stimulation. To reduce these stimulations, an HF alternating current is generated in the electrosurgical unit.

Thus, the currently used HF, high-voltage, and low-amperage current has no excitatory effect on the body other than at the point of contact. However, low-frequency currents can arise from stray HF currents when the HF current passes through a nonlinear circuit that is not 100% resistive.

Monopolar and Bipolar Electrosurgery

A closed circuit is necessary so that electrical current can flow through tissue from an entry (active electrode) through tissue to an exit (the return or dispersive electrode). If the entry electrode is used as the active electrode and the return electrode is inactive, the application is called monopolar electrosurgery. If both electrodes are used as active electrodes, the application is bipolar.

In bipolar electrosurgery, the electrodes are in close proximity; the tissue effect is localized, with very little flow of current into the patient beyond the immediate treatment zone; and only a small amount of tissue is affected. Therefore, the total power required to affect the tissue is small compared with that required for monopolar electrosurgery, in which current must flow through the body to the ground electrode. Although bipolar electrosurgery provides the safest and most controlled desiccation method using electrosurgery and more effectively controls stray current, it has a disadvantage in that it can only be used in the desiccation mode. This limitation is overcome in part by bipolar scissors that allow tissue desiccation with bipolar technology and tissue cutting with mechanical shearing.

When bipolar electrodes are used, the tissue must be grasped where the electrodes are uninsulated to allow the current to pass through tissue (Figure 3.4). Standard bipolar electrodes should not be squeezed together too tightly because the jaws of the bipolar instruments may touch one another and create a short circuit (Figure 3.4).

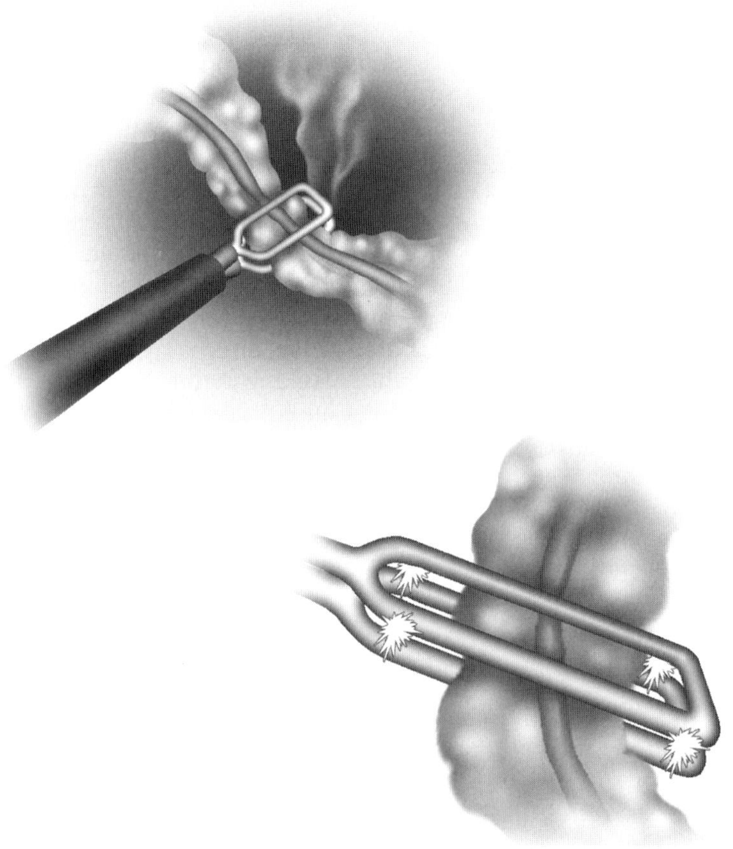

Figure 3.4. Application of bipolar electrosurgery to a mesenteric vessel. Inset: short circuit of the current between applied paddles of a bipolar unit can lead to ineffective coagulation of the tissue.

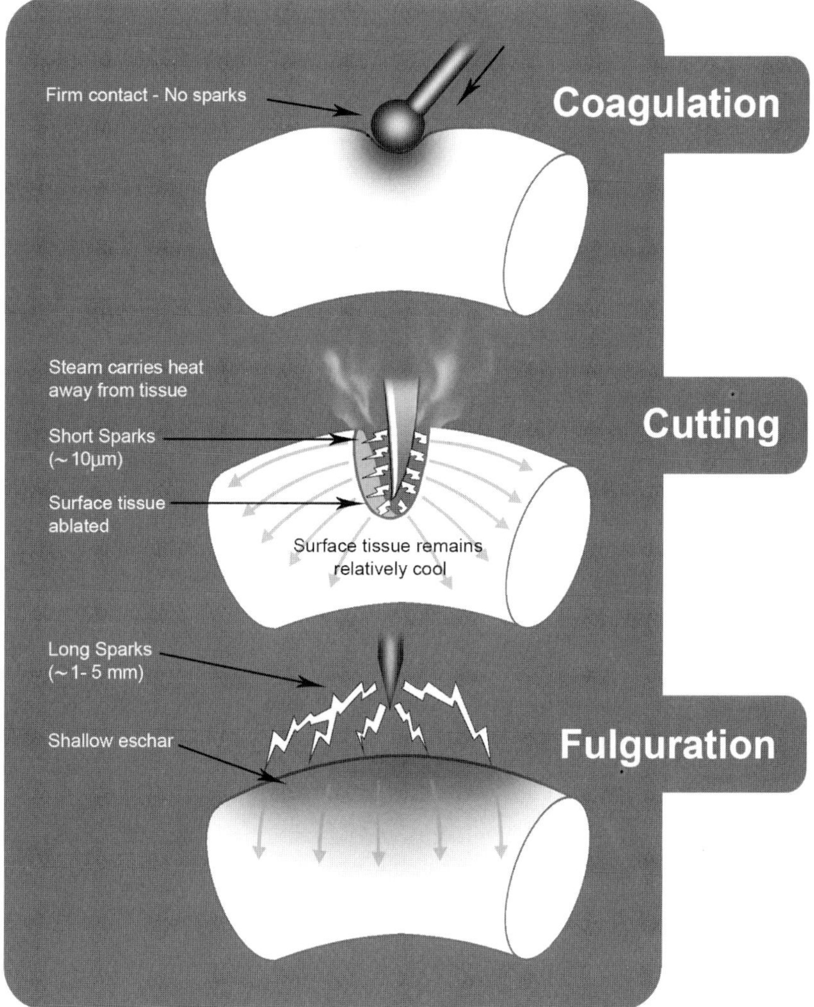

Figure 3.5. Effects of coagulation, cutting, and fulguration.

Electrosurgical Techniques

Electrosurgical modes are related to the current and voltage of a specific waveform because the effect on tissue depends on the energy applied over time and whether an arc between the electrode and tissue through air is created. In general, tissue can only be cut if the tissue temperature increases rapidly above 100°C so that water vaporizes and cells explode. When tissue is heated above 50°C, protein denatures, leading to coagulation.

HF current can be applied to affect tissue in three different ways (Figure 3.5):

- Cutting
- Fulguration (black coagulation)
- Desiccation (white coagulation)

Cutting

Cutting is usually achieved with a continuous waveform and a HF current flow. Applying the active electrode in the cutting mode creates a steady stream of arcs less than 10 μm long with a temperature of about 4000–5000 K that rapidly increases temperature in the immediately adjacent tissue. Each arc strikes a cell along the leading edge of the incision, rapidly heating the intracellular fluid so that the membrane bursts and the intracellular fluid and its contents vaporize. Because the cell contents vaporize, as the electrode is moved, it "rides" smoothly in a steam envelope; thus, cutting is not a true contact mode and gives the surgeon no true tactile feedback.

With the cutting mode, tissue vaporizes so quickly that heat conduction is minimized, and the depth of tissue necrosis is lessened to 200 μm or less.[7] Cutting current confines damage to a very small area under the scalpel electrode. Only cells adjacent to the active electrode are vaporized, and cells a few layers deep essentially are undamaged. Therefore, electrical cutting can be very clean, but it is not generally accompanied by any hemostasis.

If the pure cutting electrical waveform is interrupted and the voltage increased to deliver the same wattage, then heat conduction is promoted, resulting in improved hemostasis because small vessels are coagulated. In this combination mode, the slightly interrupted waveform increases the thermal spread so that cutting is achieved with moderate hemostasis.

Fulguration

For fulguration, the active electrode is positioned usually 5–10 mm above the tissue, and a tree-like cluster of arcs is discharged onto the tissue surface. Fulguration is a high-impedance modality with relatively high voltage, low current, and a highly damped interrupted waveform. The peak-to-peak voltage is high enough to ignite and sustain longer than 1 mm. The arcs may have a temperature more than 5000 K, and they rapidly carbonize the superficial cell layers. Because the current density is relatively low in the target tissue, little desiccation occurs below the surface eschar.

Most of the energy delivered dissipates to heat the air around the active electrode. Because air is an insulator, a high-voltage current is necessary to ignite and sustain an effective arc. To reduce voltage and increase the arcing effect, an argon beam coagulator has been introduced to dry large oozing surfaces. Because the argon's arc ignition voltage is 20% less than that of air, the arcs scatter less, instead following in the laminar argon gas flow. Thus, they can be directed more precisely and over a greater distance than the random arc strikes associated with fulguration in air.

The disadvantages of fulguration are not only that the desiccation is superficial but also that the electrode tends to absorb heat, thus bonding with tissue it inadvertently touches. If the eschar is then pulled up, bleeding will start again.

Because electrofulguration is a noncontact mode, it produces hemostasis without the probe adhering to the coagulated tissue. It is most often used to seal broad areas of capillary oozing or ablate a rectal tumor.

Fulguration is used in sealing large areas of capillary bleeding. Because it requires much more voltage than electrosurgical cutting or desiccation, the surgeon must be especially cognizant of the risk imposed by capacitive or direct coupling during fulguration.

Desiccation

Desiccation is the only true contact mode of electrosurgery. The tissue temperature is increased to the point at which proteins denature and form a rigid coagulum. Although proteins start to denature at about 45°C, a temperature of at least 55°C is required to form a coagulum. The amount of tissue coagulated depends on the volume of tissue increased above the threshold temperature.

Because desiccation is accomplished without an arc, no energy dissipates into the air, and because the electrode is in contact with the tissue, less power is needed for desiccation than for fulguration or cutting. The impedance is low as desiccation begins, so desiccation can be achieved with low voltage and high current. As tissue dries and proteins denature, molecules with the potential to become ionized become immobilized in the coagulum matrix, and the tissue impedance increases.

Electrosurgery in Laparoscopic Surgery

Both monopolar and bipolar electrosurgery are currently widely used in laparoscopic surgery. Although bipolar electrosurgery is safer than monopolar, its application is limited to tissue desiccation, so most laparoscopic surgeons still prefer monopolar electrosurgery. The combination of bipolar electrosurgery with an endoscopic scissor is used by some surgeons. Monopolar electrosurgery for laparoscopic procedures is advantageous because: 1) it is a familiar dissecting method, 2) it provides excellent hemostasis, 3) it is universally available in operating suites, and 4) it is inexpensive. The disadvantages of monopolar electrosurgery are extensive smoke development and risk of thermal injury during dissection.

Smoke development can be extensive in laparoscopic colorectal surgery because of the unique need to dissect through the fatty mesentery. Because smoke evacuators and rapidly recirculating gas insufflators are not usually used, the smoke-filled gas is flushed out of the abdominal cavity through an open cannula site. Whether the smoke created represents an inhalation hazard for patients or operating room personnel is unknown but is of some concern.

The smoke may have biologic as well as chemical effects. Heating biologic tissue results in the formation of molecules with aromatic ring structures and unsaturated radicals that may be harmful when inhaled. Electrosurgery smoke has been shown to be mutagenic in vitro to the TA98 strain of Salmonella[8] and to negatively affect the lungs in rats (muscular hypertrophy of vessel walls, alveolar congestion, and emphysematous changes).[9] These effects have also been seen in smoke generated by CO_2 laser application.[9,10]

Human immunodeficiency virus (HIV) proviral DNA with a median aerodynamic diameter of 0.31 μm (range 0.1–0.8 μm) has been reported in the laser plume of vaporized HIV-containing tissue.[11] Matchette et al.[12] found viable bacteriophages in CO_2 laser plume, but the events were rare in their study. Because most of the viable particles were large (at least 7.5 μm in aerodynamic diameter), these particles should be easily filtered with a recirculating insufflator. The significance of these scientific reports remains to be determined. No epidemiologic evidence exists that operating room personnel or patients have been harmed when exposed to electrosurgery smoke or laser plume. Nonetheless, we recommend taking simple measures to reduce the exposure to smoke, such as using an insufflator with a filter larger than 0.2 μm to recirculate CO_2 gas or one that is equipped with a smoke evacuation line connected to a suction circuit (Olympus). These measures will not only reduce the risk of any harmful effects of smoke but also improve visibility during use of electrosurgery in laparoscopic surgery.

Extent of Tissue Damage

The tissue temperature many centimeters from the operative area may increase substantially when using proper electrosurgical techniques. If tissue is desiccated and the current has to pass through a duct-like structure on its way to the dispersive electrode (Figure 3.3), the cross-sectional area of its pathway is reduced, so the current density will increase at this point. Thus, the tissue desiccation may occur far from the primary active electrode. This concept is quite important when duct-like structures, such as the appendix, pieces of the greater omentum, or adhesions are cut or desiccated.

Although bipolar instruments may help confine the effects of electrosurgery to the structures grasped, extensive coagulation may also damage surrounding tissue. For instance, ureter injuries have been reported after using bipolar electrocoagulation near the ureters in gynecologic surgery.[13]

In laparoscopic surgery, closely monitoring the effect of electrical current on tissue is mandatory because the laparoscope provides only a limited view during dissection. Inadvertent injuries using monopolar electrosurgery occur primarily at the active electrode and the return electrode.

Near the active electrode, injuries can occur in any part of the instrument: the handle, the insulated shaft, or at the uninsulated tip. These inadvertent injuries occur for three primary reasons: 1) insulation failure, 2) direct coupling, or 3) capacitive coupling (Figure 3.6A and B).[14]

Insulation failure occurs most often at the distal shaft as a result of repeated heating of the instrument or because of damage to insulation when the instrument is inserted in the cannula. Insulation failures near the instrument tip can be recognized immediately if the tip is in view during the application of electrical current. Also, all exposed metal at the tip of the instrument being used must be visible in the laparoscopic field. The insulation on the shaft of the instrument rarely fails, but is potentially dangerous because it is usually not recognized during laparoscopic procedures.

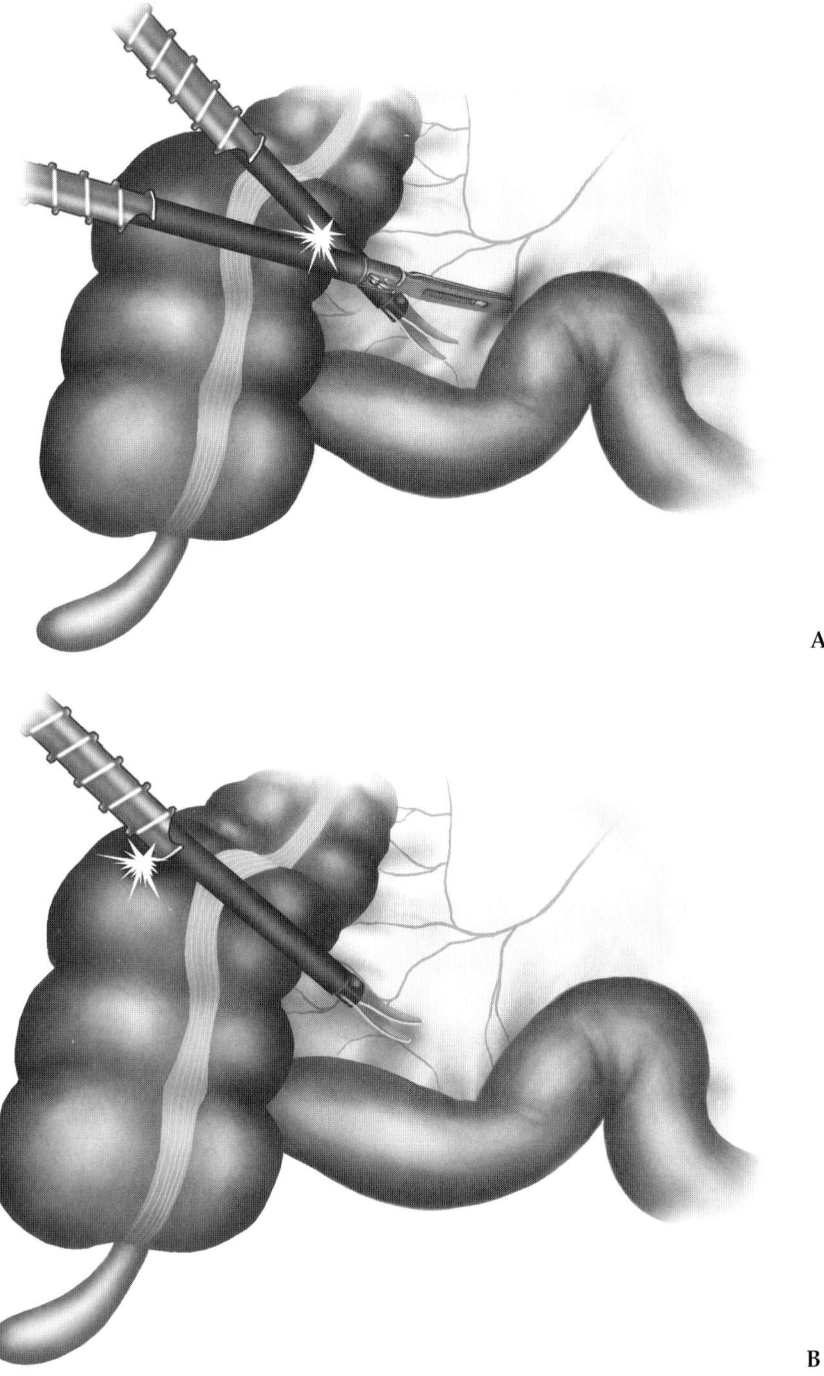

Figure 3.6. Insulation failure can occur by two major means when performing electrosurgery. **A** Direct coupling between two instruments. **B** Capacitive coupling when the charged instrument is being used with a metal cannula that is insulated from the abdominal wall by a nonconducting anchoring device.

Direct coupling describes any inadvertent contact between the active instrument and other metal instruments or cannulae in the abdomen. Whereas the metal instrument tip is free and ready to be used for coagulation or cutting, the more proximal metal parts can touch other instruments; this contact may lead to accidental coagulation or cutting without insulation failure. Thus, during the application of cutting or coagulating current, the entire instrument blade must be visible in the laparoscopic field.

The third important mechanism of inadvertent tissue damage during monopolar electrosurgery is capacitive coupling. Capacitance is the ability of an electric nonconductor to store energy. A capacitor consists of two conductors separated by an insulator. Capacitive coupling can occur if an instrument with insulation failure along the shaft is used in a metal cannula with a plastic abdominal wall anchoring device; the plastic anchoring device prevents the current from flowing through the metal cannula into the abdominal wall and onto the dispersive electrode.[14,15] In general, 10%–40% of the power of the electrosurgical unit may be coupled, or transferred, from the isolated shaft to the active electrode to the cannula. As long as the current can pass through a low power-density pathway and return to the dispersive electrode, it will not harm the patient. If the path to the dispersive electrode is blocked through a high-resistance, nonconductive anchoring device, however, capacitive coupling can occur.

Stray currents produced during capacitive coupling may produce inadvertent burns on intraabdominal structures. When a metal cannula (or instrument with insulation failure) touches any organ or intraabdominal structure when stray current is stored in the cannula, this electrical energy may be discharged from the metal cannula to any structure touching it, including those outside the field of vision of the surgeon. Capacitive coupling can occasionally be recognized by neuromuscular stimulation of the abdominal wall.

Direct coupling and capacitive coupling rarely cause electrical injury. Unfortunately, they are seldom recognized during a procedure because they usually occur outside the view of the laparoscope[14,15]; however, such injuries can be prevented. Capacitive coupling can be prevented if the anchoring device and the cannula are both made of plastic or metal.

Although alternating current has the potential to cause an effect at both the active and the return electrodes, the effect usually occurs at the active electrode because the current density is much higher at the active electrode because it is smaller, and tissue temperature is directly proportional to the square of the current density. The alternating current delivered at the active electrode is identical to that at the return electrode; therefore, if the current density is the same at the return electrode as at the active electrode, the same thermal effect will occur at both. Monopolar electrosurgery is frequently used with a return grounding electrode, which allows any current flow through the body to safely disperse. The maximum temperature attained under a dispersive electrode depends on the maximum current density, the duration of activation, and the relative cooling from tissue perfusion.

The distribution of the current under the dispersive electrode depends on the design of the electrode and the anatomic distribution of tissue under it.

Resistive and capacitive contact electrodes can be used as dispersive electrodes with a low risk of inadvertent thermal injury if the electrode is applied correctly and not accidentally dislodged. Resistive electrodes usually are gel pads or a conductive adhesive and are in resistive contact with the tissue. Capacitive electrodes have a nonconductive film between a metallic plate and the skin surface, so that a capacitor is formed and a type of capacitive coupling is used to prevent injury. Although resistive dispersive electrodes, in contrast to capacitive electrodes, have a nonuniform heating pattern because the current is more concentrated at the electrode edges, both types of dispersive electrodes appear to be equally safe in surgery.

To prevent burns at the return electrode, manufacturers have incorporated electronic sensors with circuit breakers (contact-quality monitoring electrodes) in the electrosurgical unit that monitor the quality of the connection between the dispersive electrode and the patient as well as between the cable and connector when no surgical current is in use. The change in contact impedance during the procedure is determined by a microprocessor, and if impedance increases, the electrosurgical unit will shut down. These safety features, together with the proper use of dispersive electrodes, have substantially reduced the number of burns at the return electrode.

Bipolar Electrosurgery

A closed circuit is necessary for all electrical energy to be used in surgery. If both electrodes are used as active electrodes, the application is bipolar.

Bipolar electrosurgery has been used for decades in both open and laparoscopic surgery. Earliest uses were in tubal ligation procedures using such devices as the Kleppinger machine. Because the electrodes are in close proximity, tissue effects are localized. Total power required to affect the tissue is small compared with that required for monopolar electrosurgery, where current must flow through the body to the ground electrodes.

Recently, important adaptions have been made in bipolar electrosurgery technology, resulting in the LigaSure™ Vessel Sealing System (Valleylab, Boulder, CO), which is a bipolar electrothermal device using a high-amperage, low-voltage current. Developed for both open and laparoscopic procedures, it is capable of sealing vessels up to 7 mm in diameter. By grasping the tissue with the device and activating the energy source, both physical pressure and electrothermal energy are delivered to the vessels. The elastin and collagen of the wall of the vessel are partially denatured, and then allowed to cool briefly as a seal intrinsic to the vessel wall forms. The newly sealed tissue, which is often transparent, can then be divided using a cutting knife built into the LigaSure™ device (Figure 3.7). In our experience, this device has helped make laparoscopic surgery immensely easier, especially in the handling of mesentery and omentum.

The LigaSure™ device has a similar appearance to other energy devices. There is a generator box that houses the energy source for the tissue sealing as well as the hardware responsible for sensing the changes in tissue density that indicate a seal. A cord connects either the 5-mm (LigaSure V™) or the 10-mm device (LigaSure Atlas™) to the generator. A major advantage of the new instruments is the ability to cut the tissue at the same time after sealing it. After tissue sealing has taken place, a trigger can be depressed, deploying a cutting mechanism that bisects the sealed area of tissue.

A tissue-response feedback mechanism on the device measures the density of the tissue and calculates the appropriate amount of electro-thermal energy to be delivered. The generator then provides an audible tone when the sealing process is complete. Depending on the thickness of the tissue, we find that the sealing time varies between about 2 and 10 seconds. Subsequently, the cutting mechanism of the laparoscopic tool can be triggered, and the sealed tissue bisected. Depending on the thickness of the pedicle that is to be ligated, and the presence or absence of major vessels, multiple firings can be done before division. We typically use two to three applications per major vascular structure or with thicker bites of tissue, dividing the tissue at its distal-most seal (Figure 3.8). These multiple applications provide an increased length of tissue seal, and also allow for direct inspection of the sealed area, which is often translucent, adding confidence in the hemostasis before cutting.

The vessel seal created by the LigaSure™ provides bursting strengths that are well above physiologic range. In an in vitro model using

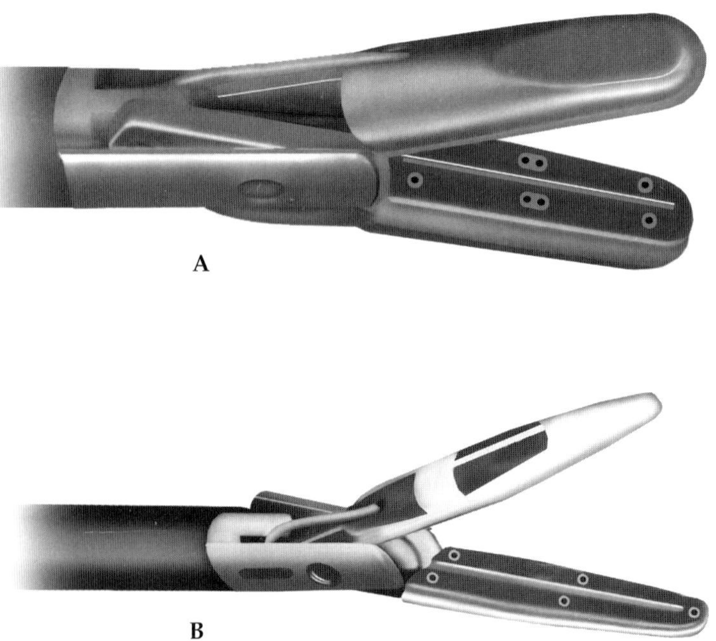

Figure 3.7. Vessel sealing devices (LigaSure™) **A** 10 mm and **B** 5 mm, each with a cutting mechanism.

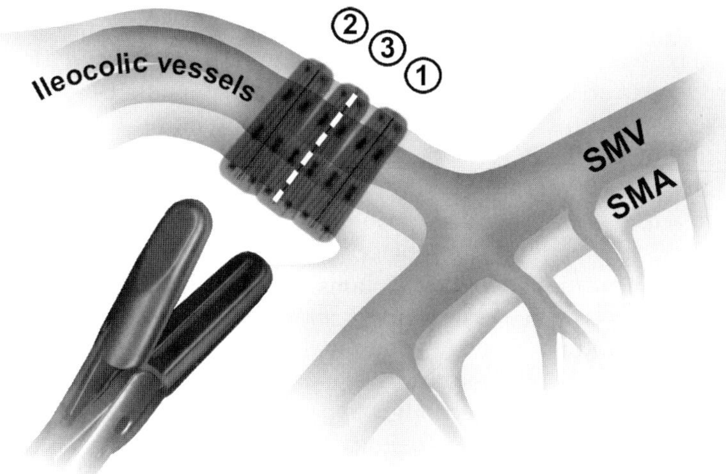

Figure 3.8. Ligation of the ileocolic vessels using the LigaSure™ 10 mm instrument.

porcine renal arteries, bursting strengths were demonstrated to be greater than 400 mm Hg – comparable to clips and ligatures, and superior to ultrasonic and bipolar devices.[16] Furthermore, the seal created is permanent, and intrinsic to the vessel itself. The surgeon does not need to rely on a luminal clot and does not need to fear a clip becoming dislodged or a tie being too loose on an edematous tissue pedicle.

The quality of hemostasis is demonstrated again in the reliability of the device. In a study involving a variety of open and laparoscopic general surgical cases, with over 4200 applications of the LigaSure™, Heniford et al.[17] demonstrated a 0.3% rate of post-application bleeding that required alternative hemostatic techniques. In 98 cases studied, they had no postoperative bleeding complications. We have had similar success at our institution, only encountering difficulty with hemostasis in the infrequent setting of a heavily calcified vessel, and finding exceptional benefit in the setting of Crohn's disease. Further discussions in its use will come in the procedure chapters.

Ultrasonic Energy

The high-power ultrasonic dissection devices have become an integral part of current laparoscopic surgical instrumentation.[18–21] They carry undoubted advantages over HF electrosurgery in that they do not generate smoke, while maintaining good cutting and secure tissue coagulation at dissection. Currently, three systems are commercially available: UltraCision Harmonic Scalpel™ (Ethicon Endo-Surgery, Cincinnati, OH), Autosonix™ (USSC, Tyco Healthcare, Norwalk, CT), and SonoSurg™ (Olympus, Tokyo, Japan). Each system consists of an ultrasonic generator, a foot switch, a hand piece, and various types of minimally invasive instruments. The generator supplies an electrical signal to the hand piece through a shielded coaxial cable. A piezoelectric ceramic element in the hand piece expands/contracts rapidly (up to 55 kHz) when electrically activated. This mechanical energy is then transduced to an imperceptibly moving blade that oscillates to produce heat secondary to friction and shear when coupled to the tissue. The vibration of the blade also causes cavitational fragmentation to separate the tissue ahead of the blade. Coagulation is also accomplished by conversion of ultrasonic energy into localized heat in tissue, which causes collagen molecules in adjacent tissue to denature. Because the scalpel itself is not heated, it does not become very hot. Thus, there is no smoke production (it produces a water vapor "mist"), no charring, no accumulation of debris on the blade, and thermal injury can be minimized. In general, lower power causes slower tissue heating and thus more coagulation effect. Higher-power setting and rapid cutting is relatively nonhemostatic. In these regards, ultrasonic surgery is similar to other forms of energy-induced hemostatic modalities. Aside from the power setting, hemostatic tissue effect can be enhanced by blade configuration and tissue traction in a manner analogous to electrode design for electrosurgery.

Blade configuration has a significant effect on device performance. Currently available blades include a single-blade scalpel (hook, ball, spatula) and a coagulating shears. A single blade is used in a similar manner as the monopolar electrosurgical appliances. If the sharp edge of the blade is used, good cutting is achieved. If the blunt side of the blade is pressed on tissue, good coagulation can be obtained. These "single-bladed" ultrasonic scalpels are useful for rapid incision/dissection on avascular planes such as lateral attachment of the ascending/descending colon. For colorectal surgical use, however, our recommendation is the shears-type instrument, sometimes so called "Laparoscopic Coagulation Shears" (LCS). It consists of a stationary portion that supports the tissue and a vibratory blade that transmits the ultrasonic energy to the tissue (Figure 3.9). The tissue is grasped with the shears and clamped. The blade is then activated to coagulate the tissue. The blade can also be used in a manner similar to the ultrasonic scalpel to cut or coagulate. Because of its tip configuration, the LCS-type instrument can also be used as an effective dissector when its blade is inactivated. Our experience has shown that the 5-mm LCS-type instrument provides the best surgical flexibility in colorectal surgery and reduces the instrument traffic through the working port during the operation.

Previous studies have shown that small- to medium-size arteries can be appropriately occluded and divided by LCS-type ultrasonic dissection devices.[18–20] Kanehira et al.[20] compared the bursting pressure of 3- to 3.5-mm porcine arteries occluded by SonoSurg™, laparoscopic clips, or silk ligatures, and reported the comparable performance of SonoSurg™ to clips and ligatures. Another study demonstrated that porcine arteries up to 5 mm in diameter can be divided safely by 10-mm UltraCision LCS™ if the blunt side of the blade is used.[19] These data suggest that when used alone, the ultrasonic dissection device can securely occlude small arteries in humans, if the device is used

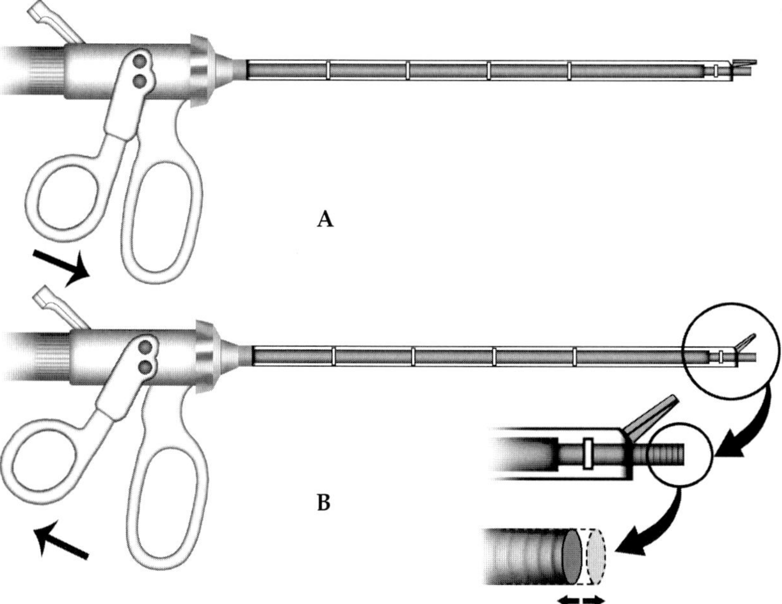

Figure 3.9. Longitudinal cut-away view of Ultrasonic Shears™ in the opened **A** and closed **B** position. In **B** note rapidly vibrating tip.

appropriately. This is valuable in colorectal laparoscopic surgery, especially when dissecting fatty tissue such as mesentery or omentum.

Reduced heat production has been known as another advantage in ultrasonic dissection.[18] Less energy to surrounding tissue during activation can lead to a reduced propensity for lateral thermal damage. Kinoshita et al.[1] studied the change in temperature around the blade of conventional electrocautery and ultrasonic dissecting device: the temperature of the tissue adjacent to the SonoSurg™ blade increased gradually and remained below 150°C; by contrast, with electrocautery at 30 W, the tissue temperature increased rapidly and exceeded 350°C within only a few seconds. They also investigated the width of the area where the tissue temperature reached 60°C or more, and reported the final width of 10 mm for SonoSurg™, as compared with 22 mm for electrocautery. These data demonstrate that ultrasonic surgery may cause fewer thermal alterations in adjacent tissue compared with conventional electrosurgery.

One well-known disadvantage of the ultrasonic dissection device is that the tissue coagulation or cutting takes more time compared with the conventional electrosurgical devices. A serious "vapor" (mist) production during the procedure is another disadvantage of LCS, although the vapor vanishes more rapidly than smoke.[22] Although one study indicated that very few morphologically intact and no viable cells were found in the vapor,[23] the aerosol created by the ultrasonic scalpel has not been well studied and no consensus exists regarding its composition.

In summary, the ultrasonic dissection device is a useful tool in laparoscopic colorectal surgery. Less thermal spread is practically valuable when dissecting significant structures from fatty tissue: e.g., taking down the ureter and gonadal vessels below the inferior mesenteric pelvic artery pedicle, and skeletonizing the vascular pedicle during pelvic lymph node dissection.

References

1. McKenzie AL. A three-zone model of soft-tissue damage by a CO_2 laser. Phys Med Biol 1986;31:967–983.
2. Walsh JT, Flotte TJ, Anderson RR, et al. Pulsed CO_2 laser tissue ablation: effect of tissue type and pulse duration on thermal damage. Lasers Surg Med 1988;8:108–118.
3. Zweig AD, Meierhofer B, Muller OM, et al. Lateral thermal damage along pulsed laser incisions. Lasers Surg Med 1990;10:262–274.
4. Hemingway A, McClendon JF. The high frequency resistance of human tissue. Am J Physiol 1932;102:56–59.
5. Zheng E, Shao S, Webster JG. Impedance of skeletal muscle from 1 Hz to 1 MHz. IEEE Trans Biomed Eng 1984;31:477–481.
6. Kanai H, Haeno M, Sakamoto K. Electrical measurement of fluid distribution in legs and arms. Med Prog Technol 1987;12:159–170.
7. Schroder T, Brackett K, Joffe SN. An experimental study of the effects of electrocautery and various lasers on gastrointestinal tissue. Surgery 1987;101:691–697.
8. Gatti JE, Bryant CJ, Noone RB, et al. The mutagenicity of electrocautery smoke. Plast Reconstr Surg 1992;89:781–784.
9. Wenig BL, Stenson KM, Wenig BM, et al. Effects of plume produced by the Nd:YAG laser and electrocautery on the respiratory system. Lasers Surg Med 1993;13:242–245.
10. Baggish MS, Poiesz BJ, Joret D, et al. Presence of human immunodeficiency virus DNA in laser smoke. Lasers Surg Med 1991;11:197–203.
11. Baggish MS, Baltoyannis P, Sze E. Protection of the rat lung from the harmful effects of laser smoke. Lasers Surg Med 1988;8:248–253.
12. Matchette SL, Vegella TJ, Faaland RW. Viable bacteriophage in CO_2 laser plume: aerodynamic size distribution. Lasers Surg Med 1993;13:18–22.
13. Grainger DA, Soderstrom RM, Schiff SF, et al. Ureteral injuries at laparoscopy: insights into diagnosis, management, and prevention. Obstet Gynecol 1990;75:839–843.
14. Voyles CR, Tucker RD. Education and engineering solutions for potential problems with laparoscopic monopolar electrosurgery. Am J Surg 1992;164:57–62.
15. Tucker RD, Voyles CR, Silvis SE. Capacitive coupled stray currents during laparoscopic and endoscopic electrosurgical procedures. Biomed Instrum Technol 1992;26:303–311.
16. Kennedy JS, Stranahan PL, Taylor KD, et al. High-burst-strength, feedback-controlled bipolar vessel sealing. Surg Endosc 1998;12:876–878.
17. Heniford BT, Matthews BD, Sing RF, et al. Initial results with an electrothermal bipolar vessel sealer. Surg Endosc 2001;15:799–801.
18. Emam TA, Cuschieri A. How safe is high-power ultrasonic dissection? Ann Surg 2003;237:186–191.

19. Ninomiya K, Kitano S, Yoshida T, et al. The efficacy of laparosonic coagulating shears for arterial division and hemostasis in porcine arteries. Surg Endosc 2000;14:131–133.
20. Kanehira E, Omura K, Kinoshita T, et al. How secure are the arteries occluded by a newly developed ultrasonically activated device? Surg Endosc 1999;13:340–342.
21. Kinoshita T, Kanehira E, Omura K, et al. Experimental study on heat production by a 23.5-kHz ultrasonically activated device for endoscopic surgery. Surg Endosc 1999;13:621–625.
22. Barrett WL, Garber SM. Surgical smoke: a review of the literature. Is this just a lot of hot air? Surg Endosc 2003;17:979–987.
23. Nduka CC, Poland N, Kennedy M, et al. Does the ultrasonically activated scalpel release viable airborne cancer cells? Surg Endosc 1998;12: 1031–1034.

Chapter 4

Patient Preparation and Operating Room Setup

Kiyokazu Nakajima, Jeffrey W. Milsom, and Bartholomäus Böhm

Preoperative Preparation of the Patient

The preoperative evaluation and preparation procedures for patients undergoing laparoscopic colorectal surgery are identical to those for conventional surgery – only the access to the operative site differs.

Patients should have preoperative blood testing, endoscopic and radiographic examinations, bowel preparation, and receive perioperative antibiotics exactly as if they were undergoing conventional surgery. We usually administer 90 mL of sodium phosphate solution in two divided doses (45 mL each), each mixed with a large glass of water, the day before surgery, to cleanse the bowel.

In patients with colorectal cancer, the liver should be thoroughly examined, either using preoperative computed tomography with both intravenous and oral contrast dye or using intraoperative ultrasonography, because liver palpation cannot be performed during laparoscopic surgery. We also recommend endoluminal ultrasonography be done in all patients with rectal cancer. The size, depth of wall penetration, and precise relationship of the tumor to other organs can be accurately determined in almost 90% of patients. Additionally, larger pelvic or presacral vessels can sometimes be identified by preoperative endoluminal ultrasonography and avoided during pelvic dissection.

The Operating Room Setup

A clearly defined setup for all laparoscopic colorectal procedures is recommended. Because laparoscopic surgery requires complex equipment, it is advisable to organize the operating room to facilitate each step of the procedure, increase efficiency, and shorten anesthesia time. A laparoscopic surgical procedure should be initiated only if all equipment is functional and has been calibrated immediately before the scheduled operation. There should also always be backup instruments to replace a broken or dysfunctional component. Successful troubleshooting with rapid replacement of components if the equipment malfunctions must be possible during every laparoscopic procedure. It is also advisable to have a trained member of the team available during the operation who can troubleshoot during the operation.

The general setup of the operating room for laparoscopic colorectal surgery involves three major steps:

- Assembling the basic instrumentation
- Preparing the patient in the operating room
- Positioning the personnel and laparoscopic equipment

Assembling the Basic Instrumentation

These basic instruments (see Chapter 2) should be available on the sterile equipment table for the preliminary evaluation, which may be done for diagnosis or to determine if the planned laparoscopic procedure will be possible:

- Scalpel handle equipped with no. 15 blade
- Scalpel handle equipped with no. 10 or no. 20 blade
- Fine long curved hemostats (e.g., tonsil clamps)
- Kocher grasping hemostats
- Electrosurgical unit
- Veress needle (or equivalent) if blind entry into the peritoneal cavity is considered
- Initial cannula for laparoscope (5 or 10 mm)
- Laparoscope with camera and light cable and carbon dioxide
- Insufflation tube

All surgical equipment necessary to perform a rapid laparotomy, if required, should be available.

If laparoscopic surgery appears to be feasible after the initial evaluation, the following laparoscopic instruments should be available on the equipment table to begin the procedure:

- Endoscopic dissecting device (for cutting and coagulation)
- All necessary cannulae and body wall anchoring devices
- Endoscopic scissor
- Endoscopic dissector
- Endoscopic graspers
- Finally, we believe that a colonoscope should be available at all times in the operating room if any clarification of the site of the target lesion becomes necessary. Cardon dioxide (CO_2) should be considered as the insufflating gas, to avoid bowel distension during the procedure.

Preparing the Patient

To initially position the patient, we have found that a modified lithotomy position works well for most laparoscopic colorectal surgical procedures. A moldable "bean bag" or a specialized body-length gel pad is placed under the patient's body on the table. The bean bag primarily is placed under the torso, and shoulder braces do not need to

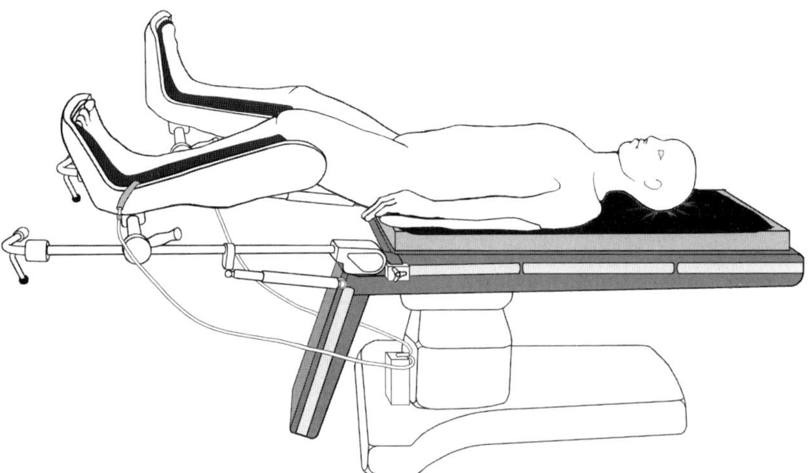

Figure 4.1. A modified lithotomy position, with legs placed in the padded adjustable stirrups and intermittent pneumatic compression system.

be used. Such a setup helps to keep the body from sliding during the steep head-down and side-to-side positions often called for in laparoscopic surgery.

The patient must be positioned so that the pelvis is just above the break at the lower end of the operating table – this position gives the surgeon free access to the perineum for intraoperative endoscopy, pelvic manipulation, or transanal anastomosis. The legs are placed in padded, adjustable stirrups (we prefer OR Direct Stirrups, Acton, MA) so that the surgeon can stand between the legs when necessary (Figure 4.1).

We initially wrap each calf or entire leg with pneumatic compression stockings. The use of intermittent pneumatic compression systems is highly recommended to prevent deep vein thrombosis. The legs are positioned in a 20° to 25° abducted position with the thighs only minimally elevated above the abdomen because higher thigh elevation may not allow the surgeon to freely move the instruments. We usually attempt to elevate the heel of each leg slightly above the knee to maximize venous outflow from the legs and minimize the risk of intraoperative venous stasis. After induction of anesthesia, an orogastric or a nasogastric tube should always be placed to empty the stomach of air and secretions. To empty the bladder and decrease the risk of inadvertent injury during the first phase of laparoscopy, a Foley urinary catheter should be placed.

In all procedures involving the left colon or rectum, rectal irrigation is performed just before skin preparation and draping. If laparoscopic surgery is to be performed to resect a colon or rectal tumor, endoscopy should be done preoperatively, and the bowel wall should be marked 2 cm below the distal tumor margin using India ink and a sclerotherapy needle passed endoscopically. In case of a tumor of the colon, either pre- or intraoperative colonoscopy or preoperative barium enema may be necessary to confirm the tumor location.

Positioning the Personnel and Laparoscopic Equipment

The positions of the personnel are determined by the location of the pathology. The surgeon generally stands on the side opposite the site of pathology, but between the legs when mobilizing either colonic flexure. When possible, standing to the patient's right side is usually preferred when performing pelvic surgery because sigmoid mobilization will be easier. The first assistant should stand opposite the surgeon or on the side opposite of the pathology when the surgeon stands between the legs. The second assistant (camera person) should stand next to the surgeon when the surgeon stands alongside the patient or next to the first assistant so that the operating team views the monitors from the same vantage point, which will facilitate guidance of the laparoscope (Figure 4.2).

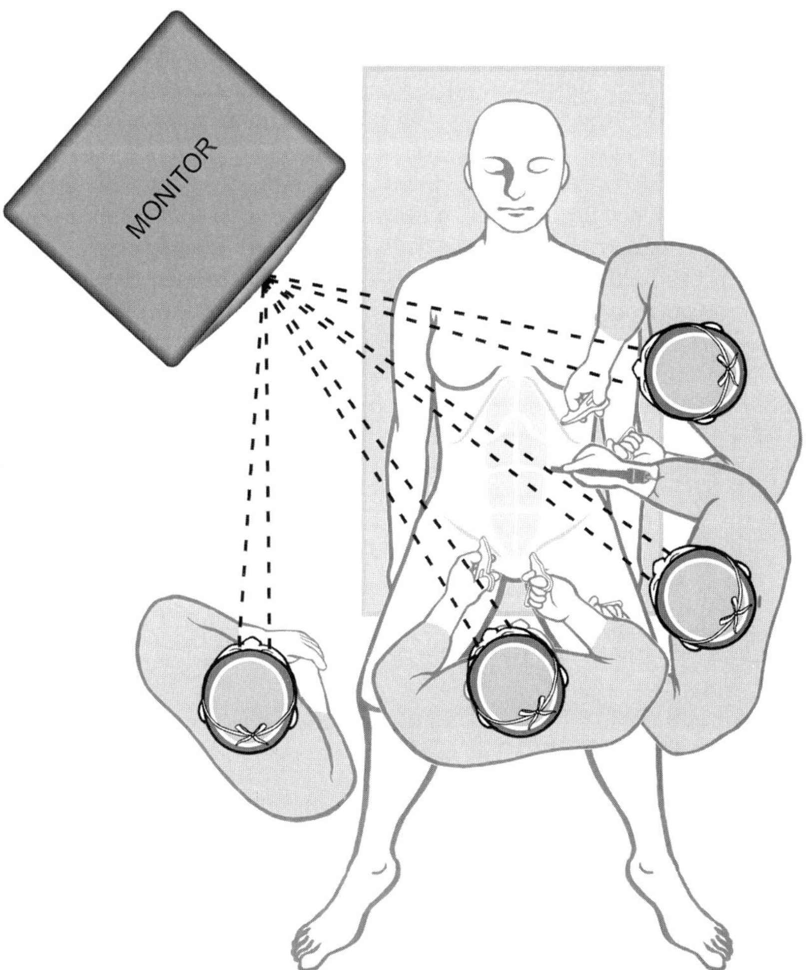

Figure 4.2. The ergonomic positioning of the surgical crew and laparoscopic monitor, which provides the same vantage point from each personnel.

The nurse should stand so that both the instrumentation table and the operative field are easily accessible. This is usually near the knee or foot of the patient usually on the left side. This position not only facilitates instrument passage but also enables the nurse to help the surgeon by performing such tasks as stabilizing the cannula while the surgeon exchanges instruments.

Depending on the area available in the operating room and the size of the equipment and instruments, the laparoscopic team should design a single setup that can easily be adapted for the most common procedures; having one setup will allow the equipment to be more quickly arranged. In addition, a backup set of equipment components must be available to avoid delay or termination of the procedure if a component fails. Because such failure is unpredictable, a plan should be developed that all team members understand so that components can be rapidly replaced. To increase efficiency, all members of the surgical team should learn the specified setup for each operation and be trained according to this setup.

The number of carts for the laparoscopic equipment should be kept to a minimum. In general, laparoscopic colorectal surgery calls for two mobile carts: they should either have wheels or be mounted on booms suspended from the ceiling. On one cart, a video monitor, light source, video system, and insufflator are placed on the patient side that is opposite to the first assistant so that the insufflator display can be seen during the entire procedure – high intraabdominal pressure, low gas flow, or an empty gas tank can thus be detected quickly. The second cart is positioned on the patient side opposite to the surgeon, and the irrigation suction unit, a video monitor, and the electrosurgical unit are placed on it.

The instrument table should be placed toward the lower end of the patient so that the nurse can easily work from it and assist the surgeon during all phases of the procedure.

Chapter 5

Anesthetic Management

Panchali Dhar

The creation of a pneumoperitoneum and positioning changes result in intraoperative cardiovascular and pulmonary changes that are uniquely different in laparoscopic compared to open surgical procedures. Proper monitoring and understanding of the physiologic changes during laparoscopic surgery are essential for safe and efficient anesthesia.

Anesthetic Techniques, Monitoring, and Positioning

Most anesthesiologists prefer general anesthesia during laparoscopic colorectal surgery. Muscle relaxation allows controlled ventilation compensating for the various changes in respiratory mechanics. The majority of general anesthetics are delivered through a cuffed endotracheal tube. Anesthetic gases may also be delivered with the laryngeal mask airway. Positive pressure ventilation up to inspiratory pressure of 40 cm is possible with the Proseal™ laryngeal mask airway (LMA). Use of the LMA in laparoscopic surgery is highly dependent on the experience and comfort level of the anesthesiologist. The anesthesiologist must consider the changes in respiratory mechanics during laparoscopy, and the potential for gastroesophageal reflux. The LMA does not protect against aspiration.

Concomitant neuraxial blockade with an epidural may be used with general anesthesia. Intraoperative epidural local anesthetic administration permits a decrease in the amount of inhalational anesthetics, narcotics, and muscle relaxants used. Spinal sympathetic outflow is blocked by application of local anesthetic through an epidural. As a result, the unopposed parasympathetic tone promotes bowel contraction and easier visualization. It is well known that N_2O tends to diffuse into closed airspaces causing bowel distension. In a double blind study of bowel distension during laparoscopic cholecystectomy with either isoflurane 70% N_2O-O_2 or isoflurane-air-O_2, the surgeon was able to identify the use of N_2O correctly 44% of the time.[1] However, in the absence of N_2O, carbon dioxide (CO_2) can also diffuse into close airspaces causing bowel distension that is indistinguishable from N_2O although it is absorbed much faster.[2] The combination of an orogastric tube and epidural anesthesia aids in bowel contraction and visualization.

Routine intraoperative monitors include standard five-lead electrocardiogram, systemic blood pressure with automated oscillometry, pulse oximetry, and capnography. The anesthetic machine must have an indicator for inspiratory airway pressures. A urinary bladder catheter and nasogastric tubes are introduced to decompress the viscera, and avoid injury to the intraabdominal contents during trocar insertion. The increased abdominal pressure and gradual diffusion of CO_2 into the stomach can place a patient at risk of regurgitation. Therefore, the orogastric tube should be placed on intermittent suction. The decision to place an invasive arterial monitor for all laparoscopic procedures is controversial. Arterial blood gas measurement certainly allows more accurate monitoring of oxygenation and ventilation. It is necessary in patients with severe cardiopulmonary disease or hemodynamic instability. Additional invasive monitoring with a pulmonary artery catheter or transesophageal echocardiography may be considered in patients with severe cardiopulmonary disease (American Society of Anesthesiologists class III–IV).

The insufflation of CO_2 into the peritoneal cavity results in increased level of dissolved CO_2 in the blood. The end-tidal carbon dioxide ($ETCO_2$) is generally used by anesthesiologists as a noninvasive substitute for the arterial carbon dioxide level ($PaCO_2$). The $PaCO_2$ is generally higher than the $ETCO_2$ by a 5- to 10-mm Hg gradient during general anesthesia. In laparoscopic surgery, the continued insufflation of CO_2 and systemic absorption elevates $PaCO_2$ resulting in respiratory acidosis. Levels increase rapidly at first, then plateau between 15 to 35 minutes later despite continued low flow insufflation. As CO_2 redistributes from well-perfused areas to less perfused tissues, the $ETCO_2$ begins to underestimate the $PaCO_2$. The anesthesiologist overcomes the increase in $ETCO_2$ by increasing minute ventilation. However, the physiologic response to continued CO_2 insufflation may not be equal in all patients. In healthy, mechanically ventilated patients undergoing laparoscopic cholecystectomy, equal and proportional increases in $ETCO_2$ and $PaCO_2$ were observed after CO_2 insufflation.[3] No significant changes occurred in minute volume and peak inspiratory pressure after CO_2 insufflation. In contrast, patients with preexisting cardiopulmonary disease were noted to have significant increase in $PaCO_2$ and decrease in pH after CO_2 insufflation, which are not reflected by comparable increases in $ETCO_2$.[4] These patients also had inspiratory pressures that were significantly higher than baseline values after CO_2 insufflation. Low cardiac output (CO) increases dead space ventilation, which is reflected by a wider arterial-to-$ETCO_2$ gradient. Additional factors such as long duration of laparoscopy, intraabdominal pressure (IAP) greater than 15 mm Hg, or subcutaneous emphysema can elevate $PaCO_2$. Radial artery cannulation for the purpose of frequent blood gas monitoring should also be considered in situations of intraoperative hypoxemia, profound elevation of $ETCO_2$, and high airway pressures.

The appearance of skin color, turgor, and suffusion is influenced by patient positioning. Because the Trendelenburg (head down) promotes central venous filling, the head, neck, and chest may assume a deep purple color. The conjunctiva may become edematous after such prolonged positioning. Addition of lithotomy adds to the increase in central venous return and abdominal pressure. Flexion of the thighs, especially in obese patients, may also compress the abdominal viscera. Resumption of the supine position or reverse Trendelenburg position can decrease elevated blood pressure caused by venous pooling in the lower extremities.

Pulmonary

Changes in respiratory physiology during laparoscopy are from the combined effects of pneumoperitoneum, positioning, ongoing CO_2 absorption, and patient body weight. The basic principles of respiratory physiology that apply to a routine general anesthetic remain pertinent under laparoscopy (Figure 5.1). In the awake state with spontaneous ventilation, a gravitational gradient promotes greater blood flow, and greater intrapleural pressure surrounding the basilar alveoli. The alveoli at the lung base are more compressed in size because of higher intrapleural pressure. As a result, the dependent (basilar/down) portion of the lungs lies on a steeper part of the pressure volume curve allowing greater expansion during inspiration. Consequently, alveoli in the dependent (basilar/down) part of the lung are better perfused, and better ventilated. Conversely, apical alveoli have less perfusion, are larger in resting size, lie on the plateau of the pressure volume curve, and expand less with inspiration (Figure 5.2). General anesthesia, supine positioning, and muscle relaxation decrease the difference in ventilation between the apical and basilar alveoli. The supine position decreases functional residual capacity (FRC) 10%–15% and the

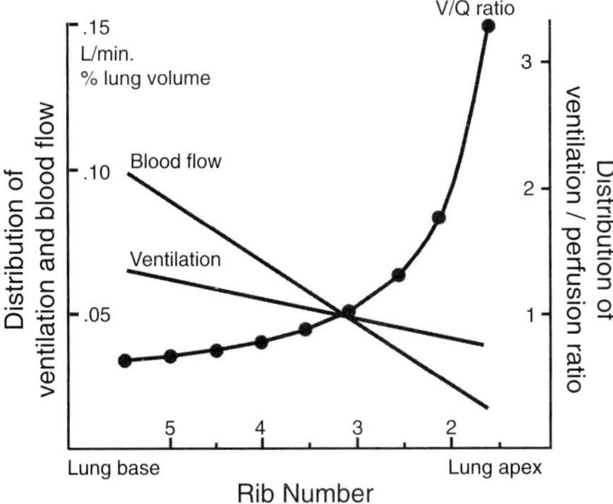

Figure 5.1. The basic principles of respiratory physiology that apply to a routine general anesthetic remain pertinent under laparoscopy.

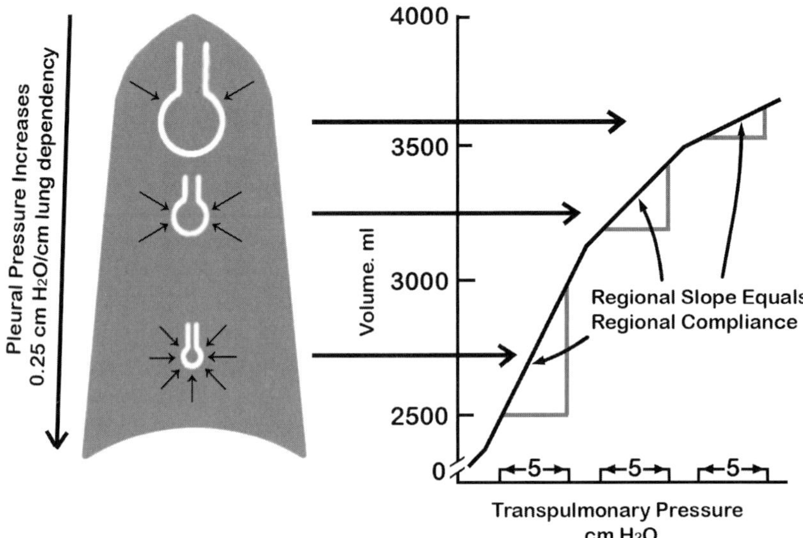

Figure 5.2. Alveoli in the dependent (basilar/down) part of the lung are better perfused, and better ventilated. Conversely, apical alveoli have less perfusion, are larger in resting size, lie on the plateau of the pressure volume curve (figure at right), and expand less with inspiration. (Reprinted with permission from Johnson ME., Factors Affecting Pulmonary Ventilation and Perfusion In Faust, RJ *Anesthesiology Review.*, 3rd edition; New York, Churchill Livingstone; 2002:9).

induction of general anesthesia further decreases FRC an additional 20%. Anesthesia and paralysis cause the reduction of lung volume through a continuum related to the body mass index (BMI).[5] A reduction in lung compliance with BMI is simply the reduction in FRC, with the intrinsic mechanical characteristics of the lung being approximately normal. Oxygenation expressed as PaO_2/PAO_2 ratio also decreases with increasing BMI. The major cause of this decrease is likely related to the reduction in FRC. Under anesthesia, the nondependent (apical/up) lung receives greater ventilation as it moves to a steeper part of the pressure volume curve (Figure 5.2). Supine positioning, muscle relaxation, cephalad displacement of the diaphragm, and compression by the abdominal contents create microatelectatic areas in the dependent part (basilar/down) of the lung and small airways collapse. This phenomenon results in true intrapulmonary shunting and ventilation perfusion mismatch.

Pneumoperitoneum and positioning changes during laparoscopic surgery add to the effects of general anesthesia and muscle paralysis. The pneumoperitoneum shifts the diaphragm cephalad, reduces diaphragmatic excursion, and stiffens the diaphragm/abdomen part of the chest wall.[6] The decreased chest wall compliance and increase in intrathoracic pressure, limits lung expansion. The restricted lung expansion elevates peak and plateau airway pressures and decreases oxygenation (PaO_2). Controlled ventilation allows the anesthesiologist to increase minute ventilation overcoming the decreased thoracopulmonary compliance and hypoventilation. In normal-weight patients, pneumoperitoneum causes a 47% decrease in lung compliance, a 50%

increase in peak airway pressure, and an 81% increase in airway plateau pressure.[7] Morbidly obese anesthetized supine patients have 30% lower static respiratory system compliance and increased inspiratory airway resistance compared with their normal-weight counterparts.[8] Laparoscopic surgery causes more severe deterioration in gas exchange in obese patients compared with normal subjects, who show a milder abnormality in alveolar-arterial oxygen difference.

Alterations such as increased tidal volume (TV) or the addition of positive end-expiratory pressure (PEEP) do not reliably improve PaO_2.[8] Increasing the TV (1000–1200 mL) often fails to improve oxygenation in both normal-weight and morbidly obese patients, suggesting that poorly ventilated, but perfused, areas of the lung are not consistently recruited.[8] In morbidly obese patients, ventilation with large TV, especially during pneumoperitoneum, results in high end-inspiratory (plateau) pressures. The end-inspiratory pressure is a measure of parenchymal stretch during ventilation. The acceptable upper limit is approximately 35 cm H_2O.[9] Prolonged increases in inspiratory pressures may lead to barotrauma of the lung parenchyma. The addition of PEEP is not a reliable tool for improving gas exchange. The addition of 10 cm of PEEP can reduce or eliminate areas of microatelectasis.[10] It may also overstretch alveoli, decrease CO, and worsen V/Q mismatch. The use of PEEP in morbidly obese patients may slightly improved PaO_2 (from 110 to 130 mm Hg) compared with normal-weight subjects.[11] The decline in pulmonary arterial oxygenation during laparoscopy is primarily the effect of patient weight, which correlates with decreased thoracopulmonary compliance.[8] Increasing the inspired oxygen concentration may be the most reliable treatment for hypoxemia in overweight and morbidly obese patients.

Laparoscopic colectomy usually requires the patient to be placed in steep Trendelenburg position. The head down position pushes abdominal contents upward additionally impairing diaphragmatic excursion and lung expansion. Vital capacity (VC) is reduced because of the increased weight of the abdominal viscera against the diaphragm. Prolonged placement in the Trendelenburg position can lead to edema of the airway including the larynx. Despite the appearance of a positive trend, a 30° reverse Trendelenburg position does not have significant beneficial effects on breathing mechanics.[12] Inspiratory resistance is increased both in the Trendelenburg and reverse Trendelenburg positions if minute ventilation is manipulated (Figure 5.3). This change in inspiratory airway resistance with position applies to both normal-weight and obese patients. There is also a potential for inadvertent right mainstem bronchial intubation, and hypoxemia with Trendelenburg positioning.[13]

The CO_2 continually insufflated into the abdomen dissolves in the blood elevating arterial CO_2, and consequently alveolar CO_2. This is reflected as an increase in $ETCO_2$. Spontaneous ventilation, especially in patients with diminished pulmonary reserve, would result in profound respiratory acidosis. Because general anesthesia allows controlled ventilation, it permits the anesthesiologist to increase the minute ventilation either by increasing the TV and/or respiratory rate. Usually, an increase in the respiratory rate is sufficient to overcome hypercarbia.

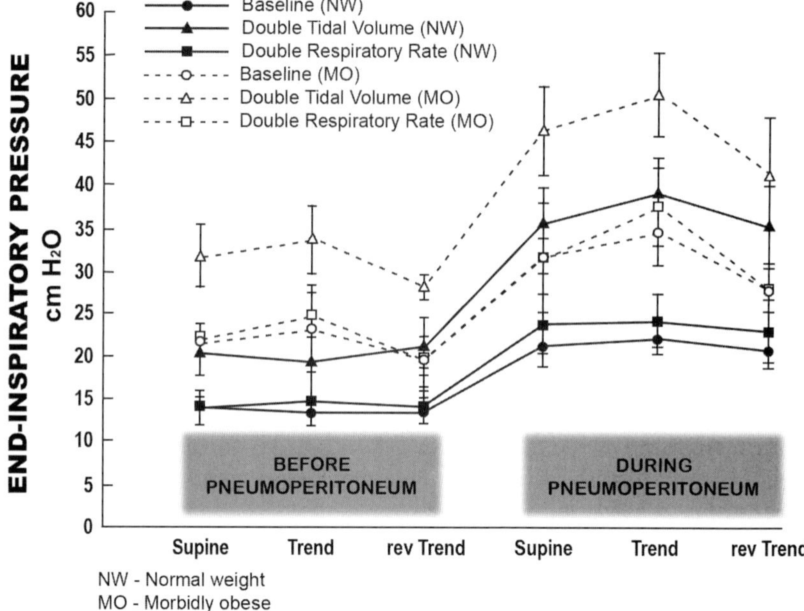

Figure 5.3. Pneumoperitoneum increases inspiratory pressures and resistance in both the Trendelenburg (Trend) and reverse Trendelenburg (rev Trend) positions. (Reprinted with permission from Sprung J, Whalley DG, Falcone T, Wilks W, Navratil JE, Bourke DL: The Effects of Tidal Volume and Respiratory Rate on Oxygenation and Respiratory Mechanics During Laparoscopy in Morbidly Obese Patients *Anesthesiology Review*; 2003:07:268–274.)

Abdominal distension may not allow an increase in TV without further increase in inspiratory airway pressures. Controlled ventilation throughout laparoscopic surgery helps prevent hypercarbia and respiratory acidosis.

After open abdominal surgery, the VC is reduced by 40%–50% of preoperative values. The VC is gradually restored over the next 5–7 days. FRC is reduced by 70%–80% of preoperative values. Gradual restoration of lung volumes begins on the second to third postoperative day. Full restoration to preoperative status may take as long as 1 week. These postoperative effects in FRC and VC are attributed to pain and reflex diaphragmatic dysfunction.[13] Patients undergoing laparoscopic procedures are noted to have better postoperative pulmonary mechanics than those undergoing open procedures.[14] A 20%–25% postoperative improvement in forced expiratory volume in 1 second, forced VC, and forced expiratory flow in patients undergoing laparoscopic cholecystectomy versus an open procedure is likely attributable to minimal abdominal wall disruption, leading to less postoperative pain.[14]

The maintenance of adequate ventilation and oxygenation during laparoscopy is a challenge for the anesthesiologist. The decrease in pulmonary compliance, lowered lung volumes, and continued absorption of CO_2 leads to hypoxia and hypercarbia. Ventilatory adjustments are continued throughout surgery to maintain oxygen and CO_2 content near the physiologic norm.

Cardiovascular

The hemodynamic changes that occur during laparoscopic surgery are a conglomeration of factors: anesthetic, mechanical, neurohumoral, and positioning. Their combined effects are difficult to separate. For example, anesthetics such as inhalational agents depress the myocardium, lower the system vascular resistance (SVR), mean arterial blood pressure, and cardiac index. In laparoscopic surgery, the artificial effects of increased IAP and positioning are additional. Healthy patients can generally compensate for the effects described below. However, patients with underlying cardiac disease, hypovolemia, anemia, or hemodynamic instability may not be able to as readily. The anticipated hemodynamic changes can be divided into separate periods surrounding the pneumoperitoneum: formation, maintenance, and release.

The formation of a pneumoperitoneum increases IAP to 12–15 mm Hg. Greater levels of IAP may be required to improve reduced visibility in obese patients caused by the weight of the abdominal wall. The increase in IAP has complex effects on the cardiovascular system. Increased IAP compresses the abdominal venous and arterial vasculature. Aortic compression contributes to an increase in SVR and afterload, which can decrease cardiac output. Venous compression causes a transient increase in venous return, followed by a decline in preload as flow through the IVC is reduced. Although venous return decreases and ventricular volumes are not increased, central venous pressure (CVP) and pulmonary capillary wedge pressure (PCWP) rise during abdominal insufflation. This is a response to a cephalad shift of the diaphragm combined with an increase in IAP and intrathoracic pressure. The rise in CVP and PCWP following establishment of the pneumoperitoneum in either the head-up or head-down position is not an accurate reflection of ventricular filling.[15] The degree of hemodynamic change is directly dependent on the patient's intravascular volume status. Volume loading with crystalloid 10–20 mL/kg can replete the intravascular volume and help minimize these cardiovascular changes in healthy patients.[16] In healthy patients, ejection fraction (EF) is maintained despite a decrease in CO.[13] If left ventricular contractility is impaired, filling pressures increase with volume load, but stroke volume decreases. The net result is a decline in ejection fraction.[17]

Circulatory responses are complex and often contradictory after the pneumoperitoneum is established. Cardiac index is decreased as much as 50% of preoperative values 5 minutes after the beginning of insufflation.[18] Further changes in CO are also influenced by patient positioning. The head-down or Trendelenburg position is critical for visualization of abdominal contents in laparoscopy. It promotes central venous return, increases pulmonary blood volume, left ventricular end-diastolic volume, and therefore, CO. The head-up position decreases central venous volume, and subsequently CO. In addition to the effect of IAP and positioning, an increase in SVR also affects the CO. In laparoscopic surgery, the SVR is sustained by mechanical and neurohumoral factors. An increase in IAP increases mechanical resistance in capacitance vessels and compresses the abdominal aorta. The effect is an increase in cardiac afterload (SVR), and a decrease in preload. The pneumoperitoneum, and continued systemic absorption of CO_2 are stimuli for sympathoadrenal outflow. Humoral factors such catecholamines, the renin-angiotensin system, and vasopressin contribute to increase SVR.[18] A fivefold increase in vasopressin levels has been noted in 60% of patients when IAP was increased to ±10 mm Hg.[18] Some studies have found no significant increase in circulating catecholeamines during laparoscopic surgery.[15] Echocardiographic evidence has documented no significant change in the transmural right atrial pressure (RAP) (RAP minus extracardiac pressure) with elevated IAP. The transmural RAP is a more accurate measure of central blood volume than directly measured RAP. A decline in stroke volume with minimal change in the transmural RAP suggests a shift in the ventricular function curve (Frank-Starling's law) to the right, perhaps secondary to the increase in afterload or SVR.[18] The increase in SVR is the primary cause of the decline in CO. It is less the result of increased sympathetic tone as a response to a decline in CO. Only an increase in SVR can explain the increase in mean arterial blood pressure observed after insufflation despite reduction in CO. In patients with underlying cardiac disease, ventricular dysfunction may be induced by an acute increase in SVR after peritoneal insufflation. In these patients, a reduced rate of insufflation and limiting IAP to a minimum may prevent dramatic changes in preload and afterload of the heart. Sympathetic blockade with epidural local anesthetic can counteract the increase in SVR. The effects of abdominal pressure, sympathetic outflow, position, intravascular volume, and anesthetic agents used cannot be separated, but must be considered together.

At the end of surgery, release of the pneumoperitoneum results in reversal of the circulatory changes described. Several events coupled together are responsible for an increase in CO and EF, and a decline in SVR. A decrease in surgical stimulation requires a decreased amount of anesthetic for maintenance of general anesthesia. A change from Trendelenburg to supine position, a decline in mechanical compression of abdominal vessels, and reduction of sympathetic stimulation contribute to a decline in the SVR. Central venous return is augmented resulting in increased CO and ejection fraction. These changes are gradual and take several minutes after the pneumoperitoneum is released.

Renal

Laparoscopic surgery is associated with decreased urine output. The etiology can be divided into prerenal, renal, and postrenal causes. Prerenal causes include decreased systemic blood pressure, hypovolemia, positive pressure ventilation or a decline in CO secondary to PEEP. Renal causes involve neurohumoral and mechanical factors. Increased sympathetic outflow results from surgical stimulation, hypercarbia, and increased IAP. Catecholamines decrease glomerular filtration rate by shunting blood from the cortex to the medulla, and constricting renal afferent arterioles.[2] The normal increase in antidiuretic hormone during surgery also contributes to reduced urine outflow. The pneumoperitoneum may cause some physical compression of the renal vasculature decreasing renal blood flow. If IAP reaches 15mm Hg, renal cortical blood flow decreases about 60% with a reversible 50% decrease in urine volume.[2] Postrenal factors can include steep Trendelenburg positioning, which allows urine to accumulate in the dome of the bladder decreasing catheter output.

Proper anesthetic management takes these factors into consideration. Fluid resuscitation should be titrated carefully because insensible losses during laparoscopy are less than that of open abdominal procedures. Overzealous hydration to compensate for a decline in urine output can lead to fluid overload and pulmonary edema.

Pain Management

The pain and loss of function after laparoscopic colorectal surgery is significantly less, and of shorter duration compared with the laparotomy approach. Minimally invasive surgery reduces the systemic inflammatory response and has been noted to reduce postoperative ileus (PI).[19] Furthermore, earlier discharge from the hospital is possible with proper pain control, prevention of nausea, and resolution of PI. Postoperative pain occurs in the upper abdomen, lower abdomen, back, or shoulders. The greatest incidence of pain is in the upper abdomen. Shoulder pain may occur in 35%–63% of patients. Pain at any location is greatest after the operation, decreases to a low level within 24 hours, but may peak later a second or third time. The duration of pain may be transient or persist for 3 days.[20] Continued and heightened pain delays resolution of ileus, nausea and vomiting, and thus recovery. The level of pain is obviously greater with hand-assisted laparoscopic procedures.

A combined effort by the anesthesiologist and surgeon can help in prevention and control of pain. Placement of an epidural catheter before surgery allows administration of local anesthetics and/or narcotics intraoperatively. These drugs act at the level of the spinal nerve roots inhibiting efferent visceral and sympathetic pain fibers. If the procedure involves hand-assisted laparoscopy, the patient can be a candidate for postoperative patient-controlled analgesia through the epidural (local anesthetic and/or narcotic), which can ameliorate pain intensity.

A persistent pneumoperitoneum causes excitation of the phrenic nerve resulting in shoulder-tip pain. This pain can be reduced by active aspiration of the gas under the diaphragm or by application of local anesthetic under the diaphragm.[20] Pain is also caused by peritoneal inflammation. The degree of peritoneal inflammation is inversely related to the abdominal compliance at the time of laparoscopy. This component can be reduced by maintaining the lower limits of IAP feasible for surgery.

Intraperitoneal instillation of local anesthetics has been shown to be effective in postoperative pain control.[21] Local anesthetics can attenuate the visceral pain, which has its maximal intensity during the first hours and is exacerbated by coughing, respiratory movements, and mobilization. Bupivacaine is the most widely used local anesthetic for this purpose. There is no consensus regarding the dose, concentration, and site and manner of administration. Generally, it is placed under visual control through the trocars in the subdiaphragmatic area, and in the surgical incisions. Most data support the use of 0.25%–0.125% bupivacaine at a dose range of 50–150 mg. Ropivacaine (7.5 mg/mL) has also proven to be effective, and may be safer because it is less cardiotoxic than bupivacaine. Lower pain scores translate to reduced morphine administration. Opioid sparing contributes to less postoperative nausea and vomiting (PONV).

Nonsteroidal antiinflammatory drugs (NSAIDs) do not have a defined role in pain control after laparoscopy.[20] Pain control is ineffective exclusively with NSAIDs. Pain scores are not significantly improved in studies comparing NSAIDs with placebo intraoperatively. NSAIDs alone are not as effective as opioids for immediate postoperative pain, and are ineffective for shoulder pain. The pain caused by peritoneal inflammation which occurs later may be better treated with NSAIDs. Antiinflammatory agents do have a role in reducing the severity of pain, and concomitantly the amount of opioid used. The maximum benefit of NSAIDs at the end of surgery is noted when they are given an hour or more before surgery. This may increase the risk of bleeding. The anesthesiologist has to consider bleeding as more difficult to detect and control in laparoscopy than laparotomy. There is a paucity of data on the effects of NSAIDs on PI, but gastric emptying after ketorolac has been shown to be significantly quicker compared with intramuscular morphine in volunteers.[22]

Postoperative Ileus

Innovative anesthetic techniques during laparoscopic surgery may aid in faster recovery of bowel motility and earlier hospital discharge. Abdominal surgery inhibits gastrointestinal motility resulting in PI. Postoperative inhibition of bowel function is not related to the degree of intraoperative handling of the bowel.[22] Clinically, PI manifests as inability to tolerate food and fluids and a delay in the return of normal large bowel function. The return of bowel movements together with tolerance of normal oral diet remains the most accurate and clinically applicable signs of resolution of PI. The pathophysiology of PI is multifactorial. The exact mechanism by which the sympathetic system contributes to PI has not been delineated. Inhibitory sympathetic reflexes originating from the gut wall, visceral and parietal peritoneum are activated with manipulation of the bowel. Additional effects of local and systemic inflammatory mediators such as inhibitory gastrointestinal peptide, anesthetic agents, use of nasogastric tubes, and pain all act in conjunction.[19]

Some anesthetic agents contribute to PI. Gastric emptying is inhibited equally by all opioids which have a similar duration of action, e.g., nalbuphine, pethidine, and morphine. Opioids given by the intrathecal or epidural route may delay gastric emptying. Gastric emptying is also delayed with atropine and this effect is most marked in the elderly. Other frequently used anesthetic drugs such as propofol, inhalational agents, nitrous oxide, benzodiazepines, muscle relaxants, and neostigmine are not strongly associated with delayed gastrointestinal motility.[22] The goal of anesthetic management for the optimal recovery after laparoscopic colectomy is to minimize the effect of the above-mentioned factors which contribute to PI. Certain anesthetic interventions can minimize development of PI and facilitate return of bowel function. Intraabdominal instillation of local anesthetic (e.g., bupivacaine) induces a faster return of colonic propulsion. This may be the result of blockade of the afferent and/or efferent link of the sympathetic inhibitory spinal nerve reflexes, blockade of inhibitory enteric neurons, direct action on the intestinal smooth muscle, or inhibition of the inflammatory response.[23] Neuroaxial blockade with epidural local anesthetic block spinal cord sympathetic reflexes resulting in unopposed parasympathetic tone. Postoperative bowel peristalsis returns earlier after epidural administration of bupivacaine compared with epidural morphine.[24] The objective of epidural blockade is to block afferent input from the wound. This is best attained when the epidural is placed at the thoracic level. Conduction blockade of afferent input can only be attained with continuously applied local anesthetic not opioids.[19]

Postoperative Nausea and Vomiting

After laparoscopic surgery, patients may be prone to PONV. The incidence of nausea and vomiting is reported to be 25%–43% after both inpatient and ambulatory surgery.[25] Nausea may arise from a long period of increased abdominal pressure, stretching of the peritoneum, and the diffusion of CO_2 into the bowel. The role of N_2O has not been established. It may contribute to the development of nausea from gastric distension. In a study in which the effects of N_2O on operating conditions during laparoscopic cholecystectomy was evaluated, no difference in the incidence of PONV was noted with or without the use of N_2O.[1] Prophylactic drugs for PONV include ondansetron, granisetron, droperidol, Compazine, metoclopramide, and dexamethasone. No individual agent has been proven to be completely effective or superior to another. Dexamethasone is now established as an effective prophylactic agent for PONV. It can decrease the incidence of PONV after laparoscopic surgery to 23%.[26] Dose ranges from 0.15 mg/kg up to 8 mg intravenously have shown favorable results for postoperative emesis.[27] Prophylactic intravenous administration of dexamethasone immediately before induction, rather than at the end of anesthesia, is more effective in preventing PONV throughout the first 24 hours of the postoperative period.[28]

A multimodal approach is superior in efficacy compared with single-agent therapy.[29] Combinations of agents such as ondansetron/dexamethasone or granisetron/dexamethasone can achieve a complete response.[30] A complete response is defined as no emesis and no need for rescue antiemetic during the 24-hour postoperative period. Control of PONV is an important component in discharge from the postanesthesia care unit, recovery, and ultimately patient satisfaction with laparoscopic surgery.

Conclusion

Laparoscopic surgery does present a unique challenge to the anesthesiologist. The understanding of the physiologic changes associated with increased abdominal pressure and positioning changes during surgery has improved over the years. Proper anesthetic management requires cooperation with the surgical team as respiratory and cardiovascular parameters vary with each stage of surgery. Postoperative issues such as nausea and vomiting and ileus are more easily managed with preoperative planning. With proper anesthetic management, laparoscopic colorectal surgery holds the possibility of more successful complex procedures and perhaps ambulatory surgery.

References

1. Taylor E, Feinstein R, White PF, et al. Anesthesia for laparoscopic cholecystectomy. Is nitrous oxide contraindicated? Anesthesiology 1992;76:541–543.
2. Yao FSF. Anesthesiology: Problem Oriented Patient Management. Philadelphia: Lippincott; 2003.
3. Liu SY, Leighton T, Davis I, et al. Prospective analysis of cardiopulmonary responses to laparoscopic cholecystectomy. J Laparoendosc Surg 1991;1:241–246.
4. Wittgen CM, Andrus CH, Fitzgerald SD, et al. Analysis of the hemodynamic and ventilatory effects of laparoscopic cholecystectomy. Arch Surg 1991;126:997–1001.
5. Pelosi P, Croci M, Ravagnan I, et al. The effects of body mass on lung volumes, respiratory mechanics, and gas exchange during general anesthesia. Anesth Analg 1998;87:654–660.
6. Mutoh T, Lamm WJ, Embree LJ, et al. Abdominal distension alters regional pleural pressures and chest wall mechanics in pigs in vivo. J Appl Physiol 1991;70:2611–2618.
7. Bardoczky GI, Engelman E, Levarlet M, et al. Ventilatory effects of pneumoperitoneum monitored with continuous spirometry. Anaesthesia 1993;48:309–311.
8. Sprung J, Whalley DG, Falcone T, et al. The effects of tidal volume and respiratory rate on oxygenation and respiratory mechanics during laparoscopy in morbidly obese patients. Anesth Analg 2003;97:268–274, table.
9. Slutsky AS. Mechanical ventilation. American College of Chest Physicians' Consensus Conference. Chest 1993;104:1833–1859.
10. Hedenstierna G. Gas exchange during anaesthesia. Br J Anaesth 1990;64:507–514.
11. Pelosi P, Ravagnan I, Giurati G, et al. Positive end-expiratory pressure improves respiratory function in obese but not in normal subjects during anesthesia and paralysis. Anesthesiology 1999;91:1221–1231.

12. Casati A, Comotti L, Tommasino C, et al. Effects of pneumoperitoneum and reverse Trendelenburg position on cardiopulmonary function in morbidly obese patients receiving laparoscopic gastric banding. Eur J Anaesthesiol 2000;17:300–305.
13. Cunningham AJ, Brull SJ. Laparoscopic cholecystectomy: anesthetic implications. Anesth Analg 1993;76:1120–1133.
14. Frazee RC, Roberts JW, Okeson GC, et al. Open versus laparoscopic cholecystectomy. A comparison of postoperative pulmonary function. Ann Surg 1991;213:651–653.
15. O'Malley C, Cunningham AJ. Physiologic changes during laparoscopy. Anesthesiology Clinics of North America 2001;19(1):1–19.
16. Hanley ES. Anesthesia for laparoscopic surgery. Surg Clin North Am 1992;72:1013–1019.
17. Harris SN, Ballantyne GH, Luther MA, et al. Alterations of cardiovascular performance during laparoscopic colectomy: a combined hemodynamic and echocardiographic analysis. Anesth Analg 1996;83:482–487.
18. Joris JL, Noirot DP, Legrand MJ, et al. Hemodynamic changes during laparoscopic cholecystectomy. Anesth Analg 1993;76:1067–1071.
19. Holte K, Kehlet H. Prevention of postoperative ileus. Minerva Anestesiol 2002;68:152–156.
20. Alexander JI. Pain after laparoscopy. Br J Anaesth 1997;79:369–378.
21. Goldstein A, Grimault P, Henique A, et al. Preventing postoperative pain by local anesthetic instillation after laparoscopic gynecologic surgery: a placebo-controlled comparison of bupivacaine and ropivacaine. Anesth Analg 2000;91:403–407.
22. Ogilvy AJ, Smith G. The gastrointestinal tract after anaesthesia. Eur J Anaesthesiol Suppl 1995;10:35–42.
23. Rimback G, Cassuto J, Faxen A, et al. Effect of intra-abdominal bupivacaine instillation on postoperative colonic motility. Gut 1986;27:170–175.
24. Wattwil M, Thoren T, Hennerdal S, et al. Epidural analgesia with bupivacaine reduces postoperative paralytic ileus after hysterectomy. Anesth Analg 1989;68:353–358.
25. Rajeeva V, Bhardwaj N, Batra YK, et al. Comparison of ondansetron with ondansetron and dexamethasone in prevention of PONV in diagnostic laparoscopy. Can J Anaesth 1999;46:40–44.
26. Wang JJ, Ho ST, Tzeng JI, et al. The effect of timing of dexamethasone administration on its efficacy as a prophylactic antiemetic for postoperative nausea and vomiting. Anesth Analg 2000;91:136–139.
27. Liu K, Hsu CC, Chia YY. The effect of dose of dexamethasone for antiemesis after major gynecological surgery. Anesth Analg 1999;89:1316–1318.
28. Wang JJ, Ho ST, Liu YH, et al. Dexamethasone reduces nausea and vomiting after laparoscopic cholecystectomy. Br J Anaesth 1999;83:772–775.
29. Scuderi PE, James RL, Harris L, et al. Multimodal antiemetic management prevents early postoperative vomiting after outpatient laparoscopy. Anesth Analg 2000;91:1408–1414.
30. Fujii Y, Tanaka H, Toyooka H. Granisetron-dexamethasone combination reduces postoperative nausea and vomiting. Can J Anaesth 1995;42:387–390.

Chapter 6

Basic Laparoscopic Surgical Skills

Kiyokazu Nakajima, Jeffrey W. Milsom, and Bartholomäus Böhm

Establishing Pneumoperitoneum

Veress Needle Technique

Pneumoperitoneum is most often established using a Veress needle. The needle is usually inserted at the site where the primary cannula for the laparoscope will be placed. Our preference is a vertical infraumbilical incision because it overlies the location where the skin, fascia, and parietal peritoneum converge and fuse. If the patient has had prior abdominal surgery, we generally avoid the old incision scars and enter from a remote site in the upper abdomen.

After the skin is incised, the subcutaneous fatty tissue is bluntly dissected until the linea alba is visible. The linea alba is grasped using two Kocher clamps and pulled anteriorly. A "U-shaped" 2-0 or 0 fascial suture can be placed around the cannula insertion site at this time to facilitate later fascial closure, and the Veress needle is inserted perpendicular to the abdominal wall. Before using the Veress, the surgeon should check that the needle is patent and the spring-loaded safety mechanism is functioning properly. The needle should be held between the thumb and index finger not more than 3 cm from the tip to ensure it passes safely and steadily through the fascia (Figure 6.1). Steadying the heel of the needle-wielding hand on the abdominal wall will minimize the risk of uncontrolled insertion through the fascia. The needle should be advanced perpendicularly through the fascia for approximately 1 cm; then the needle should be directed toward the pelvis. As the needle's spring mechanism crosses the posterior rectus sheath and peritoneum, a definite give with a click is usually felt. Once inside the peritoneal cavity, the needle tip should feel free and move easily when the hub is moved laterally.

Once the needle is in place, its intraperitoneal location is verified with the following checks before gas insufflation:

1. A 10-mL syringe filled with normal saline is attached to the needle. Three milliliters is injected and then aspirated. No resistance should

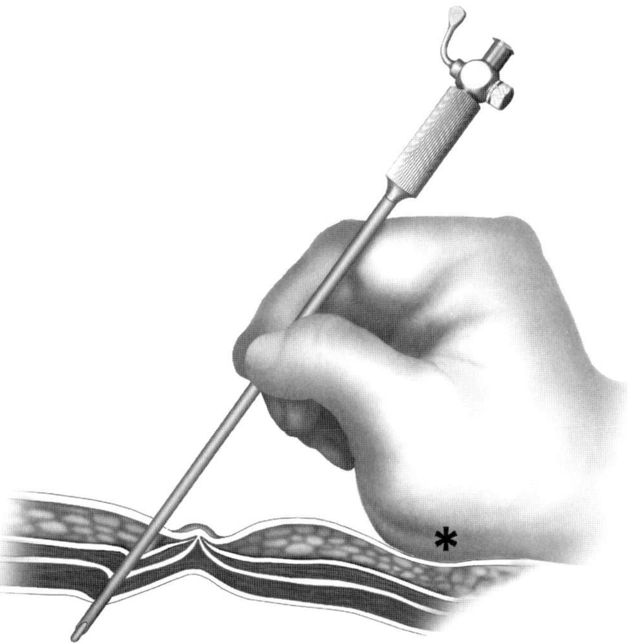

Figure 6.1. The Veress needle is held between the surgeon's thumb and index finger midway up the shaft. The risk of plunging deeply can be minimized by placing the base of hand on the body wall (asterisk).

be felt during injection. The aspirate is examined for return of blood, urine, or bowel contents.

2. The "hanging drop" test is performed, which confirms that the needle has entered a cavity. The test is done by relaxing all retraction on the abdominal wall, placing a drop of saline on the open hub of the Veress needle, then lifting up the Kocher clamps placed on the abdominal fascia. When the clamps are lifted, the saline will quickly drop into the peritoneal cavity if it has been entered.

Although these tests merely indicate whether a cavity has been entered, and may not distinguish between the peritoneal cavity and the preperitoneal space or a hollow viscera, we believe these tests should always be performed before gas insufflation.

After the syringe test and the drop test, the insufflation line is connected to the needle and CO_2 insufflation is started. The intraabdominal pressure is monitored during early gas insufflation (Table 6.1). The pressure should be less than 5 mm Hg at the beginning of CO_2 insufflation. If the pressure is greater than 5 mm Hg, the needle can be either in the abdominal wall, preperitoneal space, adjacent to or within an intraabdominal viscus, or buried in the omentum. Elevating the abdominal wall and repositioning the needle (usually by simple axial rotation) will almost always result in proper pressure readings. If the pressure remains elevated or increases rapidly over 10 seconds, the needle tip is likely misplaced, and it should be removed immediately and inserted again, or the surgeon should consider an open technique.

Table 6.1. CO_2 monitor reading – various scenarios on Veress needle insertion

Pressure	Flow	Abdominal distension	Possible etiology
Starts low ↓ Rises gradually	Low at first	Distends gradually	Normal
Starts low ↓ Stays low	Low at first Stays high	Not much	1) Leak in the system 2) Needle in hollow organs or intravascular
Starts low ↓ Stays low	Low at first Then none	Not much or no distension	Empty CO_2 cylinder
Starts high ↓ Stays high	Low or none	No distension	1) Occlusion in system 2) Needle in abdominal wall, adhesions, or intramural (organ)

Open-Hasson Technique

Although some surgeons use the "open-Hasson" technique routinely in all patients, it is still controversial whether this technique minimizes risks of injury to the abdominal viscera at the initial abdominal access.[1] However, surgeons should always readily move to the open technique when any difficulties arise using the Veress needle technique. Currently, we use this technique selectively when dense intraabdominal adhesions are suspected: e.g., cases with history of prior major abdominal surgery.

In this technique, the peritoneal cavity is opened and a blunt-tipped open "Hasson" cannula is introduced under direct vision through a mini-laparotomy. The standard open cannula consists of three pieces: a cone-shaped sleeve, a sheath with a trumpet or flap valve, and a blunt-tipped obturator. The sleeve can be moved up and down the sheath until it is properly positioned. There are two suture struts on the sleeve or the sheath to affix the cannula to the fascial and peritoneal incisions.

A 2-cm skin incision is made at the selected entry site. A longer incision will result in the major leakage of CO_2 gas during the insufflation. The subcutaneous tissue is bluntly dissected and the underlying fascia is identified and incised. This incision should be just long enough to admit the surgeon's index finger. The abdominal entry is confirmed visually and by digital palpation, to ensure the absence of intraabdominal adhesions in the vicinity of the incision. The cannula is then inserted under direct vision between two hemostats that grasp the peritoneum. Two sets of 0 or 2-0 sutures are placed on either side of the fascial incision and wrapped around the struts to firmly seat the cannula in the peritoneal cavity (Figure 6.2). Some surgeons place these fascial sutures first, use these to elevate the fascia, and then make the fascial incision. Care should be taken not to deeply open the fascia, because underlying peritoneum and viscera can be damaged in thin patients. The CO_2 line is connected to the sidearm port and pneumoperitoneum is established under continuous monitoring of the intraabdominal pressure.

Use of Optical Access Trocar

The third alternative for the establishment of pneumoperitoneum is the use of so-called optical access trocars. The trocar used in this technique (e.g., Bladeless Trocar; Ethicon Endo-Surgery, Cincinnati, OH) has a clear, tapered (bladeless) optical obturator, which provides visibility of individual tissue layers during insertion when used with an endoscope. A 0° or 30° endoscope connected to the light source and monitor is inserted into the opening at the proximal end of the obturator until it reaches the distal tip of the obturator. The obturator is then introduced through a skin incision and advanced by applying continuous but controlled pressure with a rotating motion. The penetration of the obturator tip is endoscopically monitored and the individual tissue planes can be seen as the obturator tip advances (Figure 6.3). The trocar advances by dilating the tissue planes, not by cutting. After laparoscopic verification of the intraperitoneal placement, CO_2 insufflation is started directly through the cannula. This technique is best suited for obese patients with a thick abdominal wall, where a standard "open" technique via mini-laparotomy is occasionally technically difficult.

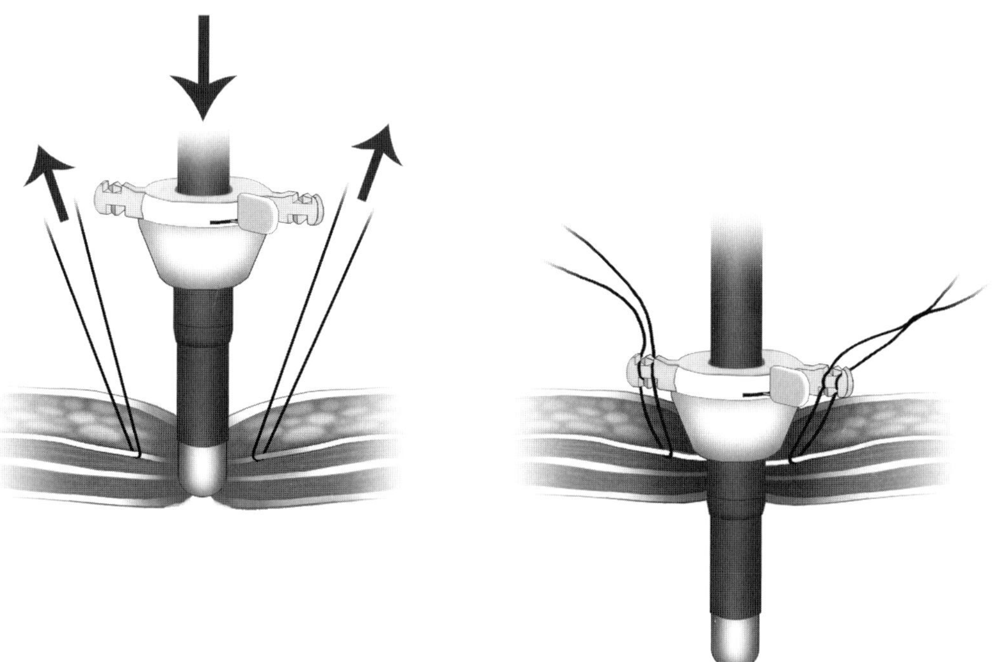

Figure 6.2. The Hasson cannula is introduced into the body wall using two fascial sutures which elevate the anterior rectus fascia. Later, these are used to secure the cannula and also to close the fascia at the conclusion of surgery.

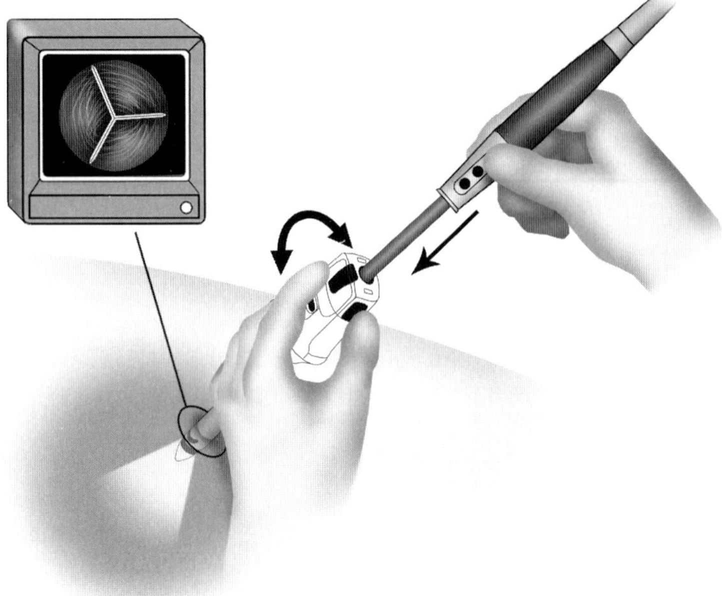

A

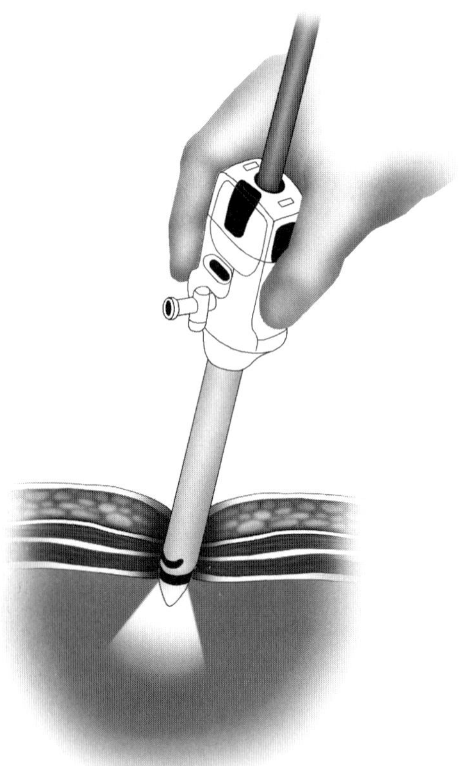

B

Figure 6.3. Optical access trocar is inserted into the abdominal wall. **A** The laparoscope is placed into the obturator while twisting the sheath, all under laparoscopic guidance. **B** A cross-sectional image of the body wall is obtained while using the optical access trocar.

Trocar Insertion and Stabilization

Trocar Insertion

In general, we place four to five cannulae for most colorectal procedures: one for the laparoscopic camera, two for the operating surgeon, and one or two for the assistant surgeon. This technique provides best surgical flexibility in all four quadrants, allowing operating and assistant surgeons to cooperate. In most instances, the operating surgeon will place the cannula opposite to the site of the pathology, which allows the greatest room to work and to visualize the pathology site. Because any abdominal wall cannula will restrict the mobility of the laparoscopic instruments, the cannula locations should also be chosen to allow the greatest mobility possible, given several additional considerations: each cannula should be placed with a distance of at least 8 cm to prevent the instruments from "sword-fighting" each other. In addition, cannulae should also be placed 6–8 cm away from the laparoscope site because closer placement impedes a clear overview of the laparoscope.

After pneumoperitoneum is established with the Veress needle, the umbilical incision is usually used for the first cannula insertion. Any kind of access systems can be used, but our current preference is an endoscopic threaded imaging port system (EndoTIP™; Karl Storz, Tüttlingen, Germany) that can be introduced under optical control. Unlike conventional trocars, the EndoTIP™ requires no trocar and minimal axial penetration force during insertion. The device has a proximal valve section and a distal cannula section with a single thread winding around its outer surface, ending in a blunt tip (Figure 6.4). The tip does not cut tissue, but is inserted by rotation, displacing structures while minimizing the risk of accidental injury. The EndoTIP™ system can be categorized into so-called "optical access" systems, and seems safely applicable for obese patients with thick abdominal wall, where a standard "open" technique is technically difficult. Ternamian and Deital[2] used the EndoTIP™ system in 234 consecutive patients including moderately and markedly obese patients, and reported that the system can be safely used for any body weight patients. Although the use of EndoTIP™ or other similar systems may minimize the risk of injuries during the first cannula insertion, the area just below the initial entry site should be inspected laparoscopically to detect possible visceral injury from the blind entry of the Veress needle.

Usually, the secondary cannulae are placed under laparoscopic guidance to avoid puncturing significant intraabdominal or retroperitoneal structures. Before insertion, the abdominal wall should be transilluminated to identify any major vessels at potential entry sites so these vessels can be avoided. The size of the skin incision for each cannula must be planned carefully. If the incision is too small, friction will develop between the skin and the cannula sleeve; consequently, greater force will be required for insertion, which will increase the risk of uncontrolled insertion and inadvertent injuries of underlying viscera. However, if the incision is too large, insufflated gas may leak out

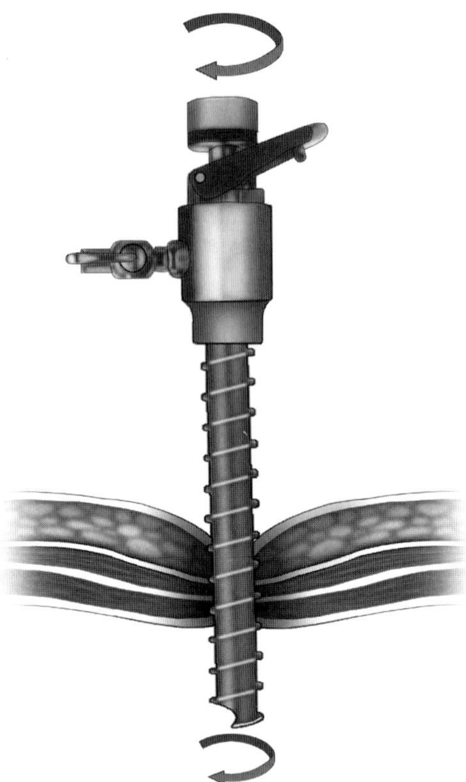

Figure 6.4. Insertion of EndoTIP™ cannula after creation of pneumoperitoneum. A laparoscope can be inserted into the cannula to monitor when the cannula enters the peritoneal cavity.

around the incision during the procedure and the cannula may dislocate more easily. It is wise to make the incision slightly too large than too small – risking an intraabdominal injury merely to save 2–3 mm of the abdominal incision is senseless and possibly dangerous.

Trocar Stabilization

The frequent slipping of the working cannula from the abdominal wall while instruments are moved in and out can cause much frustration. Once the port is out, pneumoperitoneum is lost, and the whole process must be reestablished to regain a view. This is time-consuming and potentially catastrophic when the forceps is holding an important structure or when profuse bleeding is encountered. In the case of frequent cannula dislocation, commercially available "port grippers" are used (Figure 6.5). These grippers can effectively stabilize the cannulae in the abdominal wall by a screw design; however, they usually require slightly larger skin incision for best results. Forcibly applying the grippers in the incision may damage the tissue and thus impair wound healing. An alternative is a single throw of a fixation suture (Figure 6.6).[3] A strong 0 suture is placed through-and-through the skin around the cannula entry site. The sleeve is pulled back until just enough

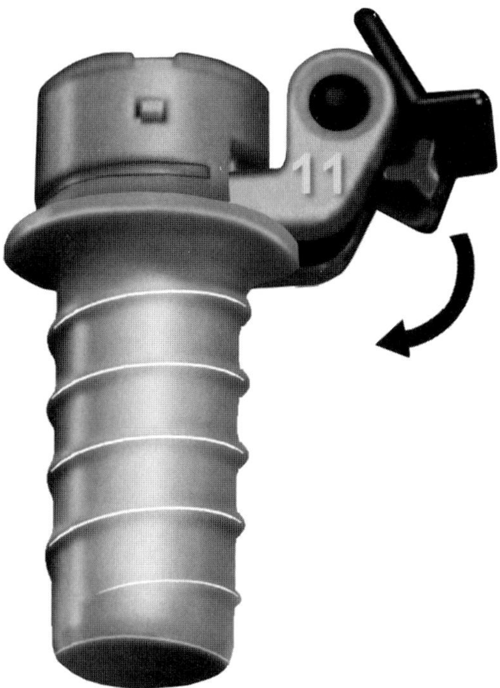

Figure 6.5. Port grippers can be used to further stabilize cannulae. Different sizes and shapes are available.

length is inside the peritoneal cavity to maintain pneumoperitoneum. The suture is secured to the cannula by wrapping it around the insufflation port. The cannula can be pushed inside the abdomen but cannot be pulled out because of the holding suture. The surgeon can easily adjust the length of the port inside the abdomen with one hand.

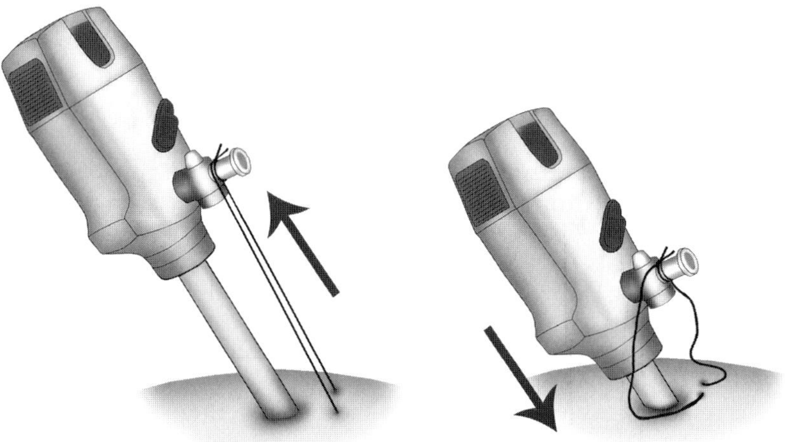

Figure 6.6. Port fixation sutures are a simple way to prevent cannulae from pulling out of the abdominal wall.

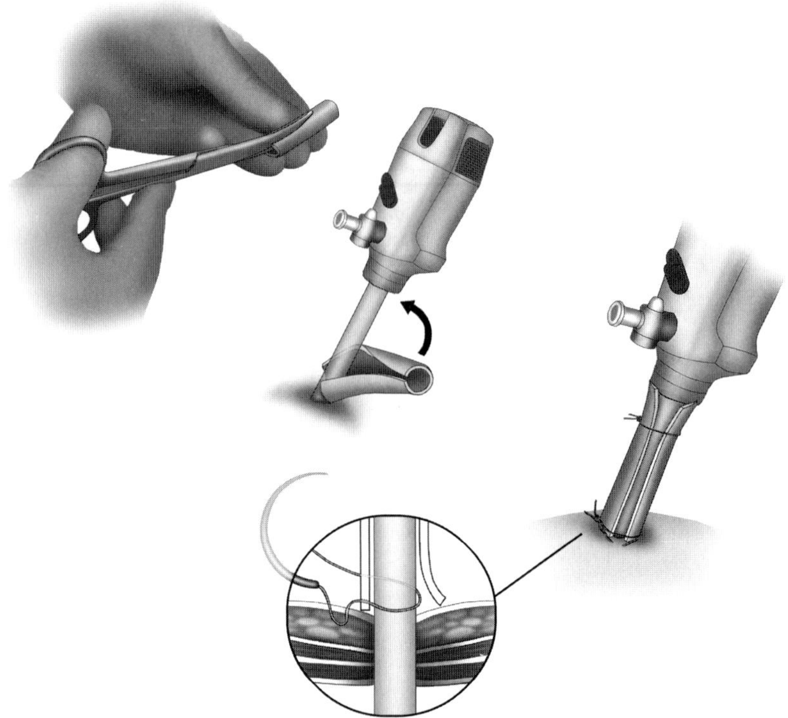

Figure 6.7. Use of a firm rubber tube is an inexpensive, easy technique for cannula fixation.

To further stabilize the cannula, we use the following technique: A tube with adequate length is sliced longitudinally and wrapped on the cannula. The length of the tube should be preadjusted so that the sleeve may be placed in the abdominal cavity with an adequate length. An abdominal U-stitch is then placed through the tube, fixing the cannula in the abdominal wall. Another suture is placed on the distal part of the tube to firmly secure the tube on the cannula (Figure 6.7).

Exposure

A good surgical exposure is always the key to success in any laparoscopic procedure. In general, this can be accomplished by the combination of:

1. adequate establishment and maintenance of pneumoperitoneum
2. appropriate positioning of the patient and the operating table to enhance gravity-induced displacement of the obstructing structures and
3. effective retraction and displacement of obstructing structures.

Adequate Pneumoperitoneum

Adequate pneumoperitoneum can be obtained under sufficient muscle relaxants with an appropriate control of the intraabdominal CO_2 insufflation. Usually, intraabdominal pressure of 10–12 mm Hg provides good laparoscopic visualization and sufficient working space. However, even after successful establishment of pneumoperitoneum, the insufflated gas can be lost from the peritoneal cavity during the instrument/laparoscope exchange, by the aggressive evacuation of smoke, and because of spontaneous gas leakage. The intraabdominal pressure should therefore be continuously monitored, and the automatic reinsufflation function is mandatory. To keep steady and quick reinsufflation, each connection to the CO_2 line should be maintained adequately through the procedure.

Appropriate Positioning

In principle, the operative site (i.e., target tissue) should be always positioned as "high" as possible in the peritoneal cavity to maximize gravitational retraction. The surrounding structures that may obstruct the exposure can be effectively displaced from the operative site with the aid of gravity. Collection of blood and tissue fluid can be also positioned away from the operative site. For this purpose, the patient should be placed adequately on the operating table so that the intraoperative rotation of the table can maximize the gravity-produced displacement. For example, to obtain good exposure of the hepatic flexure of right colon, the patient should be placed slightly in the reverse Trendelenburg position and the operating table should be turned with the right side tilted up (Figure 6.8). The operative table should be rotated appropriately as the operative site changes: In case of proctosigmoidectomy, the patient should be first placed flat or in the Trendelenburg position with the left side up to obtain good visualization of the inferior mesenteric artery pedicle, and then changed to the reverse Trendelenburg position to gain good exposure of the splenic flexure.

Effective Retraction and Displacement

In addition to the gravity-produced displacement, aggressive retraction and displacement of obstructing structures are still necessary to optimize the exposure. In colorectal laparoscopy, most of the attention is directed to the small intestine and the greater omentum, because they normally spill into all quadrants of the abdomen. Using the atraumatic laparoscopic graspers, these structures should be retracted and displaced gently to the opposite site of the pathology: e.g., in right colectomy, the omentum is to be flipped up above the transverse colon, and the small bowel loops are to be positioned to the pelvis. The instrument shafts can be safely used for this purpose. Even after repeated efforts for manual retraction/displacement, the small bowel loops may still migrate into the operative site. On these occasions, additional cannula placement should be considered, to utilize a laparoscopic retractor for effective retraction.

For bowel retraction, a one-finger or a fan retractor is not recommended, because they are originally designed to retract the liver or other more fixed organs. Intestinal loops can be trapped between the fingers of the retractor, exposing the loop to potential injury. Although there are currently no optimal retractors available for rapidly retracting the small bowel, our current preference is a paddle-type retractor (Endo Paddle

Retract™; USSC-Tyco, Norwalk, CT).[4] The device measures 12mm in diameter and 47cm in working length. It consists of a long, thin plastic tube, inside of which is housed a collapsible rectangular paddle-shaped instrument with a flat surface. Once the tube is passed inside the abdominal cavity, through a 12-mm cannula, deployment of a knob on the end of the instrument expands the paddle to a fully or partially deployed position, depending on the size of the retracting surface needed. A nylon cloth covering provides friction to the paddle, allowing for efficient retraction of the organ(s) to be moved. The Endo Paddle Retract™ is a useful tool in obese patients especially to retract the small bowel loops away from the pelvis or the inferior mesenteric artery.

Another simple technical alternative is the usage of gauze pads. A 4 × 8 inch gauze, marked with radioopaque tapes, is slightly soaked in warm saline solution then deployed through a 10- or 12-mm cannula. The gauze can be placed beneath and over loops of small bowel, especially useful in pelvic surgery or during the isolation of the inferior mesenteric artery pedicle in sigmoid colon or rectal cancer surgery (Figure 6.9).

We have also found valuable retraction using a large laparotomy pad during hand-assisted laparoscopic surgery (HALS). The hand access device, inserted through a Pfannenstiel incision, permits the insertion and handling of this large pad.[5] Use of this method in morbidly obese

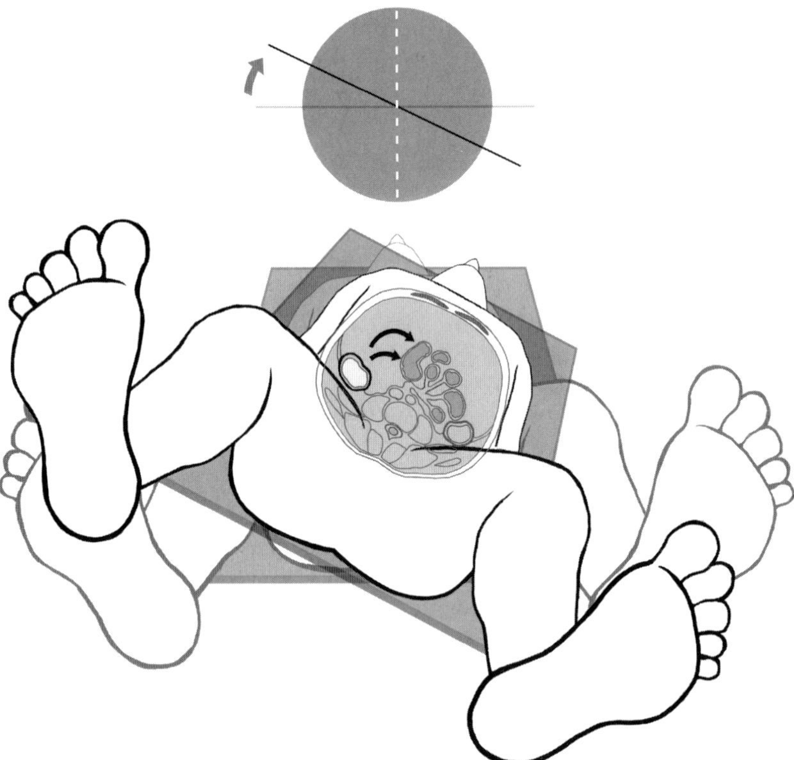

Figure 6.8. Use of gravity: Positioning of the patient by lateral tilting can be a key maneuver for moving the small intestines away from the surgical site.

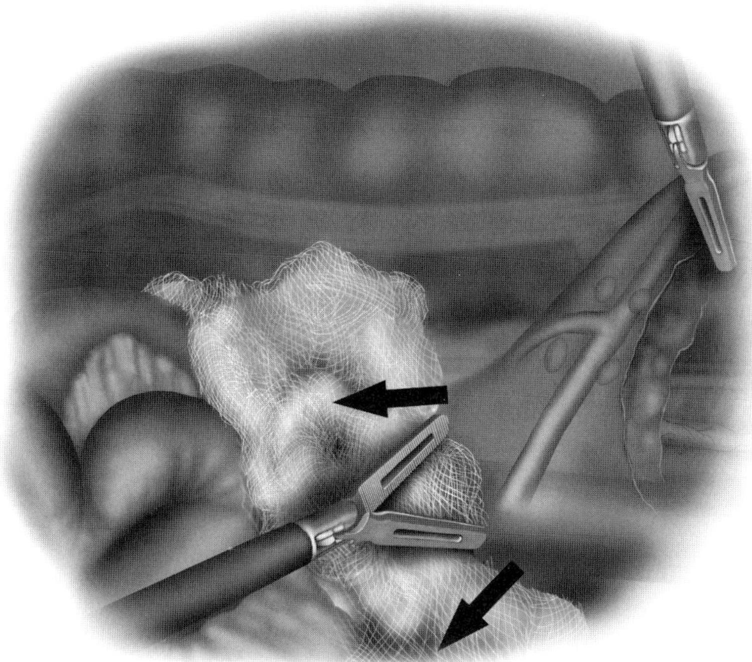

Figure 6.9. Retraction and protection of the small bowel can be easily achieved with a gauze pad, placed through a 10-mm or larger cannula.

patients may allow minimally invasive surgical techniques to be used when they would otherwise be impossible.

Tissue Triangulation

Tissue triangulation is one of the most essential techniques in colorectal laparoscopy. The tissue is triangulated between three grasping instruments, two held by the assistant and one by the surgeon (Figure 6.10). This tension allows for precise initial incision of the peritoneum and guidance in the direction of the dissection using the third grasper. Thereafter, mesenteric vessels can be palpated and isolated with a gentle, blunt sweeping maneuver of the dissecting instrument and then coagulated or clipped. With this technique, the mesentery can be divided quickly with only minor bleeding.

Separating the greater omentum from the transverse colon should also be accomplished using tissue triangulation. Any adhesions of greater omentum to the colon/mesocolon can be divided under tension using a scissor with electrosurgery, the ultrasonic scalpel, or the LigaSure™ vessel sealer. In some patients with colitis, the greater omentum may develop vascular attachments to the colon, and dissection may be difficult and require extensive coagulation. Because the greater omentum itself is usually quite flaccid, coagulation with ultrasonic scalpel is difficult. The LigaSure™ device seems preferable to us in these cases (Figure 6.11).

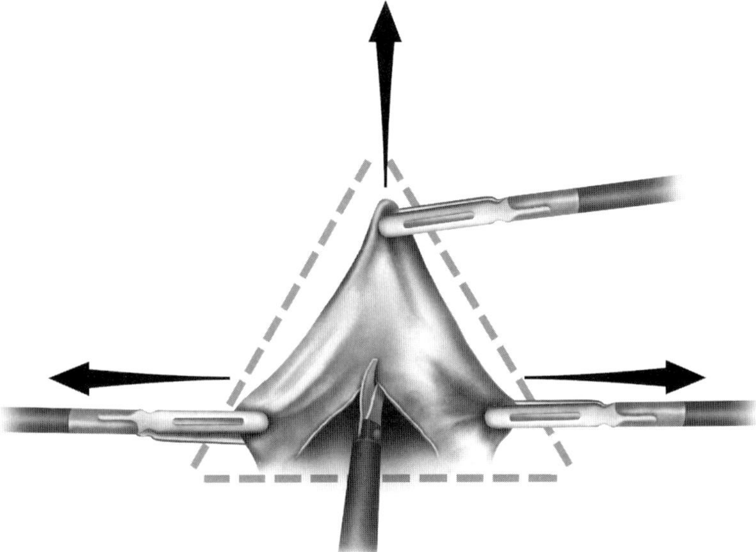

Figure 6.10. Tissue triangulation is a key component of accurate dissection during laparoscopic surgery.

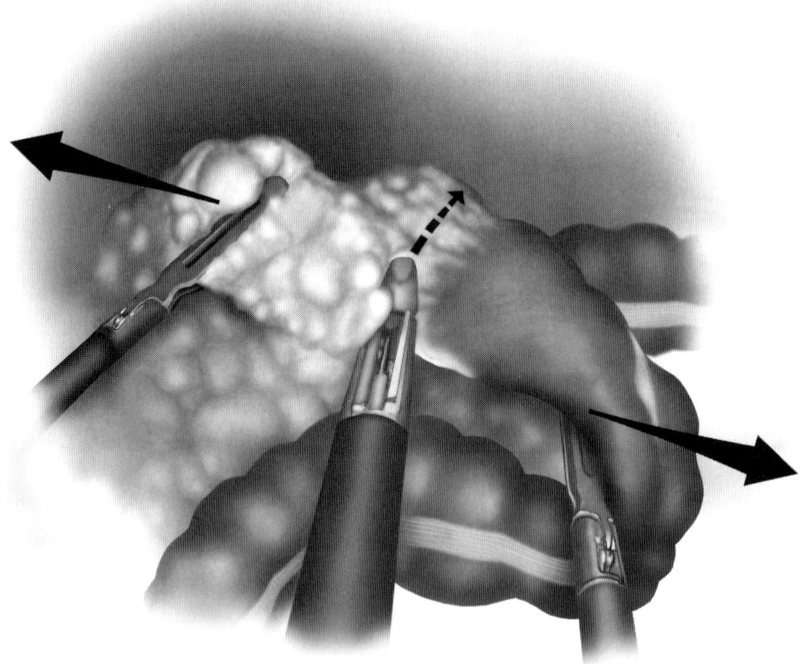

Figure 6.11. The LigaSure™ device is used to divide vascular attachments of the omentum to the colon by applying strong traction and countertraction to the tissue.

Hemostasis

Bleeding from small and moderately sized blood vessels can be controlled by grasping them with bipolar forceps or a dissecting/grasping instrument equipped with monopolar electrosurgery (Figure 6.12). Small vessels can usually be coagulated by using the tip or side of an endoscopic scissor equipped with monopolar electrosurgery. When applying electrosurgery, the cautery tip should be fully visible to avoid inadvertent tissue damage. We avoid the application of electrosurgical current directly to staples or clips. Larger vessels (>3 mm in diameter) should be clipped with endoscopic clips, stapled with endoscopic staplers, or ligated with a LigaSure™ device or Laparoscopic Coagulating Shears™.

If a moderately sized or large blood vessel is injured inadvertently and bleeding occurs, the bleeding vessel should be precisely grasped at the puncture site. This action usually stops the bleeding so that clips may be safely applied on both sides of the vessel or LigaSure™ may be applied properly. If the puncture site cannot be located precisely, the bleeding vessel is grasped on both sides of the bleeding area and the vessel temporarily occluded. Further dissection can then be performed and the vessel clipped, stapled, or sealed with LigaSure™. After hemostasis is achieved, the operative site is aspirated and irrigated. With good assistance and laparoscopic exposure, nearly all points of hemor-

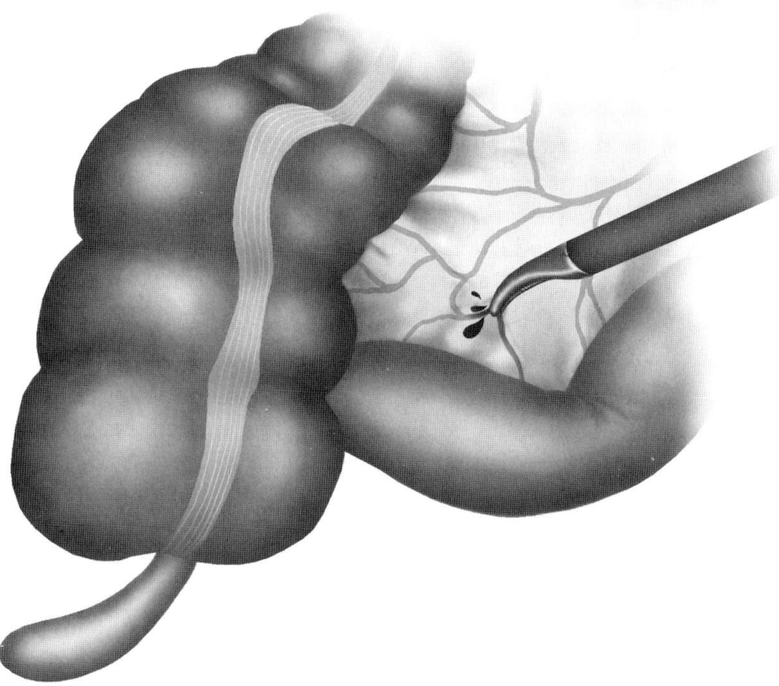

Figure 6.12. Controlling a bleeder by pin-point grasping.

rhage may be accurately identified and safely controlled. If the surgeon believes that the bleeding cannot be controlled with laparoscopic techniques, the surgeon should first grasp the surrounding tissue with endoscopic graspers to occlude the vessel temporarily before possibly converting the surgery to an open procedure. The graspers will mark the region of concern and control the bleeding vessel until a final decision as to what type (open or closed) of surgical techniques should be applied.

Suturing

Intracorporeal Technique

In laparoscopic tissue approximation, intracorporeal suturing and knot tying is the preferred method because it is highly adaptable and economical while utilizing standard laparoscopic instruments. In certain occasions, e.g., laparoscopic rectopexy, intracorporeal knotting is still feasible but extracorporeal knotting may be preferred.

The ergonomic positionings of the surgeon, laparoscope, and each of the hand instruments are crucial to facilitate the intracorporeal maneuvers. The ideal position for the laparoscope is midway between two working ports. The port positioning, relative to the proposed suture line, should provide the proper angle of access and a fulcrum for the instruments. The ideal angle between laparoscope and each-handed instrument has been reported to be 30–45°. The surgeon, target tissue (suture line), and the monitor should be positioned in line, to maximize surgeon's eye-hand coordination. This "triangulation" positioning should be preserved in unison when the surgeon attempts to suture different sites.

Laparoscopic suturing instruments have a variety of designs. The handle can have either a pistol grip or an in-line, coaxial handle, with or without a holding ring. Our current preference is the ringless in-line handle, which affords greater maneuverability even in difficult situations (Figure 6.13). The needle driver, used mostly by the dominant hand, handles the needle and suture material. The driver for this purpose should have a short shaft and a powerful and blunt tip. The assisting grasper, used by the nondominant hand, handles the tissue and is to be more curved and pointed.

The principle of needle handling and passage is similar to that of open surgery. However, a higher level of concentration is required to perform even simple needle driving maneuvers when working in a magnified laparoscopic field. The strength of the needle holder, in particular the locking and unlocking maneuver, can inadvertently traumatize the tissue, especially in thin structures such as small bowel. Handling needles outside the laparoscopic view may lead to incidental injuries to the surrounding organs. A good cooperation with laparoscopist and assistant surgeon is essential to avoid this situation.

A suture with a GI needle, less than 15 cm in length, is introduced via a 10/12-mm working port. This insertion is facilitated by grasping

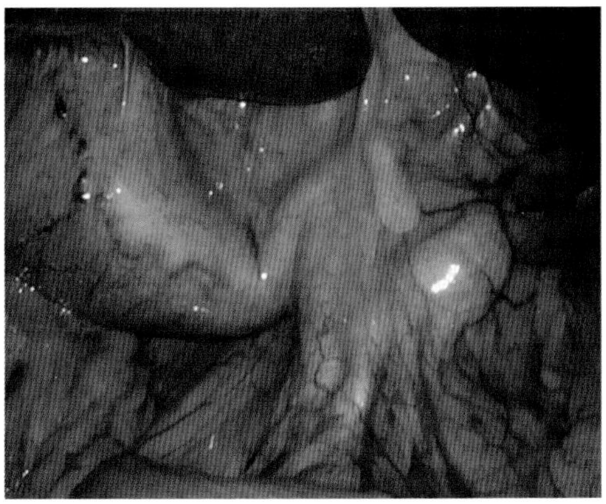

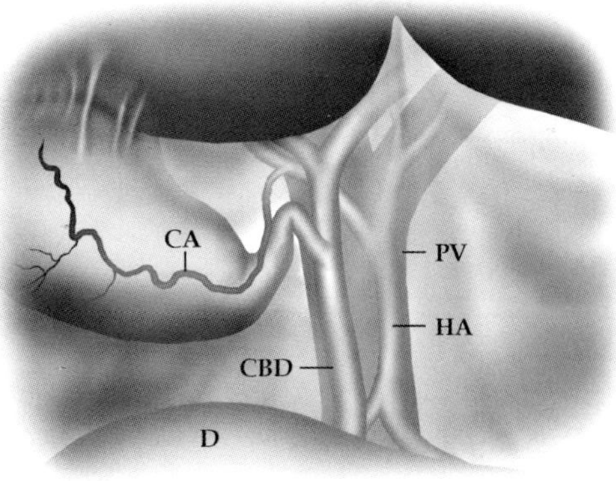

Figure 7.3. By lifting up the lower edge of the liver, the porta hepatic and the gallbladder may be seen. CA, cystic artery; CBD, common bile duct; D, duodenum; PV, portal vein; HA, hepatic artery.

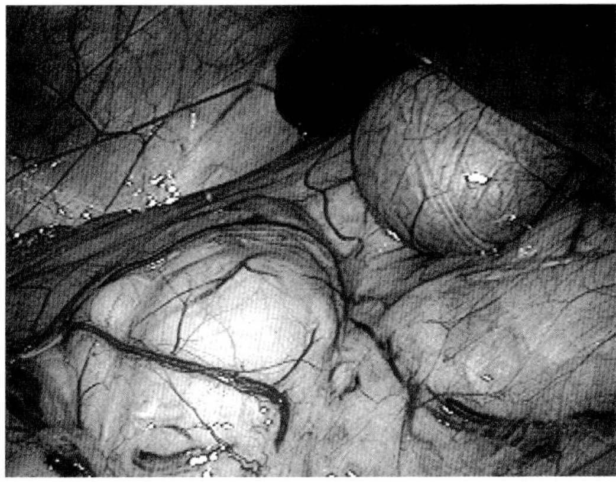

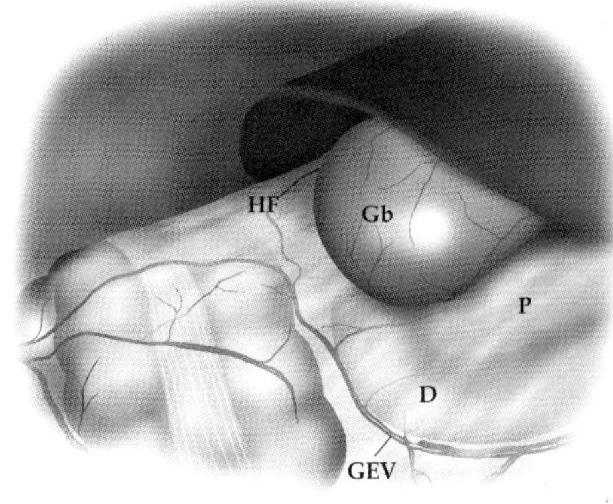

Figure 7.4. Just below the liver in a thin patient, the hepatic flexure, duodenum, and pancreatic head may be seen. HF, hepatic flexure; Gb, gallbladder; D, duodenum; P, pancreas; GEV, gastroepiploic vessels.

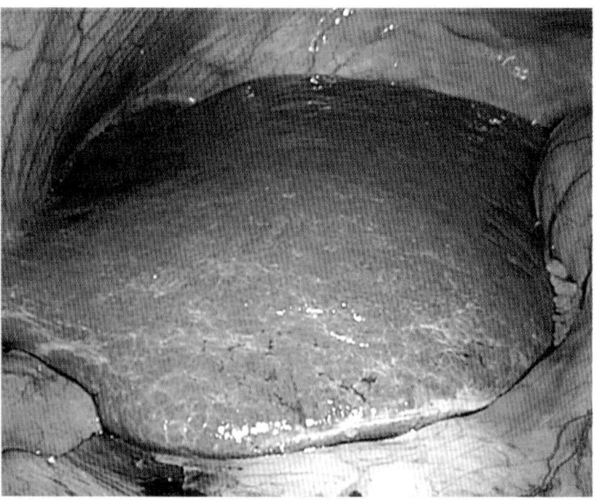

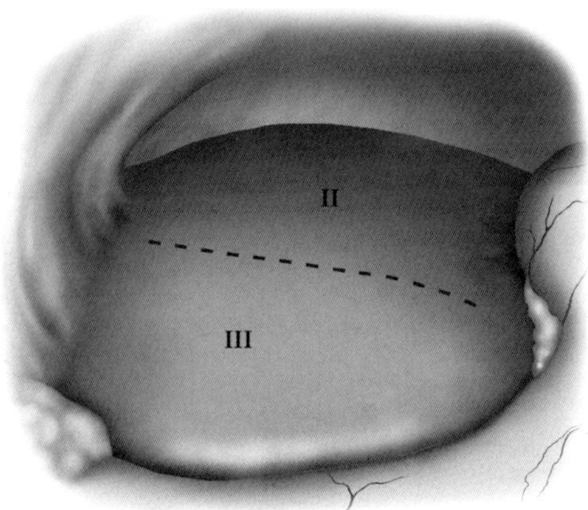

Figure 7.5. Just to the left of the falciform ligament, segments II and III are easily visualized in most patients.

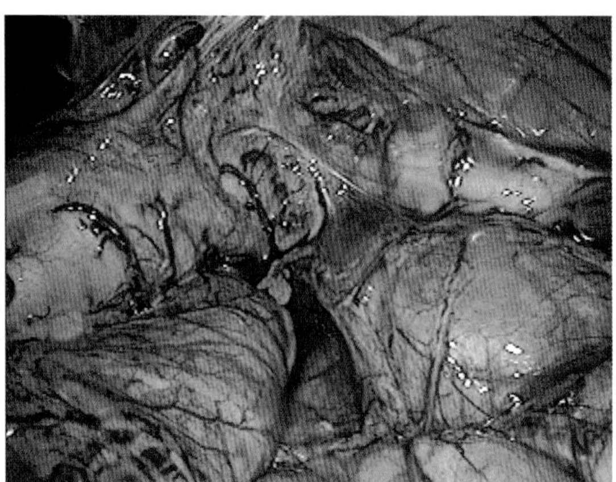

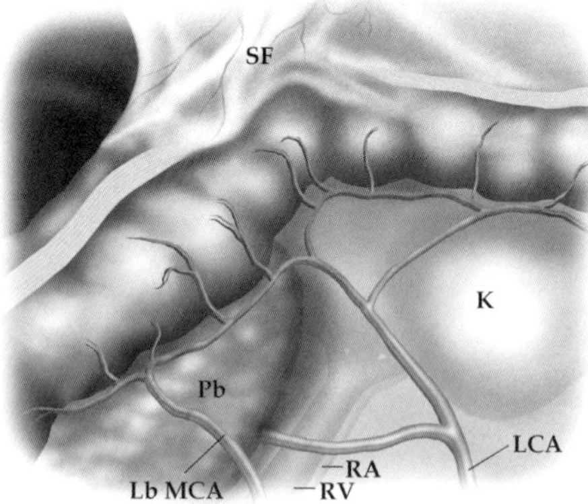

Figure 7.7. The splenic flexure may be seen by lifting the omentum cephalad. In this thin patient, many of the left colonic vessels and retroperitoneal structures are seen. SF, splenic flexure; Pb, pancreatic body; LbMCA, left branch of the middle colic artery; RV, renal vein; RA, renal artery; K, kidney; LCA, left colic artery.

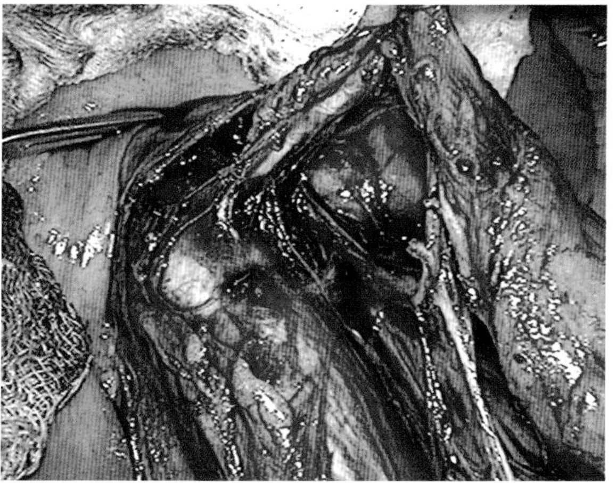

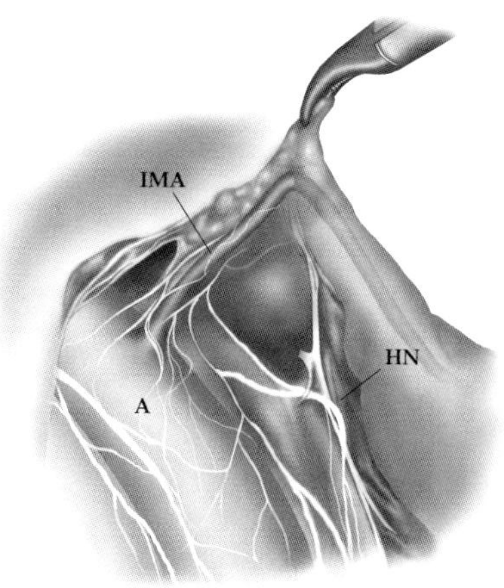

Figure 7.11. During a surgical dissection of the origin of the inferior mesenteric artery, the relationships of the hypogastric nerves and the aorta are appreciated. Note how the two branches (left and right) are straddling the aorta. IMA, inferior mesenteric artery; A, aorta; HN, left branch of the hypogastric nerve plexus.

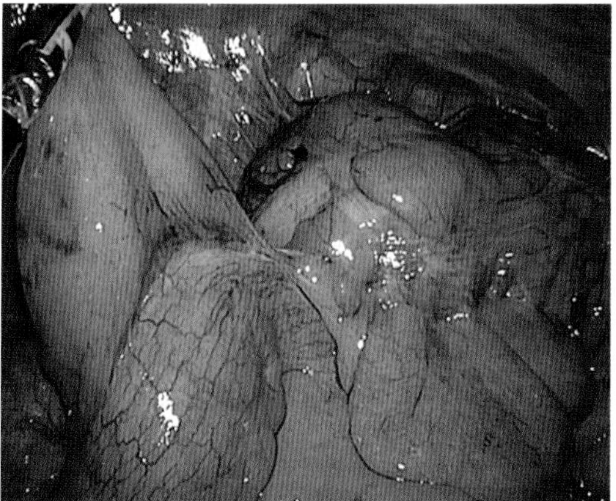

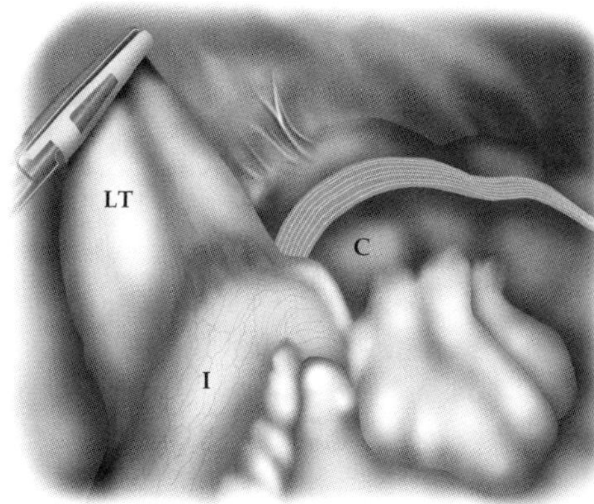

Figure 7.12. With a patient in the Trendelenburg position and the right side tilted upward, the terminal ileum, cecum, and ligament of Treitz may all be visualized. I, terminal ileum; LT, ligament of Treitz; C, cecum.

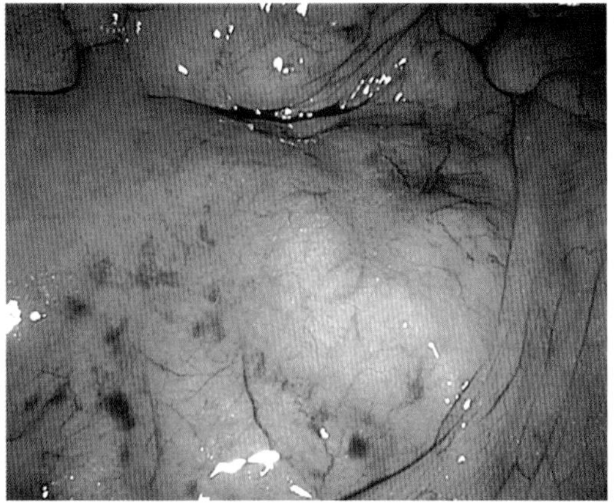

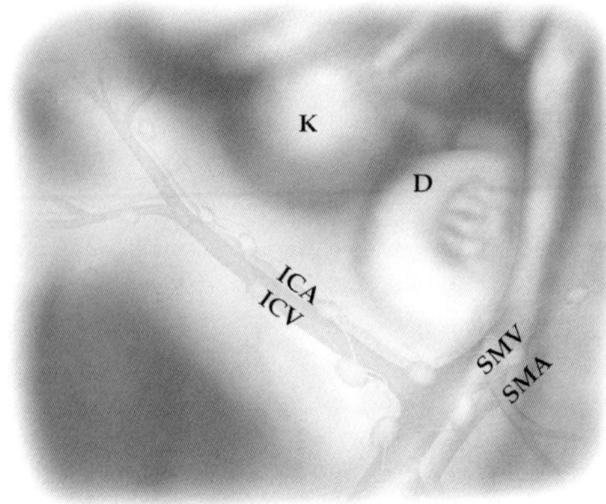

Figure 7.13. The major vascular structures of the right colon may be appreciated through the mesocolon, along with the right kidney and duodenum, with the small bowel retracted inferiorly and to the left. ICA, ileocolic artery; ICV, ileocolic vein; K, right kidney; D, duodenum; SMV, superior mesenteric vein; SMA, superior mesenteric artery.

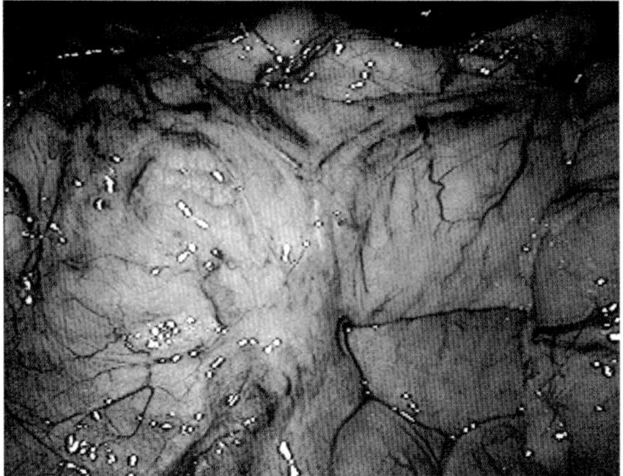

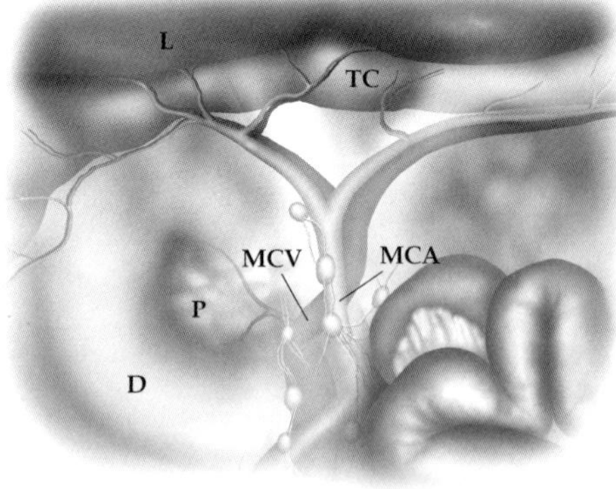

Figure 7.15. In thin patients, the vessels of the transverse colon and major structures in this region may be seen. L, inferior edge of liver; TC, transverse colon; MCV, middle colic vein; MCA, middle colic artery; D, duodenum; P, head of pancreas.

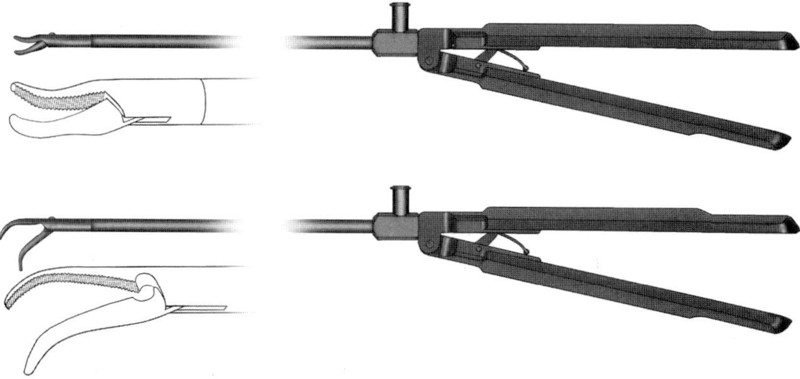

Figure 6.13. A popular laparoscopic needle driver (parrot beak) and assistant grasper (flamingo beak) (Szabo-Berci laparoscopic needle holders and graspers; Karl Storz, Tüttlingen, Germany).

the suture material 1–2 cm away from the needle. The suture is grasped by the right-handed needle holder and passed through the tissue (from right to left in this example), with a short tail left on the trailing side (Figure 6.14). The right-handed needle holder regrasps the suture immediately adjacent to the needle after the passage. The short tail should be long enough so that it cannot be pulled out accidentally from the tissue, but not so long that it compromises the following tying procedure. The right-handed instrument then holds the long tail and forms a "C-loop" (Figure 6.15). The left-handed instrument is placed over the loop. The right-handed instrument is used to wrap the long tail around the stationary tip of the left instrument. The left-handed instrument grasps the short tail under the arch in the suture, and is pulled back to the left to complete the first flat knot (Figures 6.16 and 6.17). Holding the jaws of the assistant grasper open before grasping the short tail may help prevent the loops from sliding off its tip. For the first knot, a simple square knot should be used for braided sutures and a surgeon's knot for monofilament sutures.

For the second opposing flat knot, a "reverse C-loop" is created by the left-handed instrument (Figure 6.18). The right instrument is placed over the reverse C-loop and the left-handed instrument wraps the thread around the right instrument (Figure 6.19). The tips of both instruments are moved together in unison toward the short tail, which is grasped with the right instrument. The second knot is completed by pulling back the short tail through the loop and pulling both tails in opposite directions parallel to the stitch under equal tension (Figure 6.20).

If the first knot becomes loose while beginning the second knot, the first locking square knot can be converted into a sliding knot (at least with monofilament suture material) by pulling one strand until it is

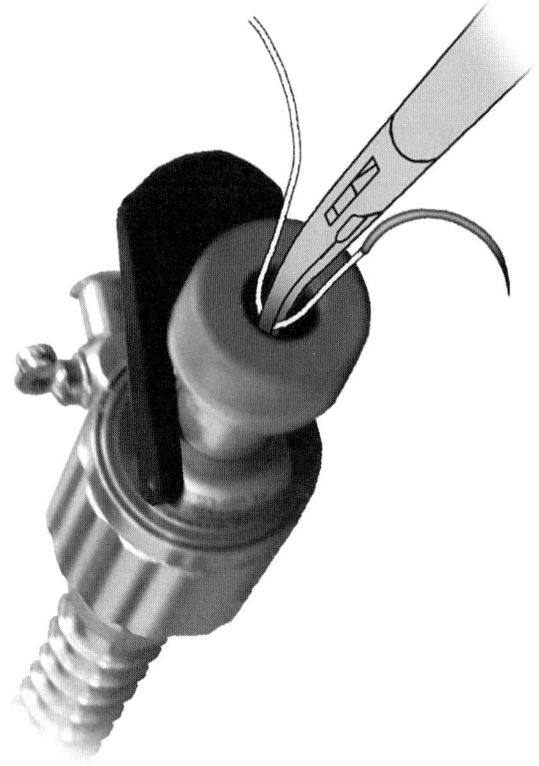

Figure 6.14. Intracorporeal suturing. Introducing the needle and suture into the abdomen through a 10-mm or larger cannula.

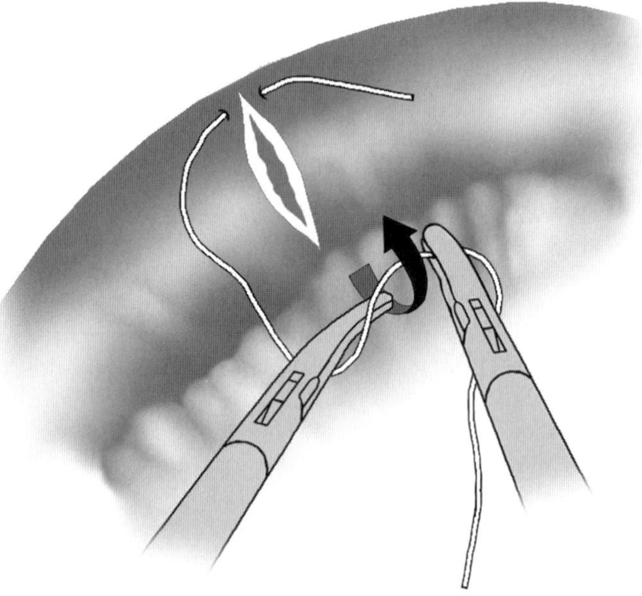

Figure 6.15. Intracorporeal suturing. To initiate the knot, wind the loop of suture (the "C" loop) around the assistant grasper.

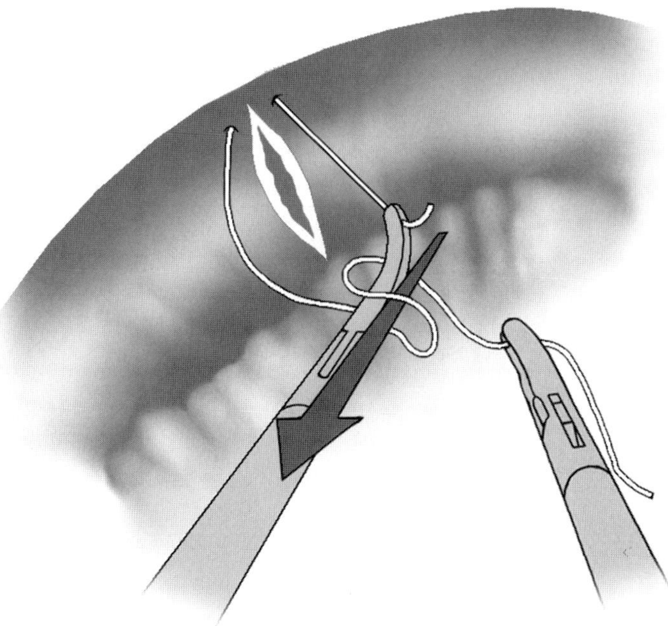

Figure 6.16. Intracorporeal suturing. Grasping the short tail and pulling it back through the C loop.

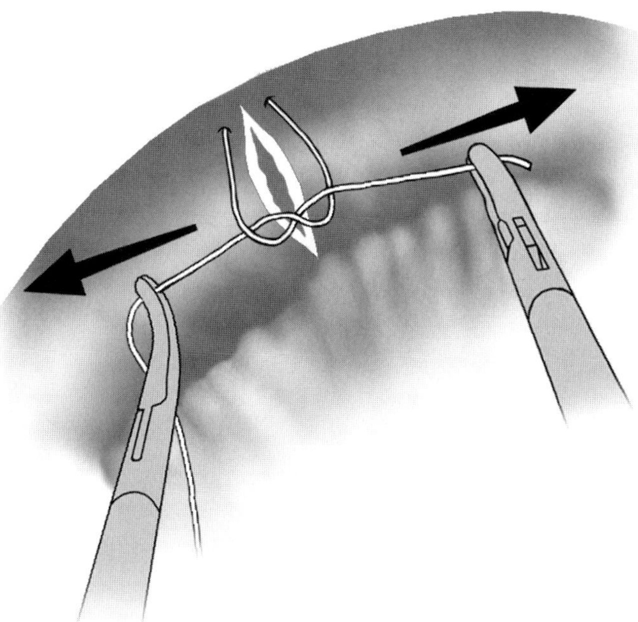

Figure 6.17. Intracorporeal suturing. Completing the initial flat knot.

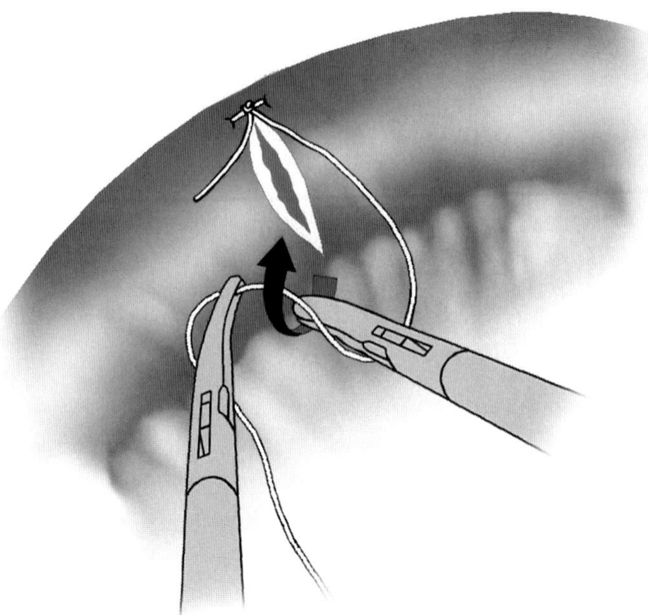

Figure 6.18. Intracorporeal suturing. Wind the loop around the right-handed instrument to create the second knot.

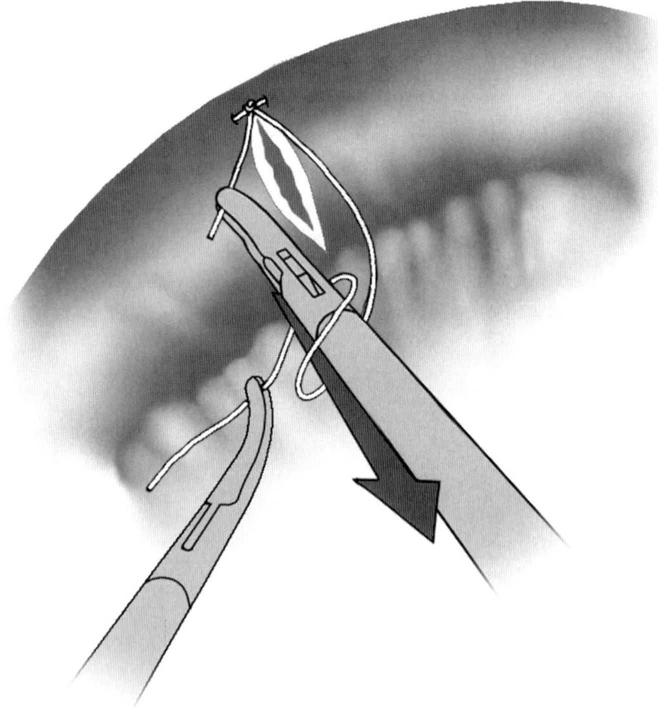

Figure 6.19. Intracorporeal suturing. The short tail is pulled back through the loop.

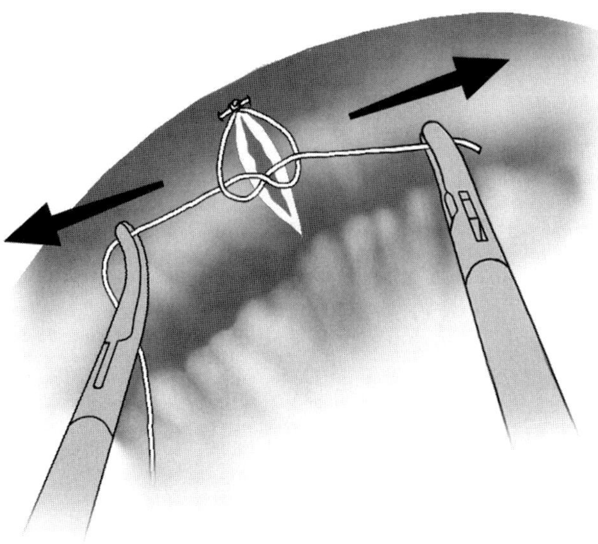

Figure 6.20. Intracorporeal suturing. Completion of the second knot.

straight (Figure 6.21). The knot on the other strand can then be pushed down to the proper position and converted back with pressure on both strands to ensure stability of the knot.

Extracorporeal Technique

In this method, a knot is tied extracorporeally on long thread and slid down to the tissue with the aid of a push rod (knot pusher). The technique seems to be relatively simpler than the intracorporeal knot tying, yet it requires a systematic, accommodative, and careful application to avoid traumatizing the tissues and damaging the suture.

A Röder knot is frequently used for extracorporeal tying. The Röder knot was originally developed a century ago as a ligating technique that used a catgut ligature loop with a slip knot for tonsillectomy in children. It was later introduced to laparoscopic practice by German gynecologist Semm with a push rod application system, before intracorporeal knotting was developed. This is the knot now used in commercially available pretied suture ligatures with an applicator tube and sheath that fits through a 5-mm cannula. A wide variety of push rod systems is also available (Figure 6.22).

A long suture is brought into the laparoscopic field, leaving its tail outside of the cannula. A stitch is placed intracorporeally, and the needle end is brought out through the same cannula (Figure 6.23). Gas leakage should be prevented by blocking the cannula with the index finger of the assistant surgeon. A Röder knot is created by tying an overhand knot and then wrapping the suture tail back around both arms of the loop three times (Figure 6.24). The suture is locked by bringing the tail back through the large loop, between the last two twists of the wrap. The knot is then slid down with a knot pusher into the operative field and secured (Figure 6.25). Care must be taken

A

B

C

D

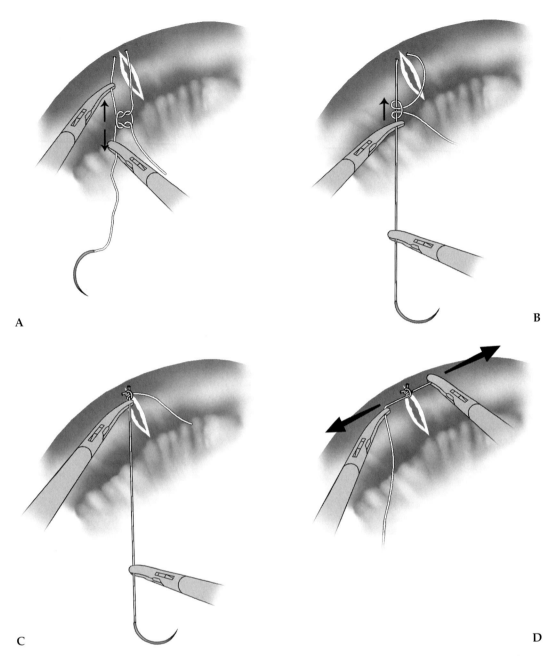

Figure 6.21. Conversion of a square knot to a sliding knot: **A** Two strands are pulled in opposite directions. **B** The knot is slid. **C** The knot is tightened. **D** Conversion back to a square knot.

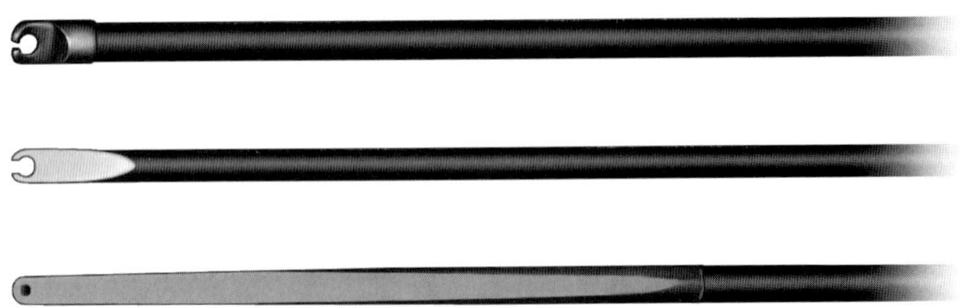

Figure 6.22. Laparoscopic knot pushers: various styles.

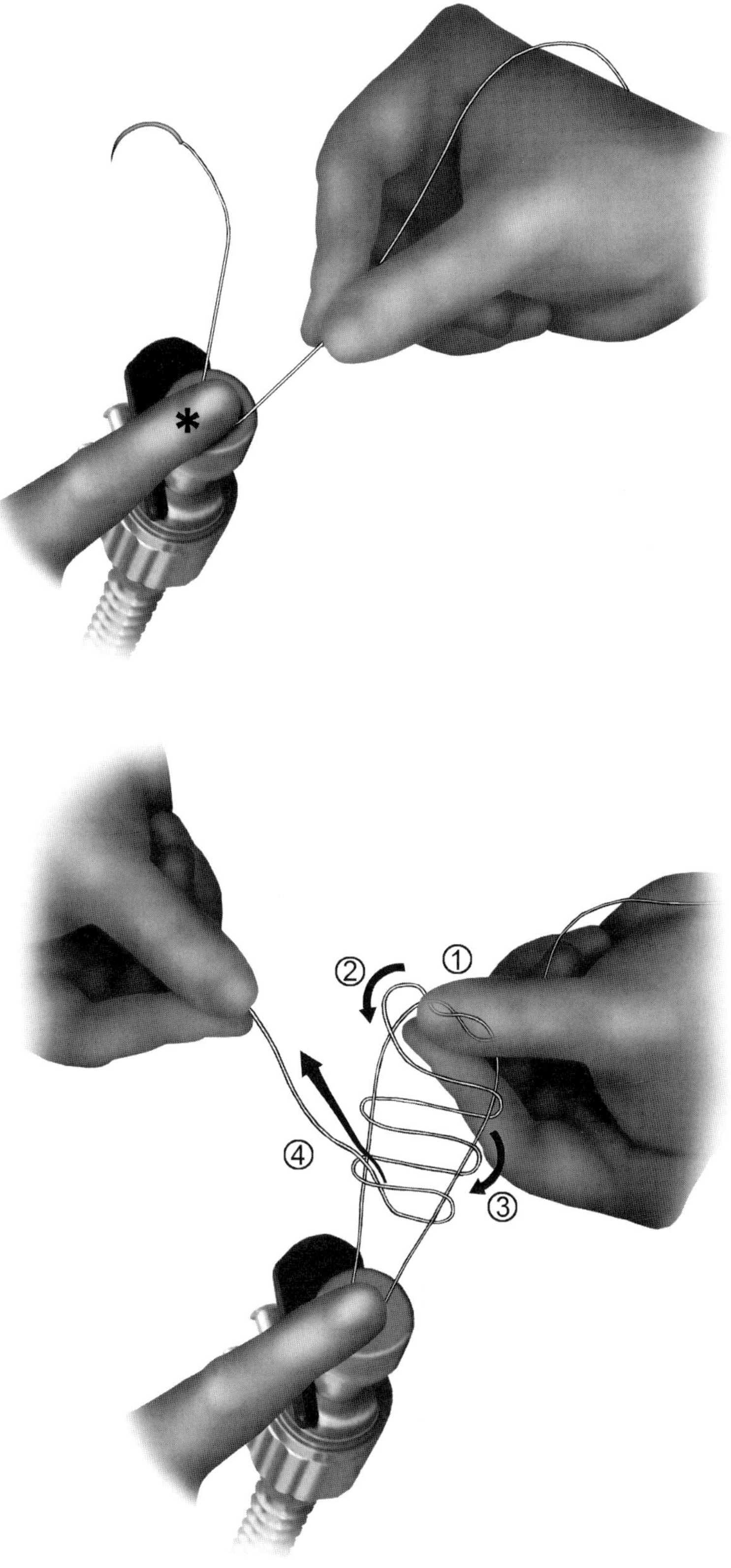

Figure 6.23. Extracorporeal suturing. The extracorporeal knot is initiated by bringing both ends of the suture back through the same cannula. The assistant uses a finger to prevent gas leakage (asterisk).

Figure 6.24. Extracorporeal suturing. The Röder knot is created extracorporeally by 1) first placing the one throw, 2) pinching it, 3) then winding one end of the suture three times around the two strands, and 4) passing it between the second and third wind and the two strands.

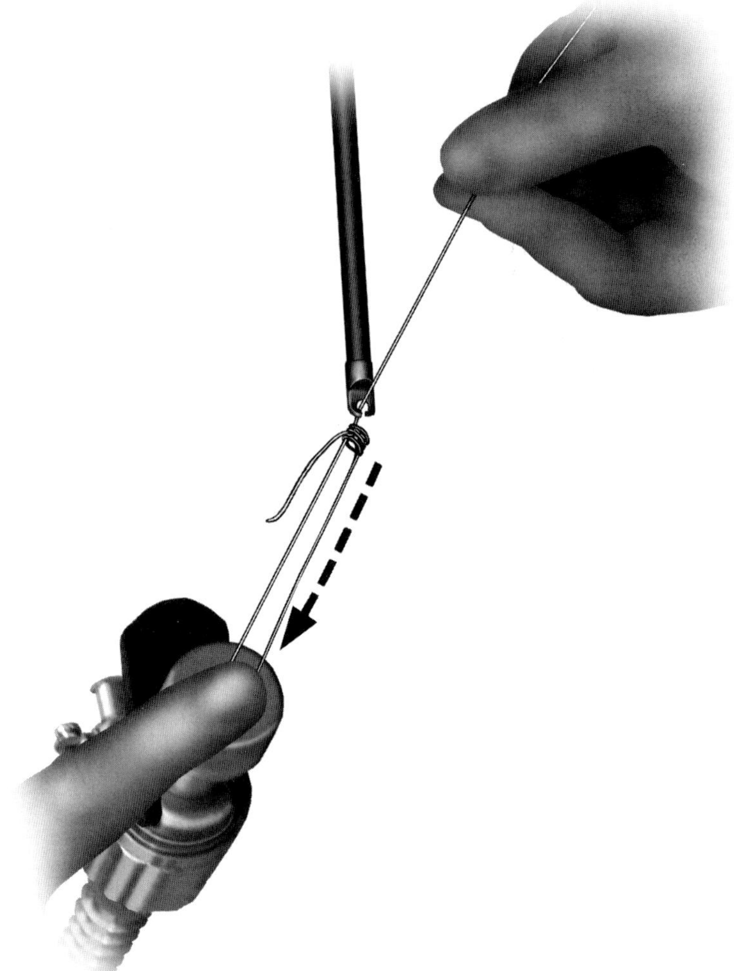

Figure 6.25. Extracorporeal suturing. The knot is pushed into the abdomen with the knot pusher and tightened.

to prevent abrasion, traction, or laceration of tissue as the slip knot is secured.

Specimen Extraction

In most cases of laparoscopic colorectal resections, specimens that are to be extracted are originally larger than the laparoscopic port site. The port site is therefore enlarged at the beginning of the extraction procedure. This wound enlargement is further justified because it also facilitates certain extracorporeal procedures, e.g., bowel anastomosis, as required. An excessive wound enlargement, however, may result in the elimination of known advantages of laparoscopic surgery such as less pain and better cosmesis. Nevertheless, an adequate specimen extraction technique including a "minimal" wound enlargement, is necessary and wound size should never compromise treatment of the disease.

In general, all colorectal specimens should be isolated in the retrieval bags before extraction, or drawn out of the abdomen with a wound protector in place, to prevent the peritoneal cavity, abdominal wound, and soft tissue from contamination with the colonic contents. It is not recommended to reduce the size of specimen by removing the contents or by cutting the specimen in pieces, because these may increase risks of infection and cancer dissemination. In addition, destruction of the specimen may also lead to incomplete postoperative pathologic evaluation.

An appropriate choice of retrieval bag is crucial for safe specimen delivery in laparoscopic colorectal surgery. Among various commercially available bags, our current recommendation is a 15-mm Endo Catch™ II (USSC-Tyco) specimen pouch (see Chapter 2). The Endo Catch™ II consists of a long cylindrical tube and a polyurethane pouch. The system seems suitable for colorectal laparoscopy, because: 1) the opening diameter (5 inches) and depth (7 inches) are sufficient for most colorectal specimens; 2) the polyurethane pouch prevents spillage and minimizes intraoperative contamination by isolating possible colonic contents coming with the specimen; 3) the pouch is maintained in an open position by a flexible metal ring, allowing for an easy placement of the specimen without the aid of additional instruments; 4) the pouch and attached string are durable enough for aggressive retrieving procedures. Although the Endo Catch™ II officially requires a 15-mm trocar sleeve for its insertion, it can be inserted via a regular 10/12-mm port site, by withdrawing the trocar sleeve and slightly enlarging the port site with surgeon's index finger, then inserting the shaft of the Endo Catch™ II without a cannula.

After completely isolating the specimen into the bag (Figure 6.26), the attached string or the shaft is pulled up with trocar sleeve (if placed) until the neck of the pouch appears outside the incision. The neck of the pouch is secured with a Kocher clamp outside the incision and the trocar sleeve is removed (Figure 6.27). At this point, the pouch is inspected to see if there is air or fluid in it. If air is trapped in the pouch, simply enlarging the neck of the pouch may allow air to escape. If fluid is entrapped, careful suction may be used to remove excess fluid. Care must be taken not to spill the fluid in the incision. The skin incision is then "minimally" enlarged to complete the removal procedure (Figure 6.28). For most colorectal specimens, a final incision length of 4–5 cm is usually required. Pneumoperitoneum is switched on and off, and the bag is pulled up gradually in rotating motion. Excessive pulling force may tear the pouch and lead to inappropriate specimen removal and wound contamination. In actuality, the Endo Catch™ bag is remarkably resistant to tearing, and permits a surprisingly small incision to be made for specimen extraction.

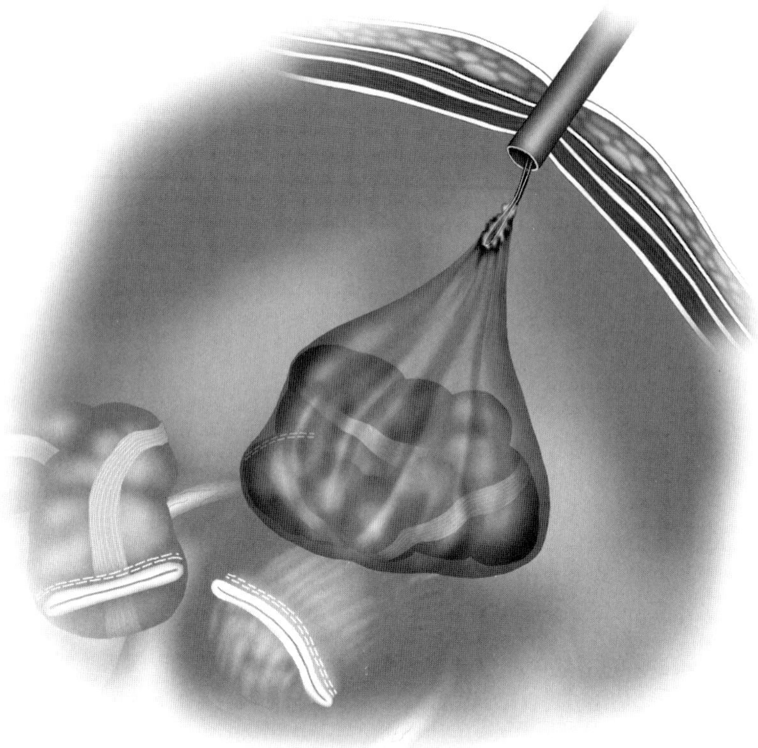

Figure 6.26. Specimen extraction using a plastic bag equipped with a draw string. The complete isolation of the specimen into the bag.

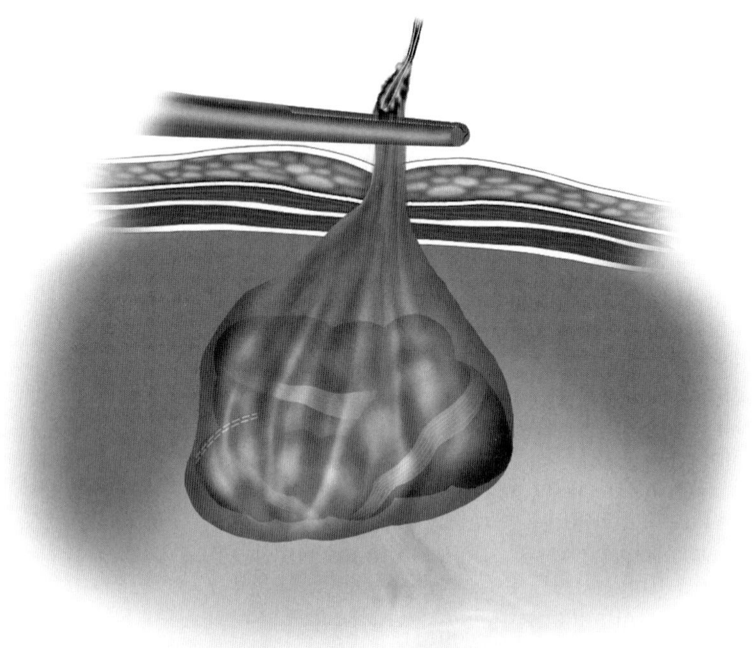

Figure 6.27. Specimen extraction using a plastic bag equipped with a draw string. The neck of the pouch is secured with a Kocher clamp as soon as it is drawn out of the abdominal wall.

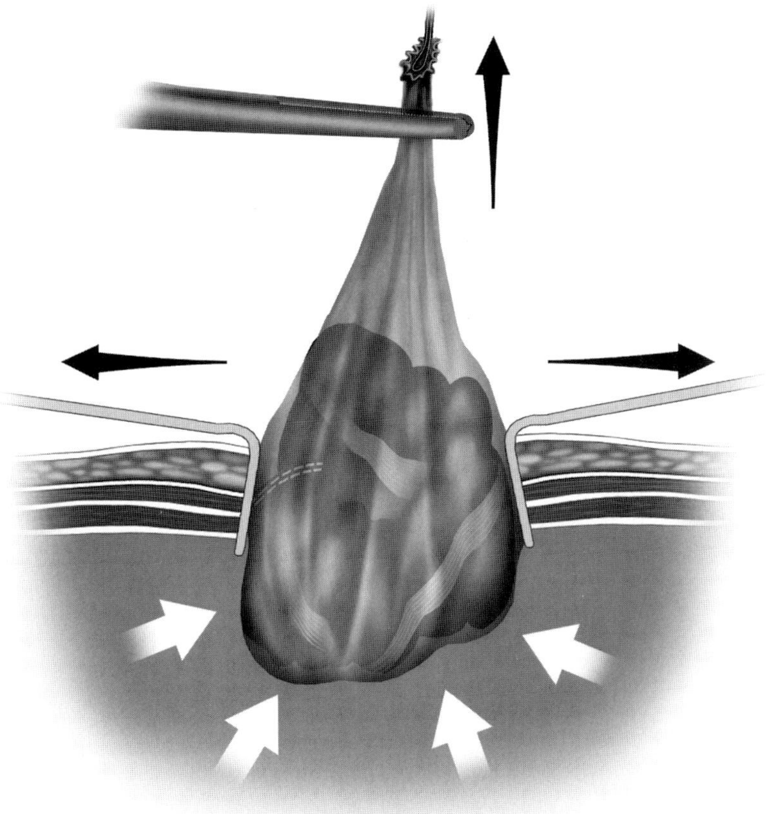

Figure 6.28. Specimen extraction using a plastic bag equipped with a draw string. The incision is minimally enlarged to allow extraction of the bag. Maintaining the pneumoperitoneum helps push the specimen out through a small incision.

Irrigation/Suction

An excellent combination of irrigation and suction systems is necessary for any laparoscopic procedure. In cases of bleeding or spilled intestinal contents, irrigation systems with a minimal flow rate of 1 L/min are essential. Adjustable suction with interchangeable 5- and 10-mm metallic suction tubes should be available to remove smoke, laser plume, fluid, clots, or other debris. Using suction tips with multiple side holes is important when irrigating and evacuating fluid or clots rapidly or in large volumes.

Intraoperative irrigation should be performed with a warmed (37°C) isotonic solution; normal saline or lactated Ringer's solution is suitable. To effectively aspirate a collection of blood or tissue fluid at the conclusion of the operation, the operating table should be rotated appropriately so that the site of collection can be positioned lowest in the abdomen (Figure 6.29). An adequate suction power should be used to avoid rapid loss of pneumoperitoneum, keeping the probe below the level of fluid to be aspirated. Often omentum, mesentery, epiploic appendages, and intestinal loops may migrate into the collection and are drawn onto the suction probe. Care must be taken to release these attached tissues before the suction probe is withdrawn through the cannula. This may be achieved by switching off the suction, transiently switching on the irrigation, and a gentle manipulation of the trapped tissue. In case of inadequate suction caused by repeated obstruction by trapped tissue structures, a surgical gauze is inserted through the 10-mm cannula, and the suction is performed upon contact with it (Figure 6.30). This technique greatly facilities the suction/irrigation procedure especially in obese patients and is of practical value in preventing tissue trauma or accidental bleeding during the withdrawal of the instrument.

In case of inadvertent bleeding, adequate irrigation/suction is necessary to precisely locate the bleeders. In contrast to the situation of the elective irrigation/suction procedure, this requires the operating table to be rotated so that the bleeding area can be positioned for optimal viewing.

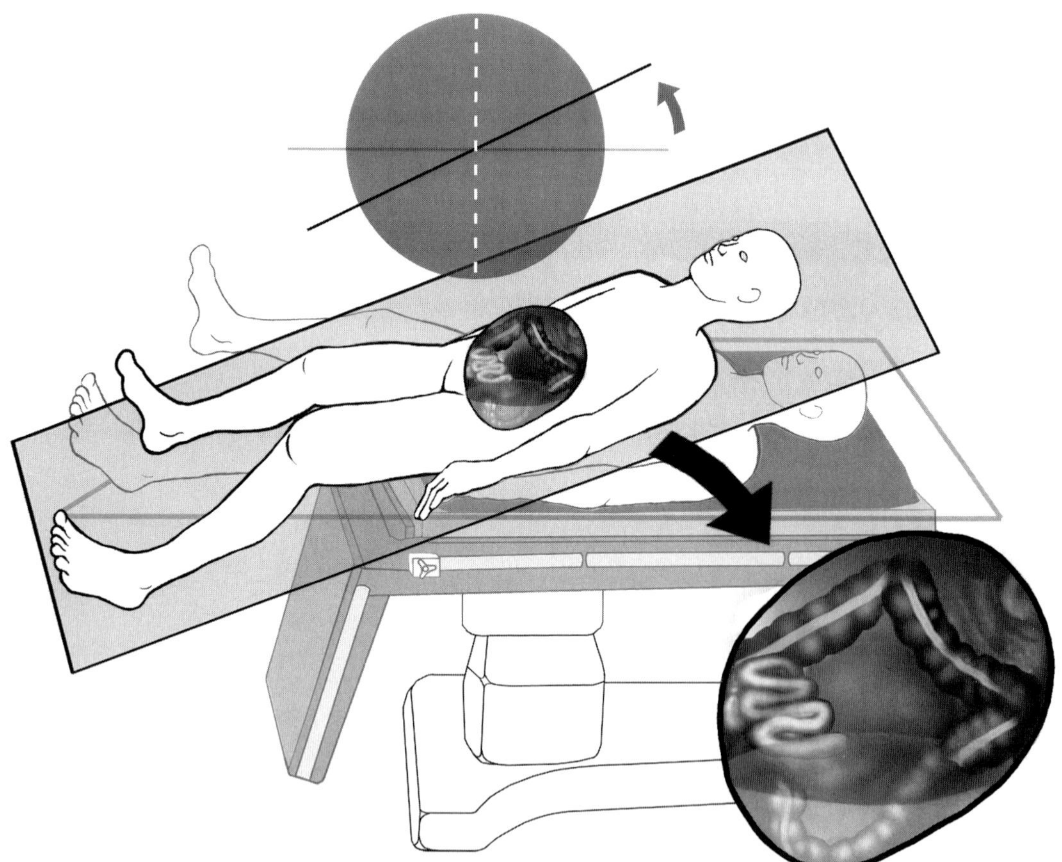

Figure 6.29. Rotating the operating table to optimize positioning for irrigation/suction.

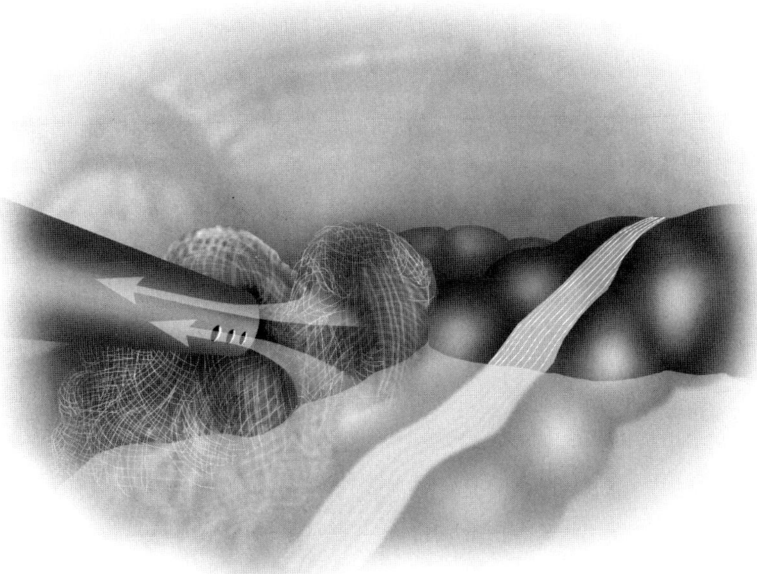

Figure 6.30. The gauze technique avoids sucking tissue into the suction cannula.

Trocar Wound Closure

At the conclusion of every laparoscopic procedure, cannulae should be removed one by one under direct laparoscopic control while the abdominal wall puncture sites are inspected for hemostasis. As each cannula is removed, an assistant should plug the puncture site with a finger to maintain the low-pressure pneumoperitoneum. After all cannulae are removed except the one housing the laparoscope, the laparoscope is withdrawn 4–5 cm into the cannula and this cannula then is slowly withdrawn from the body wall as the surgeon inspects the edges of the abdominal wall for hemostasis.

Because we have seen some symptomatic hernias through 10-mm incisions, all body wall incisions from 10/12-mm cannulae should be closed using conventional techniques or with a transabdominal suture while the cannula is still in place.[6] For this purpose, a needle is available that resembles the Veress needle except its inner blunt-tipped cannula looks similar to a crochet needle and can be extended beyond the sharp needle tip to grasp a fascial stitch (see Chapter 2). The needle is equipped with the fascial suture and then initially passed through the fascia and peritoneum about 5–7 mm from a cannula (Figure 6.31). The loop of the suture is released under laparoscopic visual control, grasped by a grasper placed at another site, and the needle is removed (Figure 6.32). The needle is then reinserted through the abdominal wall on the other side of the cannula and used to grasp the loop of the suture (Figure 6.33). The suture is pulled back up through the abdominal wall

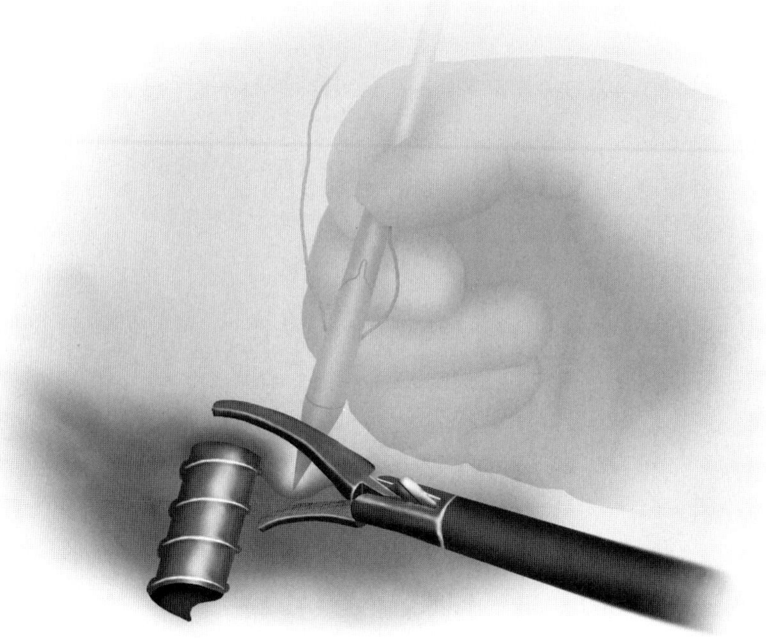

Figure 6.31. Cannula wound closure. Introducing the SuturePasser into the abdomen. Countertraction is applied by a laparoscopic instrument at the puncture site.

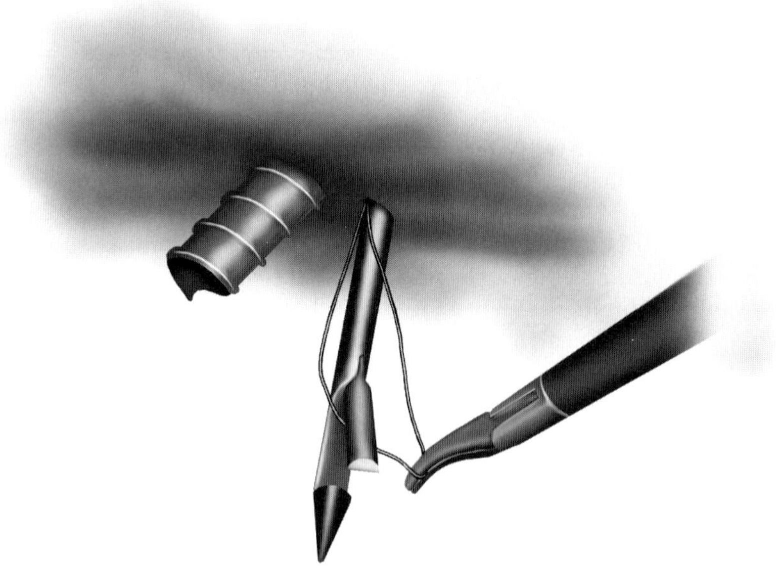

Figure 6.32. Cannula wound closure. The suture is freed up from the SuturePasser so it may be removed.

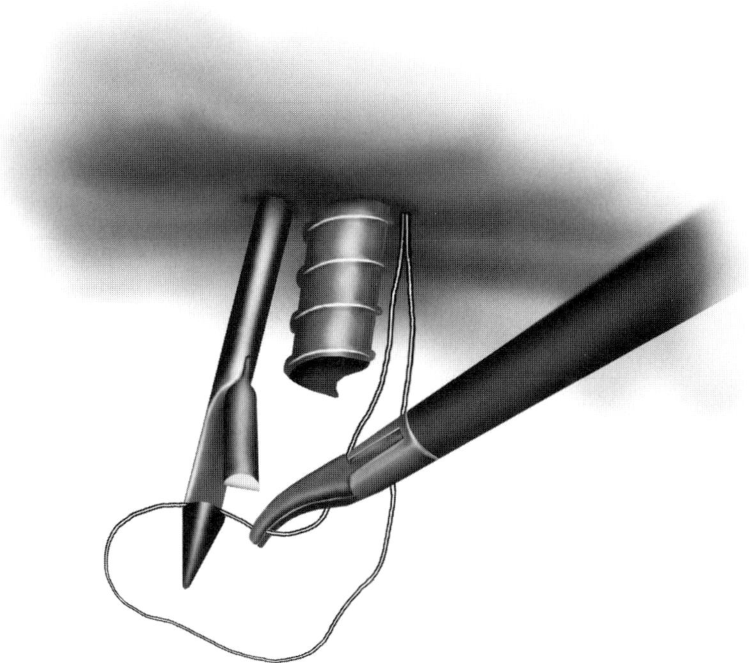

Figure 6.33. Cannula wound closure. The second puncture by the SuturePasser permits extraction of the suture and fascial closure.

with the needle, and the cannula removed, hemostasis is checked, and the suture is tied to close the peritoneum, muscle layer, and fascia en mass. When using this technique of cannula site closure, at least three cannulae should remain in the abdominal cavity until all cannula sites have had sutures placed – one site is needed for the laparoscope and one for a grasping device while the third site is being closed. We recommend placing all necessary stitches at the beginning of the operation, just after completing all laparoscopic cannulae placements (Figure 6.34). The fascial/peritoneal defects are closed by tying the previously placed sutures after desufflation of the abdomen. Lastly, the skin is closed with skin staplers, adhesive strips (such as Steri-Strips), or skin adhesives (e.g., Dermabond^{TM}; Ethicon), with/without absorbable subcutaneous sutures.

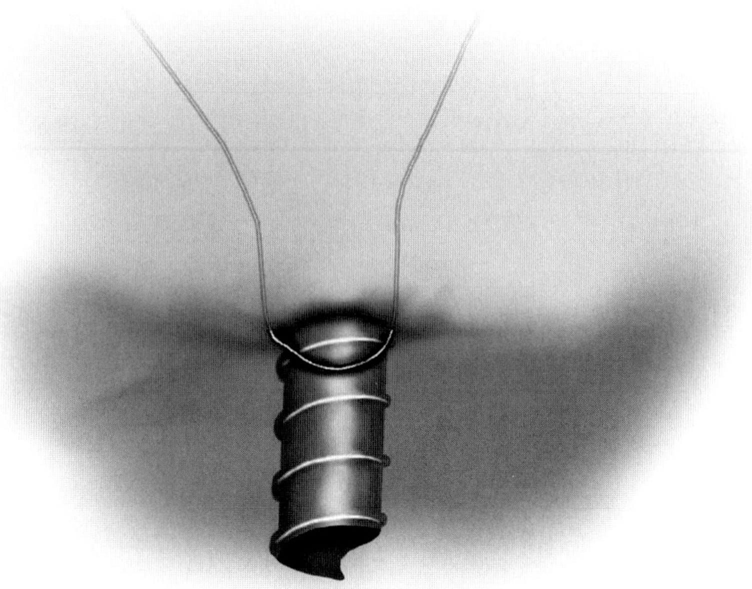

Figure 6.34. Cannula wound closure. Position of the suture should be checked before cannula removal.

References

1. Hashizume M, Sugimachi K. Needle and trocar injury during laparoscopic surgery in Japan. Surg Endosc 1997;11:1198–1201.
2. Ternamian AM, Deitel M. Endoscopic threaded imaging port (EndoTIP) for laparoscopy: experience with different body weights. Obes Surg 1999;9:44–47.
3. Lee DW, Chan AC, Kwok SP, et al. Ports, don't slip out! Surg Endosc 1999;13:628.
4. Milsom JW, Okuda J, Kim S-H, et al. Atraumatic and expeditious laparoscopic bowel handling using a new endoscopic device. Dis Colon Rectum 1997;40:1394–1395.
5. Nakajima K, Milsom JW, Margolin DA, et al. Use of the surgical towel in colorectal hand-assisted laparoscopic surgery (HALS). Surg Endosc 2004; 18:552–553.
6. Stringer NH, Levy ES, Kezmoh MP, et al. New closure technique for lateral operative laparoscopic trocar sites. A report of 80 closures. Surg Endosc 1995;9:838–840.

Chapter 7

Laparoscopic Anatomy of the Abdominal Cavity

Jeffrey W. Milsom, Bartholomäus Böhm, and Kiyokazu Nakajima

In only the past one and a half decades, the surgeon has become capable of inspecting every recess of the abdomen with extremely high resolution and magnification through a tiny incision in the abdominal wall. By placing a laparoscopic videocamera into the abdominal cavity, not only the surgeon but the entire surgical team may achieve a visual perspective heretofore not possible, thus accelerating the learning of surgery and anatomy.

The laparoscope has its limitations – the view is often confined to only one area of several centimeters – but this view has likely enhanced our understanding of abdominal anatomy in a surprising number of ways. For example, we now may see directly over the top and underneath the liver, and in colorectal surgery we can place a 15–20 X magnified view of the pelvis directly on the video screens in the operating room, or save them for digital reproduction in lectures, conferences, and texts.

More evidence that a new era for anatomy is upon us relates to educational aspects of abdominal, and particularly pelvic, anatomy. For nearly all generations of surgeons of the 20th century, only the operating surgeon and maybe the first assistant could see into the depths of the pelvis and learn about the relationships of various organs during an actual operation such as low anterior resection. In the current era, actually for the first time in the history of surgery, the entire operating team, including the nurses, anesthesia team, and all of the surgical trainees including medical students may watch an entire pelvic operation and understand the relationships of the various organs, vessels, and nerves as the surgery unfolds on the video screen. Additionally, owing to magnification, many of the smaller structures, such as the tiny branches of the pelvic nerves, can be seen clearly and reliably during each and every operation.

This chapter will provide an outline for viewing the major structures of the abdominal cavity, and will illustrate the important ones most surgeons will need to recognize during laparoscopic colorectal surgical procedures.

Overall Evaluation

The overview of the abdominal anatomy is begun using the laparoscope placed into the umbilical port. This central location permits the surgeon the best vantage point from which to perform nearly all procedures, and from this point nearly all of the illustrations/photographs of the chapter have been taken. Once successful entry into the abdomen is accomplished, we recommend a quadrant by quadrant viewing of the abdomen, to ensure that nothing significant is overlooked. We start in the right upper quadrant (RUQ), and move in a clockwise manner in order to see all quadrants and then the pelvis.

The Right Upper Quadrant

To best see in the RUQ, the patient should lie in the reverse Trendelenburg position with the body tilted with the right side up. First, the liver should be assessed overall for its shape, size, and surface texture (Figure 7.1). Also demonstrable is the under surface of the right diaphragm (Figure 7.2). Generally, the umbilical port is best for doing this, with instruments in the other ports used for lifting up the edge of the liver and looking underneath at the porta hepatis, and the gallbladder (Figure 7.3, see color plate). Also visible is the hepatic flexure of the

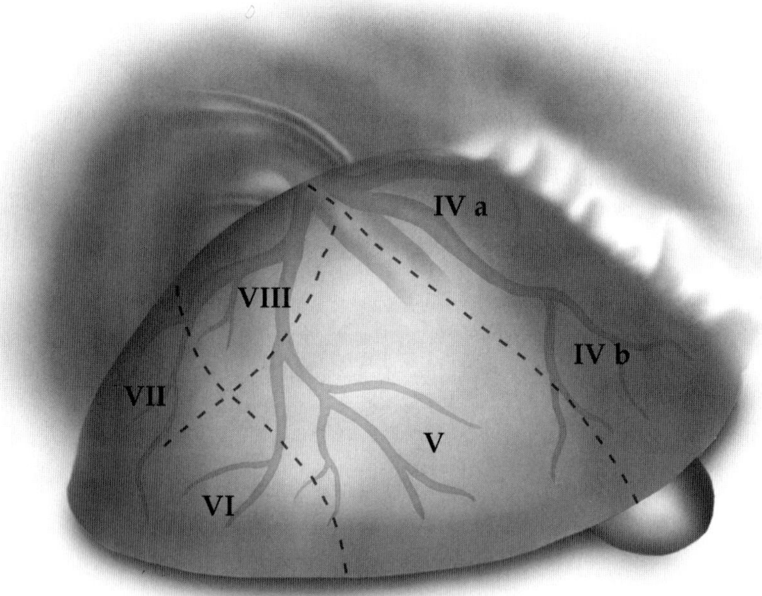

Figure 7.1. At the start of a laparoscopy, the liver to the right of the falciform ligament may be viewed broadly over its surface (hepatic segments of Couinaud and the hepatic veins are depicted in the drawing).

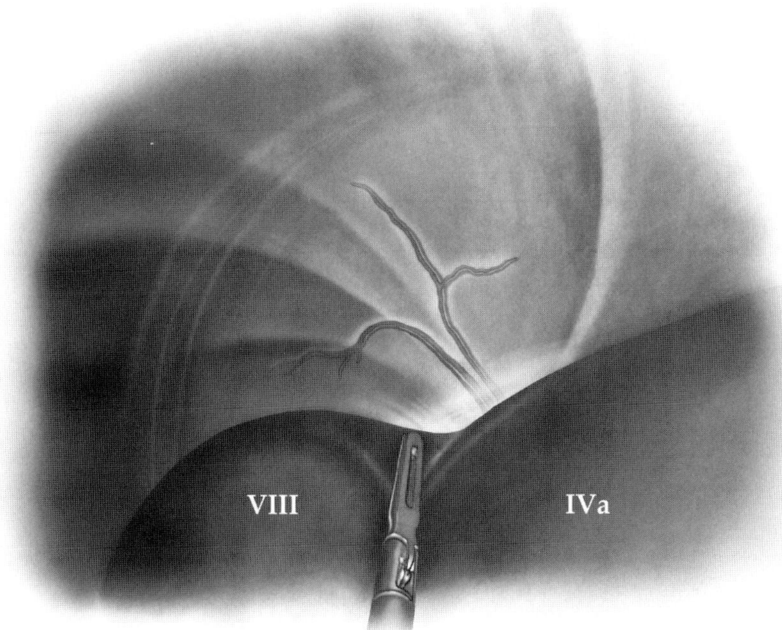

Figure 7.2. Peering above the right portion of the liver, the posterior portions of segments VIII and IVa and the undersurface of the right diaphragm may be seen.

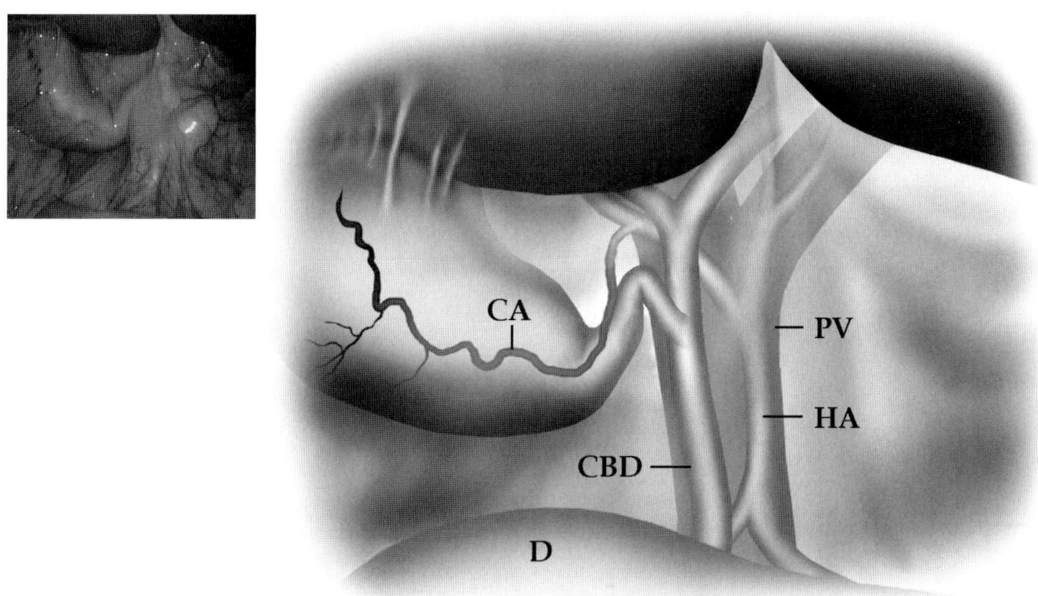

Figure 7.3. By lifting up the lower edge of the liver, the porta hepatic and the gallbladder may be seen. CA, cystic artery; CBD, common bile duct; D, duodenum; PV, portal vein; HA, hepatic artery. (See color plate.)

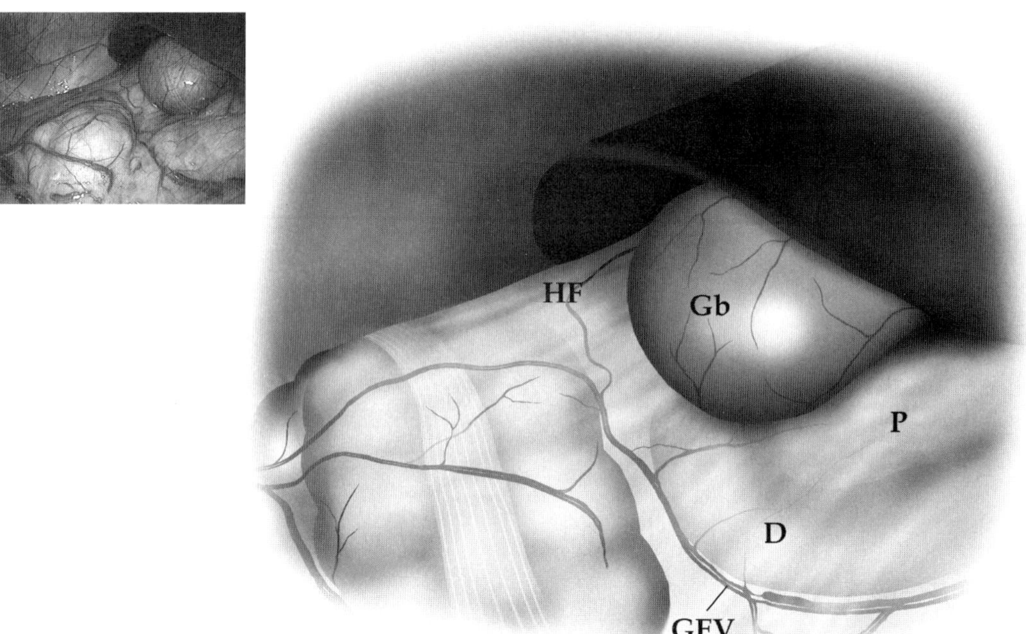

Figure 7.4. Just below the liver in a thin patient, the hepatic flexure, duodenum, and pancreatic head may be seen. HF, hepatic flexure; Gb, gallbladder; D, duodenum; P, pancreas; GEV, gastroepiploic vessels. (See color plate.)

right colon with the duodenum, in thinner patients the pancreatic head, gallbladder, and the inferior aspect of the right lobe of the liver (Figure 7.4, see color plate).

The Left Upper Quadrant

By sweeping the laparoscope across the abdomen to the left side and tilting the left side of the body up, segments II and III of the liver can be easily inspected (Figure 7.5, see color plate). The esophageal hiatus, the caudate lobe through the hepatogastric ligament, and the cardia of the stomach can be demonstrated by lifting up the left lobe with atraumatic grasper (Figure 7.6). Also demonstrable is the undersurface of the left hemidiaphragm, and the spleen. The splenic flexure, the splenocolic ligament, and the omentum may be easily visualized, along with the transverse colon (Figure 7.7, see color plate). The body of the pancreas may often be seen indenting the transverse mesocolon in the left upper quadrant (LUQ) as well.

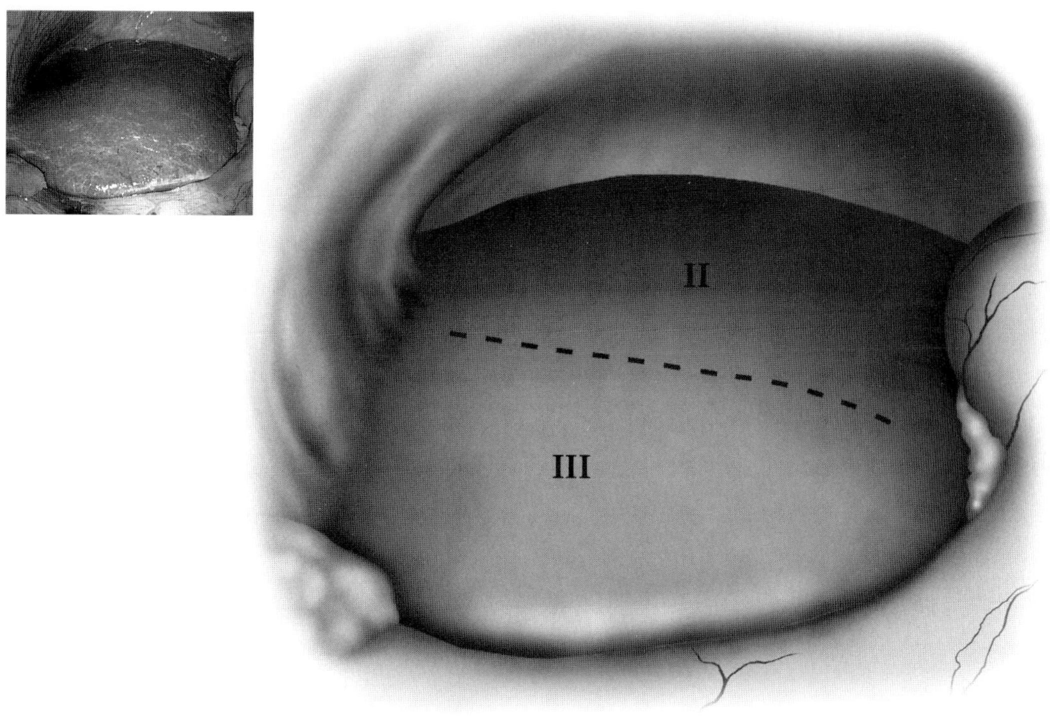

Figure 7.5. Just to the left of the falciform ligament, segments II and III are easily visualized in most patients. (See color plate.)

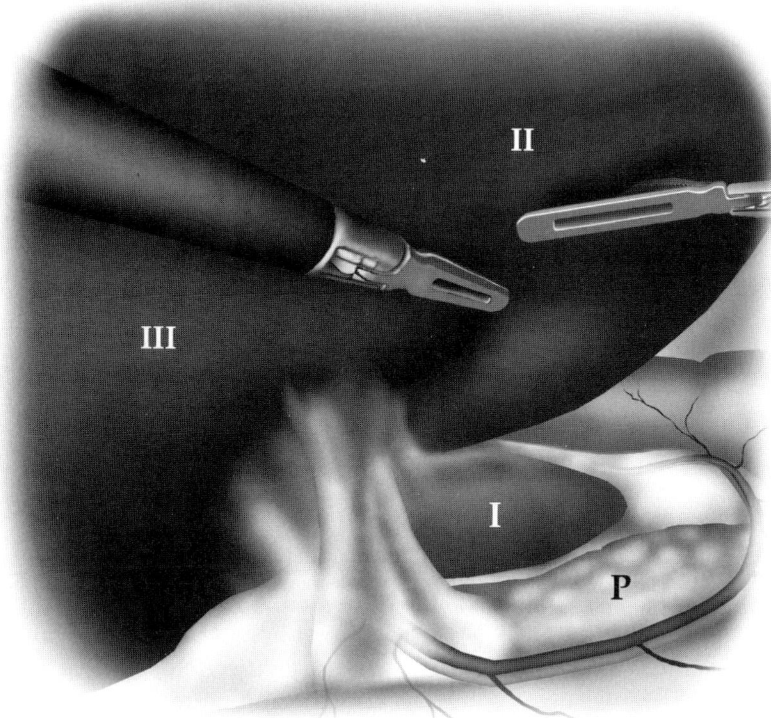

Figure 7.6. By lifting up segments II and III of the liver, the lesser sac and the caudate lobe of the liver (segment I) may often be seen in thin patients. P, pancreas.

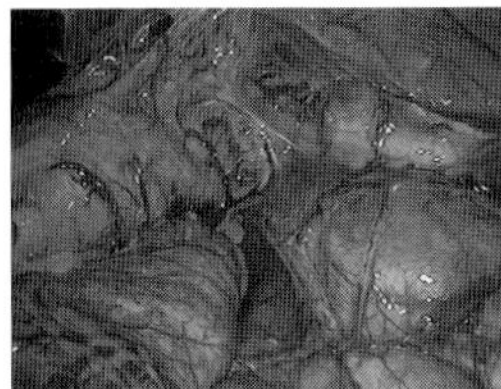

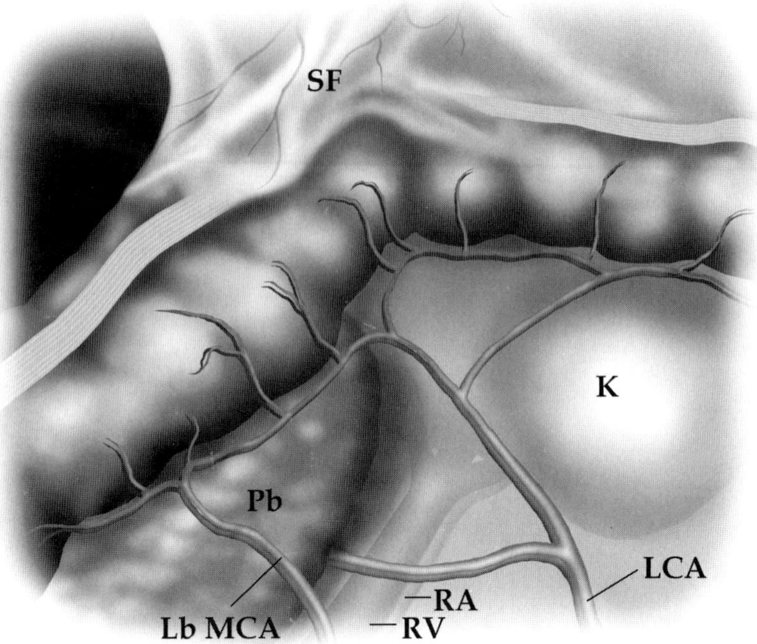

Figure 7.7. The splenic flexure may be seen by lifting the omentum cephalad. In this thin patient, many of the left colonic vessels and retroperitoneal structures are seen. SF, splenic flexure; Pb, pancreatic body; LbMCA, left branch of the middle colic artery; RV, renal vein; RA, renal artery; K, kidney; LCA, left colic artery. (See color plate.)

The Left Lower Quadrant

Sweeping the camera from the LUQ caudally, the descending colon, the ligament of Treitz, and vascular structures of the left mesocolon may be appreciated (Figure 7.8). To best see this area, the patient must be tilted with the left side up, and in some degree of Trendelenburg position. The attachments of the sigmoid colon to the lateral abdominal side wall and to the pelvis are easy to visualize, and the vessels supplying the left colon and rectum, including the inferior mesenteric artery and vein may be identified by retracting the small bowel to the right side of the abdomen (Figure 7.9). The retroperitoneal structures in this quadrant, including the left gonadal vessels, the left ureter (Figure 7.10), and the hypogastric plexus (Figure 7.11, see color plate), are all readily visualized when the left colon and sigmoid are mobilized as in a rectosigmoid cancer operation.

Figure 7.8. Just inferior to the splenic flexure, the ligament of Treitz and the main vessels of the left colon are seen. LT, ligament of Treitz; IMV, inferior mesenteric vein; IMA, inferior mesenteric artery.

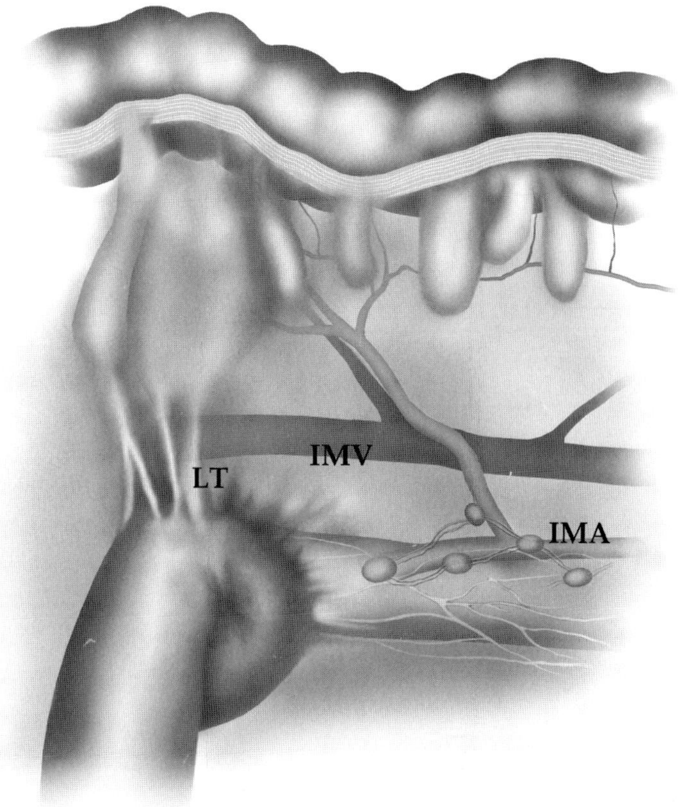

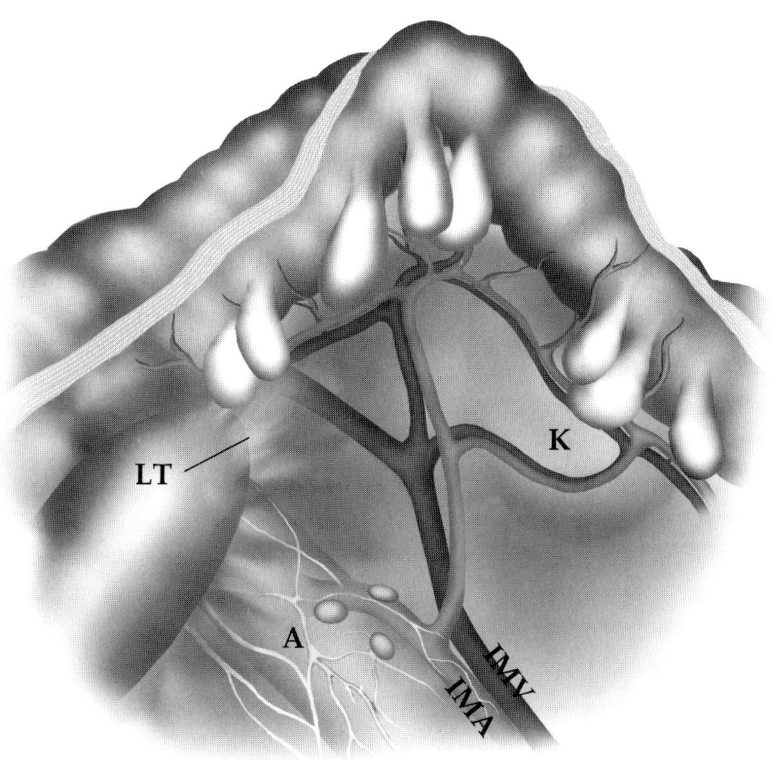

Figure 7.9. By retracting the small bowel to the right side of the abdomen, the attachments of the sigmoid colon and the main vessels of the left colon may be seen.

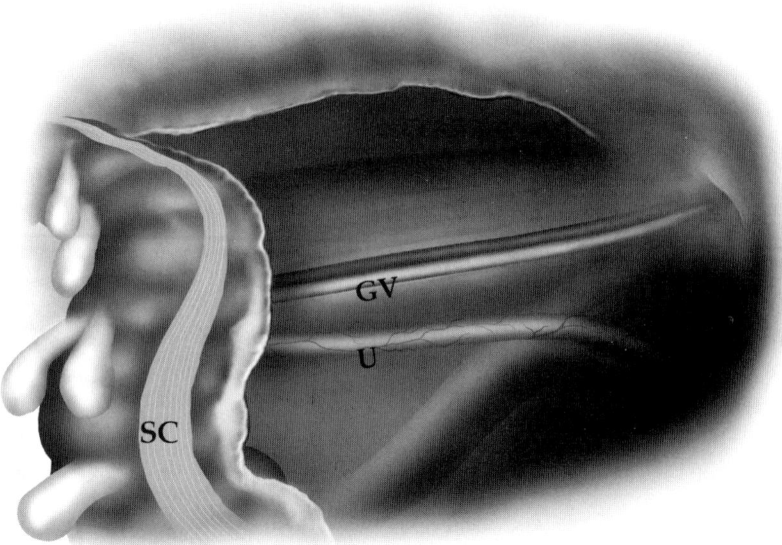

Figure 7.10. During the surgical mobilization of the sigmoid colon, the relationships of the gonadal vessels and the ureter are appreciated. SC, sigmoid colon; GV, gonadal vessels; U, ureter.

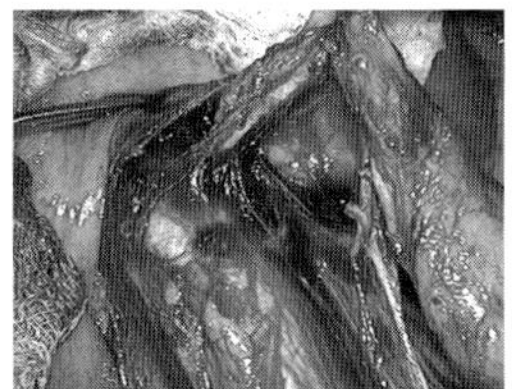

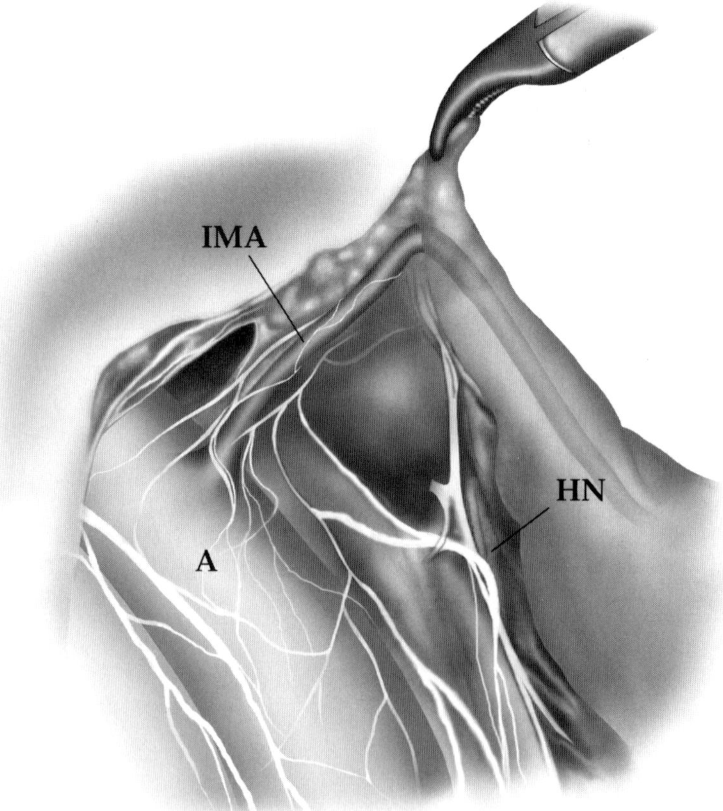

Figure 7.11. During a surgical dissection of the origin of the inferior mesenteric artery, the relationships of the hypogastric nerves and the aorta are appreciated. Note how the two branches (left and right) are straddling the aorta. IMA, inferior mesenteric artery; A, aorta; HN, left branch of the hypogastric nerve plexus. (See color plate.)

The Right Lower Quadrant

By placing the patient in the Trendelenburg position with the right side up, the terminal ileum, its retroperitoneal attachments, the cecum, and the ligament of Treitz can be visualized (Figure 7.12, see color plate). The vascular structures of the ileum and right colon may also be identified (Figure 7.13, see color plate), and their relationship to the duodenum may be appreciated. With dissection of the ileum and right colon away from their retroperitoneal attachments, then the psoas major muscle, the psoas minor tendon, and the right gonadal vessels and ureter are easily seen. The hepatic flexure is well visualized as the ascending colon is mobilized from the retroperitoneum (Figure 7.14). In thinner patients, the vascular structures in the transverse mesocolon (i.e., right and left branches of middle colic vessels) can be clearly demonstrated even before mesenteric dissection (Figure 7.15, see color plate).

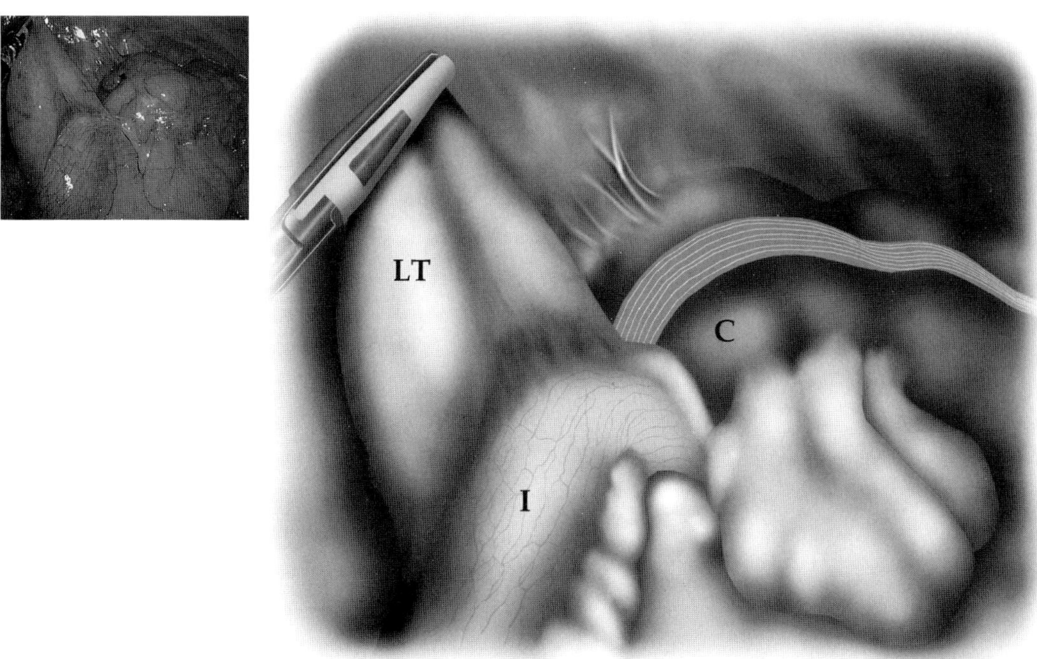

Figure 7.12. With a patient in the Trendelenburg position and the right side tilted upward, the terminal ileum, cecum, and ligament of Treitz may all be visualized. I, terminal ileum; LT, ligament of Treitz; C, cecum. (See color plate.)

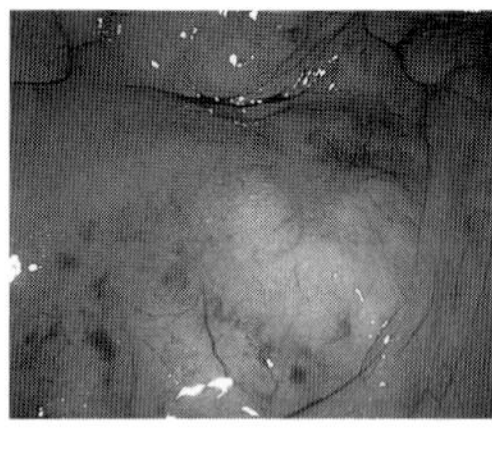

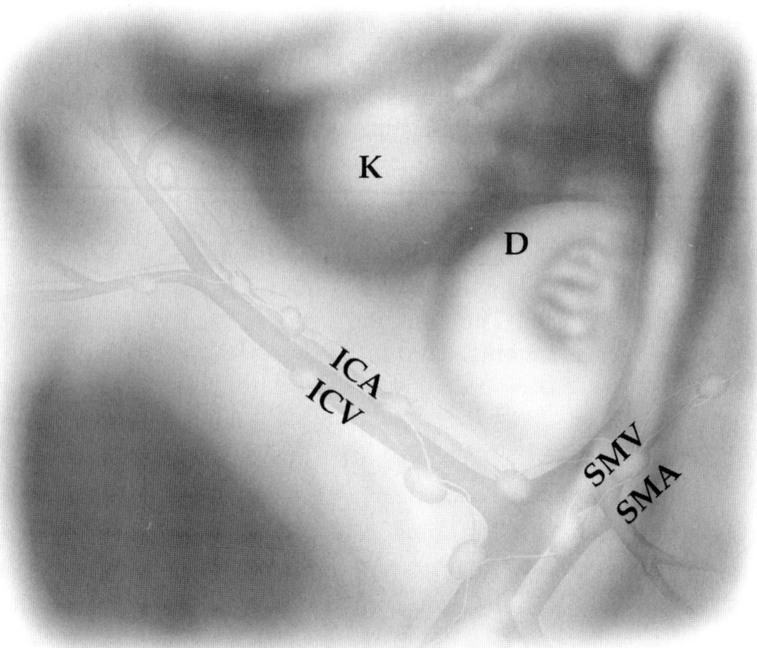

Figure 7.13. The major vascular structures of the right colon may be appreciated through the mesocolon, along with the right kidney and duodenum, with the small bowel retracted inferiorly and to the left. ICA, ileocolic artery; ICV, ileocolic vein; K, right kidney; D, duodenum; SMV, superior mesenteric vein; SMA, superior mesenteric artery. (See color plate.)

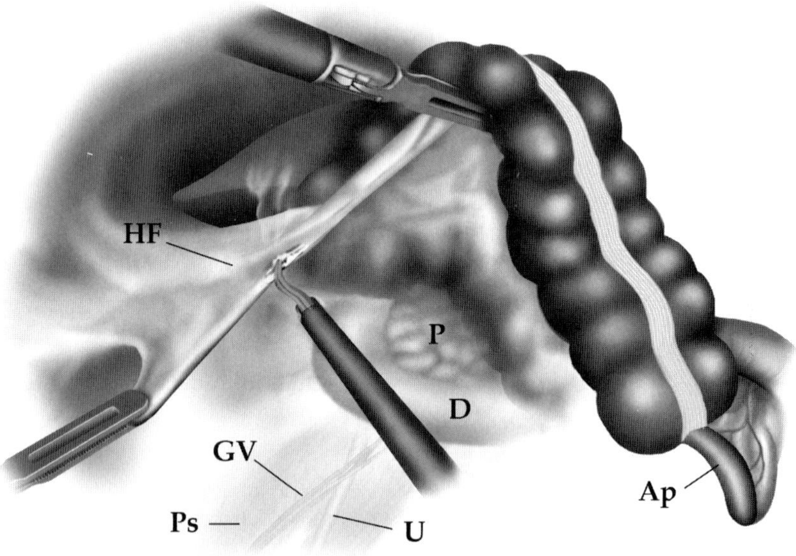

Figure 7.14. As the right colon is mobilized, the retroperitoneal structures are well seen. HF, hepatic flexure; Ps, psoas major muscle; GV, gonadal vessels; U, ureter; D, duodenum; P, pancreatic head; Ap, appendix.

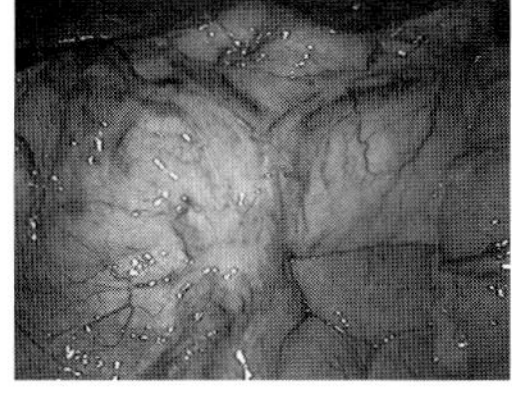

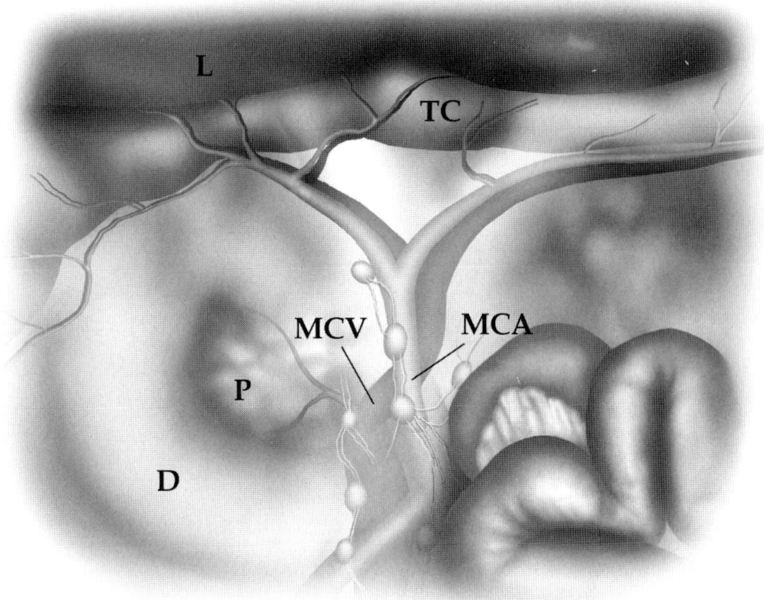

Figure 7.15. In thin patients, the vessels of the transverse colon and major structures in this region may be seen. L, inferior edge of liver; TC, transverse colon; MCV, middle colic vein; MCA, middle colic artery; D, duodenum; P, head of pancreas. (See color plate.)

The Pelvis

In the Trendelenburg position, by displacing the small bowel contents into the upper abdomen, the pelvic contents may be inspected. Often it is surprising how well the pelvis may be seen as compared with open surgery, and part of this is attributable to the distension of the pelvis from the pneumoperitoneum. The relationship of the pelvic vessels to the organs is seen, and the inguinal areas are also visualized in a manner not often appreciated during conventional surgery (Figure 7.16). In female patients, Douglas pouch can be clearly observed by gently lifting up the uterus with an atraumatic grasper (Figure 7.17). The ovary can be further inspected by lifting it with the tip of the instrument (Figure 7.18). Once the rectum is mobilized, the relationships between pelvic nerves, the ureters, gonadal vessels, and the anterior structures can be appreciated, especially in less obese patients. During rectal surgery, even the pelvic floor can be well visualized in a detailed manner not often seen with conventional surgical methods (Figure 7.19).

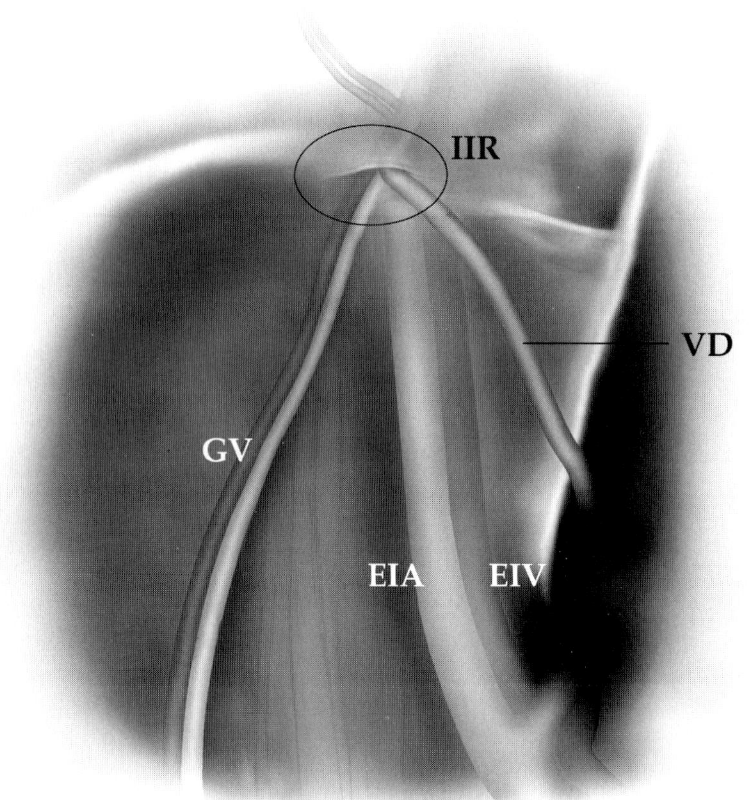

Figure 7.16. In the left inguinal region, the relationships of the gonadal vessels, vas deferens, and the major vessels exiting into the left leg are well appreciated during laparoscopy. GV, gonadal vessels; IIR, internal inguinal ring; EIA, external iliac artery; EIV, external iliac vein; Vd, vas deferens.

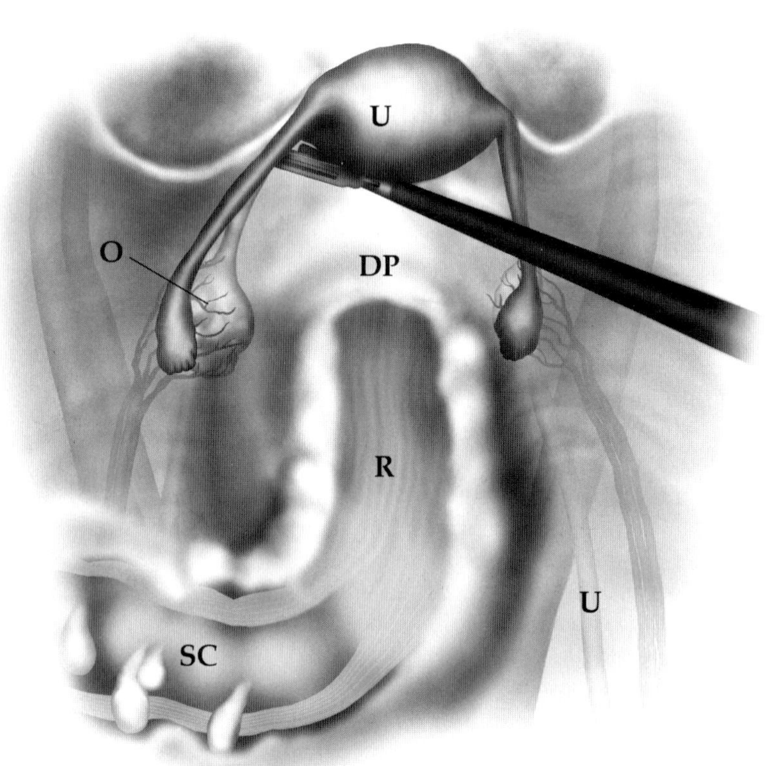

Figure 7.17. A broad view of the pelvis is seen during laparoscopy in women. U, uterus; DP, Douglas pouch; O, left ovary; R, rectum; SC, sigmoid colon; U, right ureter.

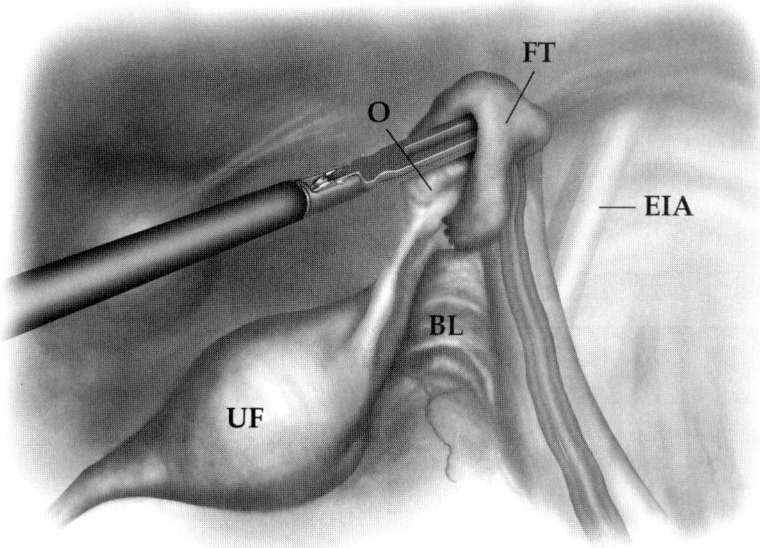

Figure 7.18. Lifting up on the right uterine adnexa permits appreciation of the relationships of these structures to the pelvis. UF, uterine fundus; O, ovary; FT, Fallopian tube; BL, broad ligament; EIA, external iliac artery.

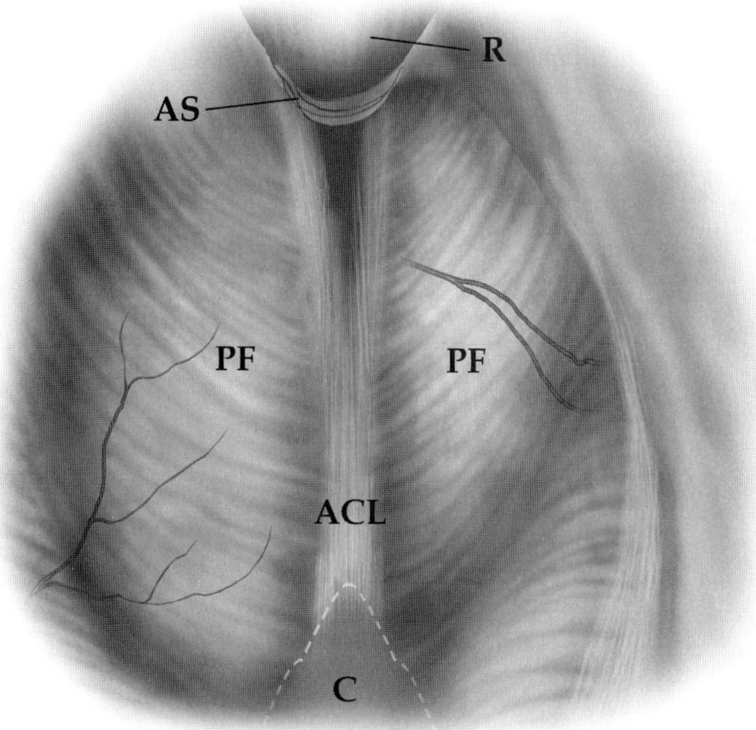

Figure 7.19. After complete mobilization of the rectum, the laparoscopic view affords excellent appreciation of some of the deep pelvic structures. R, rectum; AS, anal sphincter; PF, pelvic floor; ACL, anococcygeal ligament; C, coccyx.

Conclusions

Using appropriate positioning, retraction with simple laparoscopic tools, and meticulous dissection, excellent visualization of the important anatomic structures of the abdomen and pelvis are possible during routine colon and rectal laparoscopic procedures. Use of a flexible laparoscopic camera probably enhances the possibility to see overtop of the liver, and to obtain views in hard to reach areas including the pelvis and the LUQ. The pneumoperitoneum probably contributes to the views seen in the pelvis. By virtue of the enhanced views offered by the laparoscope, the laparoscopic surgeon has the opportunity to enhance the understanding of the anatomy of the abdomen and thereby enhance surgical outcomes.

Chapter 8.1

Small Bowel Resection

Jeffrey W. Milsom, Bartholomäus Böhm, and Kiyokazu Nakajima

Indications

A laparoscopic small bowel resection with primary anastomosis is most frequently indicated for benign diseases. These would include isolated Crohn's disease, gastrointestinal stromal tumors, benign strictures, and vascular malformations. Malignant conditions represent relative contraindications in that they are rare and if diagnosed or suspected we do not believe laparoscopic methods have a defined role in their treatment. The conduct of the operation should be in a manner very similar to that of a conventional small bowel resection.

Patient Positioning and Operating Room Setup

The patient is placed supine in a modified lithotomy position using Dan Allen stirrups. Surgery is begun in the Trendelenburg position (20° head-down tilt) and, after cannula insertion, the patient is tilted left side down for ileal surgery or the right side down for jejunal surgery.

The surgeon and assistants stand in a half circle opening toward the area of interest. Figure 8.1.1A shows the positions for ileal surgery. After cannula insertion, the surgeon stands between the legs and both assistants stand on the left side of the patient for the remainder of the procedure. The scrub nurse should stand on the right side near the knee. One monitor is placed close to the patient's right shoulder, the optimal position for viewing by the surgeon and assistants; the second monitor is placed near the left shoulder, the best location for viewing by the nurse. An alternative can be that one flat screen monitor is used, which is placed above the patient's head, for all members of the operative team to use (Figure 8.1.1B). For jejunal surgery, the setup is a mirror image of the ileal positions.

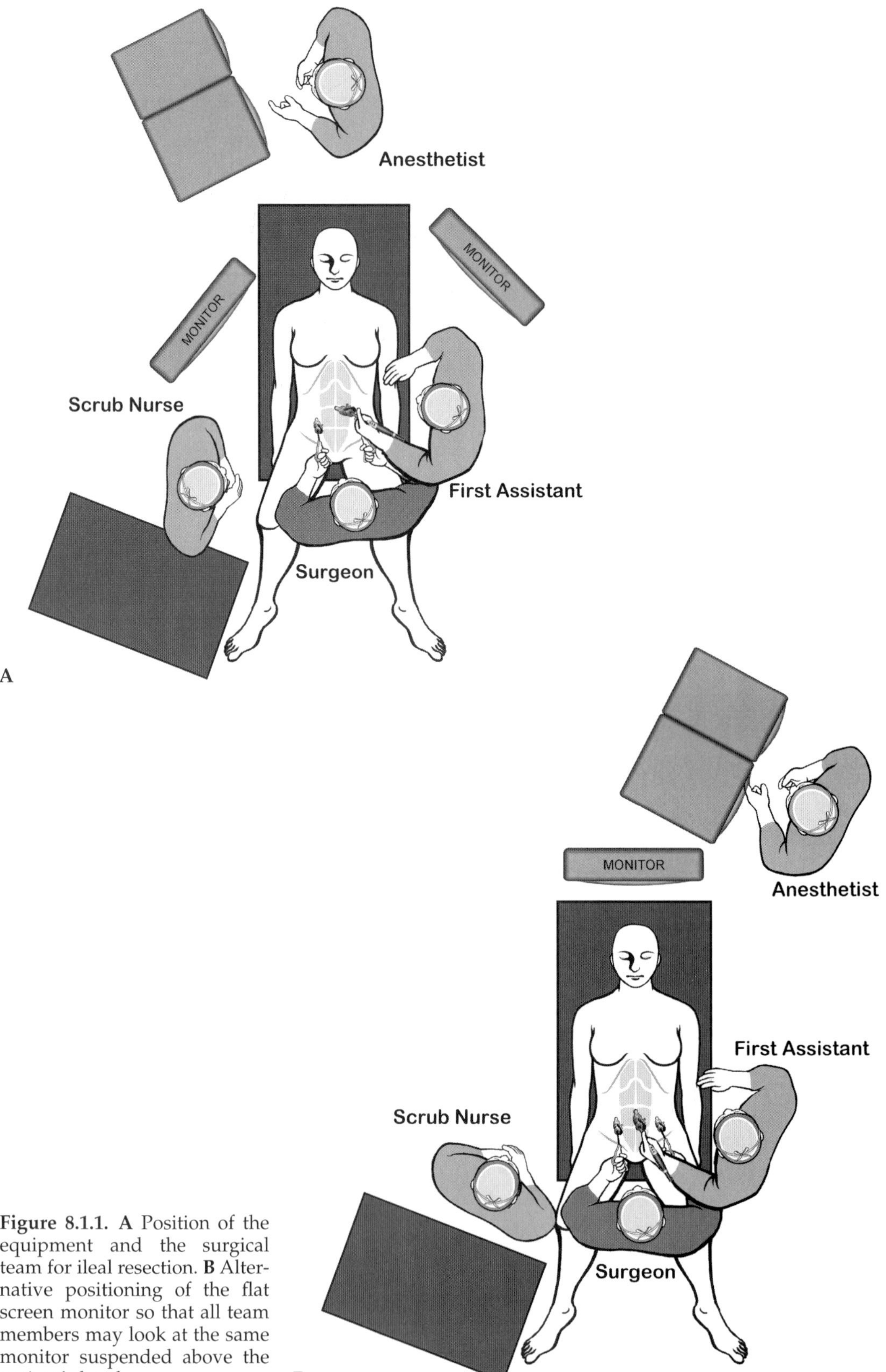

Figure 8.1.1. A Position of the equipment and the surgical team for ileal resection. **B** Alternative positioning of the flat screen monitor so that all team members may look at the same monitor suspended above the patient's head.

Table 8.1.1. Specific instruments recommended for laparoscopic small bowel resection

3–5	Cannulae (1 × 10 mm, 2–4 × 5 mm)
1	Dissecting device (i.e., LigaSure V™ or Ultrasonic Shears™ or electrosurgery)
1	Laparoscopic scissor
1	Laparoscopic dissector
2	Laparoscopic graspers

Instruments

Specific instruments recommended for small bowel resection are listed in Table 8.1.1.

Cannula Positioning

Cannulas should be positioned in a half circle or line facing toward the site of pathology. Thus, for jejunal surgery, the half circle will open toward the right upper quadrant (Figure 8.1.2), whereas for ileal surgery,

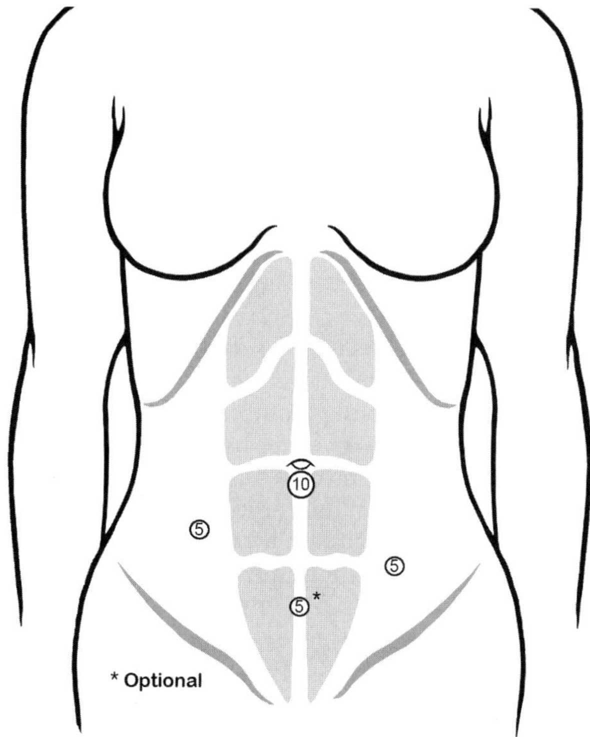

Figure 8.1.2. Position of the cannulae for ileal resection. For jejunal surgery, the left- and right-sided cannulae may suffice. For ileal surgery, it may be preferable to use the suprapubic cannula and omit the right lower quadrant one.

it will open toward the left upper quadrant. In many cases, only 2–3 cannulae are used to accomplish a diagnostic laparoscopy and to localize the pathology. A fourth cannula in the suprapubic area may be helpful in certain cases and should be placed readily if this may be helpful for retraction or exposure. Alternatively, for ileal surgery, the suprapubic cannula may be preferable and the right lower quadrant one may be eliminated.

Technique

Once the preoperative diagnosis is confirmed and the laparoscopic procedure appears feasible, the pathology is located by running the entire length of the small bowel and placing a suture just upstream of the pathology.

Running the small bowel is accomplished from proximal to distal by placing the patient on the left side up, in slight reverse Trendelenburg position until the mid small bowel is reached, then adjusting the patient to the right side up with Trendelenburg position to run the distal half of the small intestine. The surgeon should start the "running" from between the legs then switch to the left side of the patient for the distal half (or permit the first assistant to run the distal half from left side of the patient). The technique of "running" should be "hand-over-hand" (Figure 8.1.3A and B) or "hand-to-hand" (Figure 8.1.4A–C) based on the degree of freedom present within the abdominal cavity.

If it will be advantageous to divide the mesenteric vessels before delivery of the specimen through the abdominal incision, this should be done using a LigaSure V™ instrument. We currently would just ligate the main vessel supplying the affected segment, and leave the other vessels of the mesentery to be divided through the incision. This may be especially helpful in a patient with a thick abdominal wall.

Once the specimen is fully mobilized, a cannula site is enlarged to 3–5 cm. For small incisions, a transverse incision is preferred. The anterior rectus sheath is transversely incised, the rectus muscles retracted, and the posterior sheath also transversely incised. If the incision has to be larger because of a bulky tumor, a longitudinal incision in the midline is accomplished above and below the umbilicus.

The wound is protected using a plastic sheath and the loop of intestine to be resected is drawn out through the enlarged incision. Wound protection is important to reduce any contamination by tumor cells or intestine and it may also facilitate the specimen extraction. The resection and anastomosis are then made in a standard manner extracorporeally, either by a hand-sewn or stapled method. The mesenteric defect is usually closed with a running absorbable suture through the incision.

After performing the anastomosis, the abdomen is copiously irrigated with warm sterile saline solution through the incision. The fluid is removed by placing the patient in the head-up position and passing a sump suction cannula into the pelvis. After irrigation of the peritoneal cavity, the abdominal wall is closed with a running suture or a series single suture.

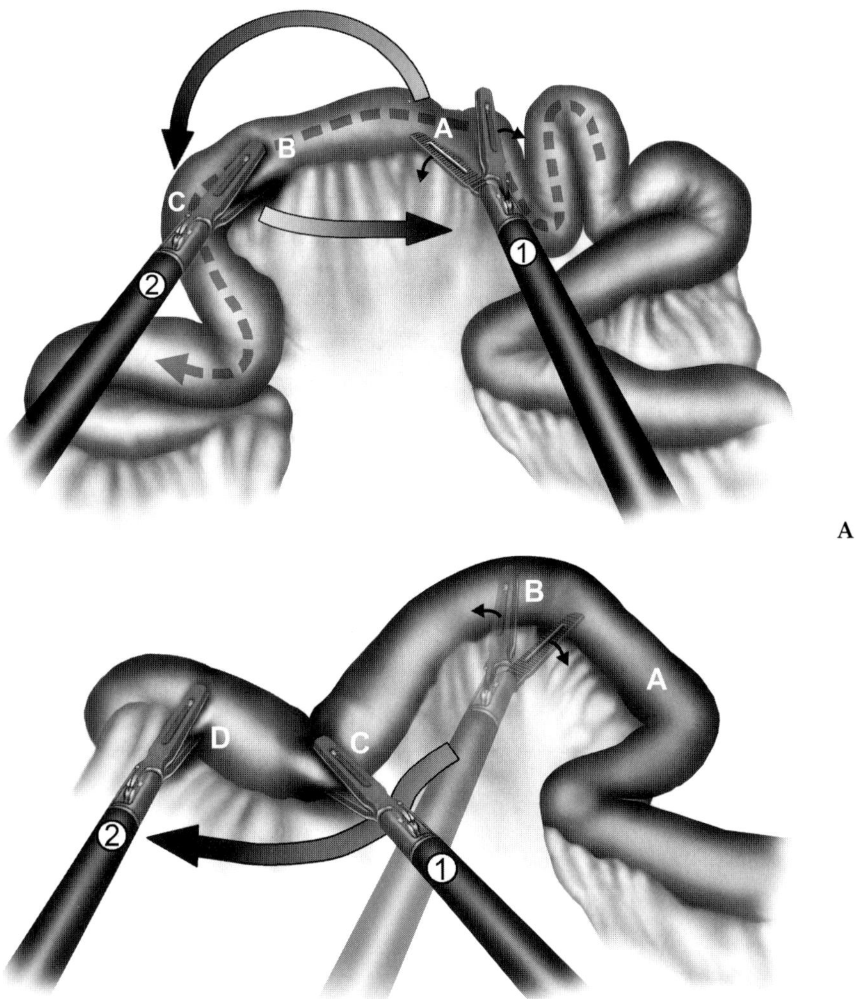

Figure 8.1.3. Running the bowel using the "hand-over-hand" technique. **A** The right-handed grasper (1) releases the bowel and prepares to move from point A on the bowel to point C, while the left handed grasper (2), at point B, prepares to slide to the right of the illustration. **B** The instruments are crossed (hand-over-hand), and the left hand (2) now releases point B on the bowel and slides beneath the right-handed grasper (1) to regrasp at point D. Next the process repeats itself.

The peritoneal cavity can then be finally inspected laparoscopically by leaving the wound protector in place, twisting it closed at the skin level, then clamping it with a Kocher clamp (Figure 8.1.5). This permits rapid reestablishment of the pneumoperitoneum, with a good seal of the specimen extraction site, for a final inspection inside the abdomen.

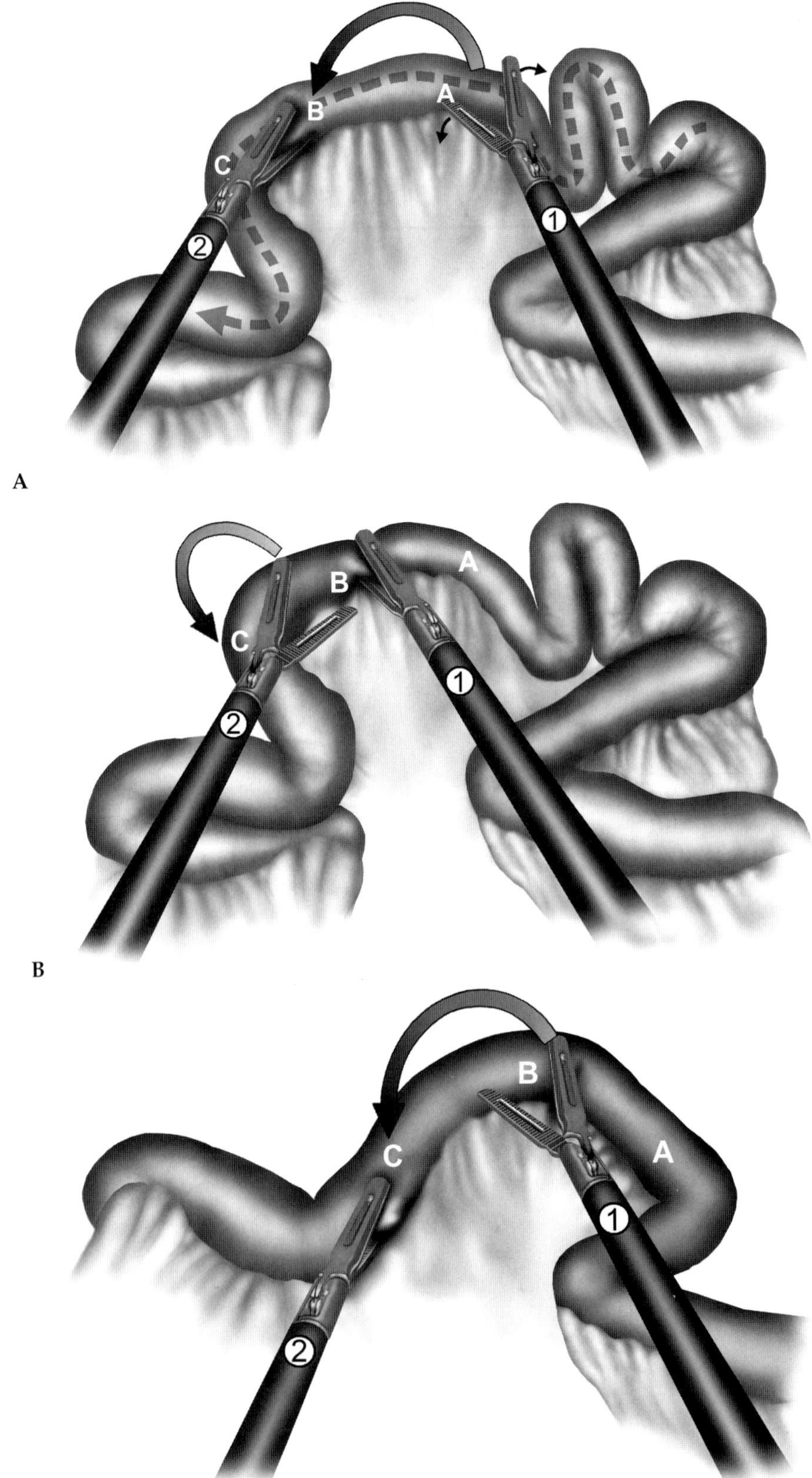
A
B
C
1
2
A
B
C
1
2
A
B
C
1
2
A
B
C

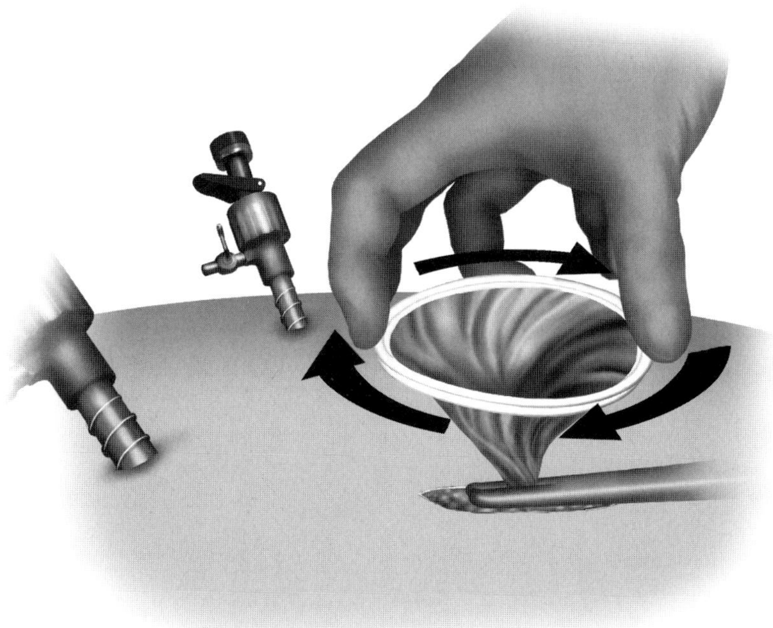

Figure 8.1.5. Twisting the wound protector and closing it with a clamp to quickly reestablish pneumoperitoneum after removing the specimen.

Special Considerations

The most important steps of laparoscopically assisted small bowel surgery are to localize and mobilize the diseased segment and deliver it through a small incision. The technique has become our procedure of choice for isolated benign small diseases. We do not believe that an intracorporeal anastomosis should be attempted at this time because most of the dissection and anastomosis can safely be performed using conventional techniques through a small incision used to remove the specimen.

The role of this approach in cancer surgery is limited. If there is diffuse spread of the disease, then it may be reasonable to consider a laparoscopic localization of the tumor in order to minimize the incision, or to consider only biopsy and no resection. Because these are rare tumors, and there is no proof of the efficacy of a laparoscopic approach,

Figure 8.1.4. Running the bowel using the "hand-to-hand" technique: **A** The right-handed grasper (1) releases the bowel and moves down from A to B next to the left-handed grasper (2). **B** The left-handed grasper releases (2) then moves downstream from point B to C grasping the bowel there. **C** The process repeats itself, the right-handed grasper (1) releasing again and moving down (2) from B to C.

caution should be exercised before applying laparoscopic methods for a resection. A laparoscopic-assisted approach could be considered, which would include a careful inspection of the entire abdomen, including the liver, then the umbilical cannula site enlarged in order to perform the appropriate mesenteric and intestinal resection. Thus, the actual resection would be done using conventional methods.

Chapter 8.2

Ileocolectomy

Riichiro Nezu

Indications

An ileocolectomy is most frequently indicated in patients with benign disease, i.e., Crohn's disease, cecal diverticulitis, intestinal tuberculosis, enteric Behçet's disease, submucosal tumors (lipoma, gastrointestinal stromal tumor, lymphoma, carcinoid, etc.), giant villous adenoma and polyps, located in the ileocecal regions. Indications are rare for performing a limited ileocecal resection for malignancies of the terminal ileum, the appendix, or the cecum. This may be the procedure of choice in palliative resection for cecal cancer.

Before the surgery for Crohn's disease, patients should have a computed tomography scan, small bowel series, and a full colonoscopy to assess the localization and dimension of any phlegmon or abscess or the presence of small bowel stricture or fistula, respectively. The preoperative computed tomography scan is also useful to evaluate periureteral inflammation and to aid in the decision to use intraoperative ureteric catheters. Preoperative enteral or parenteral nutritional support should be considered in selected patients.

Most surgeons would agree that the laparoscopic approach is contraindicated in patients with nonlocalized intraabdominal abscesses, multiple previous bowel operations with possible dense adhesions, fixed mass with multiple fistulas, acute intestinal obstruction, and perforation.

Although the entire operation can be performed laparoscopically, most surgeons prefer a laparoscopic-assisted procedure by laparoscopic mobilization and extracorporeal resection and anastomosis.

Patient Positioning and Operating Room Setup

Under general endotracheal anesthesia, the patient is placed in the supine position (Figure 8.2.1). If a need for an intraoperative colonoscopy is anticipated, the patient should be placed in a modified Lloyd Davies position with the lower extremities in Dan Allen or Levitator

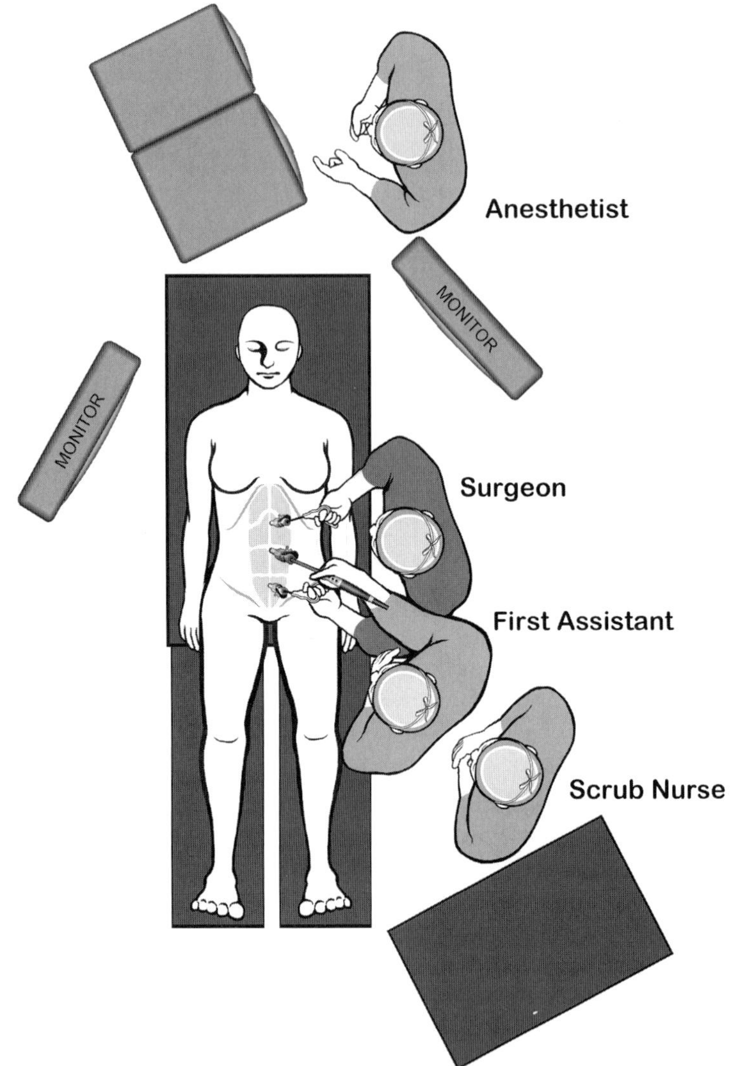

Figure 8.2.1. Position of the equipment and the surgical team for laparoscopic-assisted ileocolectomy.

stirrups (Skytron Co. Ltd., Grand Rapids, MI). A bladder catheter and a nasogastric tube are inserted, and pneumatic compression stockings are used for deep venous thrombosis prophylaxis. If utereric stents are to be placed, they are inserted with cystoscopy by a urologist after induction of anesthesia. Antisepsis and draping of the abdomen are undertaken as for laparotomy, with the exposed operative field extending between xiphoid and pubis and left and right iliac spines.

Table 8.2.1. Specific instruments recommended for laparoscopic-assisted ileocolectomy

3–5	Cannulae (1 × 10 mm, 2–4 × 5 mm)
1	Dissecting device (i.e., LigaSure V™ or Ultrasonic Shears™ or electrosurgery)
1	Laparoscopic scissor
1	Laparoscopic dissector
2	Laparoscopic graspers

Instruments

Specific instruments recommended for laparoscopic-assisted ileocolectomy are listed in Table 8.2.1.

Cannula Positioning

A 10-mm trocar for a laparoscope is inserted infraumbilically with the open Hasson technique, and 5-mm trocars are inserted in the upper midline, in the lower midline (or left lower abdomen) and the right lateral abdomen (Figure 8.2.2). When the mobilization of the colon is

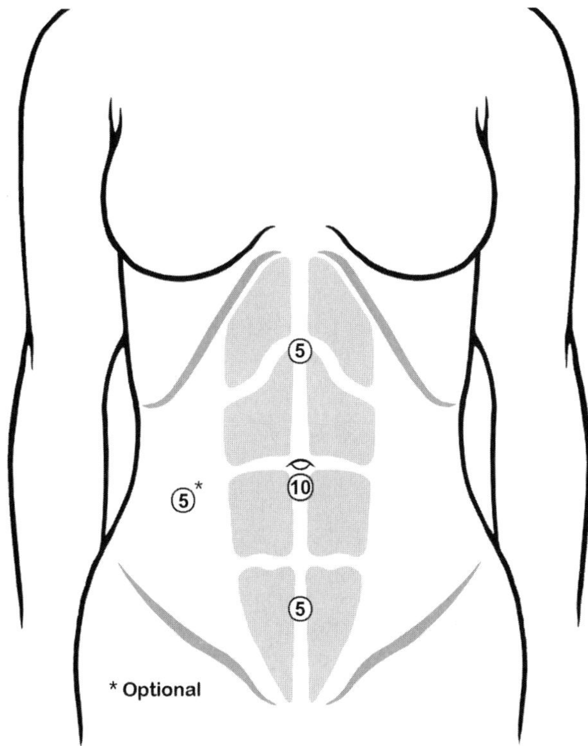

Figure 8.2.2. Positions of the cannulae for the ileocolic resection. Note that the right sided cannula is optional, but should be used with a low threshold if it will expedite the procedure.

limited from cecum up to hepatic flexure, the right lateral trocar is not necessary. In Crohn's disease, the right lower quadrant region should be spared for a future stoma creation site. If there is a scar of a previous laparotomy (e.g., in case of recurrent Crohn's disease), the laparoscope is often introduced from the left abdomen lateral to the rectus sheath with the open Hasson technique.

Technique

The patient is placed in the Trendelenburg position, and three or four trocars are inserted. For establishment of pneumoperitoneum, CO_2 is channeled through the infraumbilical trocar until the intraabdominal pressure reaches 10 mm Hg. Both the operating surgeon and camera holder stand on the patient's left side. After abdominal exploration, the operation table is rotated left side down so the small intestine falls toward the left upper quadrant.

The ascending colon is thoroughly mobilized from the base of the appendix (Figure 8.2.3) up to the hepatic flexure (Figure 8.2.4) by cutting the retroperitoneal attachments with electrosurgical scissors and laparoscopic coagulating shears, and bluntly dissecting the retroperitoneal fusion fascia and loose connective tissue. With this procedure, the duodenum, Gerota's fascia, and sometimes more inferiorly the right ureter and the gonadal vessels become visible beneath the retroperitoneal fusion fascia (Figure 8.2.5). During dissection, the direct

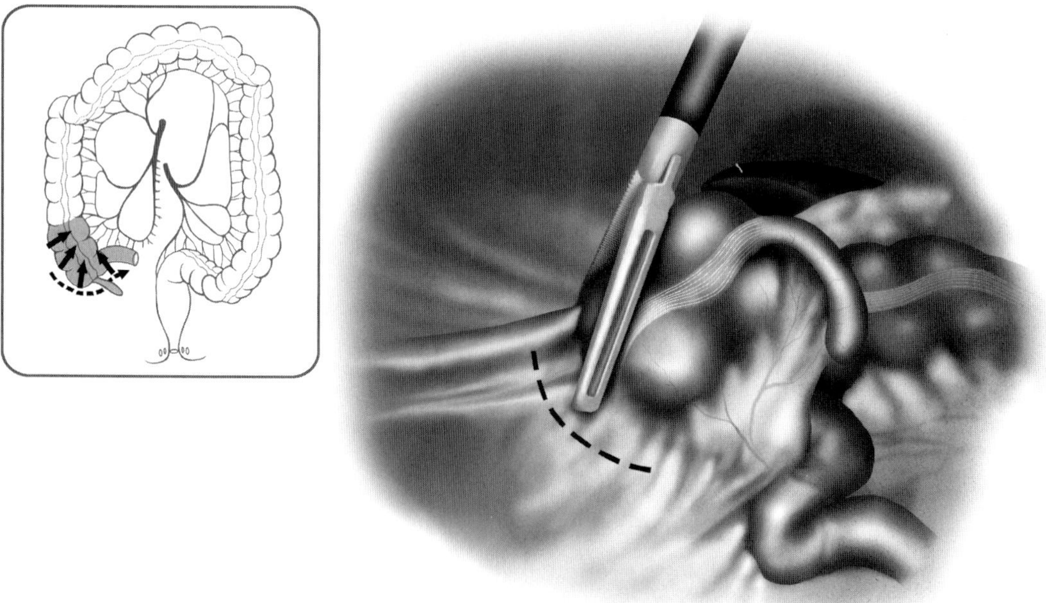

Figure 8.2.3. The initial mobilization of the bowel commences with dissection at the cecal area.

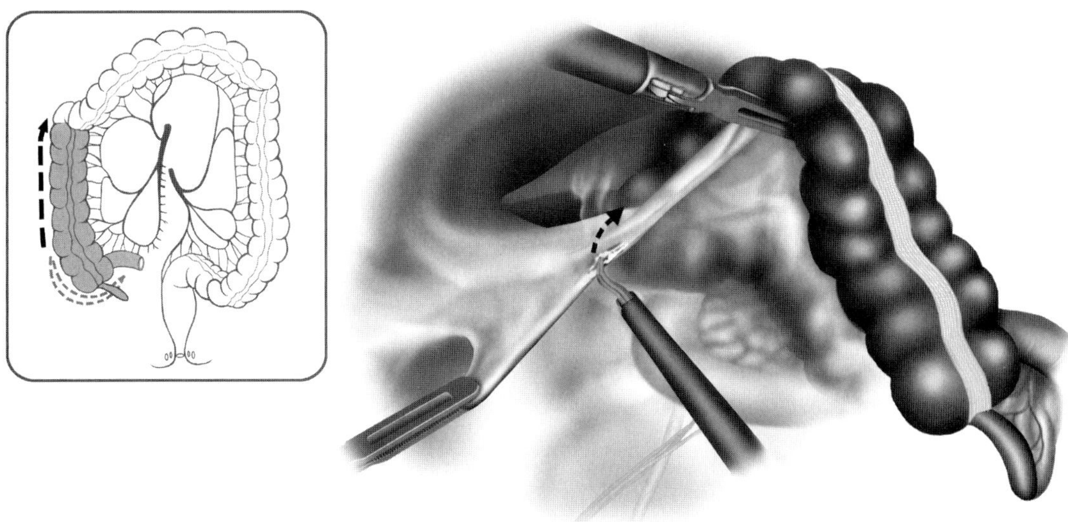

Figure 8.2.4. Freeing up the lateral attachments of the right colon after some retroperitoneal dissection.

grasping and handling of diseased bowel loops should be avoided, to prevent incidental myotomies and enterotomies.

In Crohn's disease, intracorporeal inspection of the entire small bowel is performed carefully in a hand-over-hand manner using two

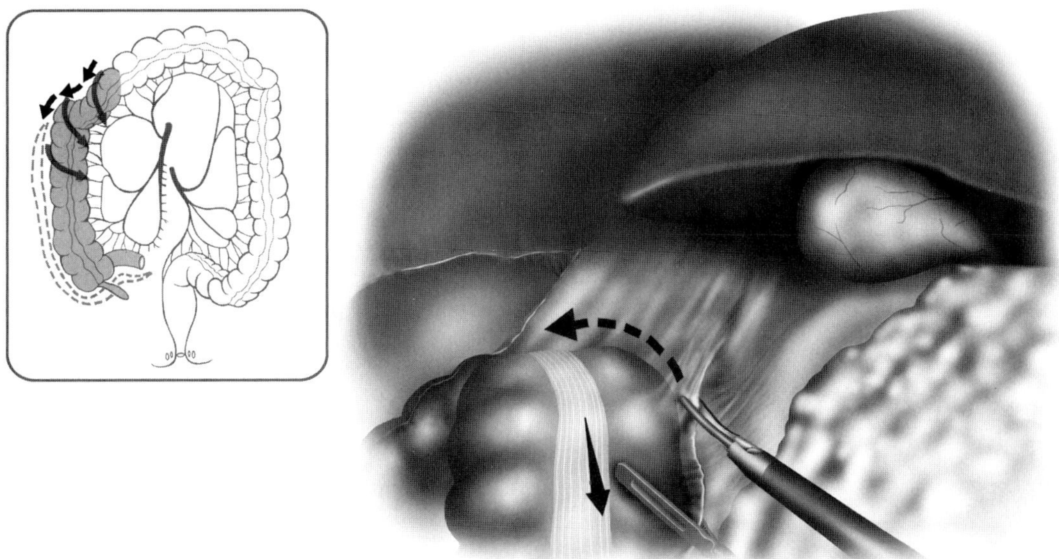

Figure 8.2.5. Freeing up the hepatic flexure so that the bowel may be drawn out through an umbilical incision. The duodenum and other retroperitoneal structures may become readily apparent.

bowel clamps following the laparoscopic colonic mobilization. In patients with ileovesical, ileorectal, and gastrocolic fistulas, division with an intracorporeal stapling device (one or two firings of the 45- or 60-mm stapler) can be done.

After mobilization of the entire ascending colon, meticulous hemostasis is made. Then, the patient is placed in a reversed Trendelenburg position temporarily and the abdomen is irrigated with warm sterile saline. The patient is placed in a flat supine position, and pneumoperitoneum is released. A small laparotomy is performed through a 5-cm-long skin incision made at the umbilical trocar site or through a Pfannenstiel incision. A wound protector is inserted and the segments of the colon are delivered through this incision. Mesenteric division, ileocolic resection, and anastomosis by Gambee's procedure using 4–0 absorbable sutures such as Vicryl® or PDS®, or functional end-to-end anastomosis using linear staplers are performed extracorporeally (Figure 8.2.6A and B). After closure of the mesenteric defect, the entire residual small bowel is examined through the incision, and the stricture plasties (either Heineke-Mikulicz or Finney type) are performed on distant skip lesions, if necessary. The omentum is laid under the wound to prevent postoperative adhesions, and the peritoneum is closed with absorbable sutures. Closed silicone drain tube is left in cul-de-sac through the right lateral trocar site if necessary, and every trocar site incision is closed with skin staplers.

Special Considerations

Patients with Crohn's ileocolitis, who have no abscess or fistula, may alternatively undergo a completely laparoscopic ileocolectomy. However, the fragility of the inflamed bowel wall, thickened mesentery, and dense adhesions may be responsible for difficulties during the procedures of mesenteric dissection, vascular isolation and ligation, and anastomosis. In laparoscopic surgery for Crohn's disease, any synchronous pathology such as strictures in skipped areas must be as reliably identifiable and treatable as it should be during laparotomy. Moreover, a small incision is ultimately necessary in order to remove the resected specimen. The size of incision is determined by the size of the specimen. Totally laparoscopic procedures with intracorporeal anastomosis are expensive, time-consuming, and provide little advantage over laparoscopic-assisted procedures.

In Crohn's disease, the mesentery is often very thick and friable, and it is the author's opinion that extracorporeal division of the mesentery is safer and more expeditious. Laparoscopic Coagulating Shears™ (LCS) cuts and coagulates by converting electric energy into ultrasonic mechanical vibrations and allows reliable, safe, and rapid hemostasis and division, except when it is used too quickly.[1] When using LCS, the position of the blade, as well as the duration of the pressure and the level of the power output, is determinant in the quality of hemostasis. Although it does not seem worthwhile to modify the direction of the blade for small vessels, coagulation of larger pedicles requires longer

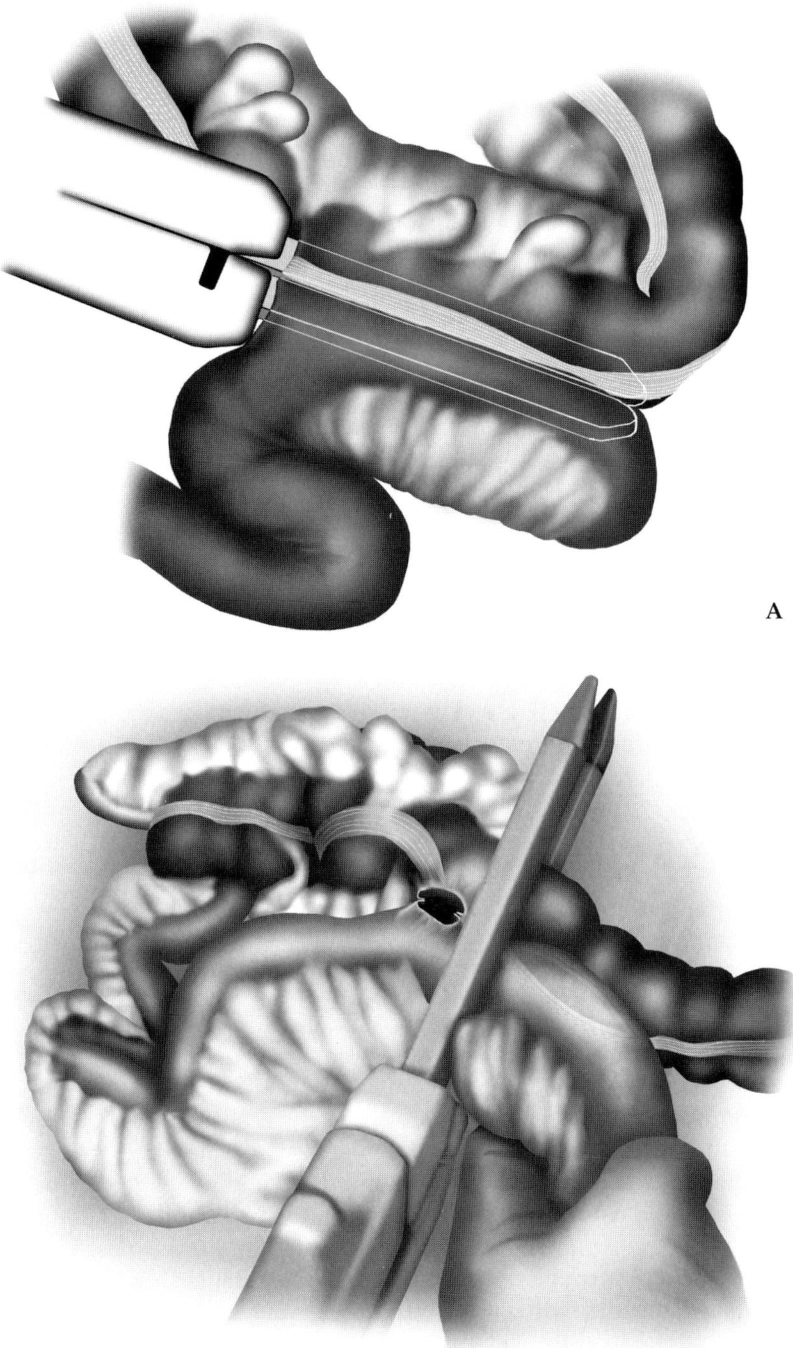

Figure 8.2.6. Creating an extracorporeal anastomosis. **A** A linear stapler is used to form a side-to-side anastomosis between small bowel and the ascending colon. **B** The anastomosis is closed using a firing of the same stapler at a right angle to the previous staple line.

application and progressive pressure with the blades in the flat position. No tension on the pedicles should be made during coagulation to avoid early division and bleeding.

To prevent the incidental enterotomy, gentle handling of the diseased bowel with endoscopic graspers is of great importance as well. The use of atraumatic instruments should be coupled with avoidance of direct grasping or handling of the diseased loop of bowel. It is also important that the dissection and mobilization should always be started in a normal area, advancing toward the diseased segment.[2]

During dissection of the ileocolic region, there is danger of injury to the ipsilateral ureter, which may be adherent to the mesentery because of the inflammatory process. Injury to the ureters may be lessened by the prophylactic placement of ureteric catheters. They should be placed in selected cases such as patients with a retroperitoneal phlegmon or abscess, or extensive inflammation manifested in the preoperative studies.[3]

Conclusions

We use a laparoscopic-assisted approach, with an extracorporeal anastomosis, rather than an entirely laparoscopic approach with an intracorporeal anastomosis. Our approach provides the benefits of laparoscopic surgery while maintaining the advantages of open vascular division and anastomosis, i.e., speed, low risk of intraabdominal stool spillage.

Editors' Comments

This chapter illustrates the most common approach to ileocolic resection, which is a common operation in Western countries, and is likely becoming more common in Eastern countries as well.

Indications: We would add that most carcinoids or carcinomas of the appendix or the ileocecal region should be treated with a formal right colectomy (see Chapter 8.3).

Patient positioning: We place patients into the modified lithotomy position, using the padded stirrups in most cases, because if there is extension of disease of the ileocolic region into the pelvis (e.g., Crohn's ileosigmoid fistula), then we can take advantage of the access to the pelvic organs offered by this position. It is rare for us to use ureteral stents, but this may be wise in certain circumstances.

Instrumentation: We often use either the LigaSure Atlas™ or more commonly the LigaSure V™, because this tool may be very useful both for thickened mesentery and all mesenteric vessels including the ileocolic pedicle.

Cannula positioning: We utilize a different setup of cannula, usually placing two on the left side (left upper and lower quadrants) and one or two on the right side (mirror image of left side). If the disease is relatively uncomplicated, then only one cannula is used on the right side. Alternatively, we might place one cannula in the suprapubic area, several centimeters above the symphysis pubis, and one in the right lower quadrant.

Technique: We run the small bowel in all patients, starting at the ligament of Treitz, then place a stitch laparoscopically at the proximal extent of disease, so that when the diseased segment is withdrawn from the abdomen, usually through a small incision, we may correlate this stitch with the laparoscopic evaluation. We also find that by ligating and dividing the ileocolic pedicle during the laparoscopic portion of the procedure, this makes it much easier to draw the specimen out through the small incision used to extract it and create the anastomosis. This pedicle tends to act like a "chordee" and impedes the ability to use a small incision.

A small wound protector (such as the Alexis model 5–9 cm; Applied Medical, Rancho Santa Margherita, CA) may expand the incision used to extract the specimen, greatly improving the ability to perform the actual bowel resection through a small incision.

When there is fistula to another organ in the pelvis, e.g., the bladder, sigmoid colon, or rectum, we advocate making a Pfannenstiel incision after laparoscopic inspection and running the bowel, permitting the surgical team to use that incision (which may be extended to 8–10 cm if necessary) to safely dissect and repair the involved organs under direct vision using conventional methods. This may also lend itself to a hand-assisted approach, as discussed in Chapter 9.

Finally, we do not use a drain for right-sided resections, and (J.M. and K.N.) do not close the mesentery unless the defect is very small (under 6–8 cm) because they believe the risk for later clinically relevant herniation is extremely low.

References

1. Msika S, Deroide G, Kianmanesh R, et al. Harmonic scalpel in laparoscopic colorectal surgery. Dis Colon Rectum 2001;44:432–436.
2. Reissman P, Salky B, Pfeifer J, et al. Laparoscopic surgery in the management of inflammatory bowel disease. Am J Surg 1996;171:47–51.
3. Wexner SD, Johansen OB, Nogueras JJ, et al. Laparoscopic total abdominal colectomy. Dis Colon Rectum 1992;35:651–655.

Chapter 8.3

Right Colectomy

Junji Okuda and Nobuhiko Tanigawa

Indications

Although benign tumors not resectable by a colonoscopic procedure and stricturing inflammatory bowel disease may be good indications for laparoscopy, they are not so common. The most common disease for right colectomy is right-sided colon cancer. Colon cancer seems to be a good indication for laparoscopic surgery if performed using proper oncologic methods, i.e., early proximal ligation of the major mesenteric vessels and wide mesenteric and intestinal resection with complete lymphadenectomy. Patients with complete obstruction caused by the cancer, cancer extensively invading adjacent organs, and bulky cancer larger than 10 cm in size should be excluded. According to these concepts, a proper oncologic approach using laparoscopy for right colon cancer is described in this chapter.

Patient Positioning and Operating Room Setup

The patient is fixed in a moldable "bean bag" form with both arms tucked in, and placed in a modified lithotomy position using Levitator stirrups. We prefer the Hasson (open) technique to safely insert the first port through the umbilicus. After establishing pneumoperitoneum, the surgeon stands on the patient's left side to expose the right mesocolon and to mark the lower border of the ileocolic vessels. Next, the surgeon moves between the patient's legs, the assistants position themselves on the patient's left side and the nurse stands near the patient's right knee (Figure 8.3.1A and B). The main monitor is placed near the patient's right shoulder to give the surgeon and the assistants optimal viewing. The second monitor is placed on the left side close to the head, a location that gives the best view for the nurse. After completing the proximal vessel ligation with lymphadenectomy and mobilization of the terminal ileum and the cecum, the surgeon moves back to the patient's left side and the first assistant stands between the patient's legs for take-down of right flexure and whole mobilization of the right colon (Figure 8.3.1A).

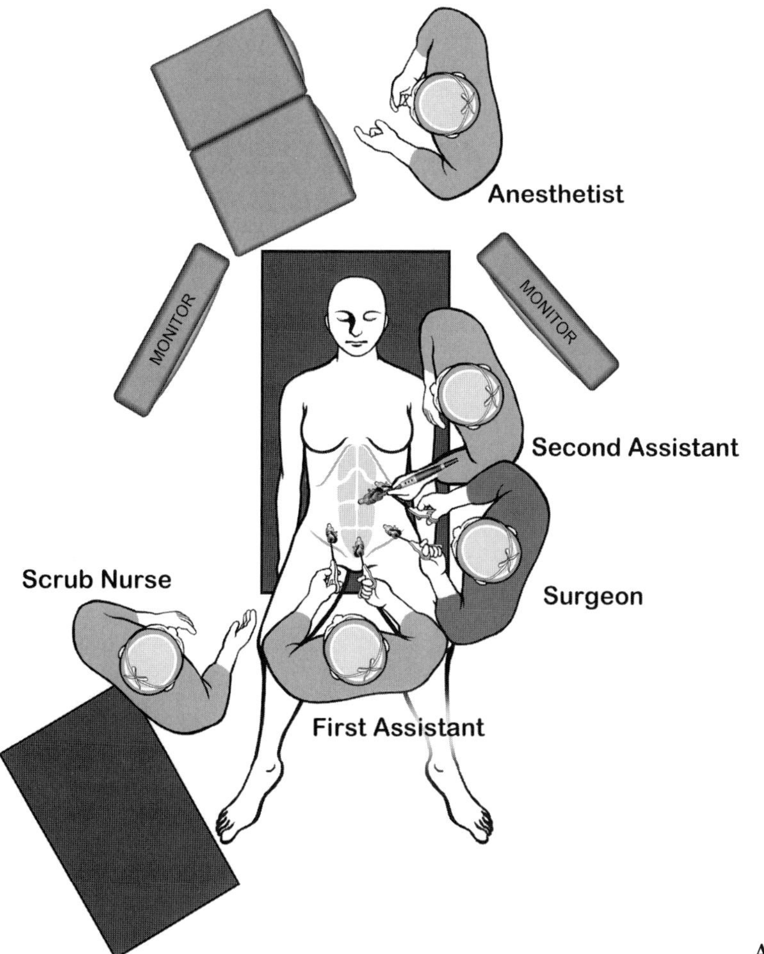

Figure 8.3.1. Positions of the equipment and the surgical team for the laparoscopic right colectomy. **A** Initially the surgeon is at the left side of the patient, and returns to this position after lymphovascular pedicle ligation. **B** The surgeon assumes a position between the legs for optimizing the approach to the dissection of the mesenteric pedicles.

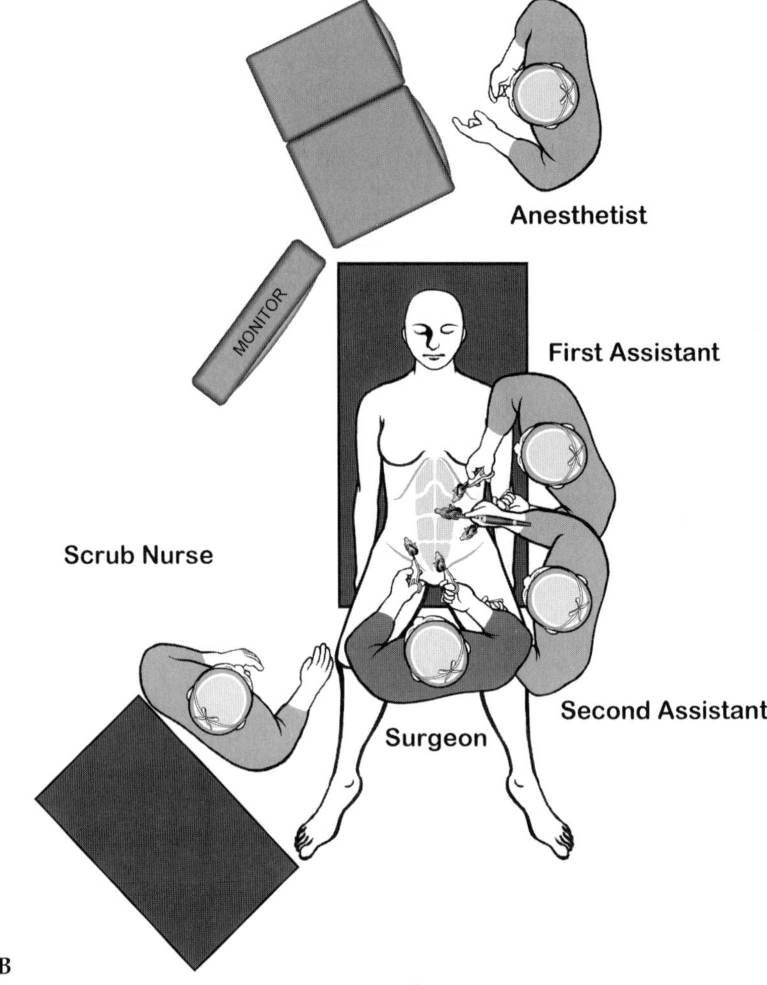

Figure 8.3.1. *Continued*

Instruments

Specific instruments recommended for laparoscopic right colectomy are listed in Table 8.3.1.

Table 8.3.1. Specific instruments recommended for laparoscopic right colectomy

3–5	Cannulae (1 × 12 mm, 2–4 × 5 mm)
1	Dissecting device (i.e., LigaSure V™ or Ultrasonic Shears™ or electrosurgery)
1	Laparoscopic scissor
1	Laparoscopic dissector
2	Laparoscopic graspers

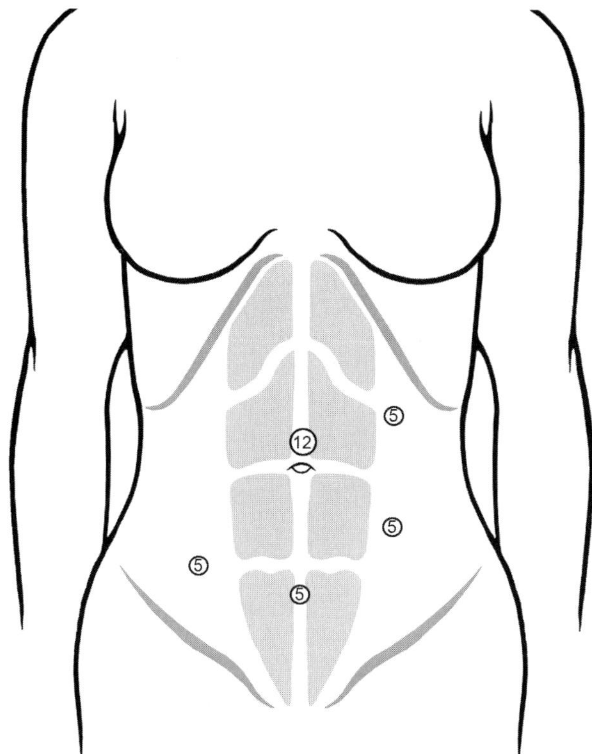

Figure 8.3.2. Positions of the cannulae for the right colectomy. The suprapubic cannula is used for the laparoscope while the lymphovascular pedicles are dissected and divided.

Cannula Positioning

Five ports are placed as shown in Figure 8.3.2. If a 10-mm laparoscope is used, a 10-mm port is positioned instead of the suprapubic 5-mm port.

Technique

The patient is placed in the modified lithotomy position to allow the surgeon to stand between the patient's legs for one portion of the operation. After establishing the pneumoperitoneum through an umbilical port, an additional four ports are placed in the left and right lower quadrant, left upper abdomen, and suprapubic area. The operating table is tilted into the slight Trendelenburg position with the left side down to move the small intestine toward the left upper quadrant. The omentum and transverse colon are moved toward the upper abdomen, the ventral side of the right mesocolon is well visualized, and the optimal operative field can be achieved (Figure 8.3.3). Before starting the dissection, the ileocolic pedicle must be definitively identified by retracting the right mesocolon (Figure 8.3.4).

Various approaches, such as lateral-to-medial (lateral approach),[1] medial-to-lateral (medial approach),[2] and retroperitoneal approach,[3]

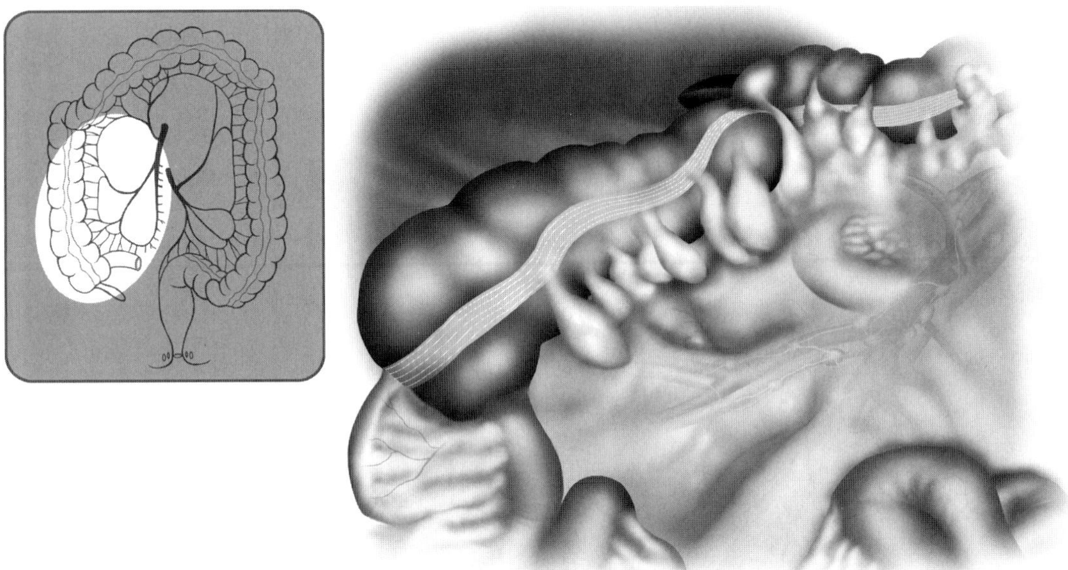

Figure 8.3.3. Good visualization of the right mesocolon is achieved by proper positioning of the patient and by placement of the omentum above the colon.

have been reported in laparoscopic colon surgery, as shown in Figure 8.3.5. The medial approach is quite effective for complete lymphadenectomy with early proximal ligation, minimal manipulation of the tumor-bearing segment, and ideal entry to proper retroperitoneal

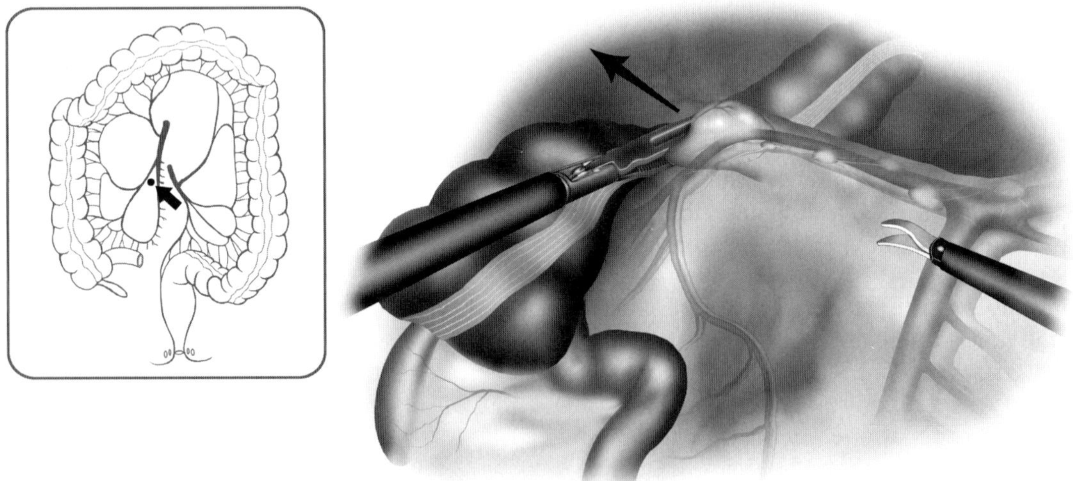

Figure 8.3.4. Definitive identification of the ileocolic pedicle is achieved by retraction at the ileocecal junction.

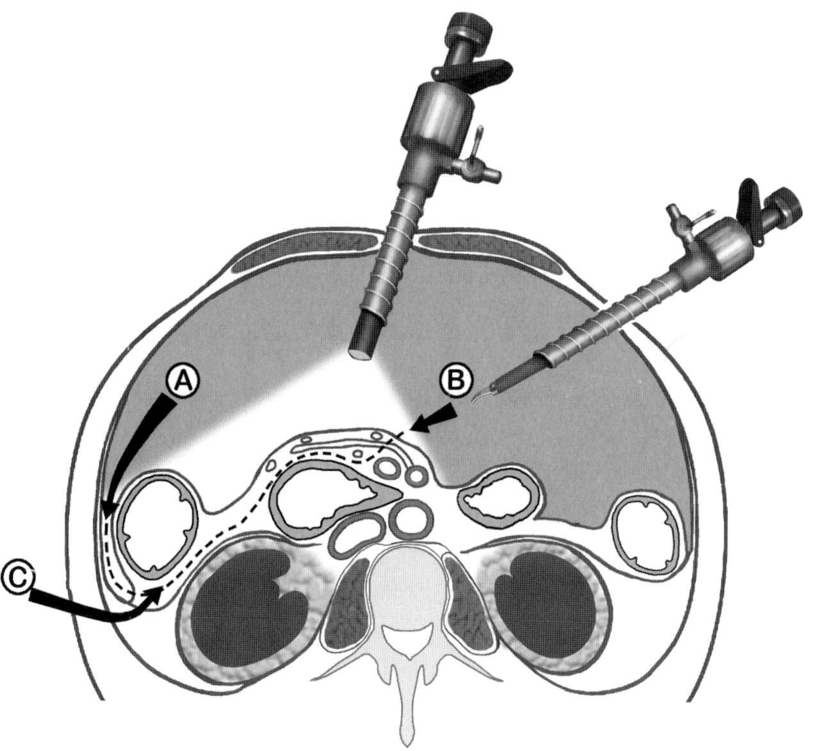

Figure 8.3.5. Various approaches to the right colon mobilization have been described. A: Lateral to medial ("classic" open approach); B: Medial to lateral (authors' preferred approach); C: Retroperitoneal approach.

plane.[4] We believe that the medial approach is optimal in order to maintain conventional oncologic principles.

First, the mesocolon near the ileocecal junction is lifted to confirm the ileocolic pedicle (Figure 8.3.4). The root of ileocolic pedicle is usually located at the lower border of duodenum. The independent right colic vessels, if present, are located at the upper border at duodenum. However, the majority of patients do not have the independent right colic vessels (vessels originating directly from the superior mesenteric artery and vein). The surgeon, first, should stand on the patient's left side to confidently know the ileocolic pedicle from the superior mesenteric vessels, and to mark the lower border of ileocolic pedicle (Figure 8.3.6).

Next, the surgeon moves between the patient's legs and the scope is inserted through the suprapubic port. The medial side of the right mesocolon is first incised starting from the previously marked region below the ileocolic pedicle, followed by the incision of the peritoneum over to the superior mesenteric vessels. This is done before mobilization of the right colon (Figure 8.3.7). With adequate traction of mesocolon toward the right upper quadrant, the ileocolic vessels are easily mobilized from the subperitoneal fascia leading onto the duodenum. Their origins are identified from the superior mesenteric vessels at the lower border of the duodenum and divided (Figure 8.3.8). We classify the

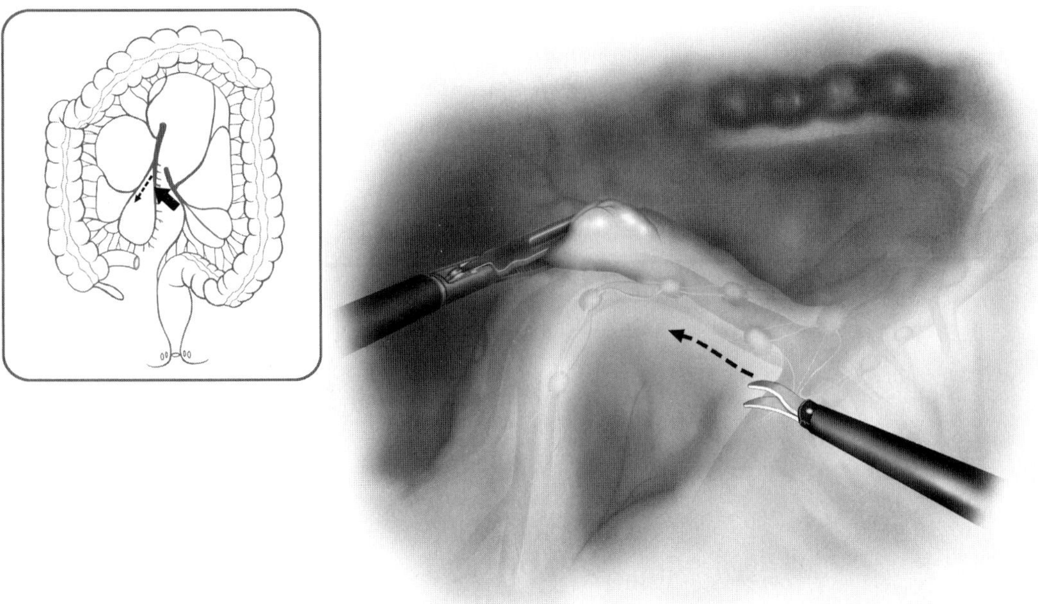

Figure 8.3.6. The surgeon's first step in the dissection is to mark the inferior border of the ileocolic pedicle.

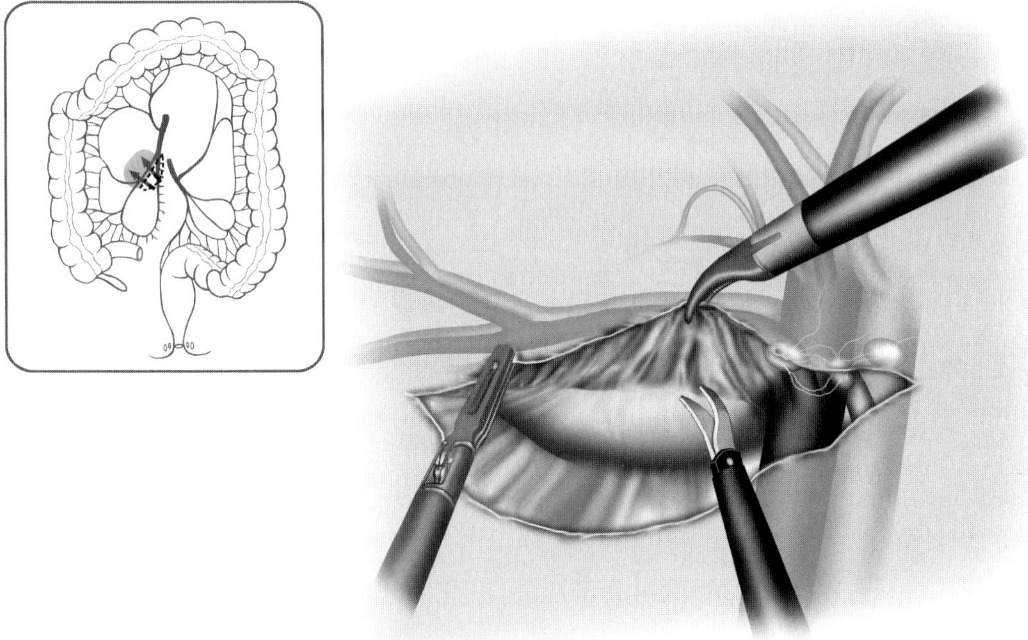

Figure 8.3.7. From between the legs, the surgeon dissects the peritoneum overlying the ileocolic vascular pedicle over to the superior mesenteric vessels.

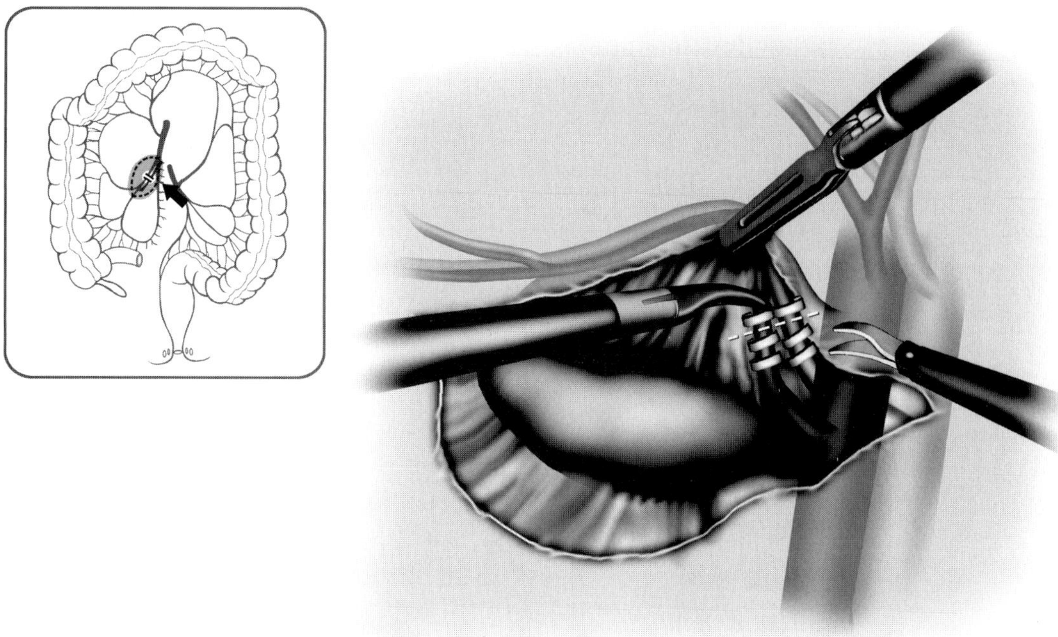

Figure 8.3.8. The origins of the ileocolic artery and vein are identified, clipped, and divided.

vascular anatomy of this area into two types (type A and type B: Figure 8.3.9A and B). Because a complete lymphadenectomy around the origin of ileocolic vessels is necessary for advanced right colon cancer, this classification is very useful to safely and effectively achieve it. In type A, the ileocolic artery is running in front of the superior mesenteric vein. After mobilization of the ileocolic pedicle from the duodenum, the dissection of the ventral side of the superior mesenteric vein leads to the dissection of the origin of ileocolic artery. In type B, the ileocolic artery is running behind the superior mesenteric vein. After mobilization and division of the ileocolic pedicle from the duodenum, the dissection of the ventral side of the superior mesenteric vein leads to a complete dissection of the root of the middle colic artery and vein (Figure 8.3.10).

Careful dissection onto the duodenum and the caudal portion of the pancreas must be exercised in the exposure of the middle colic vessels. Dissection around Henle's trunk (the truck of mesenteric veins consisting of the gastroepiploic vein fusing with the right branch of the middle colic vein or the main middle colic vein) may lead to the exposure of an accessory right colic vein. Accessory right colic vein and right branches of middle colic vessels are clipped and divided (Figure 8.3.11). However, if an accessory right colic vein is difficult to confirm in this situation, this vein may be easily detected later at the take-down of right flexure. Next, the operating table is tilted into the steep Trendelenburg position with the right side down to move the small intestine toward the right upper quadrant. After confirming the right ureter and gonadal vessels through the subperitoneal fascia at the right pelvic

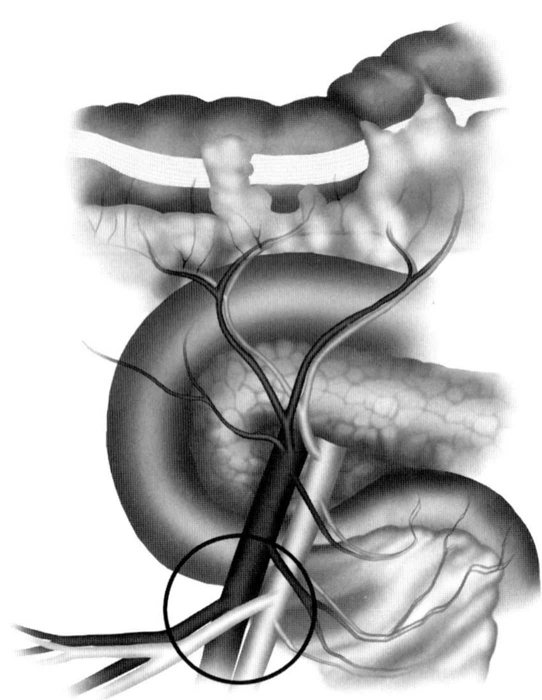

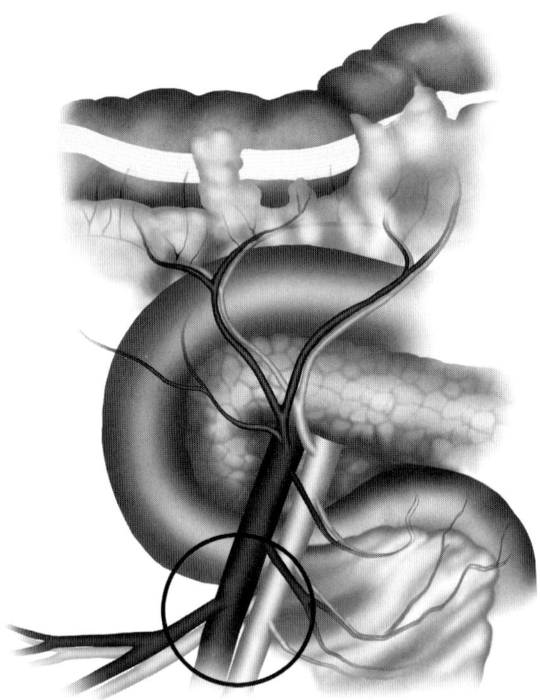

Figure 8.3.9. Anatomic variations of the origin of the ileocolic vessels. **A** The ileocolic artery runs in front of the superior mesenteric vein. **B** The ileocolic artery runs behind the superior mesenteric vein.

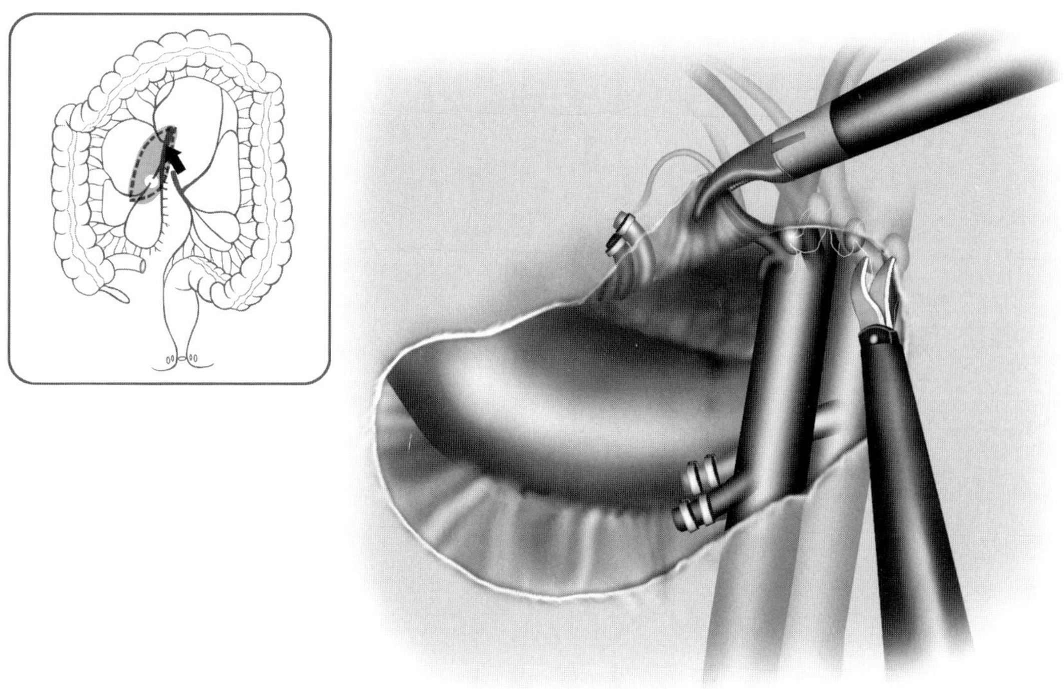

Figure 8.3.10. Dissection of the ventral side of the superior mesenteric vein permits a complete dissection of the root of the middle colic artery and vein.

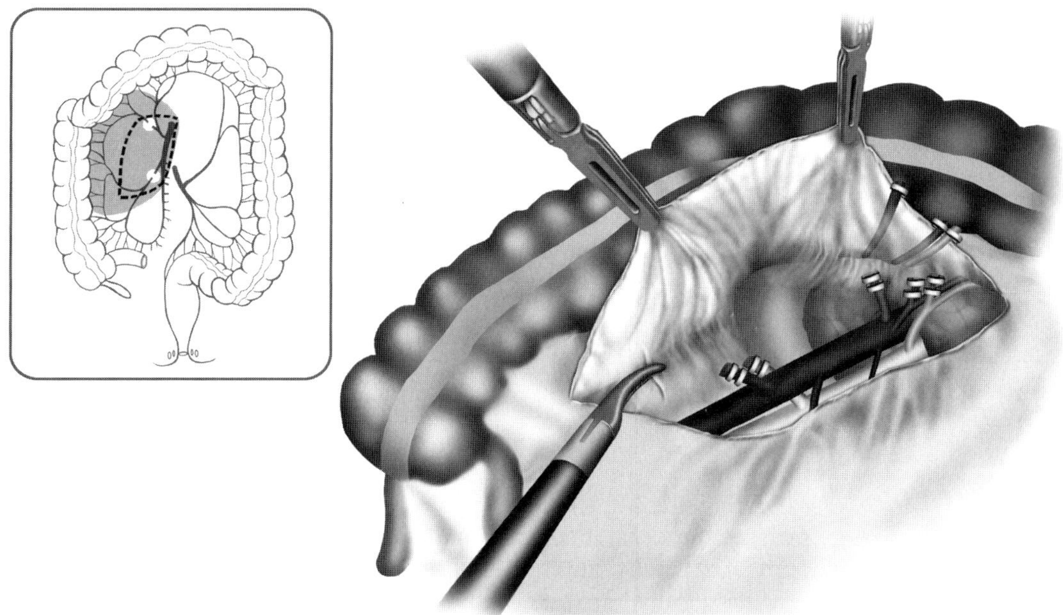

Figure 8.3.11. Accessory middle colic or right colic veins are clipped and divided. These are common.

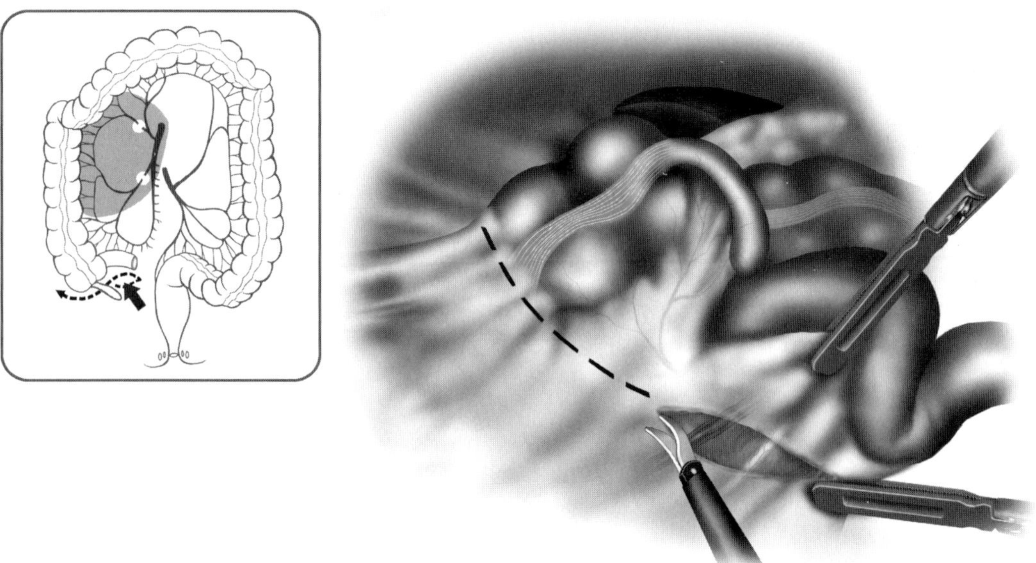

Figure 8.3.12. The peritoneum is incised along the base of the ileal mesentery upward to the duodenum.

brim, the peritoneum is incised along the base of the ileal mesentery upward to the duodenum, and the ileocecal region is mobilized medial to lateral (Figure 8.3.12).

Next, the surgeon moves back to the patient's left side and the scope is inserted through the umbilical port. The right mesocolon is mobilized from medial to lateral (Figure 8.3.13). Again, this approach allows dissection into the proper retroperitoneal plane. The right gonadal vessels and ureter are safe from injury in this plane, so exposing them is not necessary. This approach also allows the surgeon to work in a straight path from medial to lateral, without tissue to obstruct the vision that can occur working from lateral to medial. This plane connects the previous dissection plane from the caudal side.

The anatomy around the right flexure is very important to avoid inadvertent bleeding especially from around Henle's (gastrocolic) trunk (Figure 8.3.14). However, if the previous mesenteric dissection is fully performed from the caudal side and the accessory right colic vein is divided, the right flexure is easily taken down only by dividing the hepatocolic ligament (Figure 8.3.15). If the accessory right colic vein is difficult to detect at the previous dissection, it can be easily confirmed from Henle's trunk at this situation and should be divided before extracting the right colon to avoid its injury. Up to this point, the primary tumor has been minimally manipulated using medial to lateral approach. Finally, the right flexure and right colon including the tumor-bearing segment are detached laterally, which completes the mobilization of the entire right colon (Figure 8.3.16).

Once the entire right colon is freed, it is withdrawn through an enlargement of port site at the umbilicus. The wound must be covered with wound protector. The resection of ileum and transverse colon, and

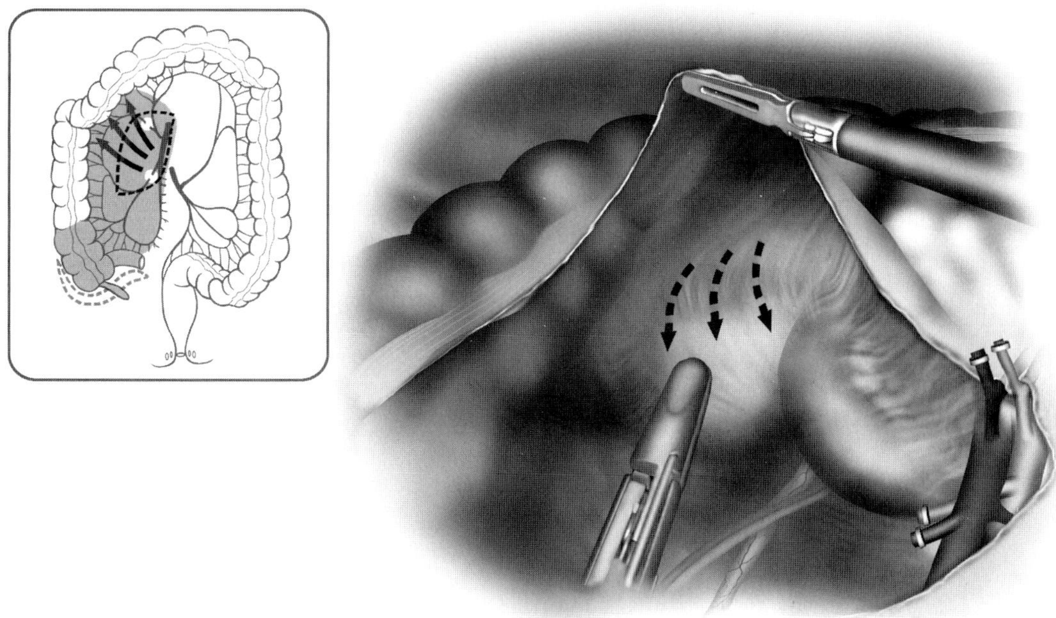

Figure 8.3.13. The right mesocolon is dissected away from the retroperitoneal structures from medial to lateral.

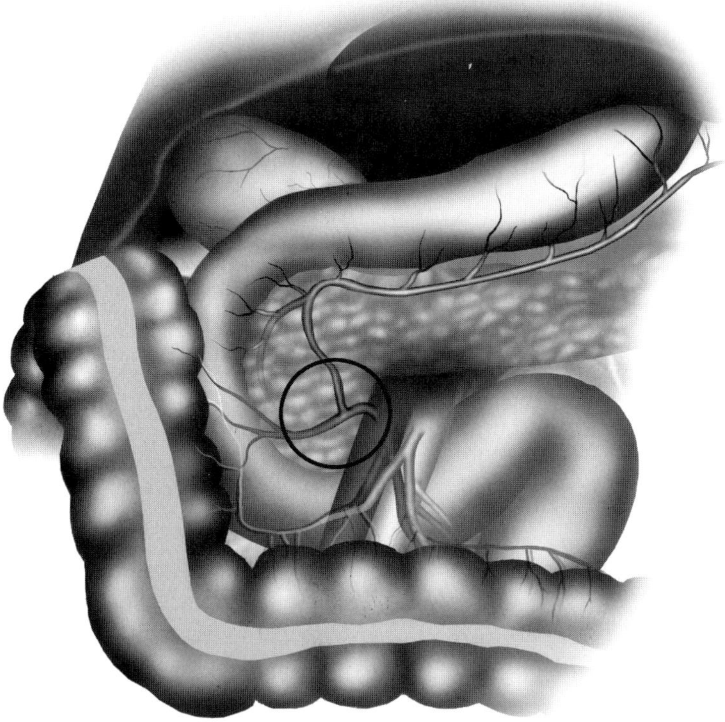

Figure 8.3.14. The venous anatomy between the hepatic flexure and the middle colic vessels has many variations, including Henle's trunk, the fusion between the gastroepiploic vein, and a branch of the right or middle colic vein.

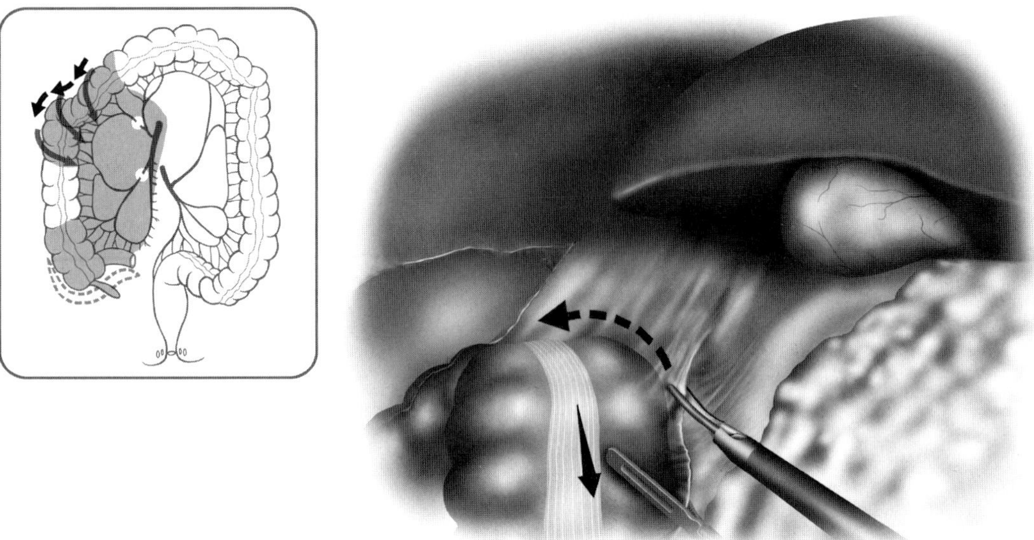

Figure 8.3.15. With earlier steps accomplished, the hepatocolic ligament is easily divided, freeing up the proximal transverse and hepatic flexure of the right colon.

the anastomosis are accomplished extracorporeally by functional end to end anastomotic method using conventional staplers or by a hand-sewn method (Figure 8.3.17). The anastomotic site is returned to the peritoneal cavity. Wounds and peritoneal cavity are copiously irrigated. All wounds are closed and operation is completed (Figure 8.3.18).

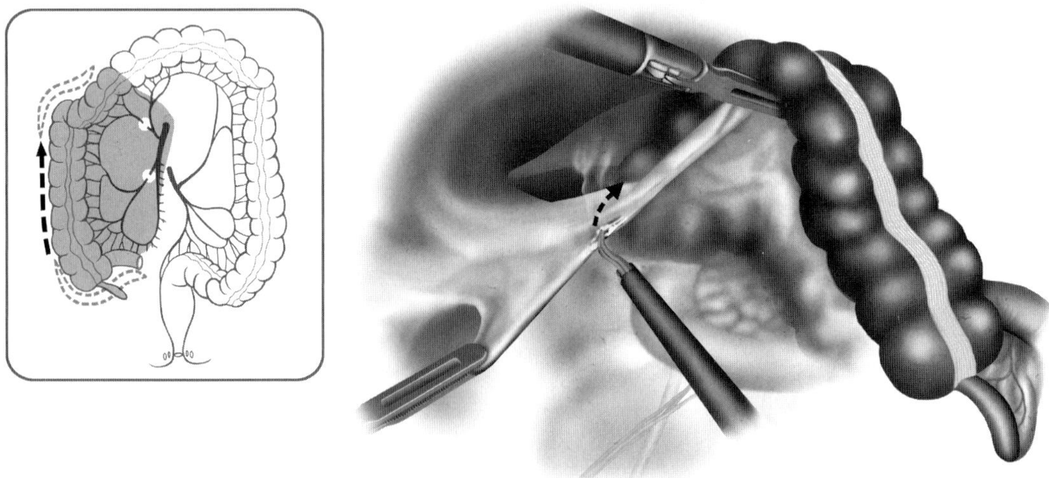

Figure 8.3.16. Finally, the tumor-bearing segment of the right colon, with its lateral attachments, are freed up, completing the right colon mobilization.

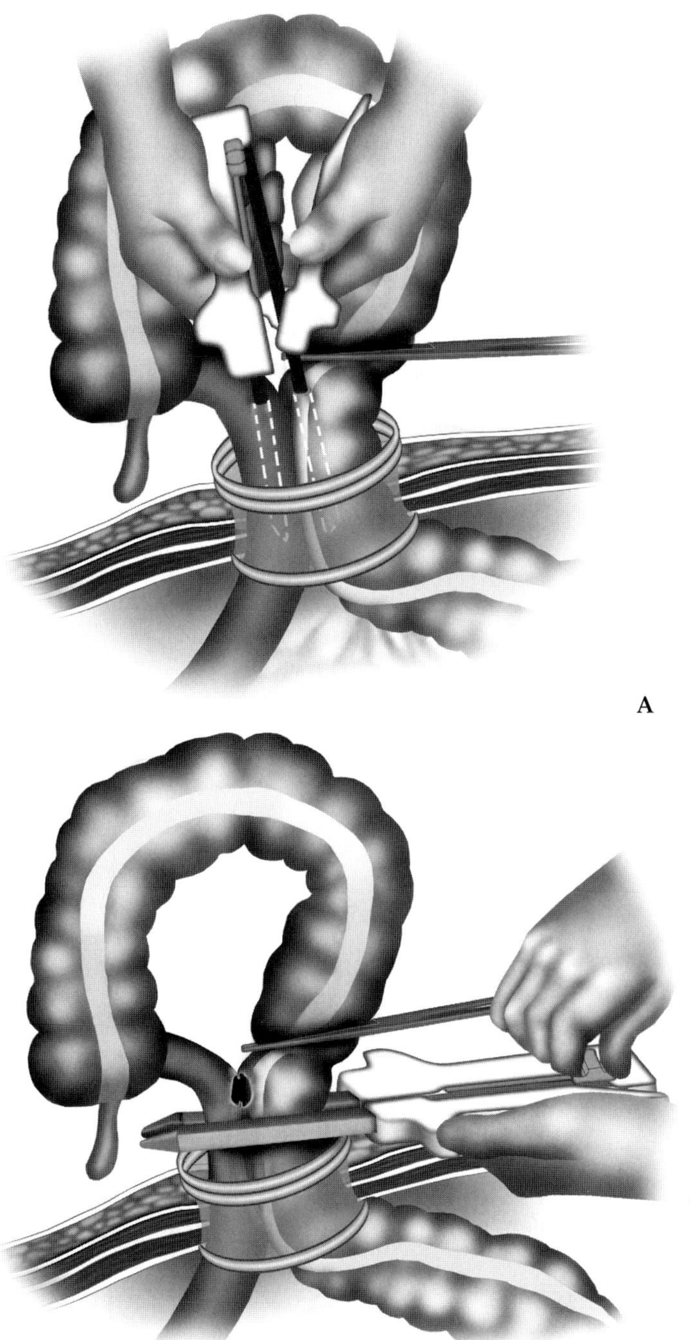

Figure 8.3.17. After drawing out the right colon using a wound protector, an anastomosis is accomplished extracorporeally. **A** A functional end-to-end anastomosis is created with a linear-cutter stapler. Note that the colon is occluded using a large Kocher clamp. **B** The anastomosis is completed with a right-angled firing of the linear-cutter stapler, completely sealing off the bowel. **C** The completed anastomosis before returning it to the abdomen.

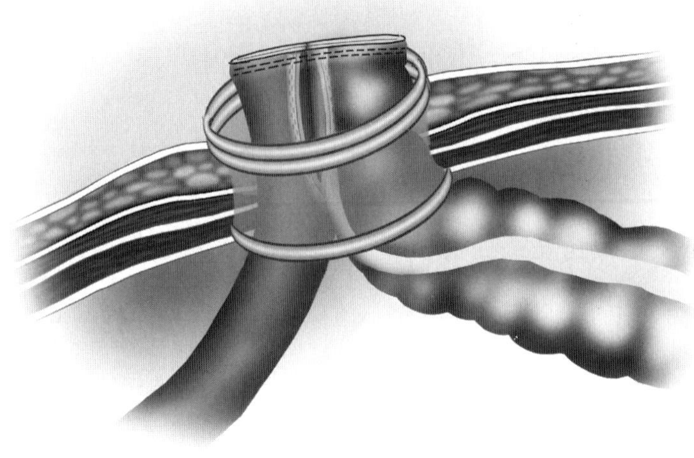

Figure 8.3.17. *Continued*

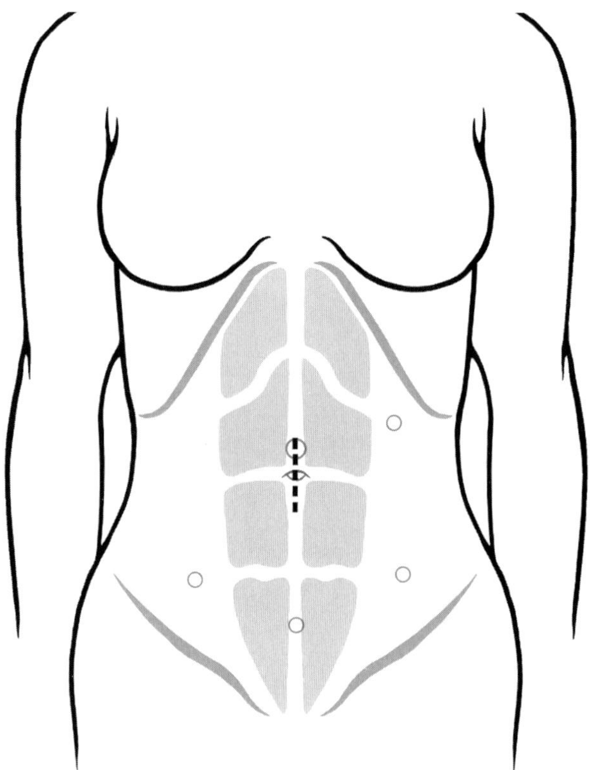

Figure 8.3.18. Appearance of the abdomen after the completion of the operation, showing the incision used to extract the specimen and perform the anastomosis (dotted line).

Special Considerations

The identification of a small tumor in the colon may be difficult even in conventional open surgery. In laparoscopic surgery, where there is no tactile sensation, pre- or intraoperative marking of the tumor is frequently needed. Various kinds of marking methods, e.g., dye injection and mucosal clip placement by preoperative colonoscopy, have been reported for the tumor localization.[5] Several reports demonstrated the usefulness of tattooing the colonic wall adjacent to the tumor with India ink in four quadrants using preoperative colonoscopy.[6,7] However, effective injection in all four points of the bowel is sometimes difficult to achieve. In some cases, we failed to achieve serosal staining visible at laparoscopy, which forced us to use intraoperative colonoscopy. This complicated the laparoscopic colon resection because of the distended bowel related to air insufflation during colonoscopy.

Preoperatively, we prefer to inject India ink into the anterior wall (antimesenteric side) of the bowel as follows: 1) A patient is placed in the supine position. 2) The tumor is irrigated with proper amount of water through the colonoscopic instrumental channel. 3) Because the water is collected in the posterior side of the bowel, the anterior wall is easily confirmed and India ink is injected precisely, which leads to optimal visualization of the lesion during laparoscopy.

In laparoscopic surgery, hemostasis is sometimes much more difficult and much more time-consuming than in open surgery. Therefore, very careful attention should be given, especially during the dissection of major vessels. In addition to skillful dissection and understanding of vascular anatomy, integrated three-dimensional computed tomography imaging is very helpful to simulate and navigate the individual patient's vascular anatomy, and to expeditiously accomplish laparoscopic dissection without blood loss.[8,9] Also, bipolar scissors and forceps are very safe and effective tools compared with monopolar electrocautery, so we prefer this to minimize the risk of inadvertent injury of vessels and/or bowels. As previously mentioned, a particular concern for bleeding in extracting right colon from the small incision is the injury of accessory right colic vein. Therefore, it should be divided before extracting right colon to avoid its injury at Henle's trunk.

Conclusions

Right-sided colon cancer can be adequately treated by proper laparoscopic procedures adherent to the oncologic principles. Port-site metastasis after laparoscopic colon cancer surgery is unlikely to be a major risk factor when the procedure is performed according to oncologic principles. We believe laparoscopic right colectomy for cancer performed by expert surgeons is accepted as less invasive surgery without sacrificing the survival benefit compared with conventional open right colectomy.

Editors' Comments

They have very well described a laparoscopic-assisted approach for the oncologic right colon resection, which is very similar to our method.

Indications: We agree with the authors regarding their indications.
Patient positioning: If available, a full-length gel pad on the operating table instead of a bean bag is more comfortable and the gel pad firmly anchors even the heaviest of patients without the risk of the above.
Instruments: We do not use the bipolar scissors, but instead substitute the bipolar LigaSure™ device (LigaSure Atlas™ or LigaSure V™).
Cannula positioning: We generally agree with their positioning.
Technique: We use a similar technique to what is described here and believe this description is excellent. We certainly believe that the laparoscopic oncologic approach described herein will accomplish an excellent cancer operation.

When intraoperative colonoscopy is indicated for precise localization of pathologies at surgery, we prefer CO_2-insufflating colonoscopy over standard colonoscopy. CO_2 is absorbed from colonic lining more rapidly than air, thus can attenuate persistent bowel distention.[10] The CO_2 feeder for colonoscopy is now commercially available (ECR, Olympus, Tokyo, Japan).

References

1. Jacobs M, Verdeja JC, Goldstein HS. Minimally invasive colon resection (laparoscopic colectomy). Surg Laparosc Endosc 1991;1:144–150.
2. Milsom JW, Böhm B. Laparoscopic Colorectal Surgery. New York: Springer Verlag; 1996.
3. Darzi A, Hunt N, Stacey R. Retroperitoneoscopy and retroperitoneal colonic mobilization: a new approach in laparoscopic colonic surgery. Br J Surg 1995;82:1038–1039.
4. Okuda J, Tanigawa N. Colon carcinomas may be adequately treated using laparoscopic method. Sem Colon Rectal Surg 1998;9:241–246.
5. Kim SH, Milsom JW, Church JM, et al. Perioperative tumor localization for laparoscopic colorectal surgery. Surg Endosc 1997;11:1013–1016.
6. Hyman N, Waye JD. Endoscopic four quadrant tattoo for the identification of colonic lesions at surgery. Gastrointest Endosc 1991;37:56–58.
7. Botoman VA, Pietro M, Thirlby RC. Localization of colonic lesions with endoscopic tattoo. Dis Colon Rectum 1994;37:775–776.
8. Okuda J, Matsuki M, Yoshikawa S. Minimally invasive tailor-made surgery for advanced colorectal cancer with navigation by integrated 3D-CT imaging. Med View 2002;86:6–13.
9. Lee SW, Shinohara H, Matsuki M, et al. Preoperative simulation of vascular anatomy by three-dimensional computed tomography imaging in laparoscopic gastric cancer surgery. J Am Coll Surg 2003;197:927–936.
10. Nakajima K, Lee SW, Sonoda T, Milsom JW. Intraoperative carbon dioxide colonoscopy: a safe insufflation alternative for locating colonic lesions during laparoscopic surgery. Surg Endosc 2005;19(3):321–325.

Chapter 8.4

Sigmoidectomy

Joel Leroy, Margaret Henri, Francesco Rubino, and Jacques Marescaux

Indications

Laparoscopic sigmoid colon resection is indicated for both benign (diverticulitis, segmental Crohn's disease, polyp unresectable by colonoscopy) and malignant (primary colon cancer) etiologies, and is one of the most common operations done by laparoscopic methods.

In chronic diverticular disease, the indications for laparoscopic sigmoid resection are the same as for open surgery. The American Society of Colon and Rectal Surgeons (ACRS)[1] and the European Association of Endoscopic Surgeons (EAES)[2] consensus statements agree that laparoscopy is an acceptable alternative to open surgery for diverticulitis, as long as the indications remain the same: Two or more attacks of uncomplicated diverticulitis, diverticular stricture, or one attack of diverticulitis in an immunocompromised patient. In acute complicated diverticulitis, laparoscopic resection may be justified in Hinchey I and II disease, if no gross abnormalities are found during diagnostic laparoscopy in the face of a large abscess not amenable to percutaneous drainage. There is no current place for laparoscopic resection in Hinchey III and IV disease. These stages of complicated acute diverticulitis should be treated with resection and colostomy (Hartmann's procedure). Although some researchers reported interesting results with simple laparoscopic lavage and drainage followed by second-stage resection and anastomosis in order to avoid the need for a stoma in patients with Hinchey III disease, these are a series of small numbers of patients; therefore, this treatment should only be performed in the setting of a clinical trial. Septic shock is an absolute contraindication to laparoscopy.

The use of laparoscopy for cancer has been very controversial for fear of port site metastases and inadequate oncologic resections. However, recent studies have shown that the rate of port site metastases is about 1%, and that laparoscopy for cancer is safe as long as oncologic rules are respected.[3] However, the presence of a large palpable malignancy suggesting a locally advanced tumor, or the suspicion of perforation represent absolute contraindications to the laparoscopic approach and should be managed by conventional open surgery.

Patient Positioning and Operating Room Setup

Patients should have a standard bowel preparation (orthograde bowel lavage) 48 hours before the operation and should receive a single-dose antibiotic dose immediately preoperatively.

For the bowel preparation, patients follow a strictly fiber-free diet 8 days before surgery, and take a sodium phosphate oral solution the day before surgery. This method is very effective because it ensures an empty digestive tract and a flat small bowel, which facilitates the layering of intestinal loops, a crucial point for achieving adequate exposure. Alternatively, polyethylene glycol can be used. In this case, administration 2 days before surgery is preferable to avoid distension of small bowel loops that may be difficult to handle during the operation.

A proper patient position is key to both facilitating operative maneuvers and preventing complications such as nerve and vein compression, and traction injuries to the brachial plexus. The patient is placed supine, in the modified lithotomy position, with legs abducted and slightly flexed at the knees. The patient's right arm is alongside the body, whereas the left arm is usually placed at a 90° angle. Adequate padding is used to avoid compression on bone prominences. A nasogastric or orogastric tube and a urinary catheter are placed.

We routinely use a heating device to prevent patient hypothermia. Adequate thromboembolism prophylaxis should be used, as preferred by the surgeon, and intermittent leg compression stockings can be used as well. The procedure is usually performed with two assistants and a scrub nurse. The surgeon is on the right side of the patient and the second assistant is also on the right side. The first assistant stands between the patient's legs and the scrub nurse at the lower right side of the table (Figure 8.4.1). The team remains in the same position throughout the entire procedure. It is advisable to use a table that can be easily tilted laterally and placed into steep Trendelenburg and reverse Trendelenburg position, in order to facilitate exposure of the pelvic space and of the splenic flexure. The laparoscopic unit with the main monitor is located on the left side of the table. It is useful to use a second monitor placed above the patient's head.

Instruments

Specific instruments recommended for laparoscopic sigmoidectomy are listed in Table 8.4.1.

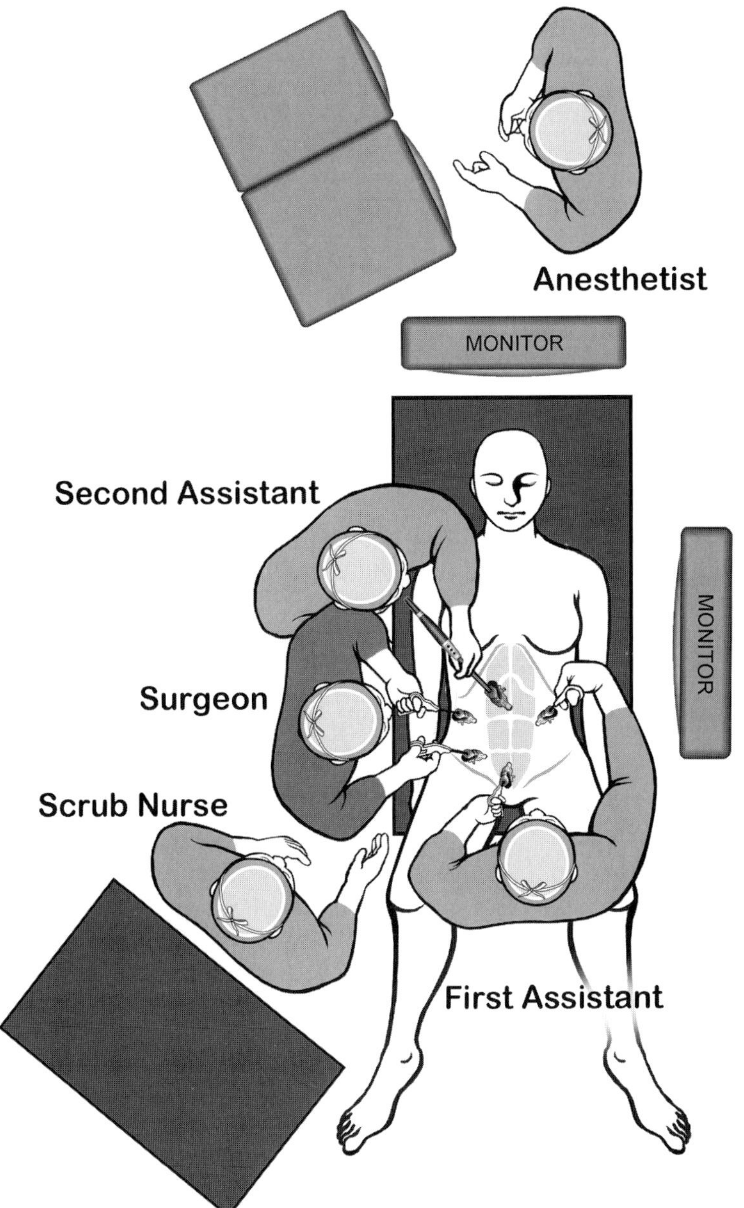

Figure 8.4.1. Positions of the equipment and the surgical team for the laparoscopic sigmoid colectomy.

Table 8.4.1. Specific instruments recommended for laparoscopic sigmoidectomy

3–5	Cannulae (2 × 12 mm, 2–4 × 5 mm)
1	Dissecting device (i.e., LigaSure V™ or Ultrasonic Shears™ or electrosurgery)
1	Laparoscopic scissors
1	Laparoscopic dissector
2	Laparoscopic graspers
1	Endoscopic stapler

Cannula Positioning

The number of cannulae, unlike their size and the length of the wound incision, has very little impact, if any, on postoperative outcomes. Although as few as three cannulae can be sufficient in uncomplicated cases, as preferred by some surgeons, we choose to standardize cannula placement and routinely use five or six cannulae for left-sided colectomies (Figure 8.4.2). This allows us to achieve an excellent exposure which may be particularly valuable at the beginning of a surgeon's learning curve. Using six cannulae allows the use of more instruments in the abdominal cavity for retraction of bowel and structures especially in the presence of abundant intraabdominal fat or of dilated small bowel, as well as during mobilization of the splenic flexure. We also believe that we are able to teach better using this approach.

Cannula fixation to the abdominal wall is important, to avoid CO_2 leakage, and in cases of malignancy, to minimize the passage of tumor cells and help reduce the incidence of port-site metastases.[4] This is mainly achieved by fitting the size of the incision to the cannula size or by fixing the cannula to the abdomen with a suture placed around the stopcock of the cannula. We no longer use screw-like cannulae, because they increase parietal trauma.

We usually perform an "open" technique for the insertion of the first cannula, which is placed at the midline, above the umbilicus, to reduce

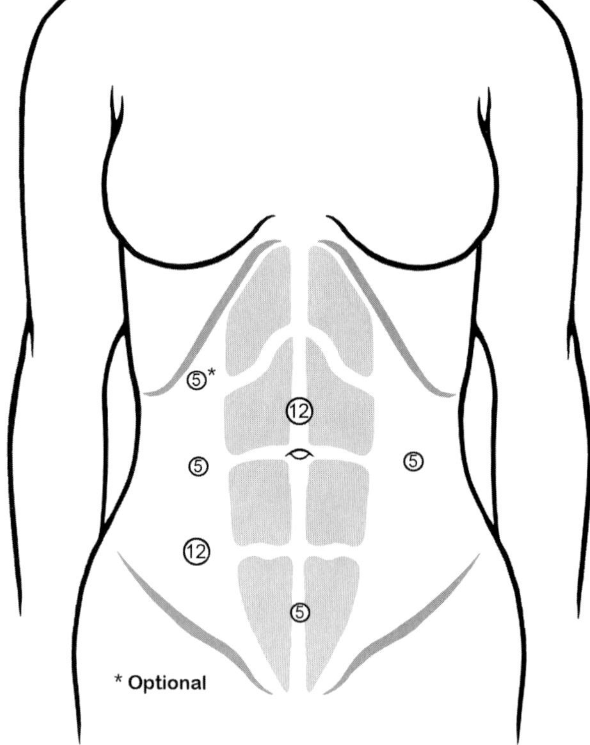

Figure 8.4.2. Positions of the cannulae for laparoscopic sigmoid colectomy.

the risk of injury of abdominal organs. With some experience, the task becomes easy and very rapid. However, in the case of previous abdominal surgery, we usually inflate the abdominal cavity using the Veress needle in the left subcostal area, in order to insert the first cannula as far lateral as possible, in the right hypochondrium, to avoid potential areas of adhesions.

As said above, the first cannula (12 mm), which is used for the optical device, is positioned on the midline 3–4 cm above the umbilicus. The two operating cannulae are introduced, one at the junction between the umbilical line and the right midclavicular line, and the other 8–10 cm inferiorly, on the same line. The latter is a 12-mm operating cannula to allow the introduction of a linear stapler at the time of bowel resection. This cannula accommodates the following: scissors (monopolar, high-frequency hemostasis device, clip, staplers), a monopolar hook, surgical loops, a suction-irrigation device, and an atraumatic grasper.

A fourth cannula is placed on the left midclavicular line, at the level of the umbilicus. This is a 5-mm cannula, which accommodates an atraumatic grasper used for retraction and exposure during the medial approach for the dissection of the left mesocolon. When performing mobilization of the splenic flexure, this cannula becomes an operating cannula. A fifth 5-mm cannula is placed 8–10 cm above the pubic bone, on the midline, and is used for retraction. For most of the procedure, it accommodates a grasper used to expose the sigmoid and descending mesocolon. At the end of the procedure, the incision at this cannula's site is lengthened to allow extraction of the specimen.

We sometimes use an additional cannula, which is a 5-mm cannula situated on the right midclavicular line in the subcostal area and accommodates an atraumatic grasper used to retract the terminal portion of the small intestine laterally at the beginning of the dissection, and to retract the transverse colon during the mobilization of the splenic flexure.

Technique

Exposure

To complete exposure of the operative field, active positioning of the bowel is usually necessary in addition to the passive action of gravity, especially in the presence of obesity or bowel dilatation (Figure 8.4.3). The greater omentum and the transverse colon are placed in the left subphrenic region and maintained in this position by the Trendelenburg tilt. An atraumatic retractor, introduced through the cannula on the left side, may also be used. Subsequently, the proximal small bowel loops are placed in the right upper quadrant using gentle grasping (Figure 8.4.3, inset). The distal small bowel loops are placed in the right lower quadrant with the cecum, and maintained there with gravity. If gravity is not sufficient, as occurs especially in the presence of abundant intraabdominal fat or dilated bowel, an additional maneuver is used. An instrument passed through the right subcostal cannula is passed at the root of the mesentery and grasps the parietal perito-

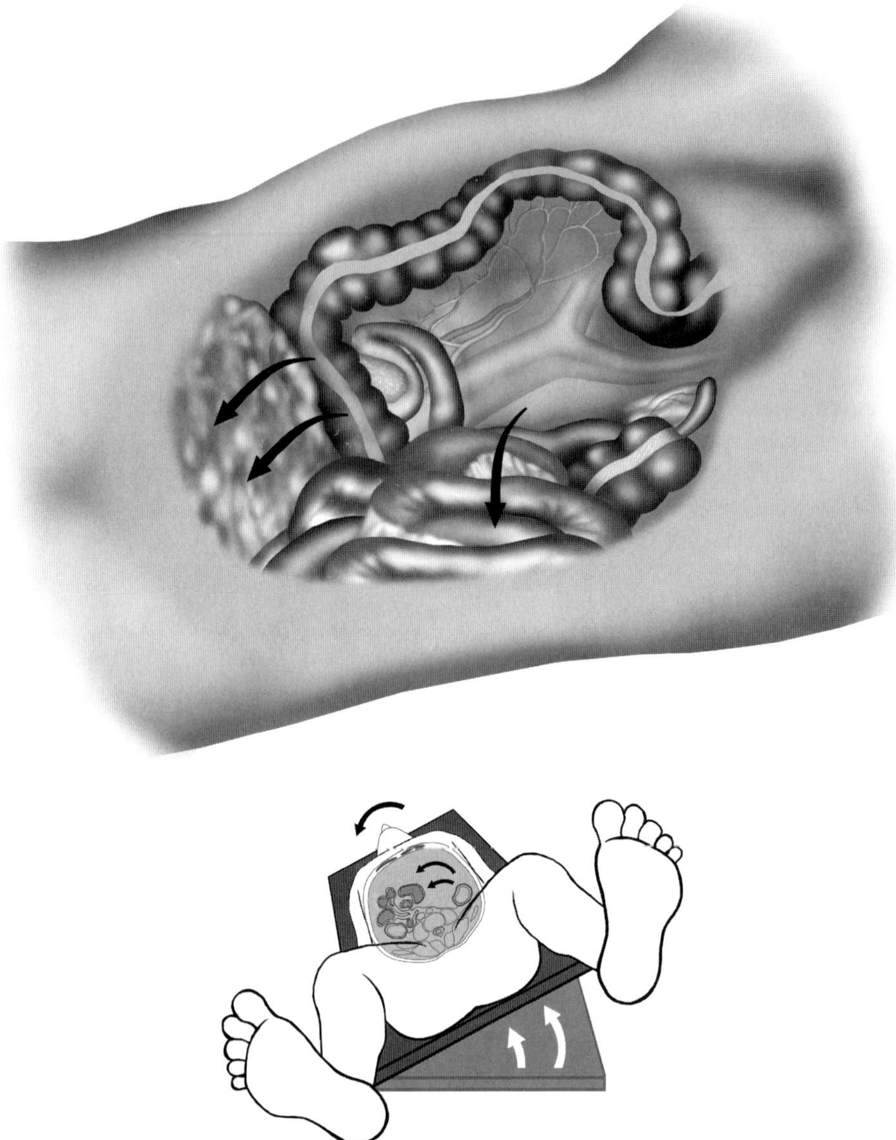

Figure 8.4.3. Active positioning using gravity produces optimum exposure. The greater omentum and the transverse colon are placed in the left subphrenic region and maintained in this position by the Trendelenburg tilt (inset). Subsequently, the proximal small bowel loops are placed in the right upper quadrant.

neum of the right iliac fossa; the shaft of the grasper thus provides an auto static retraction of the bowel loops, keeping them away from the midline and from the pelvic space. This technique of exposure provides an excellent view of the sacral promontory and of the aortoiliac axis. This particular view on the operative field is essential for the medial to lateral vascular approach that we perform routinely and will describe in the following paragraphs.

The uterus may be an obstacle to adequate exposure in the pelvis. In postmenopausal women, the uterus can be suspended to the abdominal wall by a suture (Figure 8.4.4). This suture is introduced halfway between the umbilicus and the pubis, and opens the rectovaginal space. In younger women, the uterus can be retracted using a similar suspension by a suture around the round ligaments or using a 5-mm retractor passed through the suprapubic cannula.

Very often, conversion to open surgery is caused by difficulty in exposure, not only at the beginning, but also throughout the procedure. Because we choose to perform a medial approach, time is dedicated to the perfect achievement of this exposure, which will serve not only for the initial vascular approach, but also for about half of the remaining operative time. After adequate exposure has been achieved, the following steps of the technique include the vascular approach, the medial posterior mobilization of the sigmoid, the extraction of the specimen, and the anastomosis. Additional steps include the mobilization of the splenic flexure, performed when further lengthening of the bowel is needed to perform a tension-free anastomosis.

The step of the exposure is preliminary, and it is done in a similar manner, regardless of the type of disease. The remainder of the procedure is different if the indication for surgery is a cancer or a benign disease. We will describe the two variants of the technique separately.

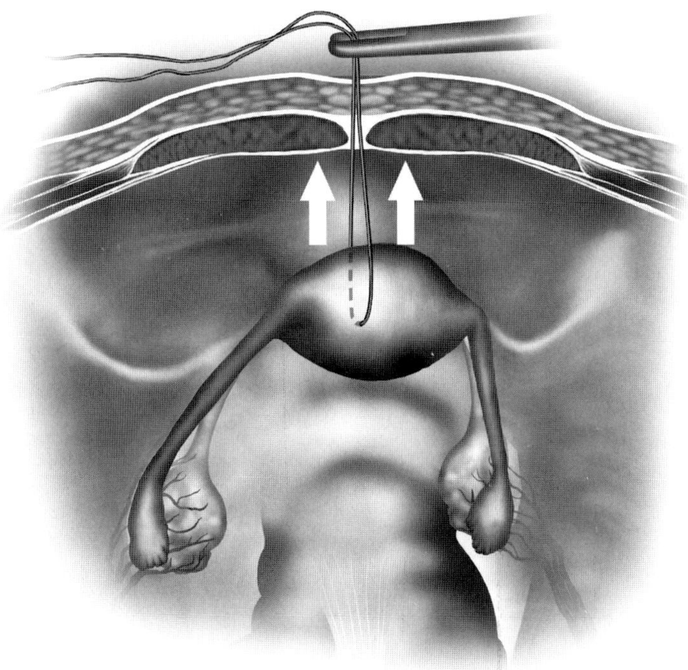

Figure 8.4.4. The uterus can be suspended to the abdominal wall using a suture placed through its fundus.

Sigmoid Colon Resection for Cancer

In laparoscopic colorectal sigmoidectomy for cancer or for benign disease, the vascular approach is the first step of the dissection. We believe that it allows us to avoid unnecessary manipulation of the colon and tumor (which may cause tumor cell exfoliation), and to perform a good lymphadenectomy following the vascular anatomy. The vessels are gradually exposed once the peritoneum at the base of the sigmoid mesocolon is incised. The medial to lateral view allows us to see the sympathetic nerve plexus trunks, the left ureter, and gonadal vessels, avoiding ureteral injuries and possibly preserving genital function.

Primary Vascular Approach (Medial Approach)

Peritoneal Incision
The sigmoid mesocolon is retracted anteriorly, using a grasper introduced through the suprapubic cannula: This exposes the base of the sigmoid mesocolon. The visceral peritoneum is incised at the level of the sacral promontory. The incision is continued upward along the right anterior border of the aorta up to the ligament of Treitz (Figure 8.4.5). The pressure of the pneumoperitoneum facilitates the dissection, as the diffusion of CO_2 opens the avascular planes.

Identification of the Inferior Mesenteric Artery
The dissection of the cellular adipose tissue is continued upward by gradually dividing the sigmoid branches of the right sympathetic trunk

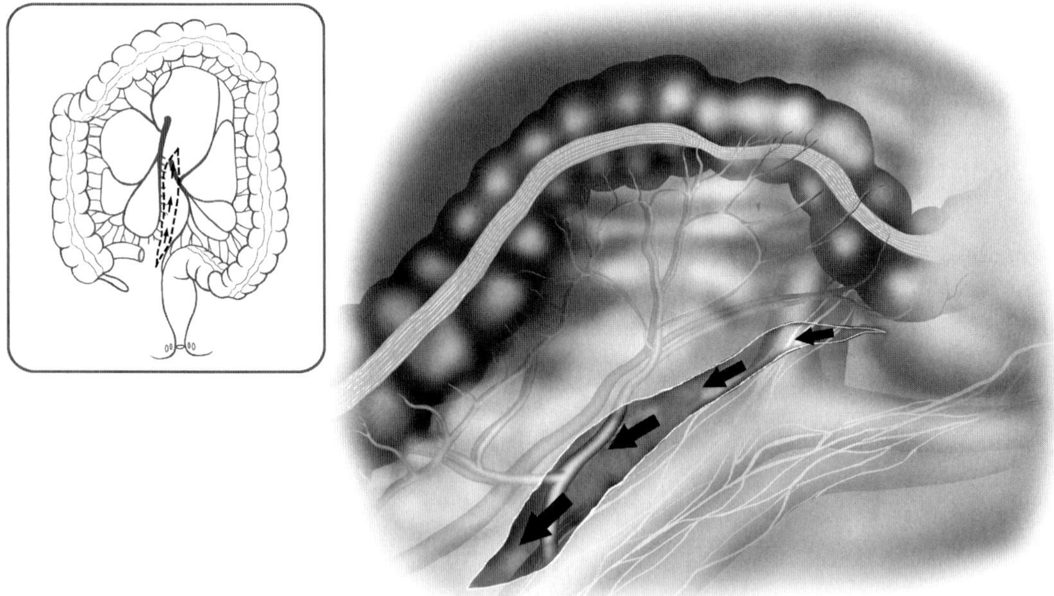

Figure 8.4.5. Initial dissection starts with an incision of the sigmoid mesentery at the sacral promontory with dissection cephalad posterior to the IMA.

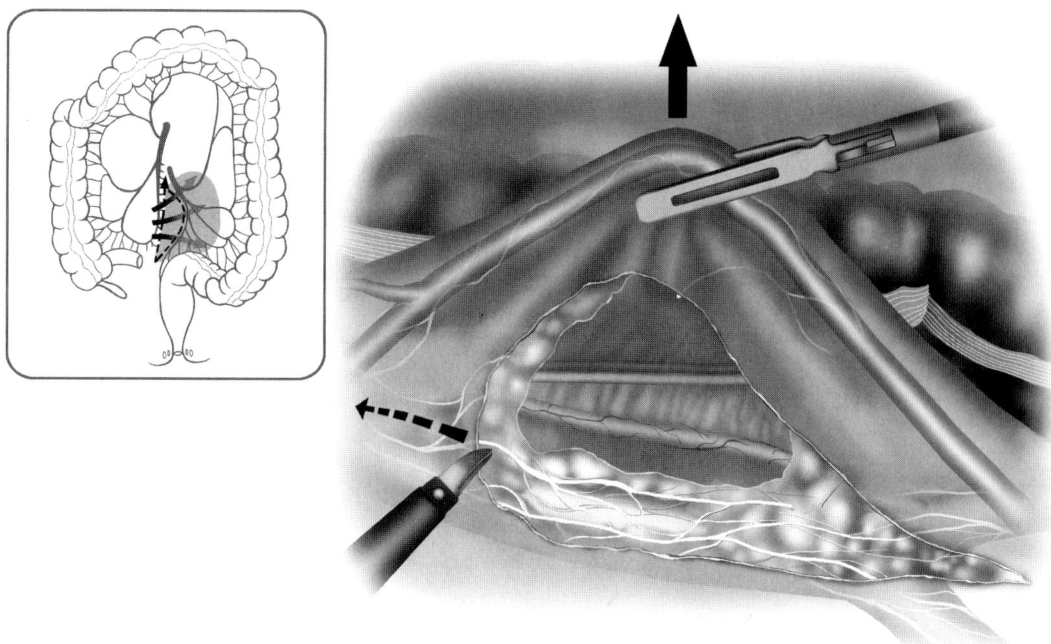

Figure 8.4.6. The dissection behind the IMA involves preservation of the main hypogastric nerve trunks, but also division of the small branches traveling to the colon.

to expose the origin of the inferior mesenteric artery (IMA) (Figures 8.4.6 and 8.4.7). To ensure an adequate lymphadenectomy, the first 2 cm of the IMA are dissected free and the artery is skeletonized before it is divided. This dissection at the origin of the IMA involves a risk of injury to the left sympathetic trunk situated on the left border of the IMA. A meticulous dissection of the artery (skeletonization) helps to avoid this risk, because only the vessel will be divided, and not the surrounding tissues. Dissection performed close to the artery also minimizes the risk of ureteral injury during the ligation of the IMA. The IMA can then be divided between clips, or by using a linear stapler (vascular 2.5- or 2.0-mm cartridges) or the LigaSure Atlas™ (Figure 8.4.8). The artery is divided at 1–2 cm distal to its origin from the aorta or after the take off of the left colic artery.

Identification of the Inferior Mesenteric Vein

The inferior mesenteric vein (IMV) is identified to the left of the IMA or in case of difficulty, higher, just to the left of the ligament of Treitz junction. The vein is divided below the inferior border of the pancreas or above the left colic vein (Figure 8.4.9). Once again, clips, or the LigaSure Atlas™ are both sure options to ligate and divide this vessel.

Mobilization of the Sigmoid and Descending Colon

The mobilization of the sigmoid colon follows the division of the vessels. This step includes the freeing of posterior and lateral attachments

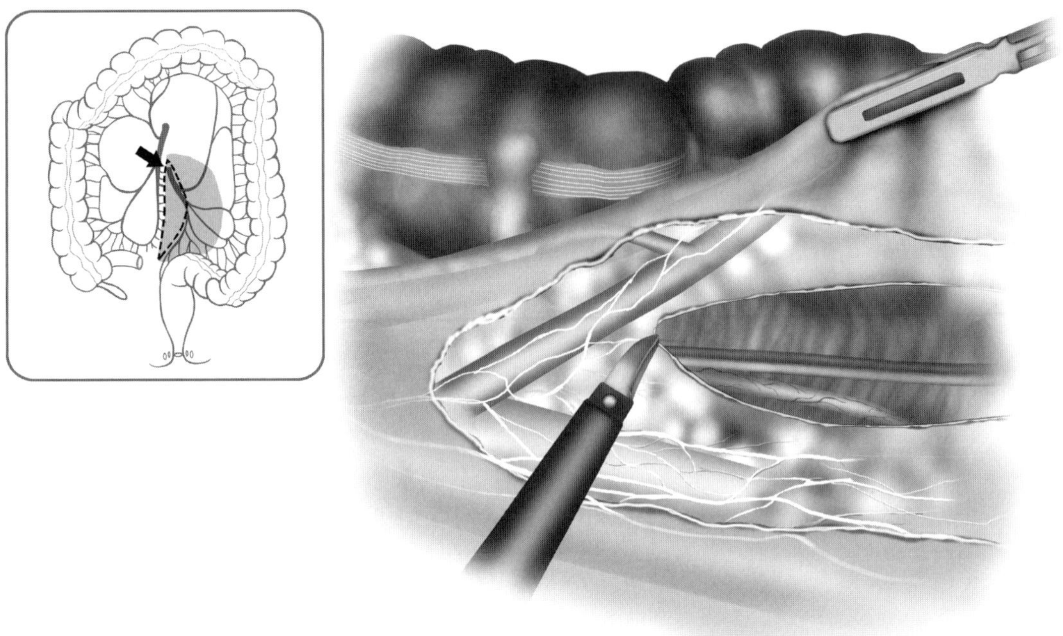

Figure 8.4.7. Radical lymphadenectomy involves exposure of the main trunk of the IMA and skeletonization, but preservation of the hypogastric nerve trunks.

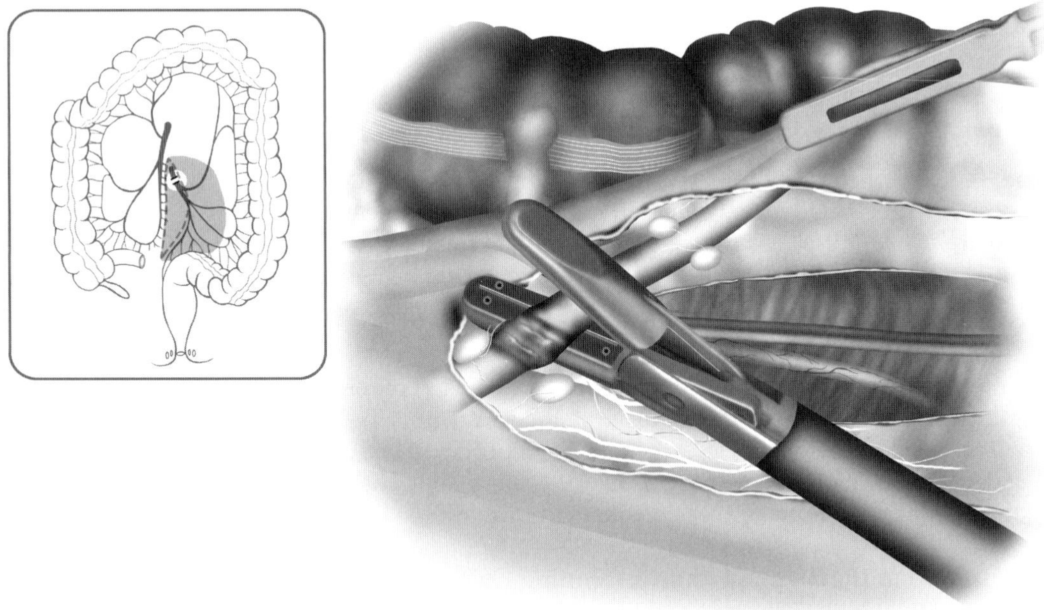

Figure 8.4.8. The IMA is divided 1–2 cm distal to its origin, or just distal to the left colic branch.

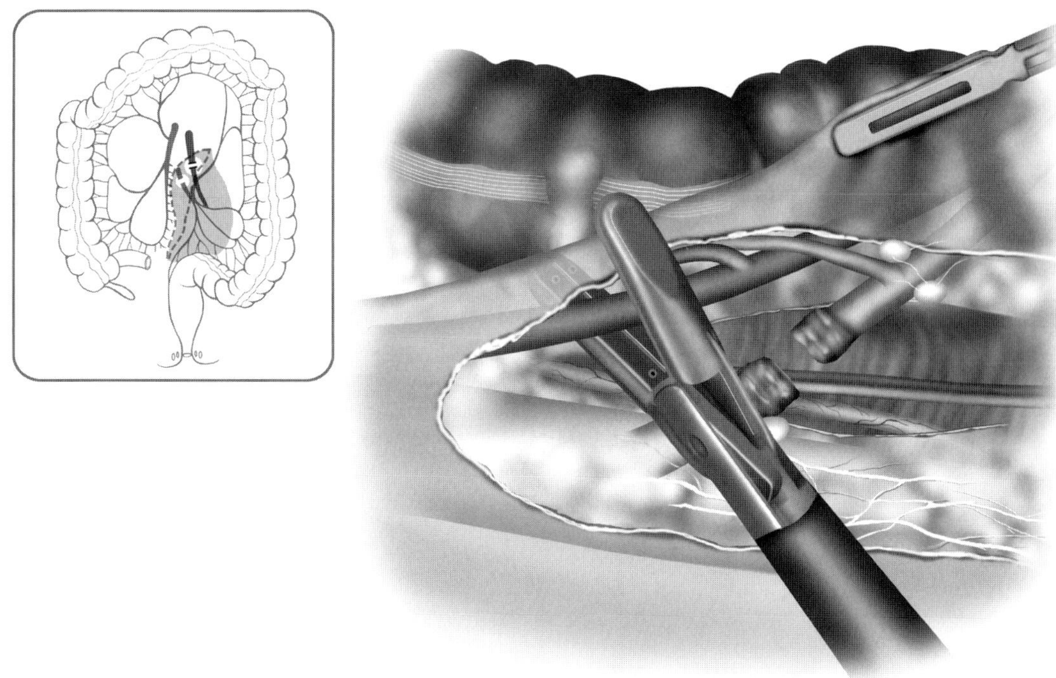

Figure 8.4.9. The IMV is divided in a safe area between the pancreas and the left colic vessels.

of the sigmoid colon and mesocolon and the division of the rectal and sigmoid mesenteries. The approach is either medial or lateral.

We routinely perform this medial-to-lateral laparoscopic dissection for all indications. The medial approach is well adapted for laparoscopy because it preserves the working space and demands the least handling of the sigmoid colon. In a randomized trial comparing the medial-to-lateral laparoscopic dissection with the classical lateral-to-medial approach for resection of rectosigmoid cancer, Liang et al.[5] showed that the medial approach reduces operative time and the post-operative proinflammatory response. Besides the potential oncologic advantages of early vessel division and "no-touch" dissection, we believe that the longer the lateral abdominal wall attachments of the colon are preserved, the easier are the exposure and dissection.

Posterior Detachment

The sigmoid mesocolon is retracted anteriorly (using the suprapubic cannula) to expose the posterior space. The plane between Toldt's fascia and the sigmoid mesocolon can then be identified. This plane is avascular and easily divided (Figure 8.4.10, including inset). The dissection continues posterior to the sigmoid mesocolon going laterally toward Toldt's line. The sigmoid colon is then completely free, and the lateral attachments can then be divided using a lateral approach.

Lateral Mobilization

The sigmoid loop is pulled toward the right upper quadrant (grasper in right subcostal cannula) to exert traction on the line of Toldt (Figure

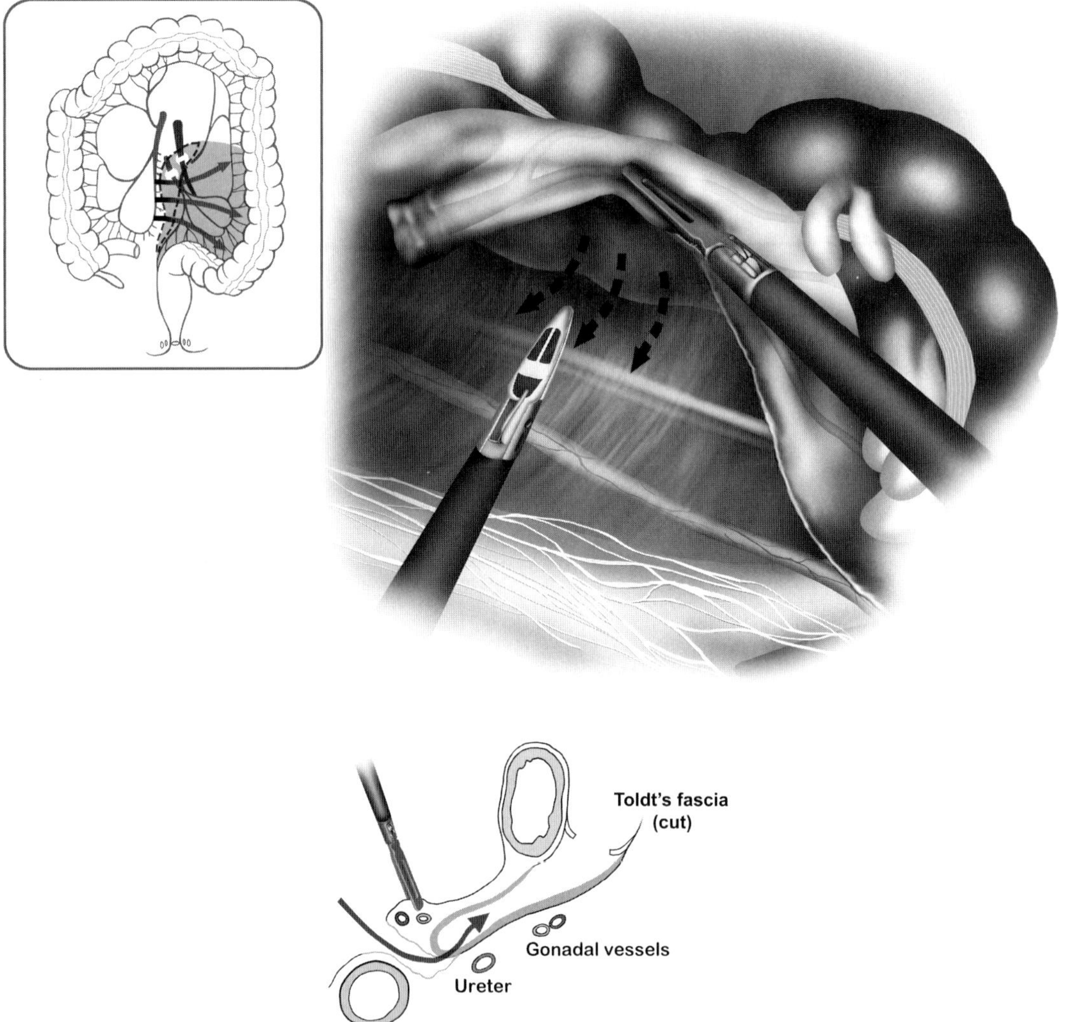

Figure 8.4.10. An avascular plane exists between Toldt's fascia and the mesocolon, which is bluntly dissected medial to lateral after IMA and IMV ligation. (Inset: Cross-sectional drawing illustrating the correct surgical plane indicated by arrow.)

8.4.11). The peritoneal fold is opened cephalad and caudad, and the dissection joins the one previously performed medially. During this step, care must be taken to avoid the gonadal vessels and the left ureter because they can be attracted by the traction exerted on the mesentery. Ureteral stenting (infrared stents) can be useful in cases in which inflammation, tumoral tissue, or adhesions and endometriosis make planes difficult to recognize.

Dissection of the Upper Mesorectum

This area of dissection should be approached with caution, especially on the left side: The mesorectum there is closely attached to the parietal fascia where the superior hypogastric nerve and the left ureter are situated (Figure 8.4.12). The upper portion of the rectum is mobilized posteriorly following the avascular plane described before, then laterally, until a sufficient distal margin is achieved.

Resection of the Specimen

Division of the Rectum

Once the upper rectum is freed, the area of distal resection is chosen, allowing a distal margin of at least 5 cm. The fat surrounding this area is cleared, using monopolar cautery, ultrasonic dissection, or the LigaSure Atlas™. Doing so, the superior hemorrhoidal arteries are divided in the posterior upper mesorectum (Figure 8.4.13). Although we do not routinely perform it, the colon may then be closed using an umbilical tape before a rectal washout is performed, which aims at reducing tumor cell implantation at the staple line. The distal division is performed using a linear stapler. The stapler is introduced through the right lower quadrant cannula. We use stapler loads (3.5 mm, 45-mm blue cartridges), which are applied perpendicular to the bowel. Articulated staplers can also be useful, although they are usually unnecessary at the level of the upper rectum (Figure 8.4.14).

Proximal Division

The proximal division site should be located at least 10 cm proximal to the tumor. It is performed by first dividing the mesocolon and subsequently the bowel (Figure 8.4.15). The division of the mesocolon is

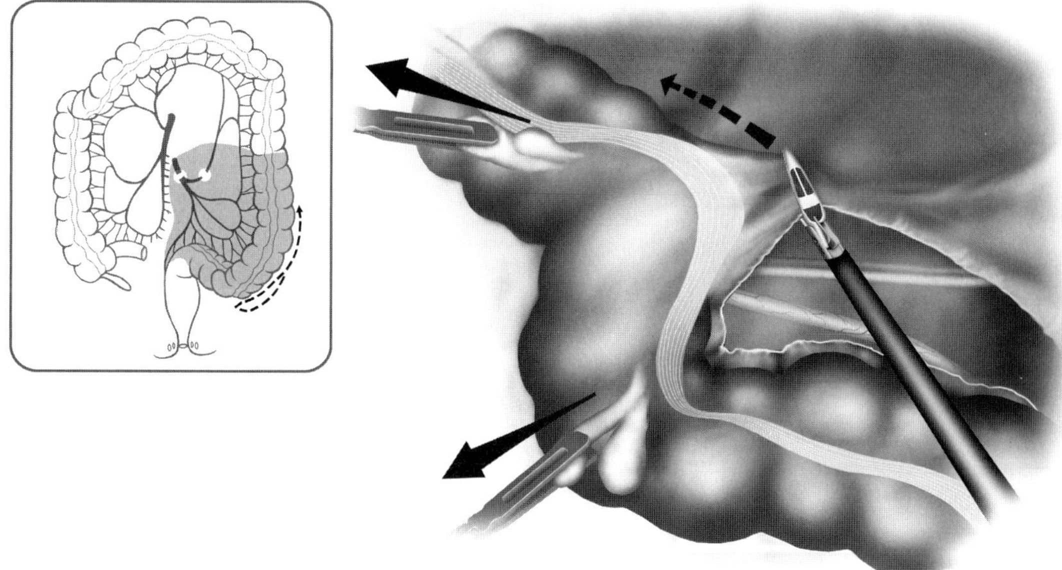

Figure 8.4.11. Lateral dissection then proceeds after the previous medical dissection.

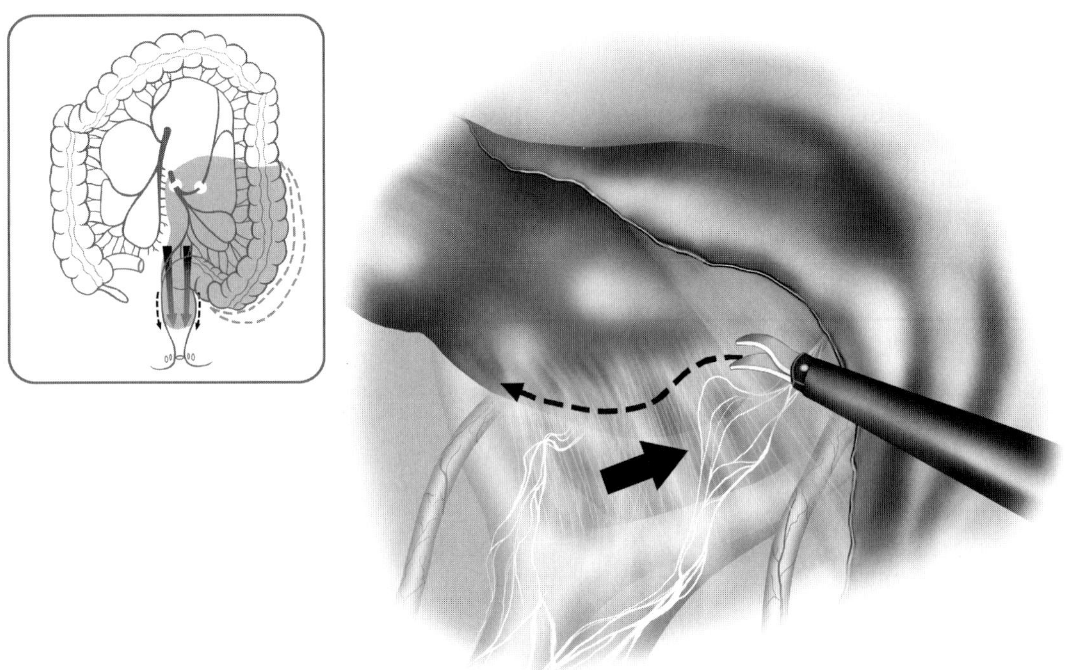

Figure 8.4.12. The dissection of the upper rectum should proceed with caution because the hypogastric nerves are tented upward and may be inadvertently injured. These nerves may be swept posteriorly before dividing the soft tissues in the area.

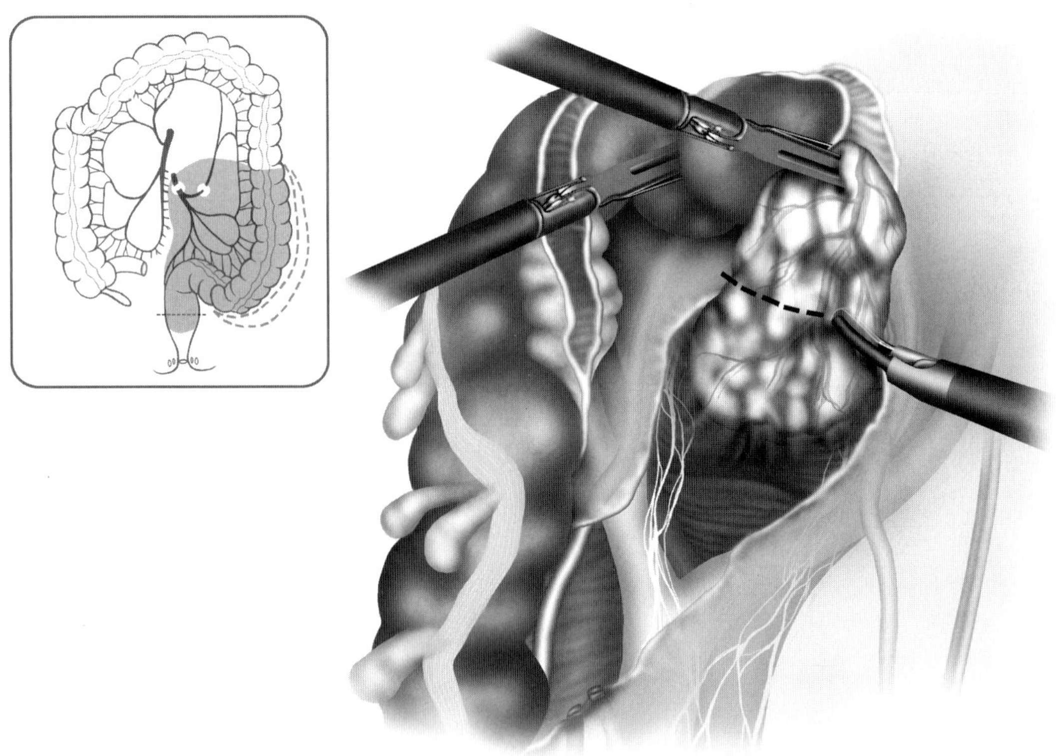

Figure 8.4.13. After upper rectal mobilization, the area of mesorectal division is chosen.

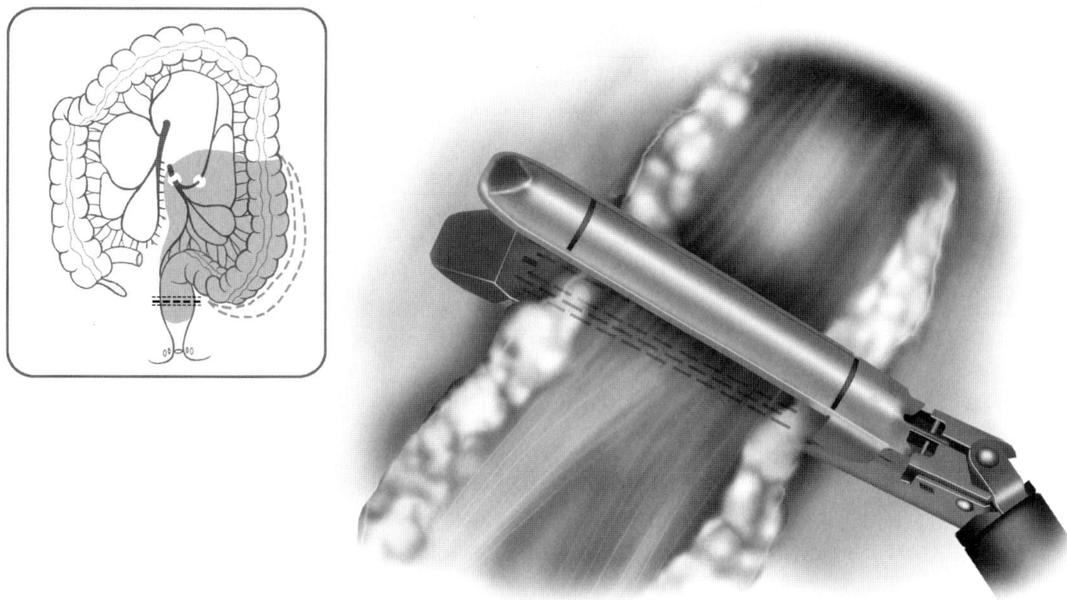

Figure 8.4.14. Distal bowel division is performed through the right lower quadrant cannula using an endoscopic stapler.

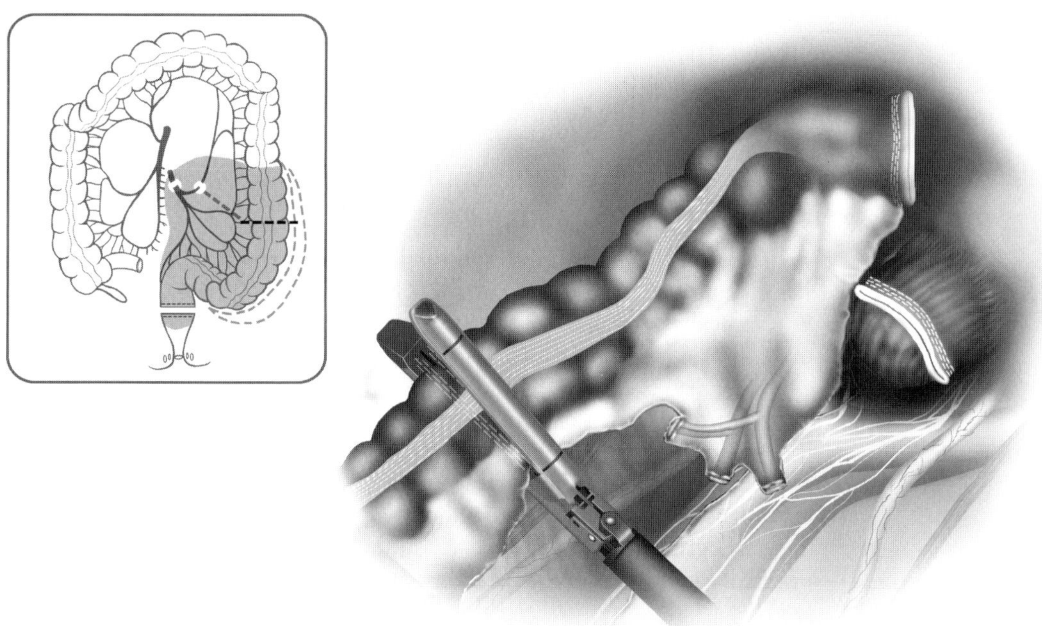

Figure 8.4.15. Proximal bowel division is performed after dividing the mesocolon up to the chosen site.

more easily performed with the Harmonic Scalpel™, or the LigaSure Atlas™, although linear staplers can also be used. The distal portion of the divided IMA is identified, and the division of the mesocolon starts right at this level and continues toward the chosen proximal section site at a 90° angle. A linear stapler is then fired across the bowel. The stapler (blue load) is introduced through the right lower quadrant cannula. The specimen is placed in a plastic retrieval sac introduced through the same cannula. This permits continuation of the procedure without manipulation of the bowel and tumor. If the resected specimen is large and obscures the operative fields, the extraction can be done before completing mobilization of the left colon.

Mobilization of the Splenic Flexure

In the frequent event that a long segment of sigmoid colon has been resected, mobilization of the splenic flexure is required. This can be achieved in different ways. It is important for the surgeon to be familiar with all approaches in order to select the most suitable approach.

Sufficient mobilization of the splenic flexure may be achieved by simply freeing the posterior and lateral attachments of the descending colon. This is begun by a medial approach to free the posterior attachments of the descending and distal transverse colon, followed by the dissection of the lateral attachments, or by doing the same task in the reverse order. A lateral mobilization is sometimes sufficient in cases of sigmoid cancer, where the posterior mobilization can be omitted.

The medial mobilization is perfectly suited to our laparoscopic approach as the surgeon, situated to the patient's right, may have an excellent view of the anterior surface of the pancreas and the base of the left transverse mesocolon, especially in obese patients (Figure 8.4.16).

In addition, division of colocolic adhesions or sometimes careful mesenteric division must be performed to achieve full mobilization and to allow adequate bowel length for a tension-free anastomosis.

Lateral Mobilization of the Splenic Flexure

This approach is often used in open surgery and can also be used in simple laparoscopic colectomies. The first step is the section of the lateral attachments of the descending colon. An ascending incision is made along the line of Toldt using scissors introduced via the left-sided cannula. The phrenocolic ligament is then divided using scissors introduced through this cannula. Retraction of the descending colon and the splenic flexure toward the right lower quadrant using graspers introduced through the right lower and suprapubic cannulae helps to expose the correct plane. The attachments between the transverse colon and the omentum are divided close to the colon until the lesser sac is opened. Division of these attachments is continued as needed, to facilitate the mobilization of the colon into the pelvis.

Medial Mobilization

This approach dissects the posterior attachments of the transverse and descending colon first (Figure 8.4.16). The dissection plane naturally

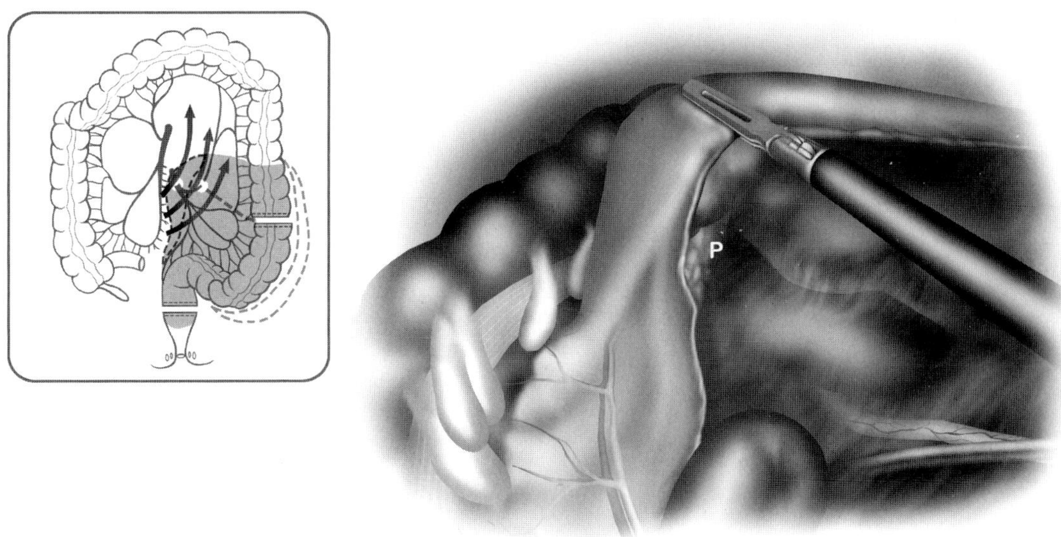

Figure 8.4.16. Medial to lateral dissection beneath the left mesocolon provides excellent views of the distal pancreas, the base of the left transverse mesocolon, and retroperitoneum.

follows the plane of the previous sigmoid colon mobilization, cephalad and anterior to Toldt's fascia. The transverse colon is retracted anteriorly to expose the inferior border of the pancreas, and the root of the transverse mesocolon is divided anterior to the pancreas and at a distance from it; we thus enter the lesser sac. The dissection then follows toward the base of the descending colon and distal transverse colon, dividing the posterior attachments of these structures. The division of the lateral attachments, as described above, then follows the full mobilization of the splenic flexure. If the mobilized colon reaches the pelvis easily, it may be safely assumed the anastomosis will be tension free as well.

Extraction

The extraction of the specimen is performed using a double protection: A wound protector as well as a retrieval sac (Figure 8.4.17). The wound protector is also helpful to ensure that there is no CO_2 leak during the intracorporeal colorectal anastomosis, which follows the extraction. This allows reduction of the size of incision and potentially minimizes the risk of tumor cell seeding.

Incision to Extract the Specimen

The size of the incision, its location, and the extraction technique take into account the volume of the specimen, the patient's body habitus, cosmetic concerns, and the type of disease. The incision is generally performed in the suprapubic region. The proximal division is per-

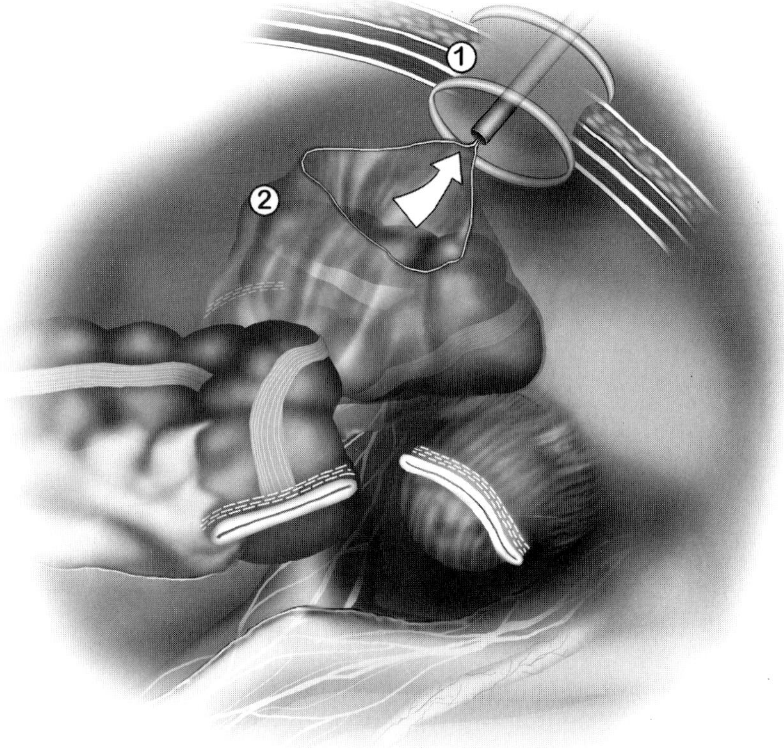

Figure 8.4.17. Specimen extraction at the suprapubic site involves double protection: 1) a wound protector; and 2) an impermeable retrieval sac.

formed intracorporeally, as described above, and the specimen placed into a thick plastic bag before being extracted through the incision at the suprapubic area.

Anastomosis

We always use a mechanical circular stapling device passed transanally to perform the anastomosis. Performing the anastomosis includes an extraabdominal preparatory step and an intraabdominal step performed laparoscopically. The extraabdominal step takes place after the extraction of the specimen. The instrument holding the proximal bowel presents it at the incision where it can easily be grasped with a Babcock clamp and pulled out (Figure 8.4.18). If necessary, the colon is divided again in a healthy and well-vascularized zone. The anvil (at least 28 mm in diameter) is then introduced into the bowel lumen and closed with a purse string (Figure 8.4.19); then the colon is reintroduced into the abdominal cavity (Figure 8.4.20). The abdominal incision is closed to reestablish the pneumoperitoneum. For an air-tight closure, it is sufficient to twist the wound protector at the level of the incision using a large clamp (Figure 8.4.21). The circular stapler is introduced into the rectum through the gently dilated anus. The rectal stump is then transfixed with the tip of the head of the circular stapler (Figure 8.4.22). In women, the posterior vaginal wall should be retracted anteriorly by the assistant passing the stapler. Once the center rod and anvil are clicked into the distal part of the circular stapler, we check for twisting of the colon and the mesentery. The stapler is then fired after ensuring that the neighboring organs are away from the stapling line. The stapler is then twisted open and withdrawn. The anastomosis is checked for leaks by verifying the integrity of the proximal and distal rings, as well as performing an air test (Figure 8.4.23). Some authors complete the evaluation of the anastomosis with a rectoscopy.

Wound Closure

The cannula sites are checked internally for possible hemorrhage. To do so, a grasper is passed through the cannula and the cannula is removed leaving the grasper in the abdomen. Because of the smaller diameter of the grasper compared with the cannula, if a bleeding was so far concealed by the tamponade effect of the cannula, it would be revealed promptly. The cannula is then reintroduced to allow maintenance of the pneumoperitoneum while performing the same check at all cannula sites.

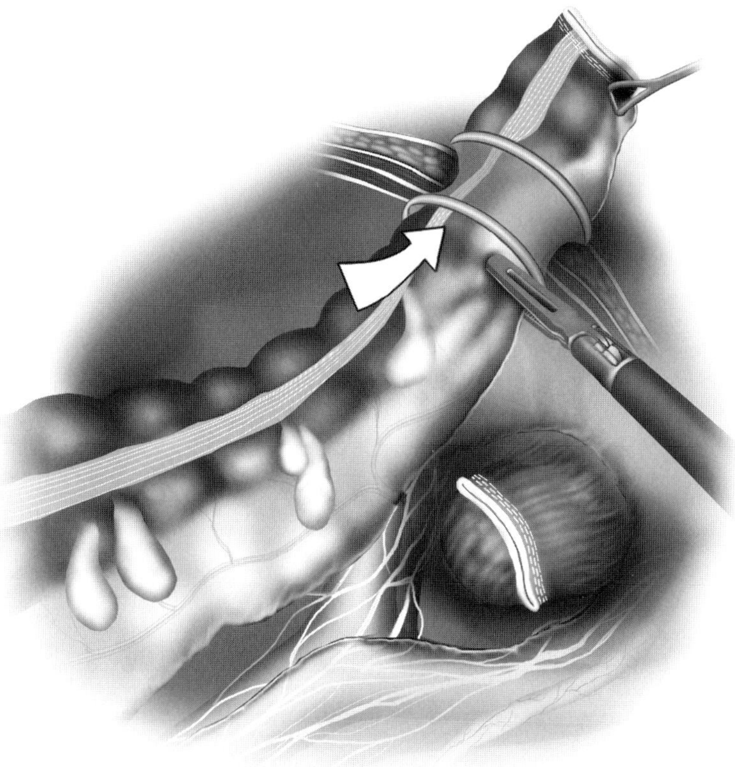

Figure 8.4.18. After specimen extraction, the proximal colon is drawn out through this site, keeping the wound protector in place.

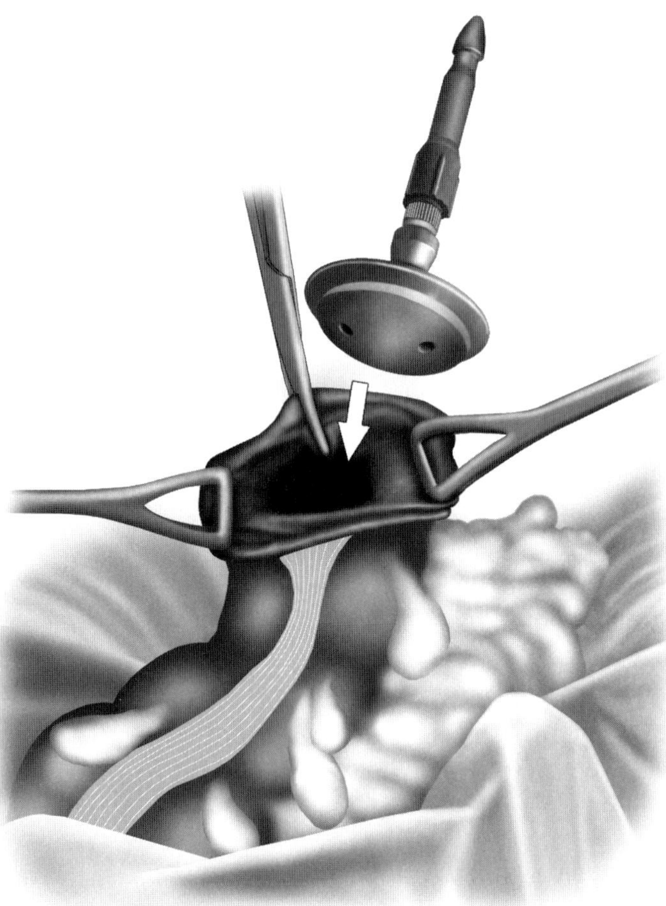

Figure 8.4.19. The anvil and center rod of the circular stapler are introduced into the bowel lumen and secured with a purse string suture.

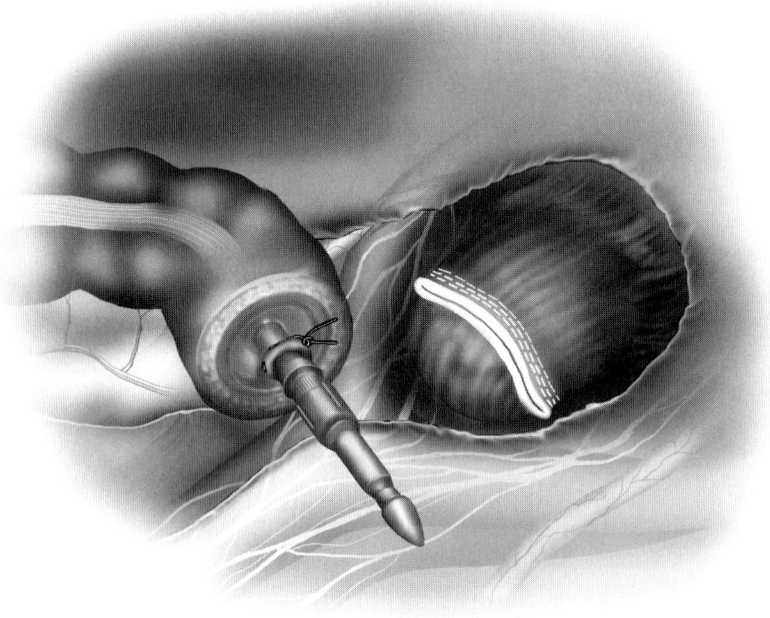

Figure 8.4.20. The bowel is reintroduced into the abdominal cavity, checking for adequate length for anastomosis. The bowel should comfortably reach the pelvis without tension.

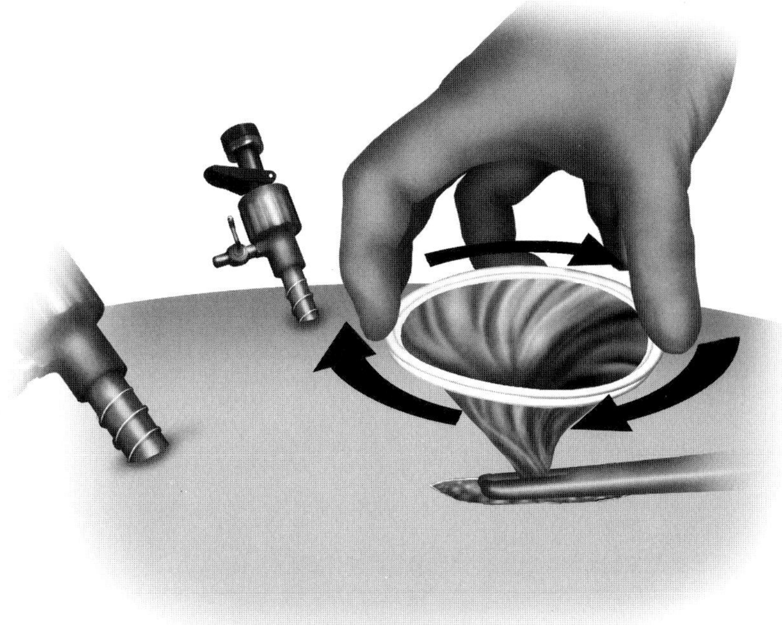

Figure 8.4.21. Reestablishment of the pneumoperitoneum can be achieved quickly by twisting the wound protector, then clamping it at the skin level with a Kocher clamp.

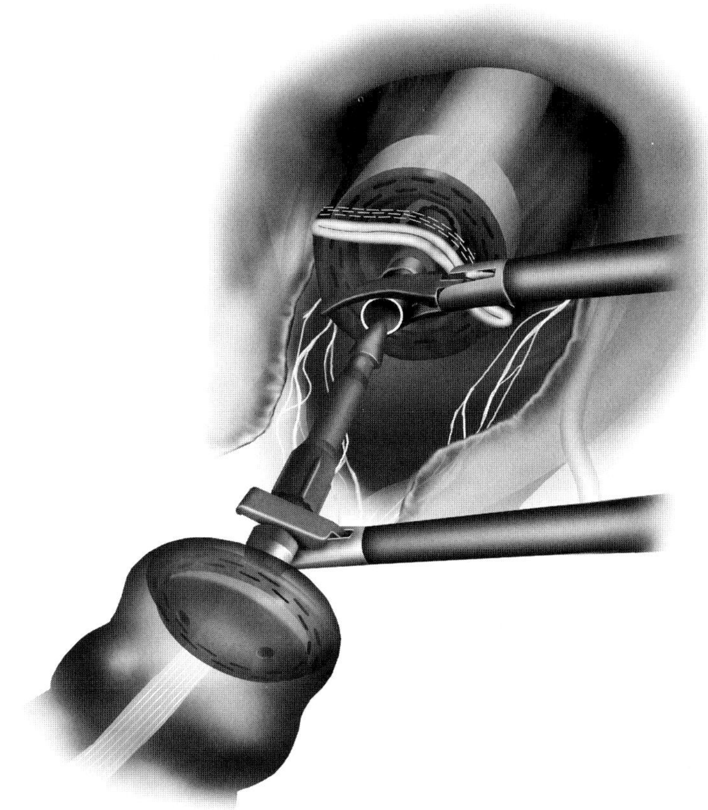

Figure 8.4.22. The anastomosis is then done under laparoscopic guidance, perforating the proximal rectal stump with the sharp spike of the circular stapler, then performing a standard double-stapled anastomosis.

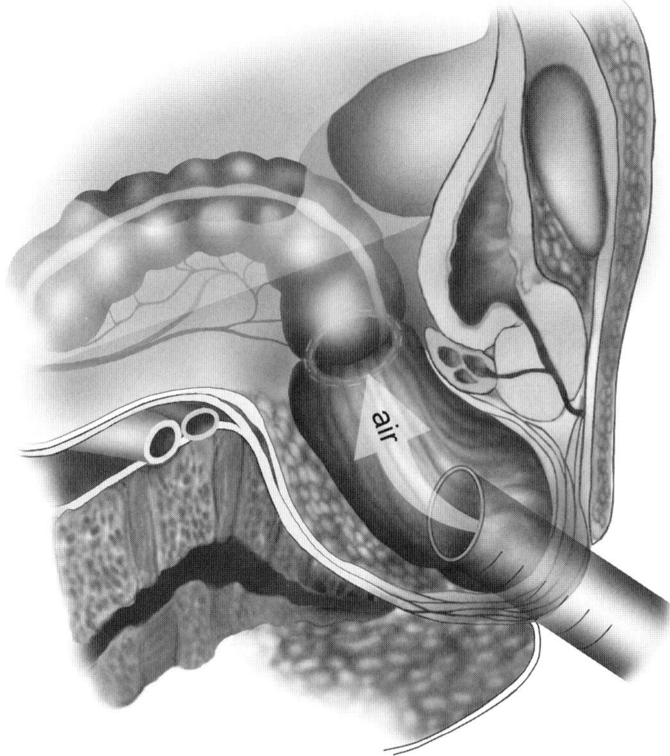

Figure 8.4.23. After firing the stapler, the anastomosis is checked by filling the pelvis with saline, then insufflating the rectum with air using a rectoscope. The bowel upstream of the anastomosis is gently occluded during this test.

When the check is completed, the CO_2 is desufflated through the cannulae and cannulae are removed. No routine drainage of the anastomotic area is performed. The suprapubic incision is closed in layers using running absorbable sutures, and all fascial defects of 10 mm and more are closed. The skin is closed with a subcuticular absorbable suture.

Sigmoidectomy for Diverticular Disease

The vascular approach for patients with benign diseases of the sigmoid colon is performed with the following steps.

Peritoneal Incision

The peritoneal incision can be similar to the cancer technique particularly in difficult cases (obesity, inflammatory mesocolon). In most cases, we try to preserve the vascularization of the rectum and the left colic vessels. The opening of the peritoneum can be limited to the mesosigmoid parallel to colon at mid distance between the colon and the root of the mesosigmoid. An initial lateral mobilization of the sigmoid can be useful in this approach. The branches of the sigmoid arterial trunk can be divided separately anteriorly to inferior mesenteric vessels (Figure 8.4.24) or together after creating windows in the mesentery to divide the various branches. A linear stapler or, better, the LigaSure Atlas™ 10-mm device can be used for this task.

Resection of the Specimen
In diverticular disease, we usually perform the distal resection of the bowel below the rectosigmoid junction. The rectosigmoid junction is located just above the peritoneal reflexion, at the pouch of Douglas. We prefer to perform the mobilization of the splenic flexure at this moment, before resection at the proximal limit, using the same principles as described above.

Extraction of the Specimen
Before extracting the colon, it is important to divide the mesocolon at the level of the proximal site of division. After adequate mobilization is achieved, the colon is extracted through a suprapubic incision, protected by the plastic drape described above, and proximal division performed externally on a compliant and well-vascularized part of the colon. The anastomosis is performed as described above for cancer (Figure 8.4.23).

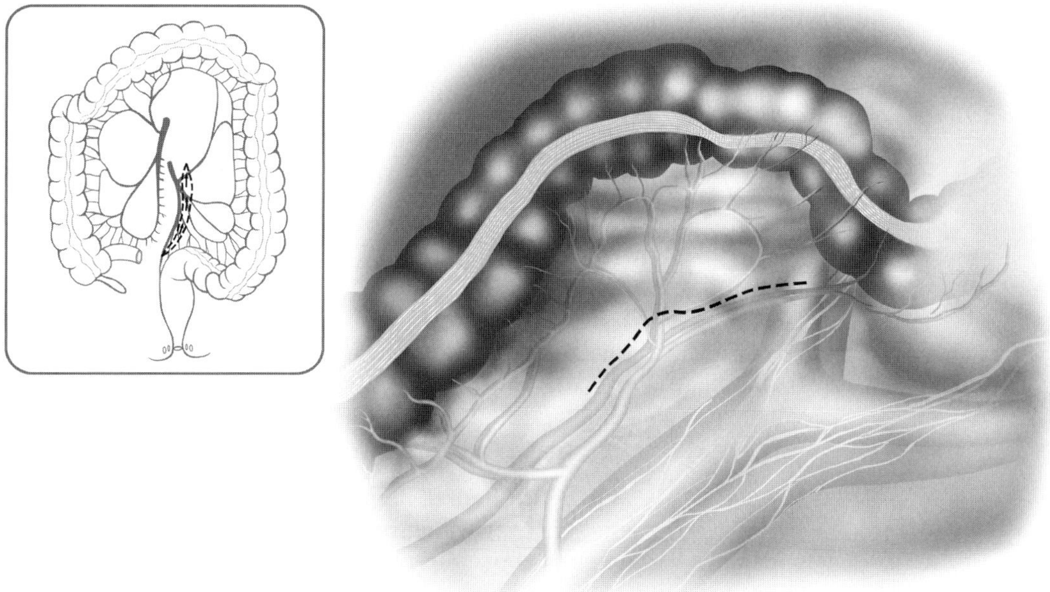

Figure 8.4.24. In sigmoidectomy for benign disease, the mesenteric division may proceed anterior to the IMA/IMV, because a less radical resection is required. This preserves more blood flow to the bowel and leaves the hypogastric nerves less subject to surgical trauma.

Special Considerations

Ureteral injuries are one of the most important complications, which can be avoided by a perfect exposure and the respect of the correct plane of dissection. Indeed, a dissection properly performed above the Toldt's fascia does not expose the ureter to accidental injury. Difficult cases, such as important inflammatory reaction, cancer invasion or adhesions, and, sometimes, endometriosis, may alter the anatomy of the region and render the identification of the ureter troublesome. In these special cases, prevention of ureteral injury may be facilitated by the use of infrared wires inserted in ureteral stents. The infrared light is cold and safe for use in close contact with the ureteral tissue, and, on the other side, makes it easy to recognize the structure under the light of an adequate laparoscope.

Conclusions

Laparoscopic sigmoid resection is presently a well-standardized technique. Whereas the open surgical approach is usually performed through a standard lateral dissection, with or without the primary vascular approach, the medial approach seems very amenable for the laparoscopic technique, and is our favored approach. Indeed, the medial approach permits a safe primary dissection and avoids manipulation of the colon.

The laparoscopic approach for sigmoid cancer is an adequate oncologic procedure in experienced hands, and is associated with a low morbidity, as well as with a risk of port-site recurrence and local recurrence not higher than what is reported in the open literature.

Even though the laparoscopic approach has not yet become a "gold standard" for sigmoid diverticulitis, it is certainly playing an increasingly important role in the surgical management of benign colonic diseases.

Editors' Comments

Dr. Leroy and his coauthors have very well described, in depth, the approach to sigmoid colon resection using laparoscopic methods for both benign and malignant diseases. Our method is very similar, and we echo their comments that an oncologic approach may be accomplished well using laparoscopic methods.

Indications: We agree with their statements.

Patient's positioning: We nearly always keep both arms at the side of the patient, because this is usually possible and may secure the patient on the bed more firmly. This also lessens the possibility of shoulder injury compared with having the arm extended during the operation. If the first assistant stands on the left side of the patients, the monitors should be positioned on both sides of the patient.

Cannula positioning: We agree that the use of multiple (up to six) cannulae matters little with the final outcome of the patient compared with the use of three or four cannulae. Thus, a proper exposure is the key to an excellent operation and not the final number of cannulae, especially if the extra ones are 5 mm.

Technique: We would consider that, especially in a distal sigmoid cancer or diverticular disease, it is important to mobilize the proximal rectum, and to carefully identify and preserve the hypogastric nerves. This is readily accomplished using the magnification afforded by the laparoscope, and careful dissection coupled with it. An alternative to the suprapubic incision may be an extension of the left lower quadrant cannula incision for extraction of the specimen. Alternatively, if the specimen is large or adherent to surrounding structures (diverticular disease), it may be useful to consider a hand-assisted approach, using a suprapubic Pfannenstiel incision of 7–8 cm (see Chapter 9.1).

In mobilizing the splenic flexure, we would also add that occasionally it is easier to commence this by opening the lesser sac in the distal transverse colon area, at the fusion of the omentum with the transverse colon in the avascular plane there. By then going back and forth, medially and laterally, the dissection of a difficult splenic flexure may be expedited. It is also a good idea to check for adhesions between the omentum and the left colon, and for adhesions between the transverse colon and the left colon, because lysing these may afford extra length to the left colon.

References

1. Wong WD, Wexner SD, Lowry A, et al. Practice parameters for the treatment of sigmoid diverticulitis: supporting documentation. The Standards Task Force. The American Society of Colon and Rectal Surgeons. Dis Colon Rectum 2000;43:290–297.
2. Kohler L, Sauerland S, Neugebauer E. Diagnosis and treatment of diverticular disease: results of a consensus development conference. The Scientific Committee of the European Association for Endoscopic Surgery. Surg Endosc 1999;13:430–436.
3. Scheidbach H, Schneider C, Huegel O, et al. Laparoscopic sigmoid resection for cancer: curative resection and preliminary medium-term results. Dis Colon Rectum 2002;45:1641–1647.
4. Balli JE, Franklin ME, Almeida JA, et al. How to prevent port-site metastases in laparoscopic colorectal surgery. Surg Endosc 2000;14:1034–1036.
5. Liang JT, Lai HS, Huang KC, et al. Comparison of medial-to-lateral versus traditional lateral-to-medial laparoscopic dissection sequences for resection of rectosigmoid cancers: randomized controlled clinical trial. World J Surg 2003;27:190–196.

Chapter 8.5

Laparoscopic Anterior Resection for Rectal Cancer

Masahiko Watanabe

Indications

Since the introduction of laparoscopic surgery, significant progress has been made in the treatment of early-stage gastrointestinal cancers.[1] Initially, the target of laparoscopic colectomy was limited to very early stages (T0 stage) in Japan. These were mainly tumors that were unresectable using colonoscopy and T1-stage tumors which were massively invasive to the submucosa. Laparoscopic colectomy was viewed as a method that would close the gap between open and colonoscopic resection.

Since then, the applications for laparoscopic colectomy for malignancy have been gradually expanded, aided by improvements in surgical technique and advances in equipment and instruments. Today, indications have expanded to include even certain T2–T4 stages for colon cancer.[2] However, large bulky tumors, cancers that involve other organs, and advanced (T3 and T4) rectal cancer are excluded from our indications in Japan.[3] The anterior resection technique described below can generally be applied to tumors that are at or just above the peritoneal reflection of the rectum.

Patient Positioning and Operating Room Setup

We fix the body with the right side of the patient lower than the left (about 15°) using the "magic bed" (bean bag moldable device) and provide lateral support on the right side. We always use intermittent lower extremity compression stockings and adjustable leg stirrups. With regard to the head, we apply a foam pad to the forehead, and fix it there to the bed with adhesive tapes. The surgeon stands to the right side of the patient, the cameraman (second assistant) stands to the left side of the surgeon, and the first assistant stands in between the legs or on the left side of the patient (Figure 8.5.1). After initial exploration within the abdominal cavity in a neutral position, the patient is tilted into a right side down position, positioning the small intestines to the

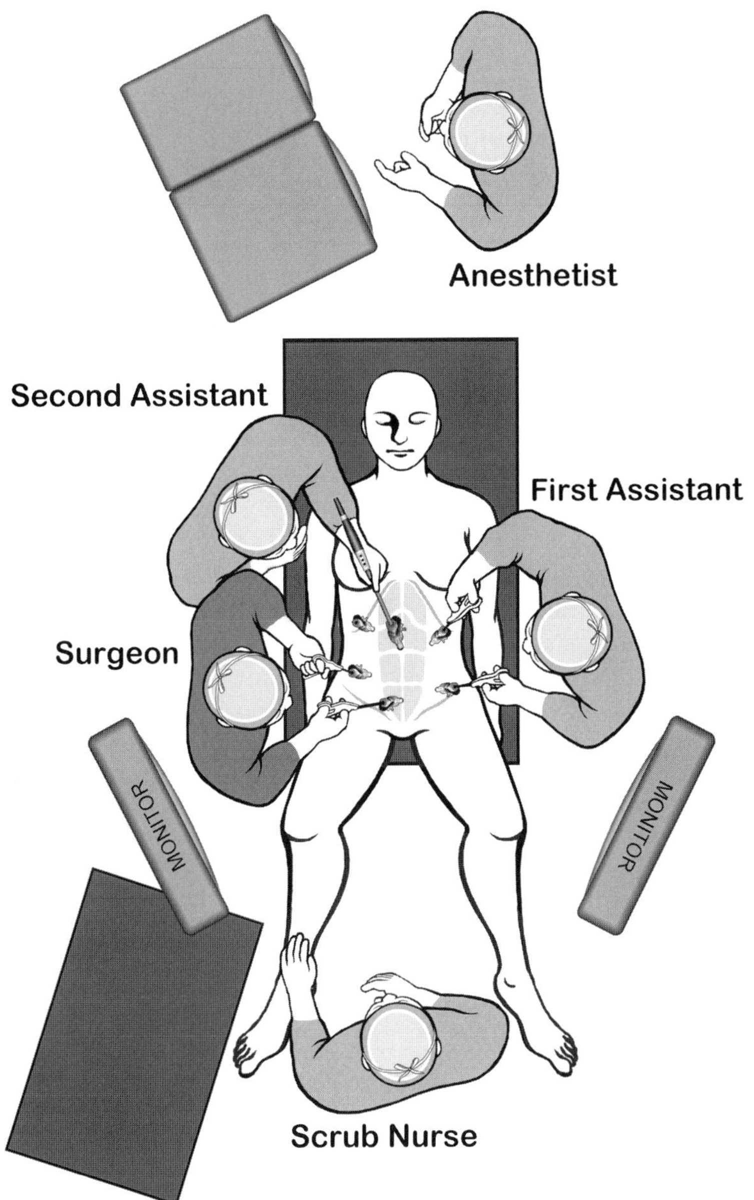

Figure 8.5.1. Positions of the equipment and the surgical team for the laparoscopic anterior resection for rectal cancer.

right upper quadrant, with confirmation of the lesion site either by visualizing the tumor or an India ink marking placed on the bowel preoperatively. The small intestines are best positioned out of the way using specialized bowel grasping forceps with rounded tips. If necessary, the patient should be positioned head down (Trendelenburg position).

Table 8.5.1. Specific instruments recommended for laparoscopic rectal resection

5	Cannulae (3 × 12 mm, 3 × 5 mm)
1	Dissecting device (i.e. LigaSure V™ or Ultrasonic Shears™ or electrosurgery)
1	Laparoscopic scissors
1	Laparoscopic dissector
1	Laparoscopic right-angled dissector
2	Laparoscopic graspers
1	Endoloop retractor
1	Endoscopic stapler

Instruments

Specific instruments recommended for laparoscopic rectal resection are listed in Table 8.5.1.

Cannula Positioning

We make an arc-shaped incision immediately above the umbilicus, introducing the first cannula (12 mm) by an open (minilaparotomy) method, performing a purse string suture of the peritoneum and fascia,

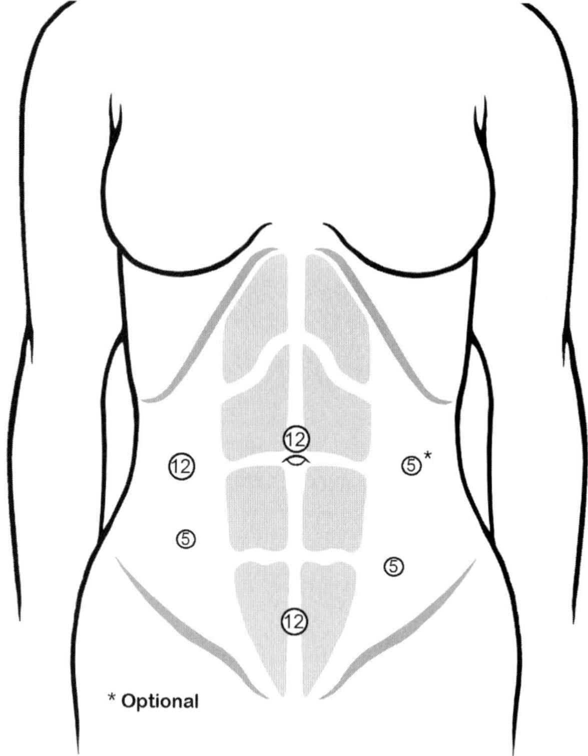

Figure 8.5.2. Positions of the cannulae for the laparoscopic anterior resection. Note that the surgeon works mainly through the right lower quadrant and the suprapubic cannulae.

fixing the cannula using a tourniquet method. After initiating a pneumoperitoneum (8–10 mm Hg), we introduce an endoscope (Figure 8.5.2). We then place cannulae in the order of: Left middle abdominal region (5 mm), the left lower abdominal region (5 mm), the midline suprapubic region (12 mm), 1–2 fingers above the pubis, and the right middle abdominal region (12 mm).

If an additional cannula is needed, a right lower abdominal cannula (5 mm) is added. The skin incision at the suprapubic site is made vertically so that open surgery can be performed at any time using a midline incision. At the remaining locations, the incision should be made horizontally for better healing from an aesthetic standpoint. We are cautious at the lower quadrant cannula sites to avoid injuring the inferior epigastric artery and vein. For the puncture in the right midabdomen, placement of the laparoscope into the suprapubic cannula will provide good visualization for a safer puncture. We usually use a flexible laparoscope to assist in visualizing the abdominal wall, but if a rigid scope is used, we advocate using an angled scope (30 or 45°).

Technique

Dissection and Detachment of the Rectosigmoid Colon

The initial step in this technique is dissection and detachment of the distal sigmoid colon and the rectum. This can be performed from either the lateral side or the medial side of the rectosigmoid (Figure 8.5.3). When the lateral approach is used, the dissection plane can be naturally exposed while the descending colon is being dissected if the operating table is tilted with the right side down. Ureter and gonadal arteries/veins are dissected without any damage if Toldt's fusion fascia, con-

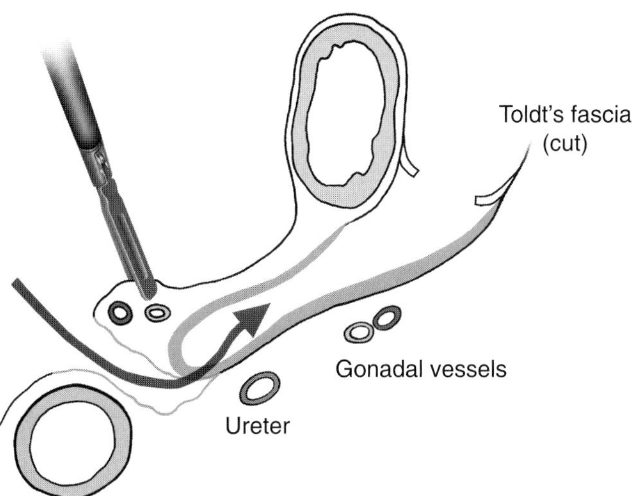

Figure 8.5.3. Dissecting plane from the medial or lateral sides of the sigmoid colon optimally involve sweeping the Toldt's fascia posteriorly (thick gray line). This safely isolates and preserves the ureter and gonadal vessels.

nected to the anterior layer of the Gerota's fascia, is exposed and the dissection performed in front of this fascia.

With the medial approach, the superior rectal arteries/veins are carefully grasped initially and lifted up ventrally along with the mesentery. Next, an incision is made in the anterior layer of the mesentery, and blunt dissection is performed between the vessels and the retroperitoneum, encountering the ventral side of Toldt's fusion fascia (Figure 8.5.4). It is always an option to perform dissection from the lateral side later, if the ureter and gonadal arteries/veins are verified and dissected on their dorsal side, also exposing the psoas muscle (Figure 8.5.5).

By introducing grasping forceps from the left lower quadrant, after detachment of adhesions at the S-D (sigmoid descending) colon junction, we next identify the Toldt's fusion fascia. It will be better not to dissect too deeply at the S-D junction, only to detach adhesions. The "white line" should be incised and the descending colon should be dissected just anterior to Toldt's fusion fascia. The assistant should introduce the intestinal grasping forceps with gauze from the left lower quadrant cannula to help confirm the proper plane. We take care at this point to not grasp the colon itself, but to attempt to hold the mesentery or an epiploic appendage.

It may be easiest to identify the gonadal vessels and ureter just beneath Toldt's fusion fascia, and this is acceptable if necessary to be sure these structures are protected (Figure 8.5.5). However, if dissection

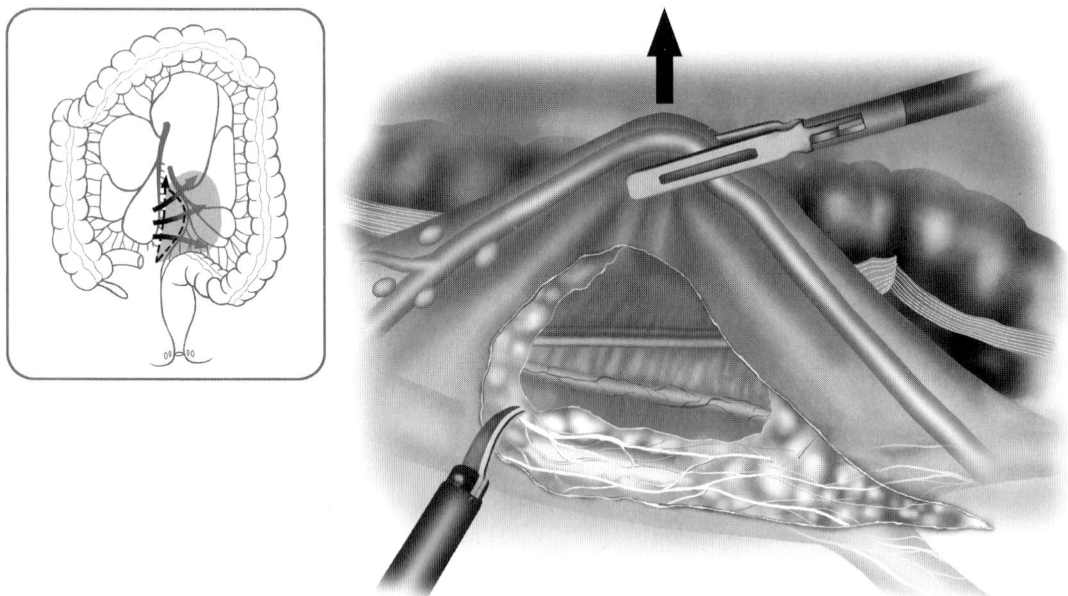

Figure 8.5.4. In the medial approach, the superior rectal (or inferior mesenteric) vessels are tented anteriorly and the plane is dissected between the vessels and Toldt's fascia.

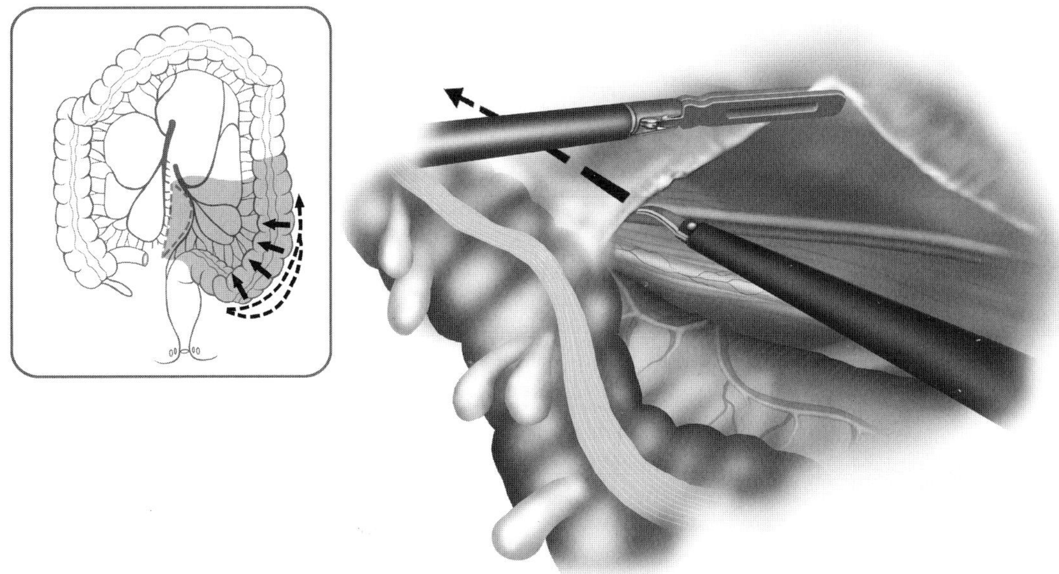

Figure 8.5.5. It is always an option to perform dissection laterally, verifying the location of the ureter and gonadal vessels.

may proceed safely just anterior to Toldt's fascia, bleeding is kept to a minimum. When arrest of bleeding is needed, we avoid irrigating with saline, and keep the plane dry by wiping the area with a small gauze introduced through the left lower quadrant cannula.

In the dissection just medial to the ureter, appreciating Toldt's fusion fascia can help to identify the anterior surface of the superior hypogastric plexus, most prominent toward the midline. Another helpful anatomic point is that the site where ureter and gonadal vein crosses is approximately the same anatomic level as the root of the inferior mesenteric artery.

The superior rectal artery and vein are delineated by retracting the mesentery of the sigmoid colon to the left and slightly ventrally (by the assistant), with forceps introduced from the cannulae of the left side and the suprapubic region. Then, a window is created just to the left of the pedicle using blunt dissection, so that the pedicle is dissected both medially and laterally. We then apply a small retractor through the left upper quadrant cannula to the window of the mesentery, drawing the pedicle ventrally, and dilate the window in a cephalocaudal manner using the forceps and electrosurgery.

Division of the Vessels

Around the root of the inferior mesenteric artery (IMA), the lumbar splanchnic nerves and lymphatic vessels arise from the right and left sides of the aorta, making the tissue in this area thick. Bleeding tends to occur readily with dissection. Thus, step by step careful dissection is required using the dissecting forceps and scissors. Exposing the root of the IMA carefully, it is possible to preserve the nerves using either electrosurgery or the Laparoscopic Coagulating Shears (LCS) (Harmonic Scalpel; Ethicon Endosurgery, Cincinnati, OH). Once the adventitious tunica of IMA is exposed, we separate it sufficiently around the vessels to perform clipping, then transection (Figure 8.5.6). We take care to only divide the nerves that branch toward the sigmoid colon by LCS, so as not to injure the aortic nerve plexus itself, especially on the left side, and furthermore, we take care to also protect the nerve bundle around the IMA on the cephalic side. After sweeping the pedicle free from the retroperitoneal structures, we then resect en masse the inferior mesenteric vein (IMV) and the left colic artery by stapling devices or LCS from the right-sided cannulae. If the instrument is introduced from the suprapubic port, the angle becomes too tangential to the vessels, leading to difficulty in proper alignment with the vessel. Thus, the pedicle of the IMV and left colic should be divided from the right-sided cannulae. We take care to identify the ureter and gonadal vessels one more time before dividing any tissues (Figure 8.5.7).

If the tumor is located in the lower rectum or if it is a T1 rectosigmoid cancer, the mesentery can be divided more distally, e.g., between the left colic artery and the first sigmoid colon artery. Then by using traction from a grasper in the left lower quadrant, by pulling the mesentery

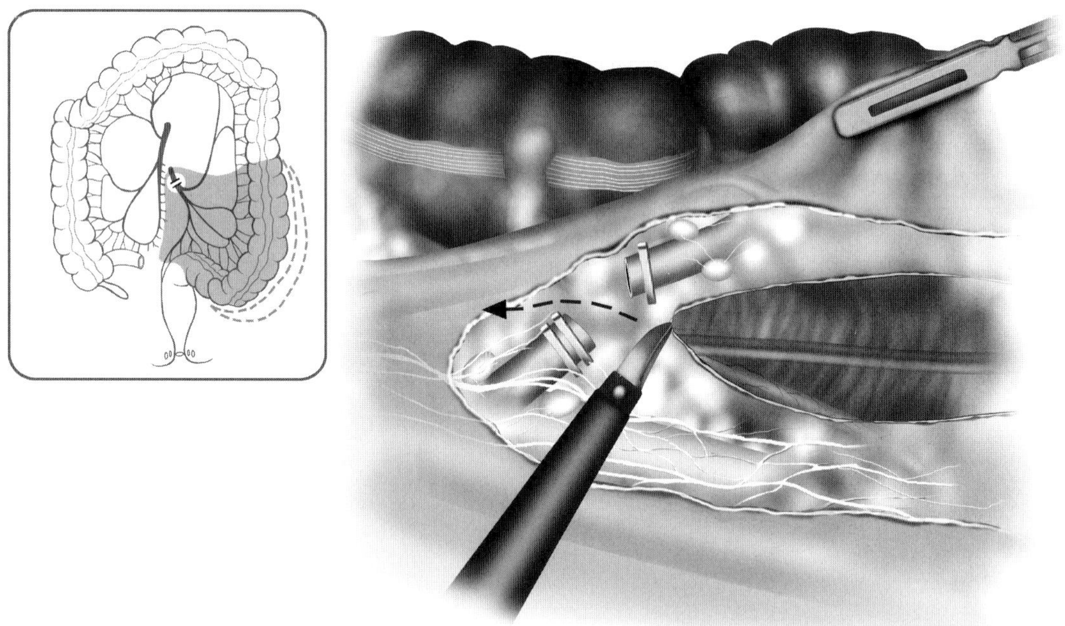

Figure 8.5.6. Once the adventitious tunica of the inferior mesenteric artery is exposed, we clip then transect it. Hypogastric nerves are exposed and preserved.

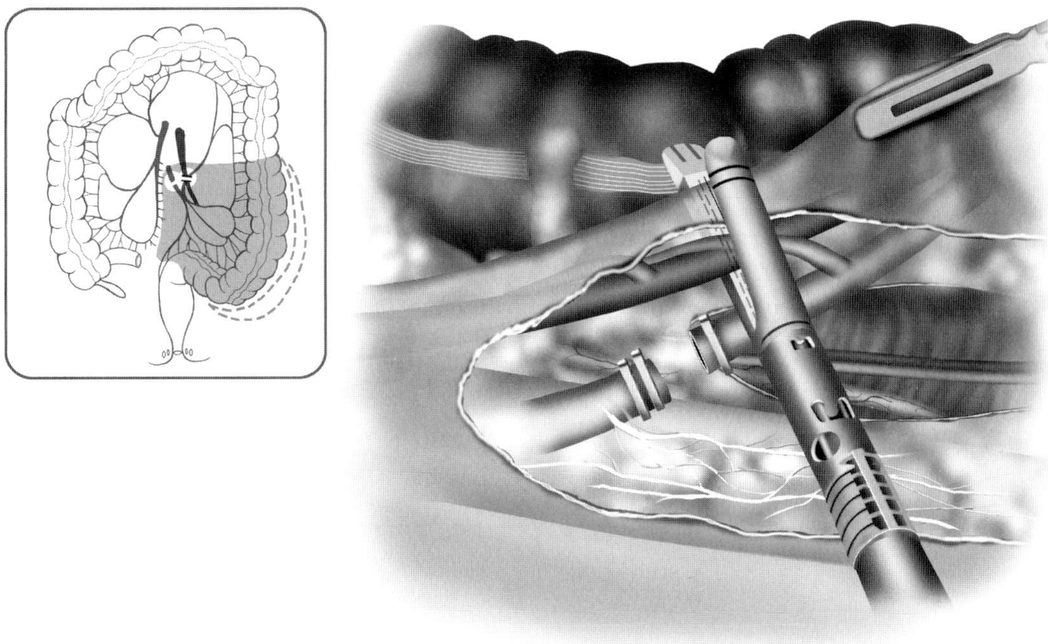

Figure 8.5.7. Next, the inferior mesenteric vein and the left colic artery can be simultaneously divided with an endoscopic stapler from the right side. Note that the ureter and gonadal vessels are clear of the stapler.

cephalad, the superior rectal artery and vein may be resected/divided using a vascular endoscopic stapler.

Dissection of the Rectum

After division of the vessels, placement of the patient into a deeper Trendelenburg position assists in retracting the small intestine out of the pelvic cavity. Placement of the left side up may also assist in keeping the small intestine well retracted. Next, we attempt to identify the right side of the rectum. The assistant should gently draw the sigmoid colon cephalad and slightly to the ventral side using the grasping forceps, drawing the mesentery near the stump of the pedicle to the left ventral side using the grasping forceps from the left upper quadrant cannula. We then bluntly separate the mesorectum (fascia propria of the rectum) from the fascia propria of the sacrum by pushing it anteriorly and identifying the retrorectal space. We adopt a dissection of the presacral space from the right to left side, recognizing the boundary between the mesorectal fascia and presacral fascia. In this manner, one may identify the hypogastric nerves and more distally the pelvic nerve plexus, and minimize potential for injury (Figure 8.5.8). In addition, meticulous dissection of fine vessels by electrosurgery minimizes bleeding into the presacral space, making the proper plane of dissection between the fascia propria of the rectum and the presacral fascia easier to identify. Once dissection proceeds distally into the pelvis to about the third

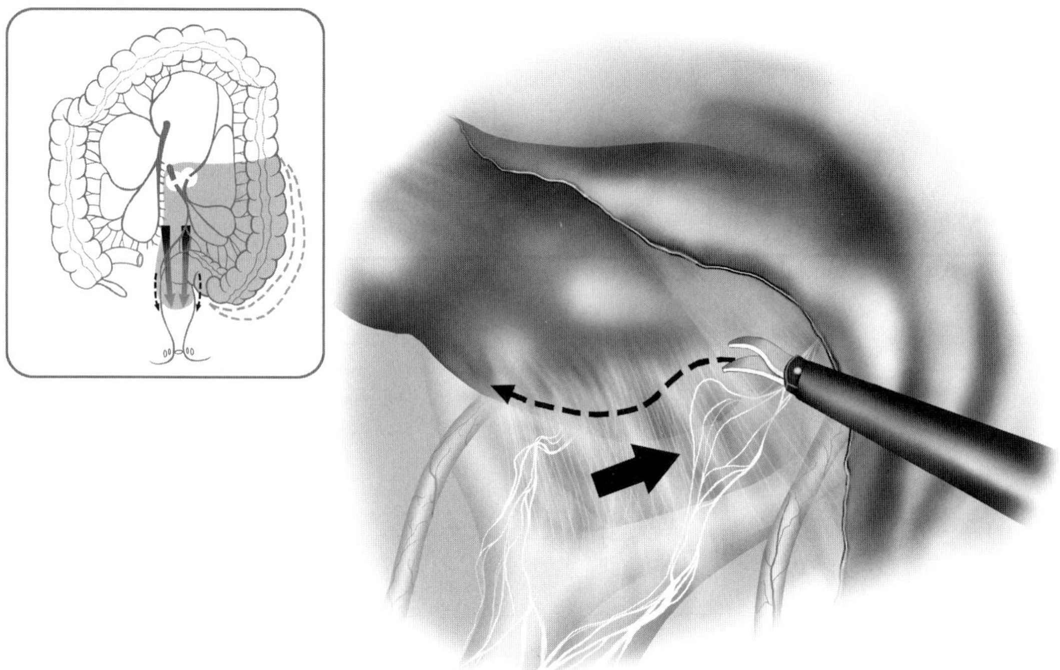

Figure 8.5.8. The rectal dissection starts from the right side, carefully identifying and sweeping down the hypogastric nerves, which can be tented upward with traction.

sacral vertebrae level, Waldeyer's fascia becomes visible as a thickening of the presacral plane. At this point, the surgeon should dissect the right side of the rectum down to the peritoneal reflection in the cul-de-sac by the assistant drawing the rectum to the left of the pelvis and by cutting the peritoneum on the right side laterally using laparoscopic mini-shears (US Surgical Corp., Norwalk, CT). Again, we take our time in this dissection, because meticulous attention to hemostasis permits better identification of the small nerve roots and branches of the pelvic nerves, and helps avoid injury to sacral venous plexus.

The next step is dissection of the left side of the rectum. The rectosigmoid is drawn to the right side of the pelvis using grasping forceps from the right upper quadrant cannula. The left side of rectum is identified and placed under tension. Because of the previous posterior and right-sided dissection, the nerves, ureter, and lateral pelvic structures are largely cleared from the dissection site. The assistant should place the mesorectum under tension by use of grasping forceps from the left upper quadrant, drawing it to the right side. Simultaneously the surgeon should hold and draw the left-sided peritoneum using grasping forceps, apply countertraction in the horizontal direction, and dissecting the boundary between the peritoneum and mesentery of the left side of the rectum using electrosurgery (Figure 8.5.9).

Once this is completed, the peritoneum is incised at the peritoneal reflection, from right to left, and gentle blunt dissection is used to define the correct plane on the anterior side of the rectum. Denonvilliers' fascia can then be exposed with identification of the vaginal wall or seminal vesicles (Figure 8.5.10). The rectum is drawn to the right upper side of the pelvis, placing the left lateral ligaments under tension, making them easier to be identified. The anterior side of this ligament is bluntly dissected with a lateral motion to define a plane between them and the lateral mesorectum, and the ligament can be divided by LCS (Figure 8.5.11). After division of the ligament, further dissection distally for several centimeters will expose the levator ani muscle and often the convex bulge of the ischiorectal fossa beneath the pelvic floor muscles. The same maneuver is repeated on the right side of the rectum, and posterior and anterior levels of dissection are checked to complete the dissection circumferentially to the pelvic floor.

Distal Rectal Transection and Anastomosis of the Rectum

By applying tension to the left side the rectum at the proposed resection line, using the grasping forceps from the left-sided cannulae, the peritoneum and mesorectum at this level are divided using the LCS (Figure 8.5.12). By using the LCS, and by striking a plane between the mesorectum and the posterior wall of the rectum, injury to the rectal wall can be avoided. Similarly, the mesorectum is dissected on the left side, exposing the rectal wall, and connecting the right and left resection

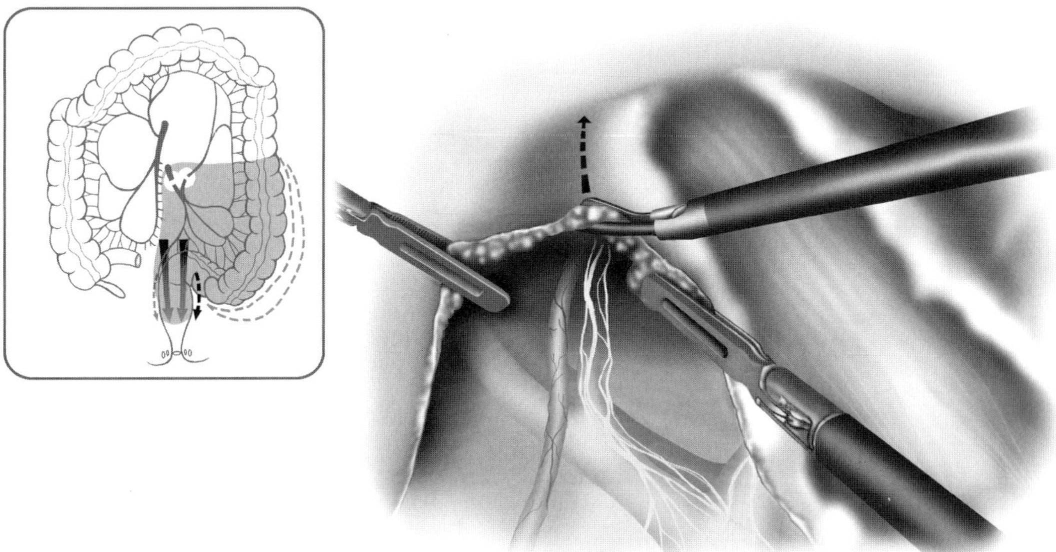

Figure 8.5.9. With careful traction and countertraction by the surgeon and the assistant, the boundary of the left side of the rectum between peritoneum and mesorectum is dissected (arrow).

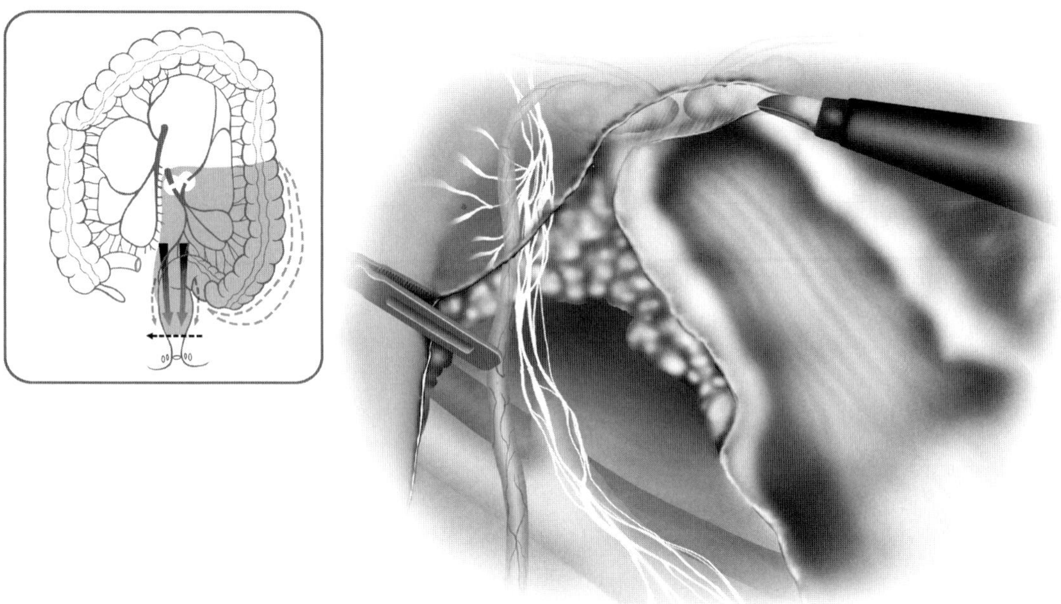

Figure 8.5.10. Next, the peritoneal reflection is incised, exposing Denonvilliers' fascia and protecting the seminal vesicles or vaginal wall.

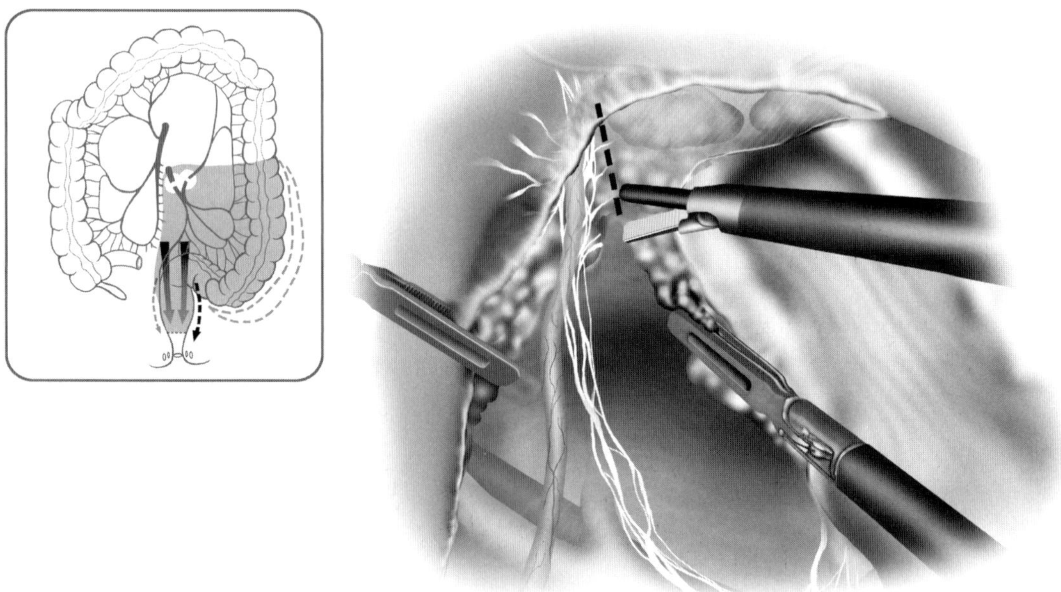

Figure 8.5.11. The lateral ligaments are placed under tension by drawing the rectum to the right side of the pelvis, then this area is dissected, carefully preserving the nerve trunks heading distally.

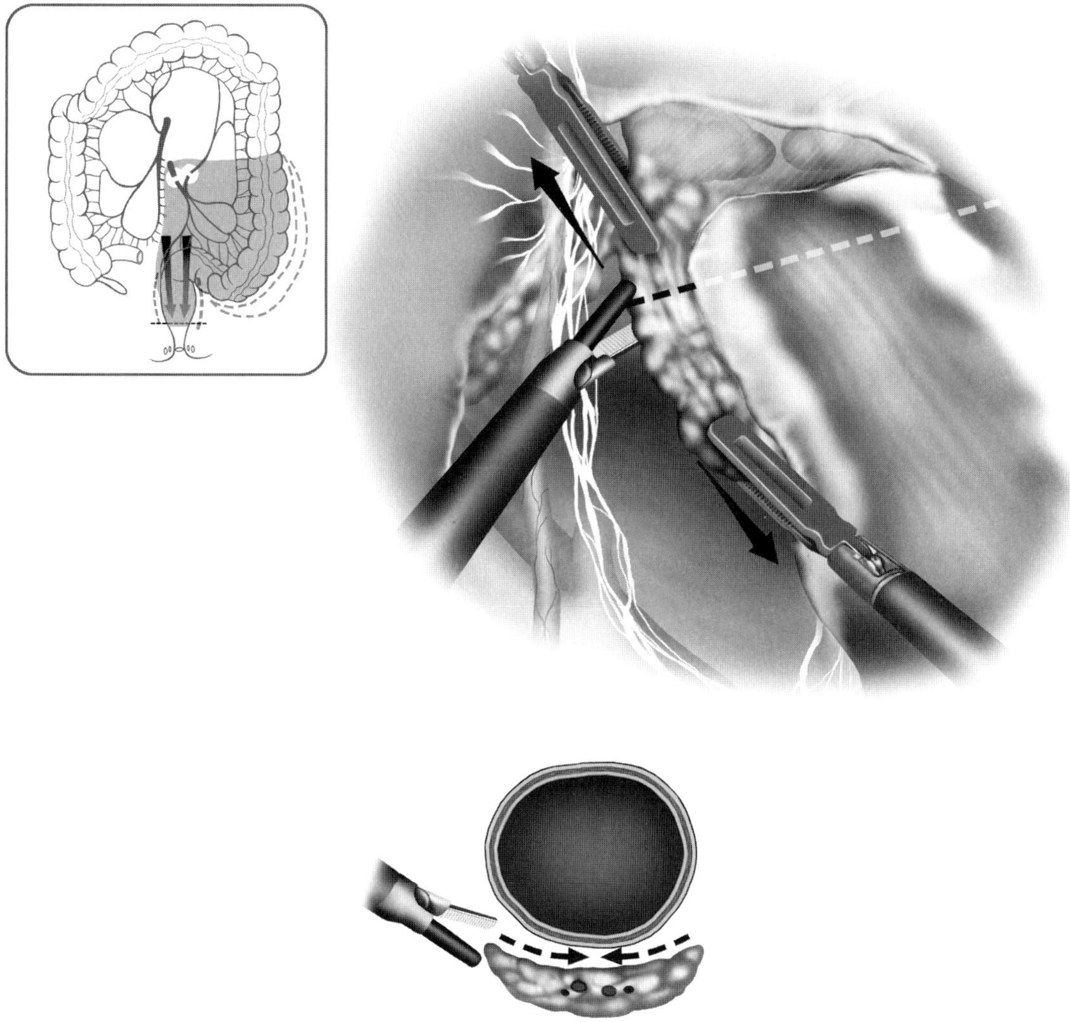

Figure 8.5.12. With tension applied to the left side of the rectum at the proposed transaction line, the mesorectum is divided using the laparoscopic coagulation shears.

lines posteriorly. We perform a distal rectal washout by grasping immediately below the tumor using a long bowel grasper, then perform rectal irrigation through a transanally placed catheter with a cytotoxic solution (e.g., 1% povidone iodine, 500 mL). Next, we introduce an endoscopic linear stapling device at right angles to the long axis of the rectum as much as possible, drawing the rectum cephalad and firing the stapler (Figure 8.5.13). If one cartridge of the stapler does not completely transect the rectum, we apply the second firing so as to overlap the initial suture line on the anal side.

Once the rectum is completely transected, the specimen side of the rectum is securely held using a grasping forceps from the suprapubic port, then this port site is incised to a length of about 3–5 cm in the

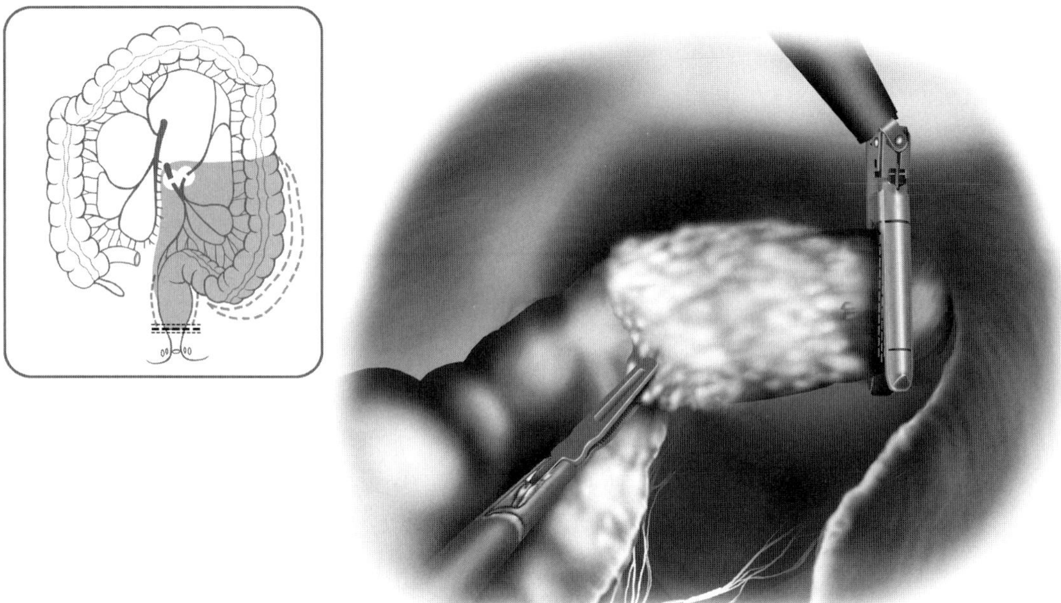

Figure 8.5.13. An endoscopic linear stapler is introduced through the suprapubic cannula and fired across the distal resection line at right angles to the bowel.

midline, and the specimen is drawn out of the peritoneal cavity after protecting the wound using a plastic ring drape or lap disk (Hakko Medical, Tokyo, Japan). The proximal resection is performed on the anterior abdominal wall using conventional techniques, and the specimen is removed. The center rod and anvil head are placed into the proximal bowel lumen and secured in place using a 2-0 polypropylene pursestring suture. The bowel is returned into the abdominal cavity, and this wound site is made airtight by placing a continuous suture on the peritoneum or by merely closing the lap disk. The pneumoperitoneum is restored in preparation for the anastomosis. The cavity of lesser pelvis is irrigated copiously, including the rectal stump. We generally use a cytotoxic solution (several 100 mL of povidone iodine 1% initially, then follow with saline). The anvil shaft is placed in the left iliac fossa, then the circular stapler is introduced from the anus. It is recommended that an experienced surgeon do this, and once the stapler is "crowning" at the top of the rectal stump, we attempt to have the spike of the stapler protrude from immediately below or immediately above the center of the suture line (Figure 8.5.14). The anastomosis must be performed very carefully so that the surrounding tissues (vagina, lateral pelvic tissues) are not caught in the anastomotic site. Before firing the stapler, we confirm that there is no torsion in the mesentery of the proximal colon, then the stapler may be fired (Figure 8.5.15). After resection, the staple line must be carefully observed to

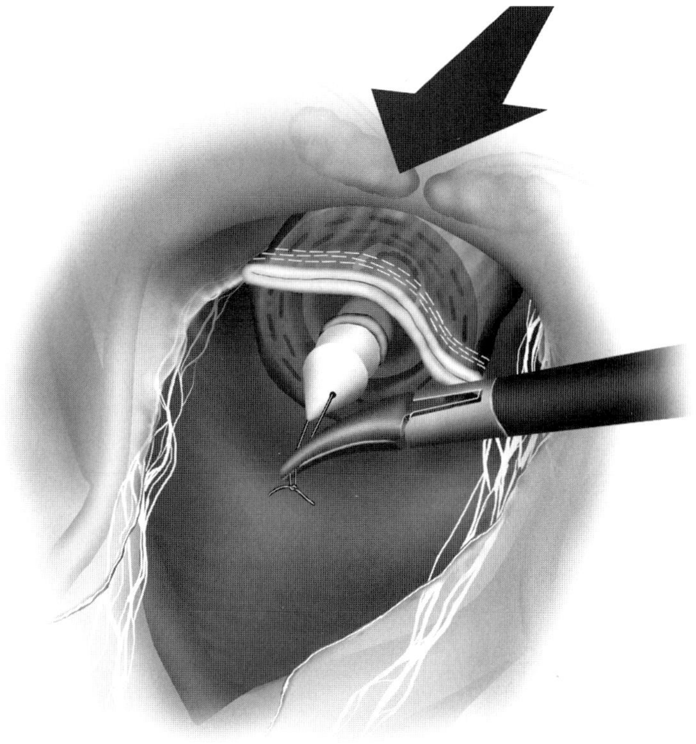

Figure 8.5.14. A transanally introduced circular stapler is placed at the top of the rectum and the spike is protruded through the wall just posterior to the linear staple line.

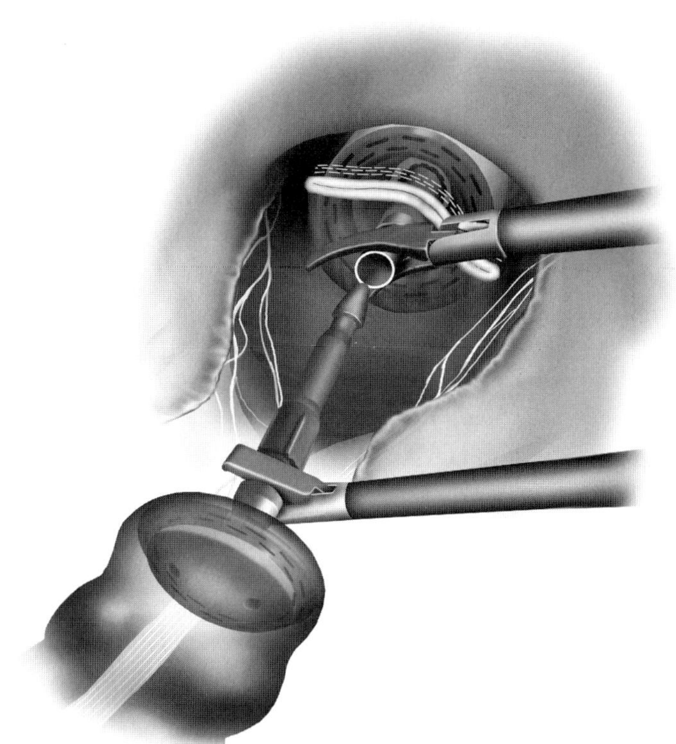

Figure 8.5.15. The double-stapled anastomosis is performed with all surrounding tissues clear of the two bowel ends.

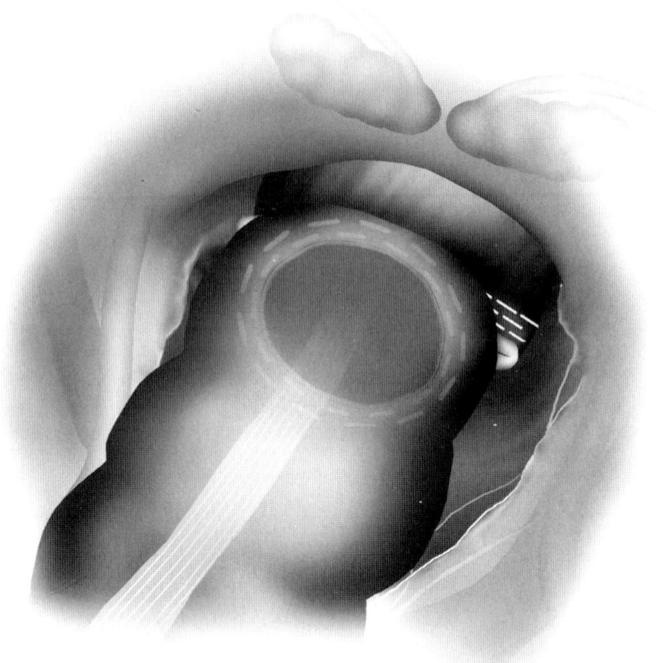

Figure 8.5.16. After resection, the staples should be evaluated to be sure there has been good "B" formation of the staples [both from laparoscopic and intraluminal (endoscopic) evaluation].

verify that the staples are aligned in a B-shape (Figure 8.5.16). The tissue rings removed by the circular stapler are inspected for completeness, then a leak test is done with air insufflation through the rectum while the pelvis is filled with saline and the bowel above the anastomosis is occluded with a bowel clamp. A closed suction drain is inserted into the pelvis from the port site of the left lower abdominal region, placing it near the anastomosis. The wounds are irrigated with saline and the wounds are closed using absorbable suture. We use a running size 0 or 1 suture for the fascia in the suprapubic area, and all cannula sites 10mm or greater are closed with size 0 sutures at the fascial level.

Special Considerations

The most important aspect of the mesenteric resection (for oncologic purposes of wide lymph node clearance) is exposure of the main mesenteric blood vessels with careful and accurate grasping/lifting of the veins/arteries. Because there is no tactile sensation, pulses of an artery must be visually verified whenever possible. Next, a shallow incision is made in the mesentery, and the adipose tissue is lifted up to explore the mesentery as the border between the adipose tissue and the blood vessels is dissected to expose the vascular wall. After this procedure, the surrounding tissue is dissected in directions parallel to and then vertical to the blood vessels. These procedures are performed so that the adventitia of the major blood vessels are finally dissected with curved forceps. This permits a length of the vascular wall to be exposed that is sufficient for safe clipping. The end of a clip must always reach beyond the blood vessel, but it is also dangerous to use a clip that is considerably larger than the vascular diameter (it may slip off). The clip applier also needs to be slightly tilted before clipping the vessel to check that a clip does not overlap another clip.

Perioperative hemorrhage can be also be a worrisome problem in laparoscopic colorectal surgery. The surgeon must be familiar with proper planes and how blood vessels run through the mesentery, and also know where hemorrhaging can easily occur in order to perform surgery with minimal hemorrhage. The proper planes that are important during dissection of the large intestine are:

1. The anterior layer of the Toldt's fusion fascia in dissection of the colon
2. The plane between the mesorectum and the presacral fascia
3. The plane between the anterior rectum and Denonvilliers' fascia in dissection of the rectum

During dissection/detachment of the colon, damage to the gonadal vessels and the ureters can be best avoided if the anterior plane of the Toldt's fusion fascia is maintained. In addition, the hypogastric plexus/hypogastric nerve/pelvic plexus can be best preserved without hemorrhaging if dissection of the rectum can be performed in the plane between the fascia propria of the mesorectum and the presacral fascia.

If the inferior mesenteric pedicle is not grasped tightly along with the mesentery, and the blood vessels slip away on the dorsal side of the mesentery that is being grasped, the isolation and ligation procedures can be dangerous. When blood vessels are handled, as much free space as possible should be created on the dorsal side as the direction of forceps-assisted dissection is alternated between the parallel and perpendicular directions in relation to the blood vessels. Even when an LCS is used for hemostasis/dissection of smaller unnamed vessels, these vessels must be coagulated several times before resection when they are large in diameter. The surgeon must also be careful not to damage blood vessels and organs with the tip of the active blade of the LCS and to keep the blade tip within the visual field. It may become quite hot with sustained use.

Blunt-tipped forceps without a ratchet mechanism should be used in handling the bowel, and the forceps should be used in a way so that the surgeon can feel the tissue using these forceps. The intestine should be grasped/pulled carefully and gently, and without straining its elasticity, so that the serosa will not be damaged. Misfire of the endoscopic stapling device during intracorporeal anastomosis must be dealt with appropriately (including the consideration for rapid conversion to an open operation), because this complication can lead to serious postoperative sequelae. A closeup visual inspection of the staple formation on the rectal stump should be undertaken each and every time by the surgeon, both right after the firing of the endoscopic stapler and when the circular stapler is placed into the rectum and pushed up to the top of the rectal stump. If the donut-shaped tissue formations contained within the circular staplers is incomplete, a leak testing should be done of the anastomosis, and additional suturing of any defect should be considered immediately, even if by laparotomy. Final consideration for the use of a proximal diverting stoma should always be considered if there is any question of the integrity of the final anastomosis.

Conclusions

Laparoscopic anterior resection is a relatively new surgical procedure that has many unresolved issues. However, improvements in surgical techniques and advances in equipment and instruments over the past 10 years have helped steadily solve the problems related to this procedure.

Editors' Comments

Indications: We agree with the author regarding his indications. Certain T3 and even T4 tumors are approachable with laparoscopic methods in our practice, but, in general, an open technique is preferable for large tumors of the rectum at this point in time.

Patient positioning: Same.

Instrumentation: We use the same instruments. A roticulating endoscopic stapler (one that can bend at the junction between the distal shaft and the stapler cartridge) is very useful in performing bowel resections in the pelvis.

Cannula positioning: We generally agree with their positioning.

Technique: There remain major unresolved issues in the low anterior resection performed by the laparoscopic method. Management of the distal rectal washout and the subsequent safe and accurate division of the rectum and low anastomosis are among the most pressing issues. What Dr. Watanabe describes is a well-illustrated technique for approaching tumors that are **not** in the distal half of the rectum. Current instruments, especially the endoscopic staplers, are often unwieldy in the deep pelvis, and we currently do not have the proper retracting tools and stapling instruments to comfortably perform many of the required steps when the resection and anastomosis are made deep in the pelvis, especially in even moderately obese patients. Because the distal rectal dissection with adequate clearance of the surrounding soft tissues (total mesorectal excision) represents one of the most critical oncologic issues for most patients, new methods and instrumentation must be developed in order to safely accomplish the laparoscopic low anterior resection by completely laparoscopic means. Currently, we often resort to the use of a hand-assisted method in order to accomplish the low resection and anastomosis (through open methods) because of these limitations (see Chapter 9.1).

The intrigue of this operation also lies in the tremendous ability to see clearly into the depths of the pelvis using the laparoscope. The need for new types of instrumentation is great, and we look forward to learning more about how to accomplish this operation completely laparoscopically as new tools emerge.

References

1. Watanabe M, Hasegawa H, Yamamoto S, et al. Laparoscopic surgery for stage I colorectal cancer. Surg Endosc 2003;17:1274–1277.
2. Hasegawa H, Kabeshima Y, Watanabe M, et al. Randomized controlled trial of laparoscopic versus open colectomy for advanced colorectal cancer. Surg Endosc 2003;17:636–640.
3. Yamamoto S, Watanabe M, Hasegawa H, et al. Prospective evaluation of laparoscopic surgery for rectosigmoidal and rectal carcinoma. Dis Colon Rectum 2002;45:1648–1654.

Chapter 8.6

Laparoscopic Abdominoperineal Resection

Jeffrey W. Milsom, Bartholomäus Böhm, and Kiyokazu Nakajima

Indications

The primary indication for the abdominoperineal resection (APR) is a malignant disease in which the tumor is encroaching on or invading the anal sphincters or the pelvic floor adjacent to them. Nearly always this will be a low-lying adenocarcinoma of the rectum, but other less common indications may be epidermoid anal canal carcinomas (squamous cell, cloacogenic, or basaloid carcinomas unresponsive to radiochemotherapy), or a gynecologic malignancy that has also proven unresponsive to chemoradiotherapy and is now invading the pelvic floor, or other rare tumors such as sarcomas. A complete excision of the rectum, with excision of the pelvic floor and anal sphincters (e.g., the APR) should not be considered in patients with benign diseases. A similar operation may be considered in certain benign conditions such as Crohn's disease in which proctectomy with intersphincteric anal excision must be done, when there is severe involvement of the anal area with the disease. In distinction to the APR, in proctectomy for benign disease, a large portion of the external anal sphincters and the entire pelvic floor otherwise are left intact.

There are no specific contraindications for the laparoscopic approach compared with open surgery, except that in certain instances, where the tumor is invading into adjacent organs extensively or where the tumor is massive in size (greater than 8 cm in greatest diameter), we would not advocate a laparoscopic approach.

Patient Positioning and Operating Room Setup

The patient is placed supine in the modified lithotomy position using stirrups. Surgery is begun in Trendelenburg position (20° head-down tilt), and after cannula insertion, the patient is tilted right side down. For the entire laparoscopic operation, the surgeon and second assistant (who acts as the camera holder) stand on the patient's right side looking at a monitor placed near the patient's left knee with the first assistant stand-

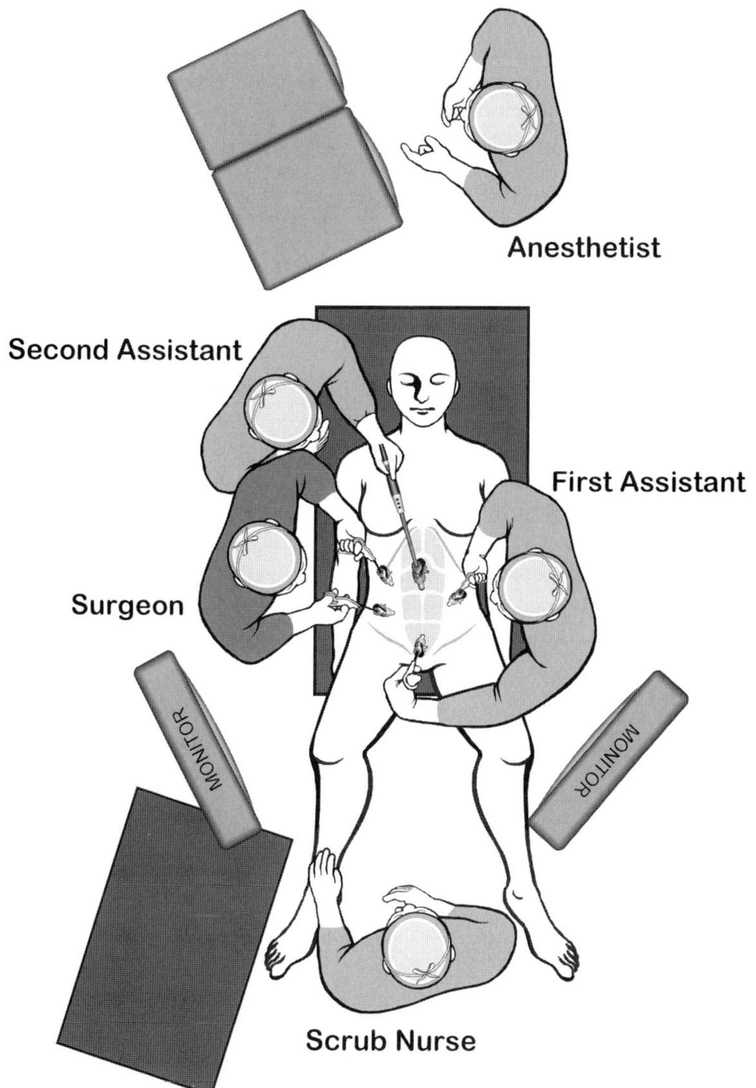

Figure 8.6.1. Positions of the equipment and the surgical team for the laparoscopic APR.

ing to the patient's left side looking at a monitor placed near the right knee (Figure 8.6.1). Alternatively, the first assistant may stand between the legs for the dissection of the inferior mesenteric artery (IMA) pedicle. The nurse may stand between the legs or just below and to the left of the left knee, with his operating table located to his left, depending on the position of the first assistant.

Instruments

Specific instruments recommended for laparoscopic APR are listed in Table 8.6.1.

Table 8.6.1. Specific instruments recommended for laparoscopic APR

5	Cannulae (1 × 12 mm, 1 × 10 mm, 2–3 × 5 mm)
1	Dissecting device (i.e., LigaSure V™ or Ultrasonic Shears™ or electrosurgery)
1	Laparoscopic scissors
1	Laparoscopic dissector
1	Laparoscopic right-angled dissector
2	Laparoscopic graspers
1	Endoscopic stapler

Cannula Positioning

The cannulae are positioned in the umbilical region (above or below, depending on the size of the patient). If the patient is thin, just below the umbilicus is usually best. If the patient has a large and dependent pannus, somewhere above the umbilicus is better, usually about 23–25 cm above the symphysis pubis. Other cannulae are placed in the right and left upper and lower lateral abdominal wall. The proposed stoma site is not used for a cannula, because this is almost always located too far medial (Figure 8.6.2).

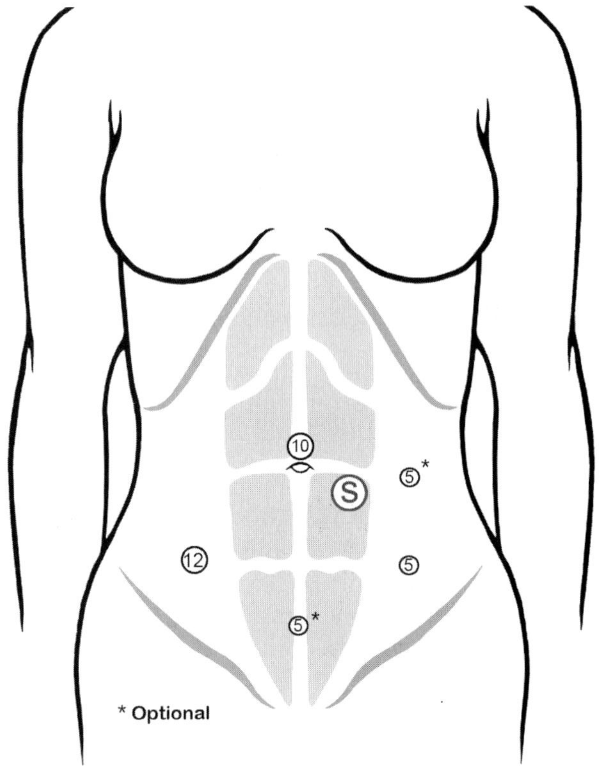

Figure 8.6.2. Positions of the cannulae for the laparoscopic APR. Note that the proposed colostomy site is *not* used as a cannula site, because it is usually too close to the (optical) port through which the laparoscope is used.

Technique

The patient is placed in a steep Trendelenburg position and the cannulae are inserted with tilting the patient to the right or left as the contralateral cannulae are placed. Sutures for later closure of the 10- and 12-mm cannulae are immediately placed using a suture passer needle device (Karl Storz, Tübingen, Germany) using a size 0 absorbable material.

Initial Exploration

A careful exploration of the entire peritoneal cavity is done, starting with the right upper quadrant, and focusing on the liver, because this is an operation done only for malignancy (see Chapter 10.1). The liver is initially examined by placing the patient in some degree of reverse Trendelenburg. Cannulae from the upper quadrants may be used to turn the inferior edges of the liver cephalad, so as to examine the undersurfaces. The porta hepatis and gallbladder are also assessed. The other quadrants and the peritoneal surfaces are next examined, and as the operation shifts to the lower abdomen, the patient is tilted into Trendelenburg position, with the right side down. This helps to shift the small intestine into the right upper quadrant. The greater omentum is retracted into the upper abdomen, above the colon if possible, and all small intestinal loops are retracted out of the pelvic area.

Dissection of the Inferior Mesenteric Artery

The dissection commences as the first assistant, either from the left side of the abdomen or alternatively from between the legs, exposes the IMA for the surgeon. This is done by retracting the mesosigmoid in a ventrolateral direction using bowel graspers from the left upper and lower quadrants. The surgeon incises the peritoneum to the right of the superior rectal artery starting at the sacral promontory (Figure 8.6.3). Under continuous traction, the peritoneum is incised cephalad toward the origin of the IMA. Using a combination of gentle spreading and electrosurgical dissection, the IMA is swept ventrally and the preaortic hypogastric neural plexus is swept dorsally to prevent injury. Small visceral branches of the nerves, supplying the colon and upper rectum, may be safely divided, while carefully preserving the main trunks leading into the pelvis, then the IMA is divided using a LigaSure device or endoscopic stapler (Figure 8.6.4).

Dissection then is continued medially beneath the artery, and the left ureter and gonadal vessels are identified and swept posteriorly (Figure 8.6.5). Tension is placed on the left colon and its mesenteric attachments by applying medial and cephalad traction with graspers, which should not be used to directly grasp the intestine, thus minimizing the chance of inadvertent visceral injury. If the left ureter cannot be identified easily from the medial approach, the lateral attachments of the sigmoid colon are incised, the sigmoid colon is mobilized left to right, and the gonadal vessels and ureter are identified and freed from the mesentery. It is helpful in this instance to place a cotton gauze sponge on top of these retroperitoneal structures (between them and the posterior aspect of the

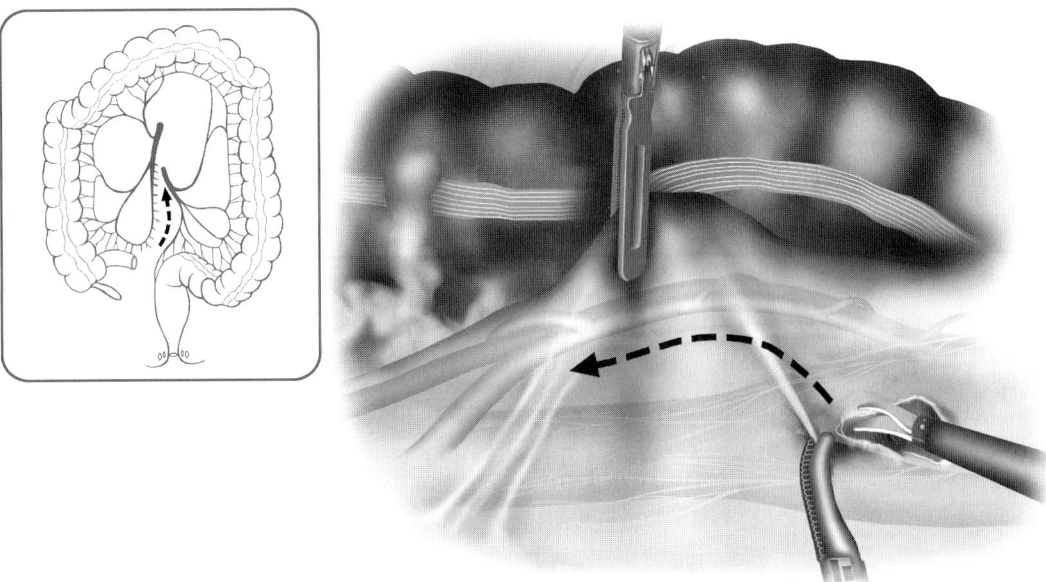

Figure 8.6.3. Initial dissection involves incising the peritoneum just to the right of the superior rectal artery just at the sacral promontory and working cephalad.

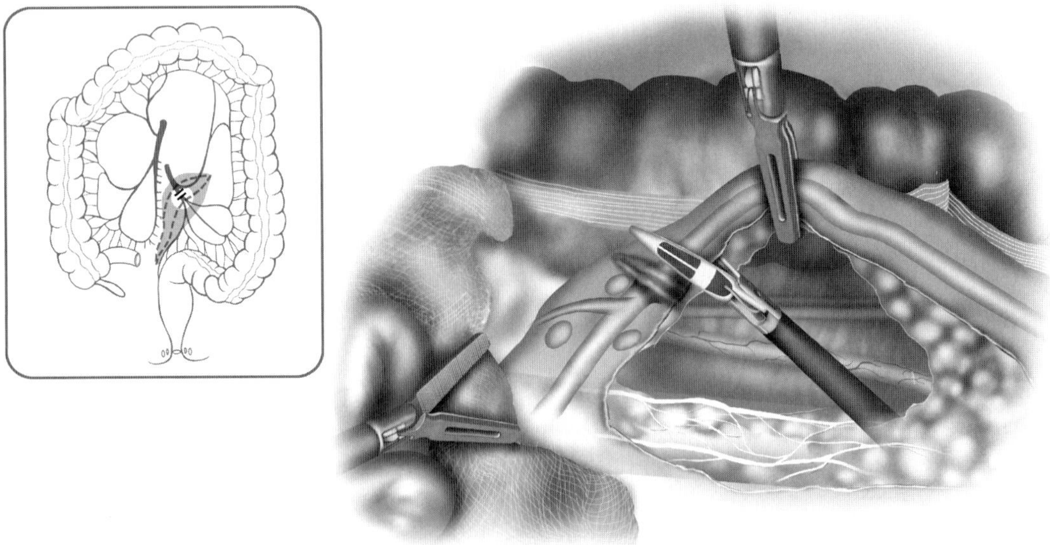

Figure 8.6.4. The IMA is divided using a LigaSure 5 mm device, dividing small visceral branches of the hypogastric nerves, but preserving the main trunks leading into the pelvis.

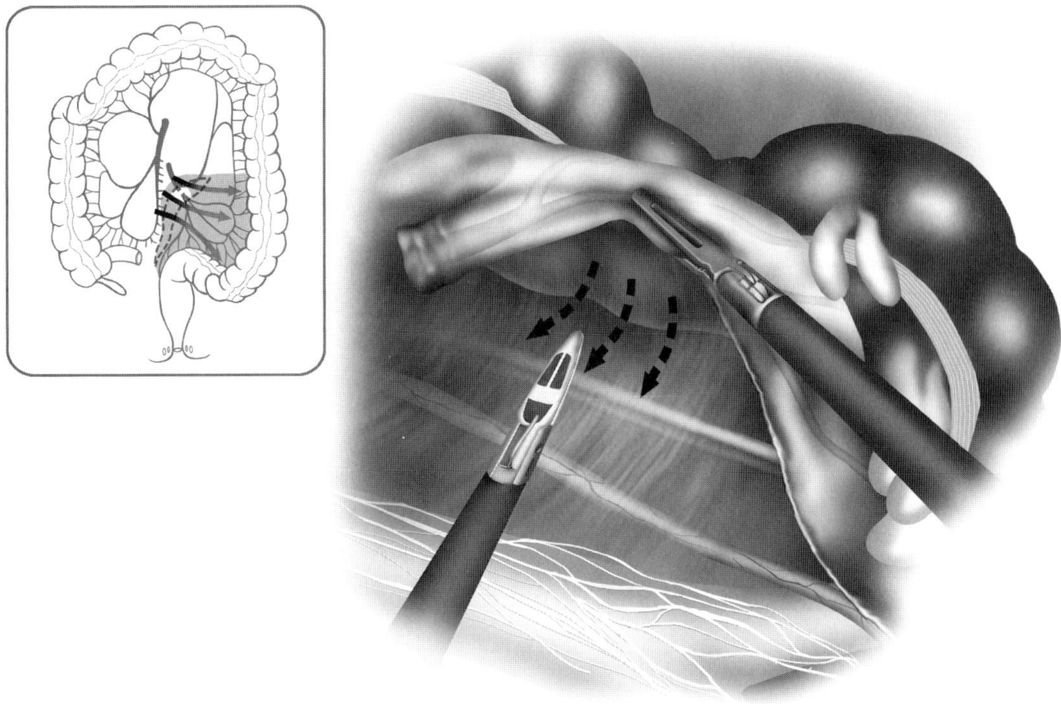

Figure 8.6.5. Dissection is then continued *medial* to *lateral* beneath the divided IMA, identifying and sweeping the ureter and gonadal vessels posteriorly.

sigmoid colon mesentery), thus when the surgical team goes back to the medial aspect of the IMA, the gauze immediately separates the ureter and gonadal vessels from the mesentery about to be divided (Figure 8.6.6 with inset).

With the IMA identified and ligated, the peritoneum is incised anteriorly over the pedicle, dissecting leftward toward the inferior mesenteric vein (IMV). Careful dissection with a right-angled dissector is used to create a peritoneal window just lateral to the IMA and IMV. This pedicle is ligated above or below the left colic artery (according to the surgeon's judgment) using a LigaSure device, but only if the left ureter can be clearly identified and retracted to avoid injury (Figure 8.6.7). We prefer to leave the IMA and IMV 1.0–1.5 cm long so that if any bleeding occurs, an additional grasping of the vessel is possible with application of another seal of the LigaSure device (or alternatively looping by an endoscopic loop can be done).

Proximal Division of the Mesentery and Sigmoid Colon

The lateral attachments of the sigmoid colon are dissected free, and the sigmoid colon is completely mobilized using a sharp and blunt dissection as in open surgery (Figure 8.6.8). Again, great care should be taken to identify and avoid any injury to the hypogastric nerves, gonadal vessels,

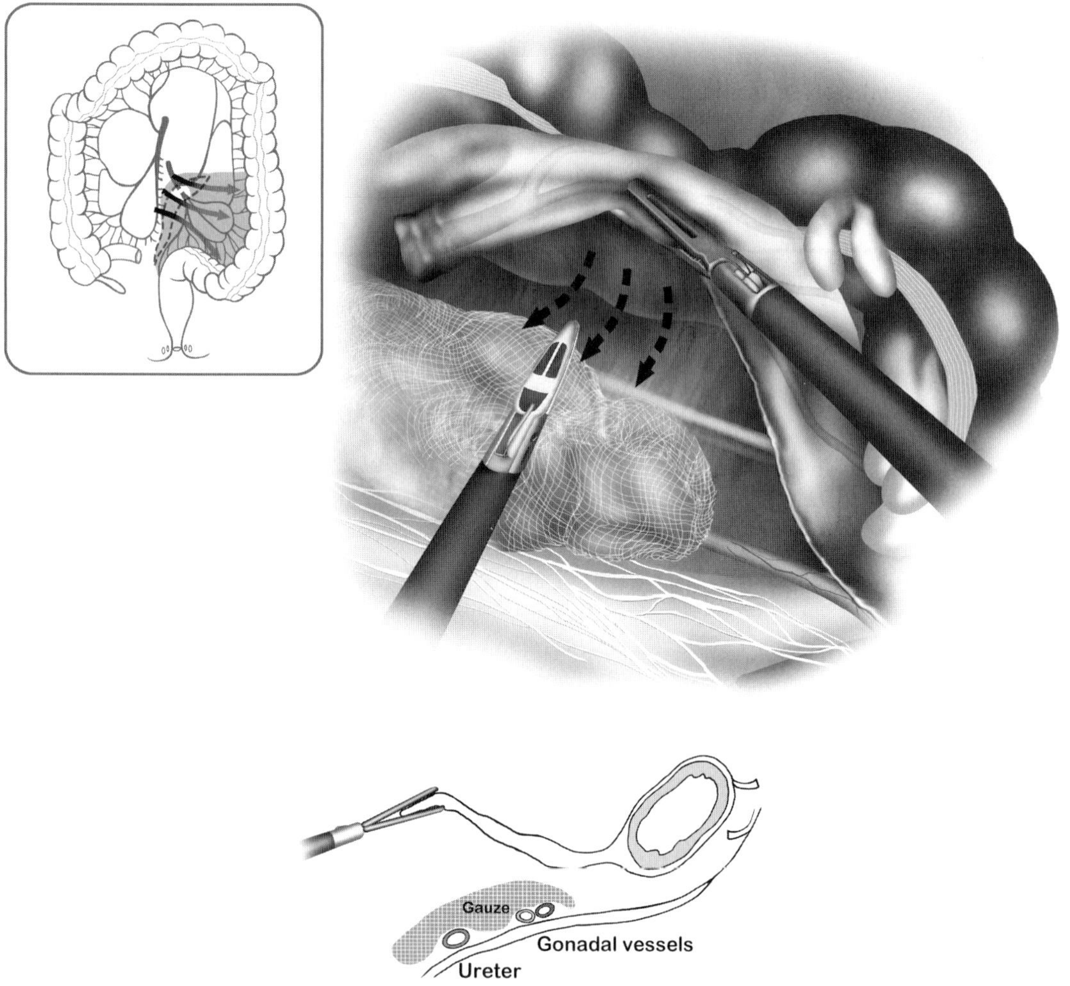

Figure 8.6.6. When the ureter cannot be easily identified on the medial side, dissection should then proceed laterally, identifying and placing a cotton gauze over the ureter. Returning to the medial side, vessel ligation may proceed with the firm knowledge that the ureter is protected beneath the gauze.

or the ureter. The mesosigmoid (or the proximal resection line just to the left of the inferior mesenteric pedicle) is held using "triangulating tension," as described in Chapter 4 and transected up to the proximal intestinal resection line. This is where the LigaSure device may be especially useful, and expeditious (Figure 8.6.9). The colon is divided with a cartridge of a 45- or 55-mm endoscopic stapler (Figure 8.6.10). The pelvic portion of the operation is now ready to begin.

Rectal Mobilization

The rectum is completely mobilized down to the pelvic floor, applying standard open total mesorectal excision (TME) surgical principles. If the first assistant was between the legs, this person now goes to the left side of the patient for the duration of the rectal dissection. The dissection is commenced with posterior mobilization, working between the fascia

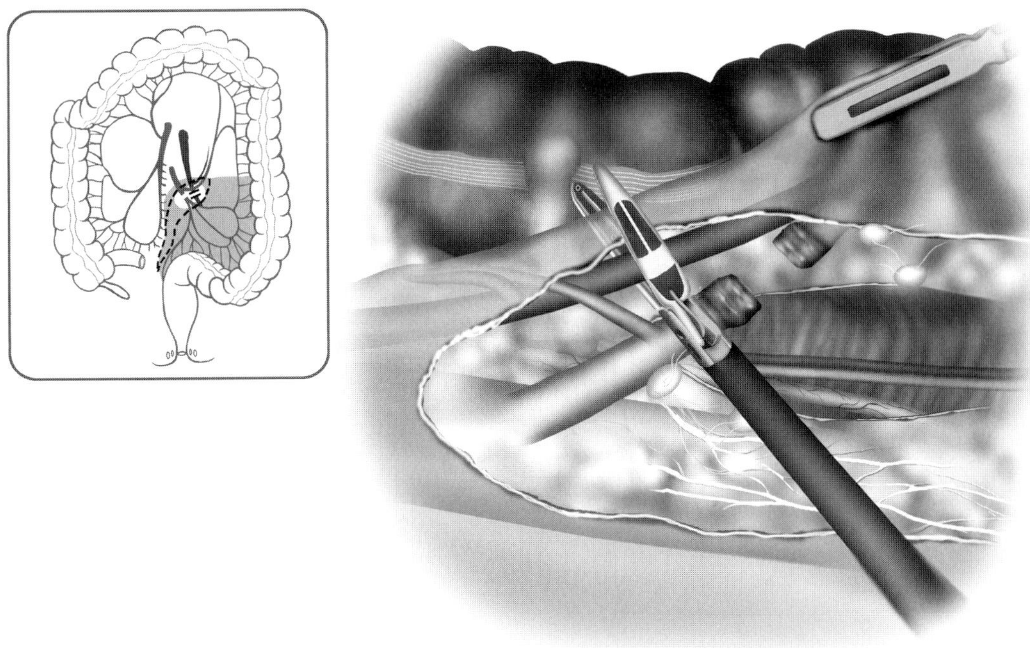

Figure 8.6.7. The IMV is ligated only if the ureter is identified and protected.

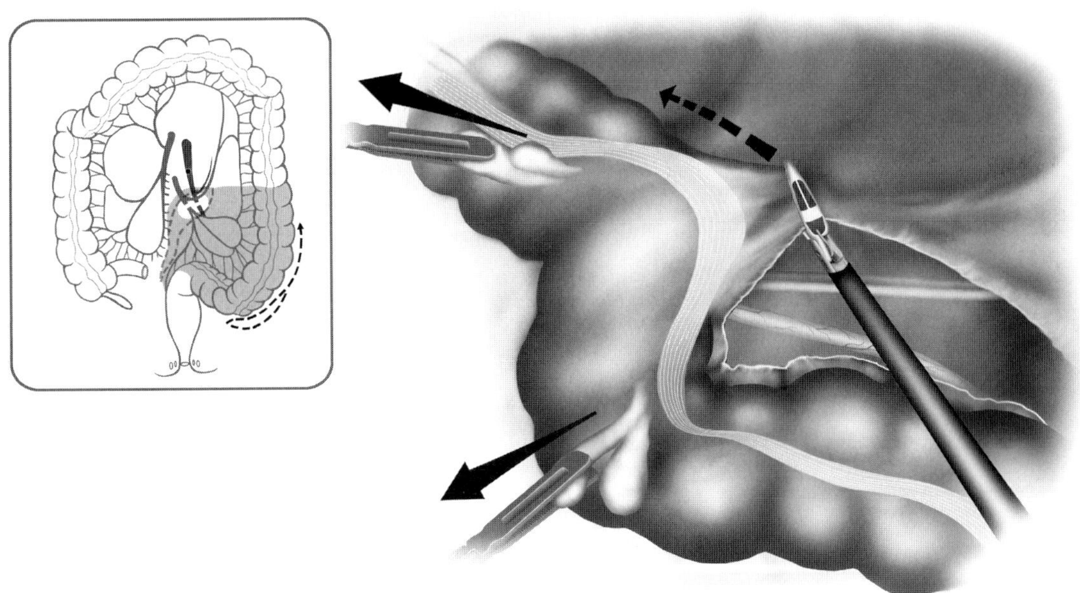

Figure 8.6.8. The lateral attachments of the sigmoid colon are next incised sharply.

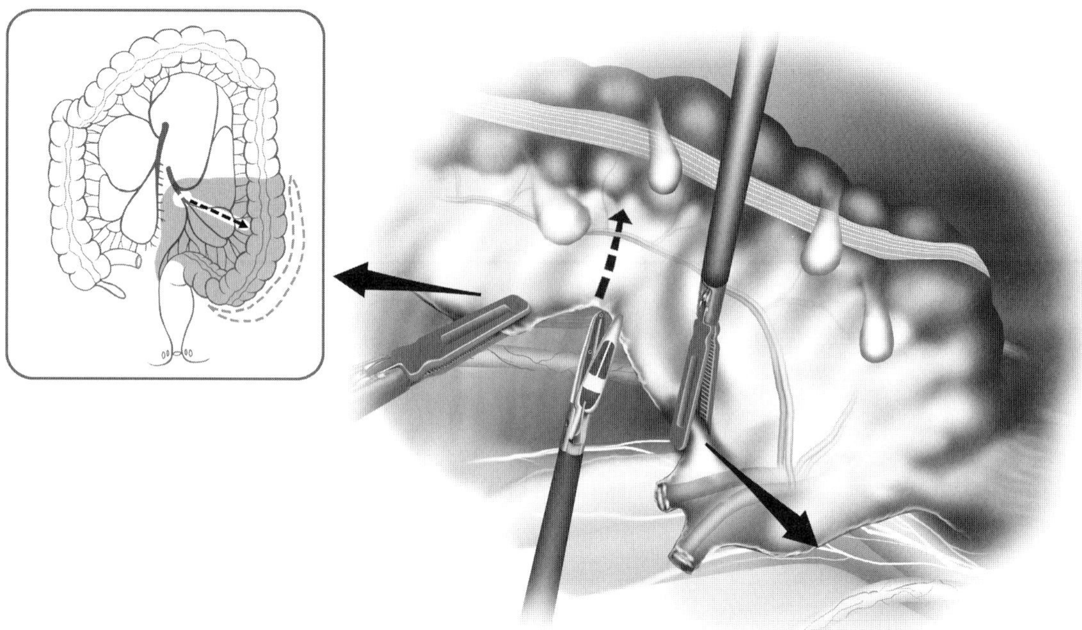

Figure 8.6.9. Using triangulating tension, the sigmoid mesocolon is incised up to the bowel edge.

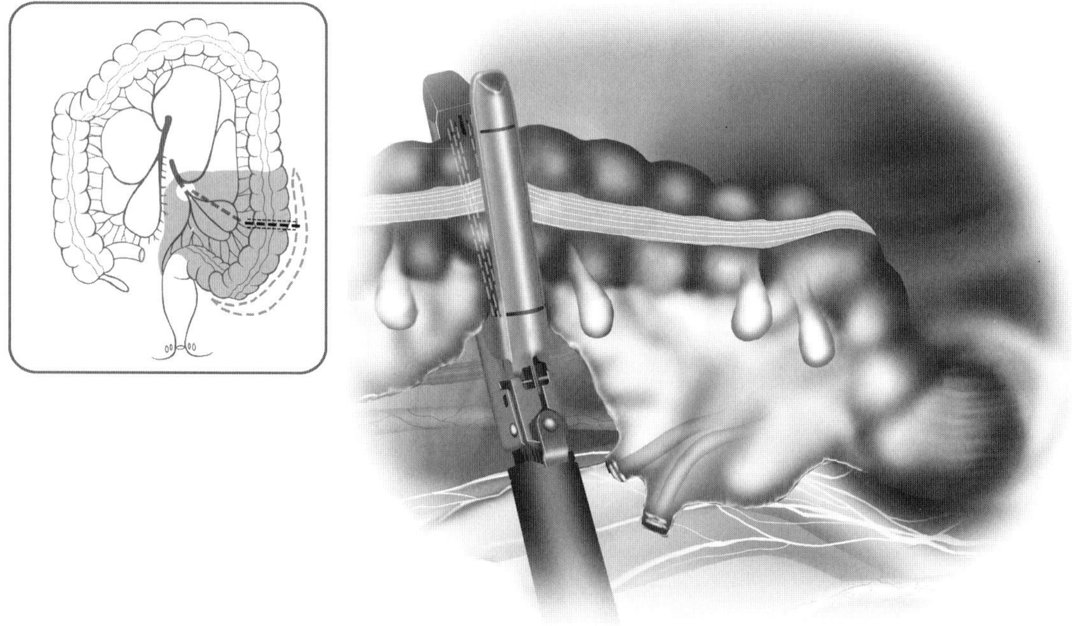

Figure 8.6.10. The proximal resection line is next incised with an endoscopic stapler.

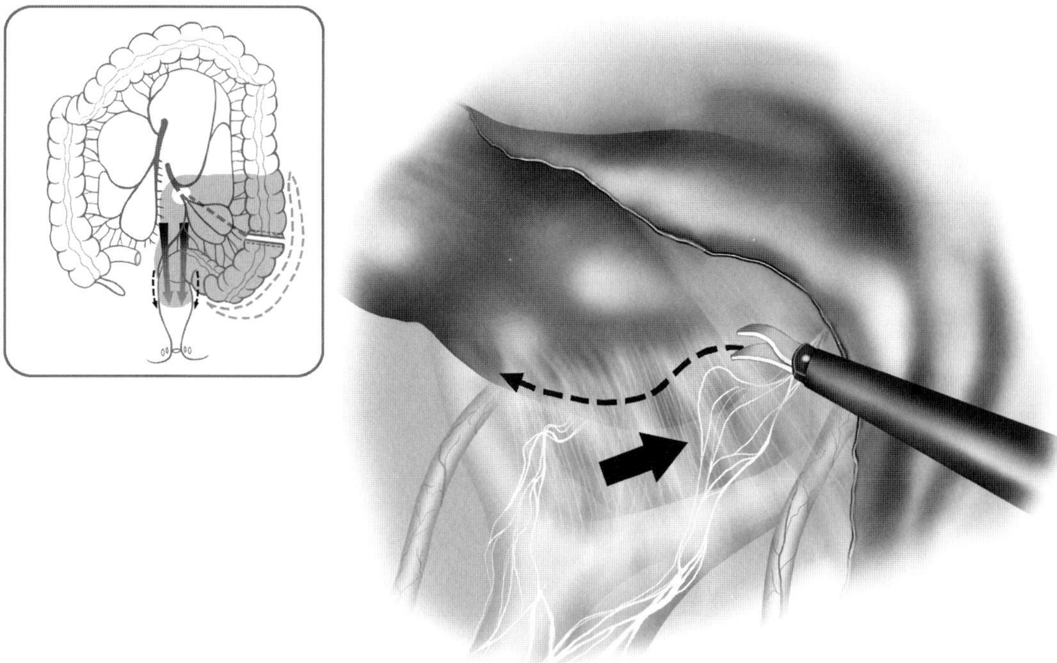

Figure 8.6.11. Posterior mobilization is initiated next at the sacral promontory, carefully sweeping off the hypogastric nerve branches which may be tented upward in the line of dissection (arrows).

propria of the rectum and the presacral fascia, initially dissecting sharply using electrosurgery, the LigaSure device, or alternatively a harmonic scalpel, as far distally as possible (Figure 8.6.11). Dissection is continued posterolaterally to the right and left sides of the rectum, dividing the flimsy peritoneum overlying the proximal rectum, carefully and continuously sweeping the hypogastric nerves trunks posteriorly and laterally. The laparoscopic magnification provided by nearly all types of scopes provides 15–20 × magnification, and this certainly affords excellent views of the pelvic structures, including theses nerves.

If the proper plane is entered posteriorly, no bleeding will occur, and the connective tissue in this plane can be divided easily (Figure 8.6.12). The assistant provides traction by using the left hand grasper to pick up the cut edge of the peritoneum on the right side of the rectum, and the right hand grasper is opened and used to lift the mesorectum anteriorly and superiorly, separating it from the anterior sacrum. The cycle of dissecting posteriorly, laterally first on the right and then on the left is repeated over and over until the tip of the coccyx and beyond is reached, without any significant anterior dissection being done yet.

The lateral stalks are most usefully divided using the LigaSure device, although the Harmonic Scalpel may also be a useful tool. Both have the advantage over standard electrosurgery in that less smoke is generated,

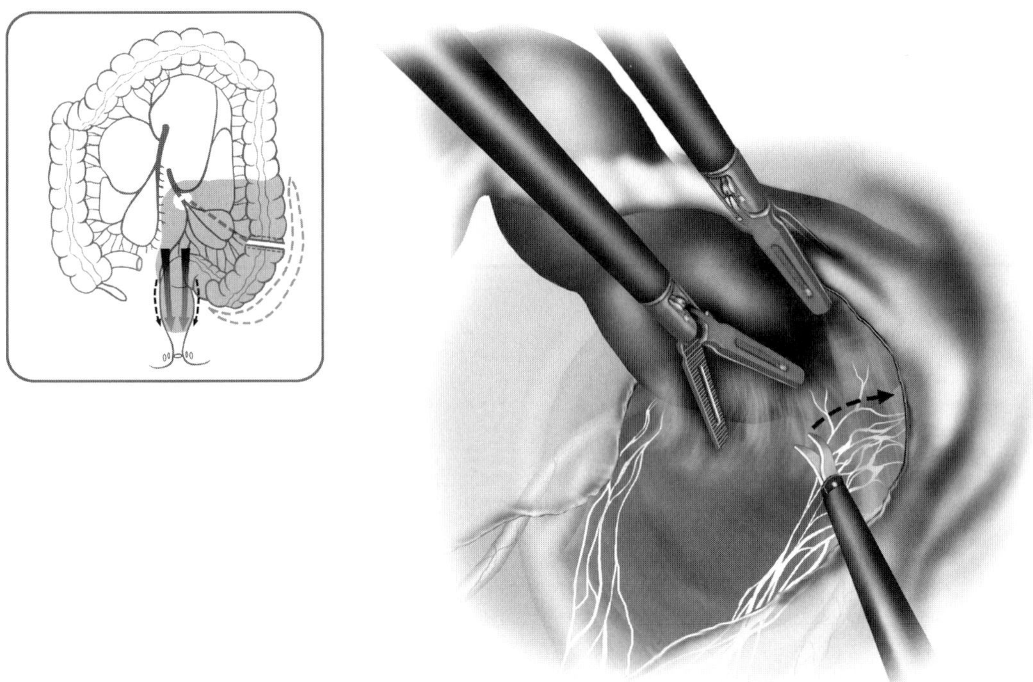

Figure 8.6.12. As the posterior rectal mobilization proceeds, the hypogastric nerves may be well visualized and protected.

and larger vessels may be closed using them. The LigaSure may be useful for nearly all vessels encountered in the pelvic dissection. Care is taken to separate the pelvic nerve plexus from the rectum at the level of the lateral stalks, unless there is suspected direct tumor invasion at this level (Figure 8.6.13).

The anterior plane, at the pelvic cul-de-sac, is struck usually after most of the posterior and lateral dissection has been completed. The first assistant uses the left hand to retract the anterior portion of the reflection anteriorly, and the right hand to retract the rectum superiorly and posteriorly, whereas the surgeon uses the left hand to retract the rectum medially (for the right side of the dissection) and the right hand is dividing tissue using the LigaSure or similar device. The key manuever is to go from "known to unknown," usually meaning posterior to lateral, and to avoid dissecting into the vagina or through Denonvilliers' fascia unless the tumor is infiltrative there. It may be highly useful to use the surgeon's doubly gloved hand, passed into the anus or vagina from the perineum, to sound out the vagina or rectum at this point, in order to remain in the proper plane at all times (Figure 8.6.14).

Once the surgical team is confident that dissection has been performed circumferentially to the pelvic floor, the surgeon should again put on a second sterile glove over the right hand, and place this hand into the rectum (and in women, the vagina) to perform bimanual palpation in order to confirm complete rectal dissection to the pelvic floor level.

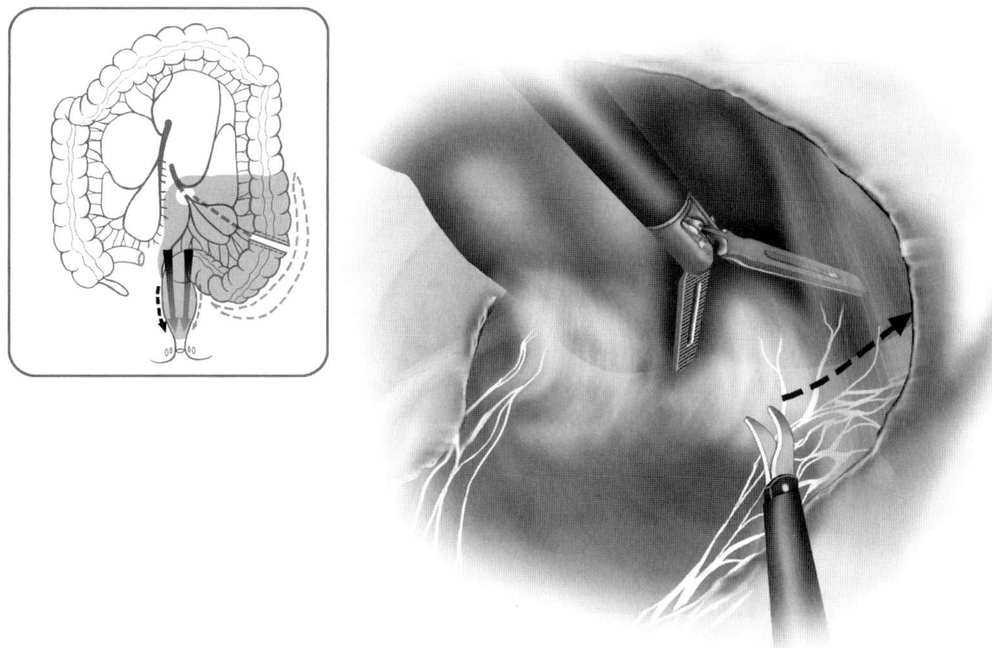

Figure 8.6.13. At the level of the lateral stalks, the pelvic plexus can be preserved unless there is direct tumor infiltration.

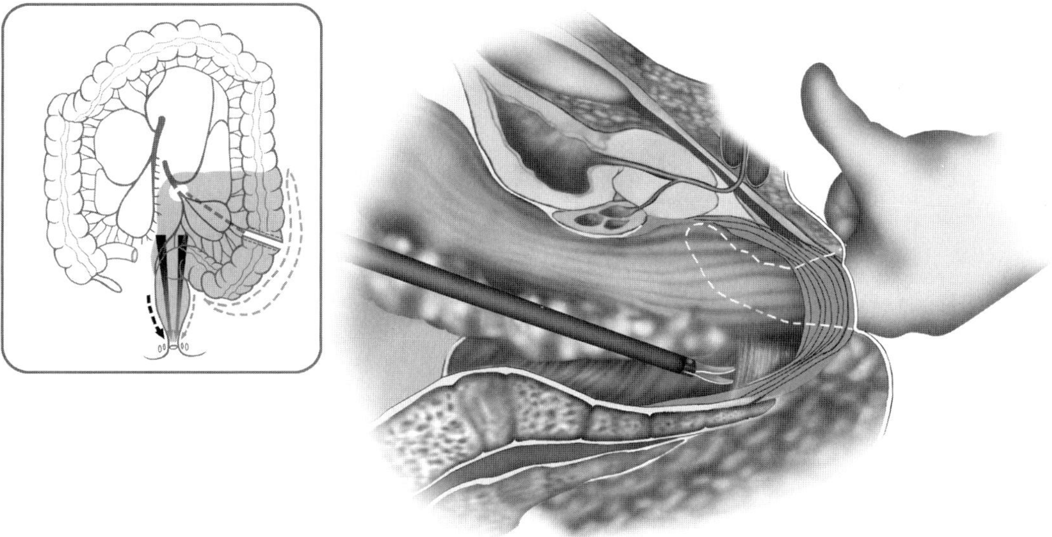

Figure 8.6.14. It may be highly useful to use the surgeon's doubly-gloved index finger to sound out the rectum or vagina in the distal rectal dissection, confirming the proper plane of dissection.

The Perineal Phase

One surgeon commences the perineal portion of the operation while the other maintains a laparoscopic control of this phase. Additionally, the CO_2 pneumoperitoneum is continued, because this actually helps alert the perineal surgeon to the proper plane as the perineal dissection proceeds (a gush of CO_2 signals the joining of the two dissections). The continued pneumoperitoneum also permits lifting of the specimen by an abdominal surgeon as the perineal surgeon dissects posteriorly, abetting the above. The abdominal surgeon may also palpate various points in the pelvis to direct the perineal dissection ("intelligent" perineal dissection).

The perineal surgeon sets up the operation by first suturing the anus closed using a large pursestring suture, then sterilely preps and drapes the patient, in keeping with oncologic principles. The adjustable stirrups are used to raise the legs, thus better exposing the perineum, but encroaching somewhat on the abdominal surgeon's field. Just as in the rectal dissection, the surgery is performed using a dissection pattern of 1) posterior, 2) lateral, then 3) anterior using an elliptical incision (Figure 8.6.15 with inset). The pelvic cavity is entered posteriorly initially, with release of the pneumoperitoneum, then perineal excision of the anus and rectum is completed out in a standard manner. Temporarily, the CO_2 insufflation is shut off. The perineal surgeon then removes the specimen, irrigation is accomplished from above and captured in a basin by this surgeon. A cytotoxic solution may be used as the initial irrigant if the surgeon desires. After irrigation, a silicon drain is passed through one of the lower quadrant cannula sites, grasped with an endoscopic grasper by the perineal surgeon, pulled into the pelvis, and properly positioned. After inspecting and securing hemostasis, the perineal surgeon closes the pelvic wound using interrupted sutures. The specimen is opened and inspected in the operating room to ensure that all margins are clear. A photodocumentation is made of the unopened and opened specimen.

The Colostomy Formation and Laparoscopic Closure

Pneumoperitoneum is reestablished. The preselected colostomy site is prepared from the skin level down to the posterior sheath in standard manner, then a 5-mm cannula is inserted. From the right side of the patient, the laparoscopic surgeon grasps the distal end of the descending colon through the right lower quadrant cannula site, and passes this up to the anterior wall beneath the stoma site. The colon is transferred to another grasper there, with a final check that there is no tension on the colon. The colostomy then is created by withdrawing the cannula from this site, dilating the fascia up to a width of two finger breadths, and then pulling the bowel end up to the skin level. After pulling the colon through the abdominal wall, the laparoscope is inserted into the right lower quadrant cannula, and the left colon is examined to ensure that it has not twisted as it passed from the left side of the abdomen to the anterior wall. The pelvis is then once again irrigated by placing the patient in the head-up position and using the right lower quadrant cannula site for insertion of an irrigation catheter. The abdominal cavity is carefully assessed lapa-

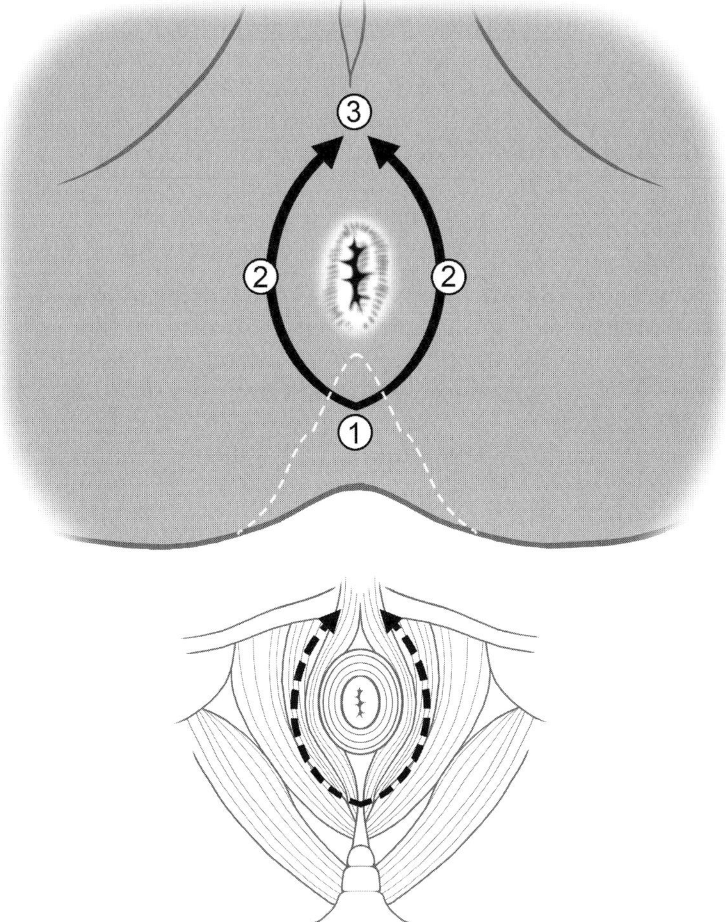

Figure 8.6.15. Just as in the rectal mobilization, the perineal phase of the operation is most safely performed in a pattern of 1) posterior, 2) lateral, and 3) anterior dissection. Inset: Anatomic view of the coccyx posteriorly and the pelvic floor and anal sphincter muscles with the perineal dissection.

roscopically for any sign of hemorrhage, particularly at all vascular pedicles and areas of dissection.

The cannula sites are closed, including at the skin level, and occlusive dressings are placed over them. The colostomy is matured in a standard manner and the operation is completed.

Special Considerations

The laparoscopic APR is remarkable in that no specimen is removed via the abdominal wall, thus the patient receives abdominal incisions only for cannulae and the stoma. The key issues relating to complications for the laparoscopic APR are similar to those encountered in the open procedure: Avoidance of injury to the hypogastric and pelvic nerves, ureters, and gonadal vessels, coupled with safe and adequate resection of the malignancy. By utilizing the above techniques and special considerations we have highlighted, the common pitfalls of this operation may be avoided. Naturally, we also advocate that any confusion or uncertainties about how to proceed laparoscopically should immediately compel the surgical team to convert to an open procedure.

Conclusions

The laparoscopic approach to complete excision of the rectum, anus, and pelvic floor including the anal sphincters is an extensive operation, but offers the patient the opportunity to avoid any large abdominal wall incisions. This may speed recovery, and decrease surgical pain, and thus is an attractive alternative to the open operation if the surgical team is experienced in these techniques. By using the above step by step method, we believe that most laparoscopic surgeons may confidently achieve a safe and oncologically sound operation.

Chapter 8.7

Total Abdominal Colectomy

Hermann Kessler

Laparoscopic total abdominal colectomy is defined by laparoscopic mobilization and removal of the entire colon from the ileocecal valve to the rectosigmoid junction at the sacral promontory.

Indications

Except for cancer, the indications for laparoscopic total abdominal colectomy are basically the same as in open surgery. For less experienced laparoscopic surgeons, however, further restrictions may apply such as previous operations with formation of intraabdominal adhesions, obesity, or fistula formation, because these conditions may make laparoscopic orientation and accessibility difficult.[1,2] This is especially true for the anatomic regions of the omentum, transverse colon, and mesocolon including its vessels. If the laparoscopic approach proves to be difficult, early conversion is recommended. In Crohn's disease, extensive colonic involvement or pancolitis with rectal sparing is an indication for total abdominal colectomy.[3–5] It may also be indicated in rare cases of ulcerative colitis with minimal rectal involvement but still carries the risk of leaving behind the principally diseased rectum with all its consequences.[6–10] In familial adenomatous polyposis, the situation is similar. If restorative proctocolectomy is not applicable, with rectal sparing and no evidence of dysplasia, with the absence of rectal cancer, and the patient's understanding of the need for future follow-up, total abdominal colectomy and ileorectal anastomosis is an option.[11,12] Assuming the failure of an aggressive prolonged conservative treatment including the trial of laxatives and fiber, in slow transit constipation, total abdominal colectomy is indicated after a thorough endoscopic, radiologic, and physiologic examination.[13–17] The indication for total colectomy in colonic cancer may occur in rare cases of two or more synchronous early carcinomas at two separate locations. In the majority of such cases, however, lymph node dissection of the middle colic vessels will also be necessary, which is technically demanding and should be undertaken only by highly experienced laparoscopic surgeons.[18,19]

Patient Positioning and Operating Room Setup

The patient is placed supine in the modified lithotomy position with the back and both thighs being at one level. Surgery is begun in the Trendelenburg position (20° head-down tilt). Cannulae are inserted and the patient is tilted right side down.

Phase I: Transection of the Inferior Mesenteric Artery and Vein, Medial Dissection of the Left Mesocolon, Pelvic Dissection, Left Lateral Mobilization of the Sigmoid Colon, and Transection of the Upper Rectum

For the first phase of the operation, the surgeon and the second assistant (who acts as the camera person) stand on the patient's right side looking at a monitor placed near the patient's left knee, and the first assistant stands on the patient's left side looking at a monitor near the right knee. The nurse stands between the patient's legs (Figure 8.7.1A).

Phase II: Mobilization of the Left Colon and the Splenic Flexure, Dissection of the Omentum

For the second phase of the operation, the surgeon stands between the patient's legs and both assistants stand on the patient's right side. The patient is moved into the reverse-Trendelenburg position (10° head-up tilt). The entire laparoscopic team looks at the monitor placed near the patient's left shoulder. The nurse moves to a position near the patient's left knee (Figure 8.7.1B).

Phase III: Transection of the Ileocolic and Middle Colic Vessels, Medial and Lateral Mobilization of the Right Colon and the Hepatic Flexure

During the third phase of the operation, the surgeon remains in the same position, whereas the first assistant and the camera person shift to the patient's left side. The nurse moves to a location near the patient's right knee, and the monitor located originally near the patient's right knee is shifted to a position near the right shoulder so the entire team can see it (Figure 8.7.1C). The patient is tilted left side down and back to the Trendelenburg position.

Instruments

Specific instruments recommended for laparoscopic total abdominal colectomy are listed in Table 8.7.1.

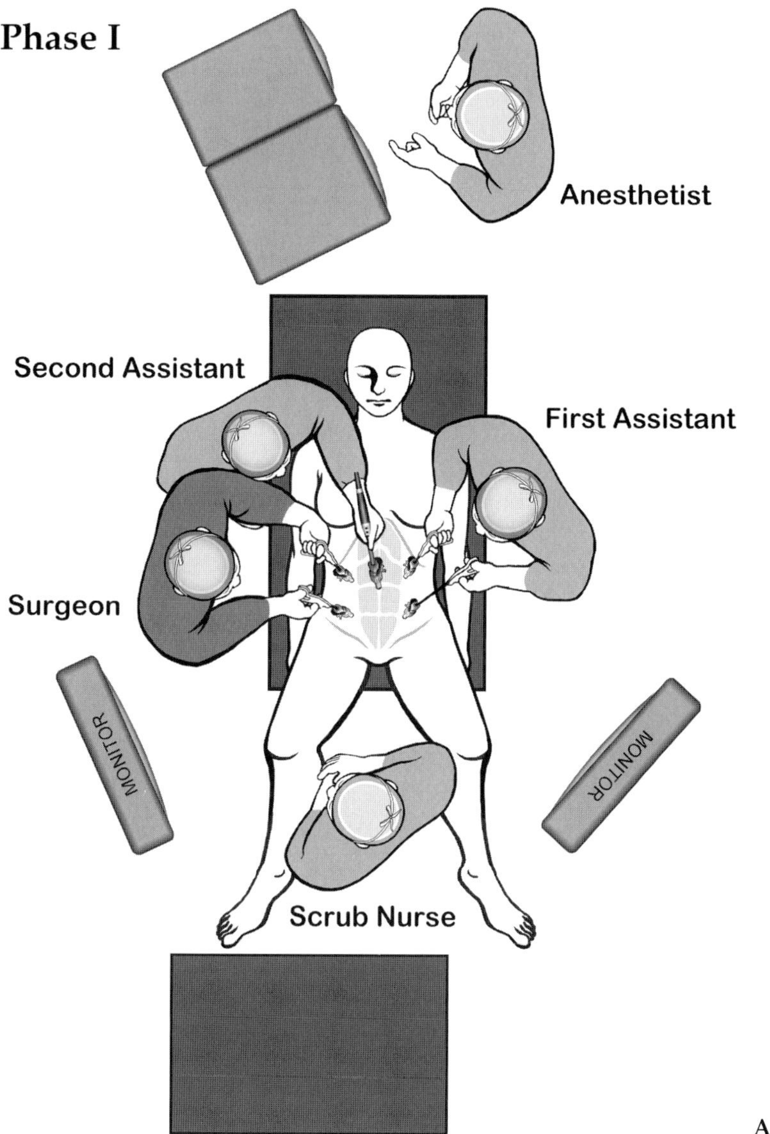

Figure 8.7.1. A Positions of the equipment and the surgical team for phase I of the laparoscopic total abdominal colectomy.

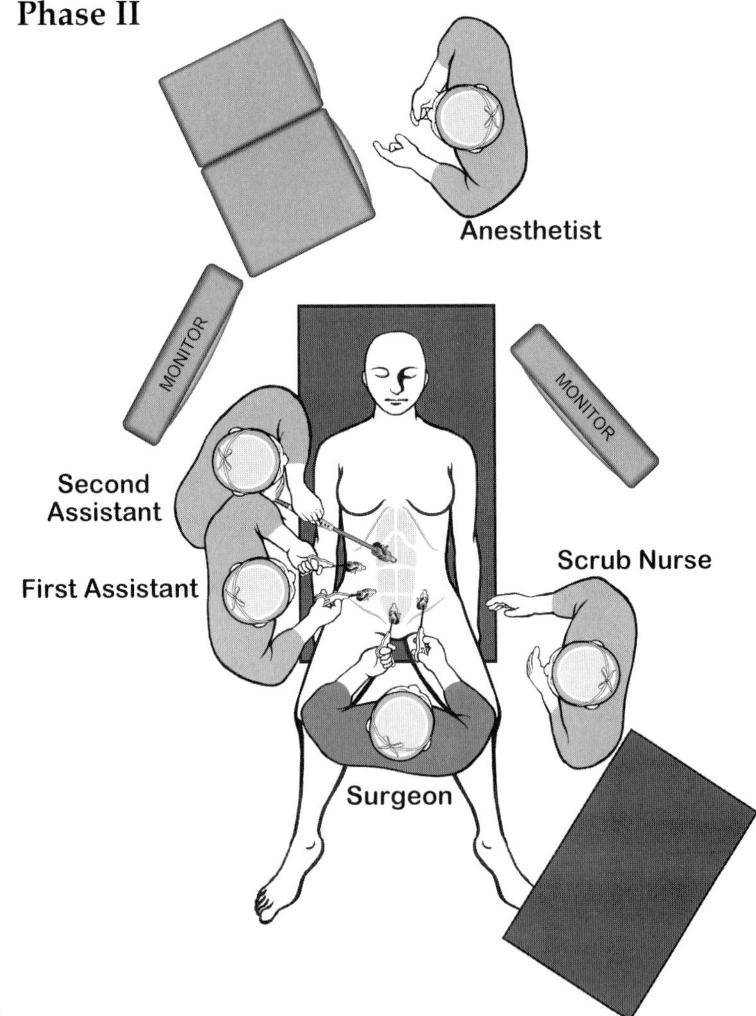

Figure 8.7.1. B Positions of the equipment and the surgical team for phase II of the laparoscopic total abdominal colectomy.

Phase III

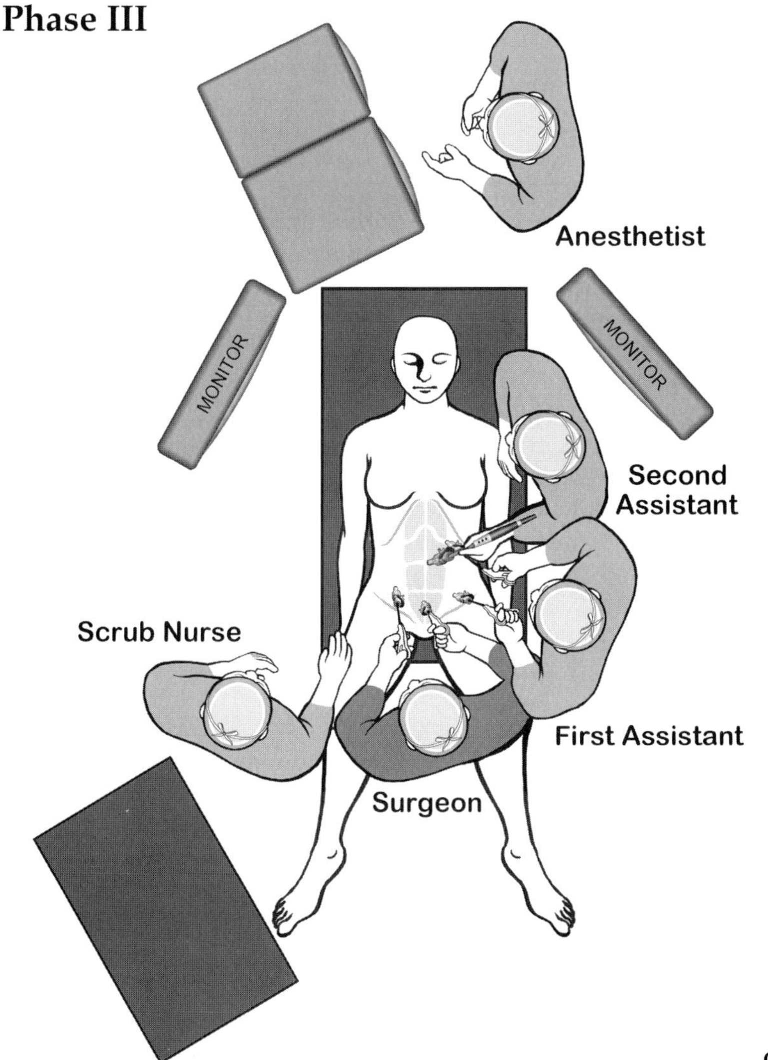

Figure 8.7.1. C Positions of the equipment and the surgical team for phase III of the laparoscopic total abdominal colectomy.

Table 8.7.1. Specific instruments recommended for laparoscopic total abdominal colectomy

6	Cannulae (2 × 12 mm, 1 × 10 mm, 3 × 5 mm)
1	Dissecting device (i.e., LigaSure V™ or Ultrasonic Shears™ or electrosurgery)
1	Endoscopic scissors
3	Endoscopic bowel graspers (5 mm)
1	Endoscopic paddle
1	Endoscopic clip applier – large size
1	Endoscopic stapler

Cannula Positioning

The cannulae are placed as shown in Figure 8.7.2.

Technique

Phase I: Transection of the Inferior Mesenteric Artery and Vein, Medial Dissection of the Left Mesocolon, Pelvic Dissection, Left Lateral Mobilization of the Sigmoid Colon, and Transection of the Upper Rectum

The procedure begins as in proctosigmoidectomy. The patient is placed in a steep Trendelenburg position and is tilted right side down so the small intestine falls into the right upper quadrant. All small intestinal loops are retracted out of the pelvis using bowel graspers. The assistant holds the mesosigmoid close to the inferior mesenteric artery (IMA) bundle under traction in a ventrolateral direction using a bowel grasper in the left-lower-quadrant cannula and a bowel grasper in the left-upper-quadrant cannula to lift up the bowel edge close to the rectosigmoid junction. The peritoneum is incised immediately to the right of the IMA, starting at the sacral promontory (Figure 8.7.3). Under continuous traction, the peritoneum is incised cephalad toward the direction of the origin of the IMA and caudally toward the right lateral rectal

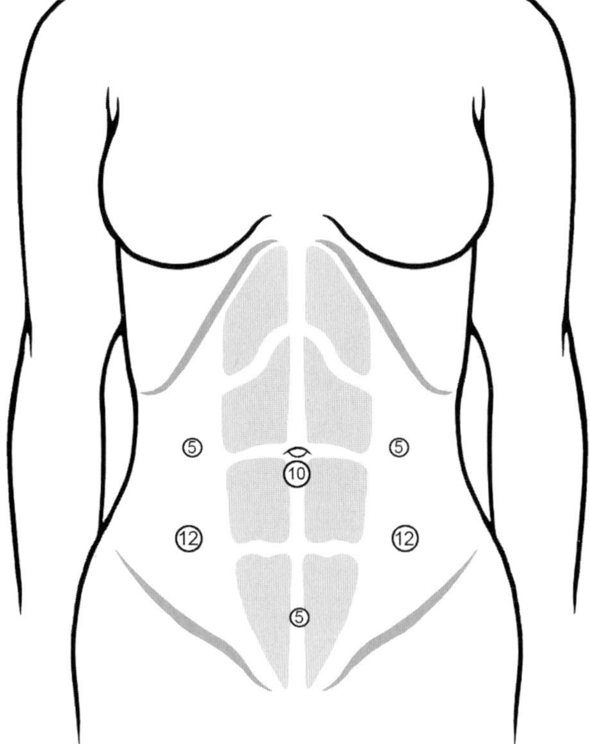

Figure 8.7.2. Positions of the cannulae for the laparoscopic total abdominal colectomy.

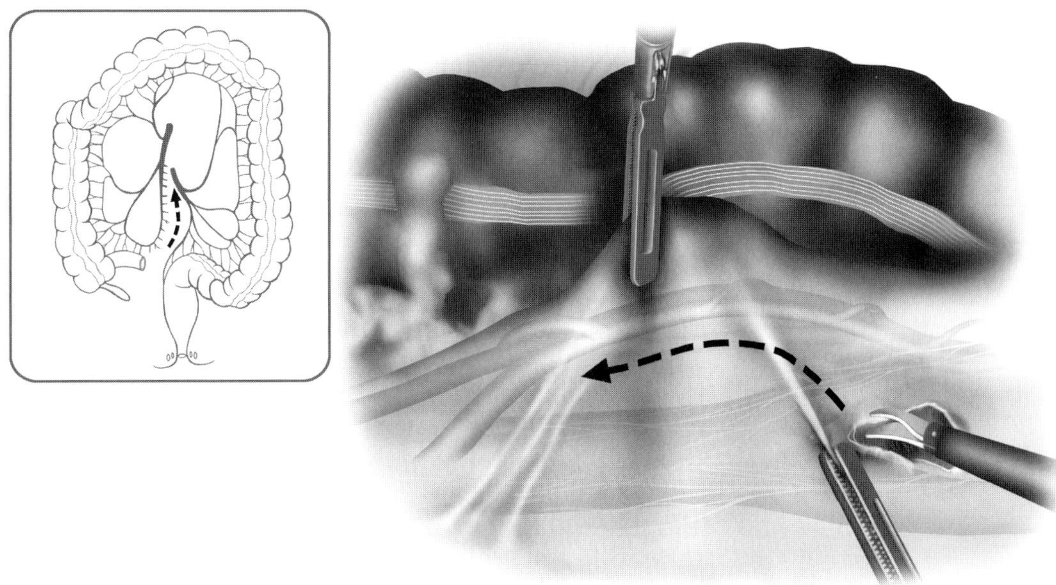

Figure 8.7.3. Dissection is commenced at the sacral promontory posterior to the inferior mesenteric vessels.

stalks. Using blunt dissection, the inferior mesenteric artery and vein are swept ventrally away from the preaortic hypogastric neural plexus, which is swept dorsally to prevent injury to it. Dissection is continued medially beneath the inferior mesenteric artery and vein; the left ureter and the gonadal vessels are identified and are swept posteriorly (Figure 8.7.4). If the ureter cannot be readily and easily identified at this point in the dissection, the lateral attachments of the sigmoid are incised, the sigmoid colon is mobilized left to right, and the gonadal vessels and the left ureter then are identified and dissected free of the mesentery.

Once the origin of the IMA is identified, the peritoneum is incised anteriorly over this pedicle and then left toward the inferior mesenteric vein. Using a combination of blunt and sharp dissecting techniques, a peritoneal window is made just lateral to the inferior mesenteric vein. The pedicle of the inferior mesenteric artery and eventually vein (if anatomically close) is ligated above or below the left colic artery (according to the surgeon's judgment) with a 30-mm endoscopic vascular stapler, but only after the left ureter has been clearly identified and retracted so it is not injured (Figure 8.7.5). We prefer to leave the IMA 1.0–1.5 cm long so if any bleeding occurs, an additional ligature can be applied to the vessel. After the stapler has been placed across the IMA (and concurrently placed across the inferior mesenteric vein if this is feasible and safe), the stapler is closed and again the ureter is checked. The tip of the stapler should be free and clearly visible, and then fired. Before the fired stapler is opened, both ends of the pedicle are grasped by surgeon and assistant so any bleeding can be easily

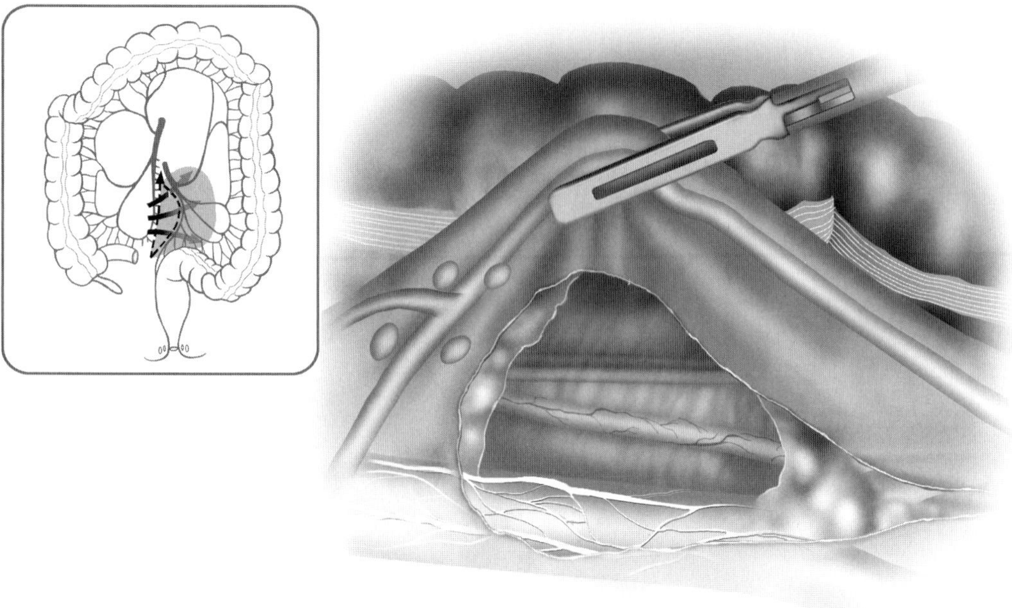

Figure 8.7.4. Dissection is continued superiorly beneath the IMA, protecting the hypogastric neural plexus.

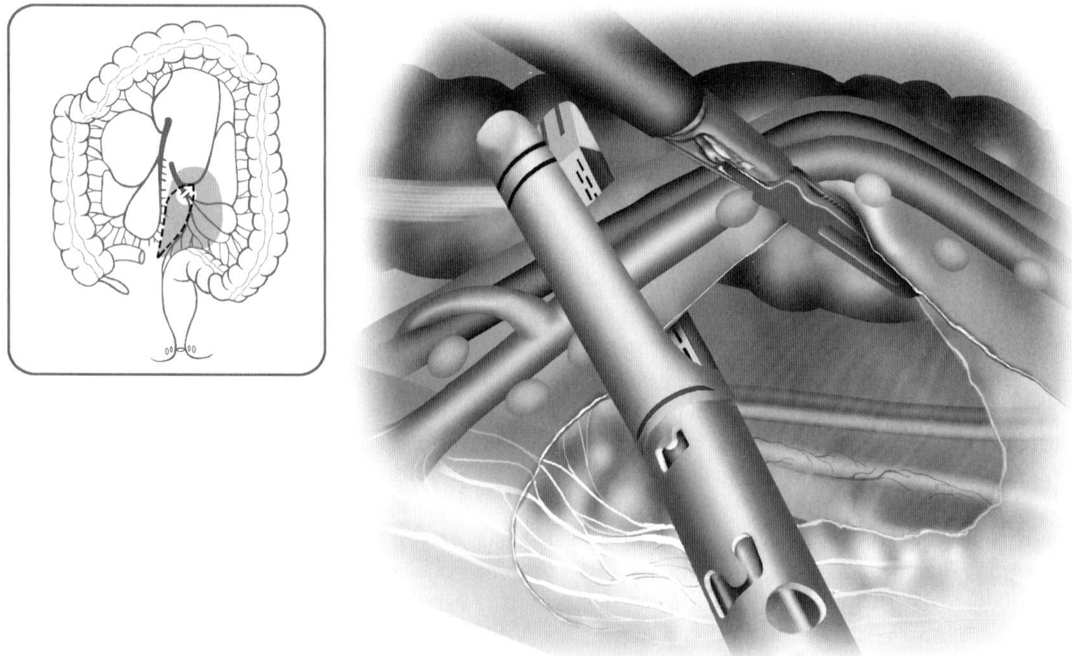

Figure 8.7.5. After creating a peritoneal window to the left of the inferior mesenteric vein, the pedicle is ligated using an endoscopic stapler. Note that the ureter is clearly isolated posterior to the pedicle.

controlled. If the inferior mesenteric vein is not simultaneously ligated by the first stapler, it is clipped or stapled separately. Next, the left colic artery must be ligated along with its accompanying vein (Figure 8.7.6). After this, the left mesocolon is dissected free posteriorly using a blunt instrument such as the endoscopic paddle, sweeping Gerota's fascia away from the posterior surface of the colonic mesentery until close to the splenic flexure and below the descending and left transverse colon (Figure 8.7.7). In thin patients, the spleen may become visible below the colonic flexure. Then, the left-lateral attachments of the upper rectum and sigmoid colon are dissected free, and the sigmoid colon is completely mobilized using sharp and blunt dissection as in open surgery. Again, great care should be taken at this juncture to identify and to avoid any injury to the gonadal vessels or the ureter. The upper rectum is mobilized. To identify the distal resection line of the bowel exactly, an experienced assistant may perform proctoscopy. At the specified point of resection (12–15 cm from the anal verge), otherwise just below the level of the promontory, the mesorectum is divided sharply, starting on the right side; the superior hemorrhoidal artery which is encountered during division is coagulated using the harmonic scalpel or may be clipped (Figure 8.7.8). If the mesorectum is difficult to dissect or if several prominent vessels must be divided, it may be most expeditious to divide the mesorectum with a 30-mm endoscopic stapler, after dissecting a plane between the posterior wall of the rectum and the anterior portions of the mesorectum. The rectum itself is then transected with one or two applications of the Endo GIA stapler (Figure 8.7.9).

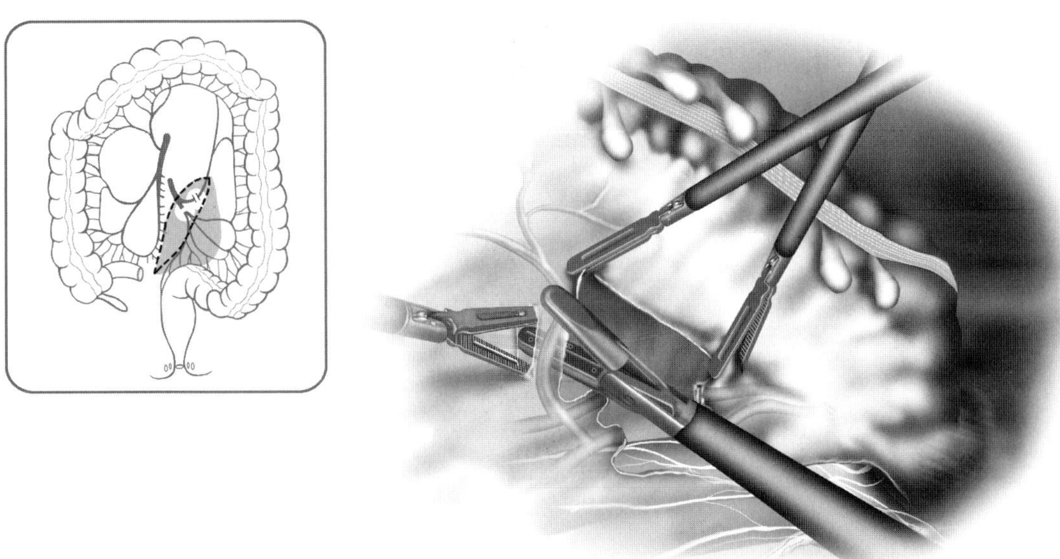

Figure 8.7.6. The left colic artery and vein are ligated separately.

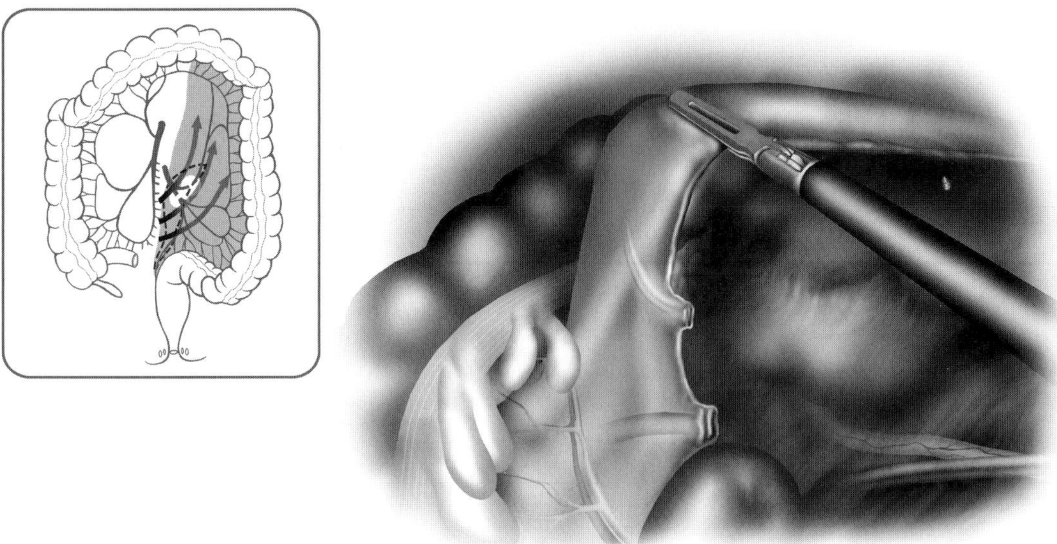

Figure 8.7.7. The left mesocolon is dissected away from the retroperitoneal structures using medial to lateral blunt dissection.

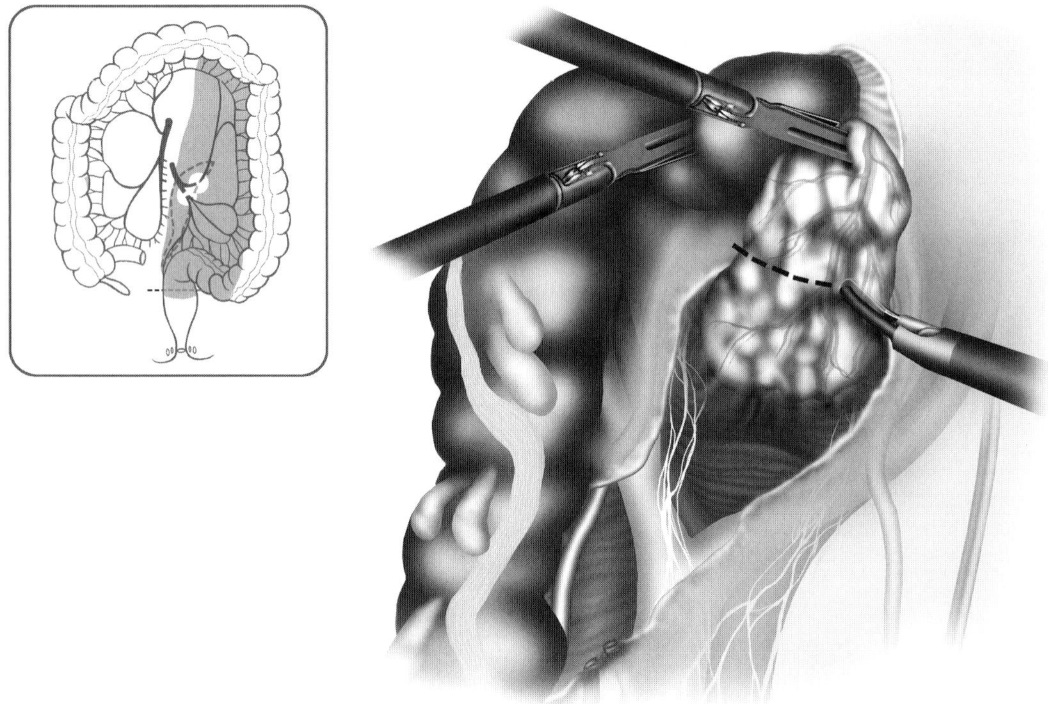

Figure 8.7.8. The mesorectum is divided sharply, starting on the right side, using a harmonic scalpel or bipolar device.

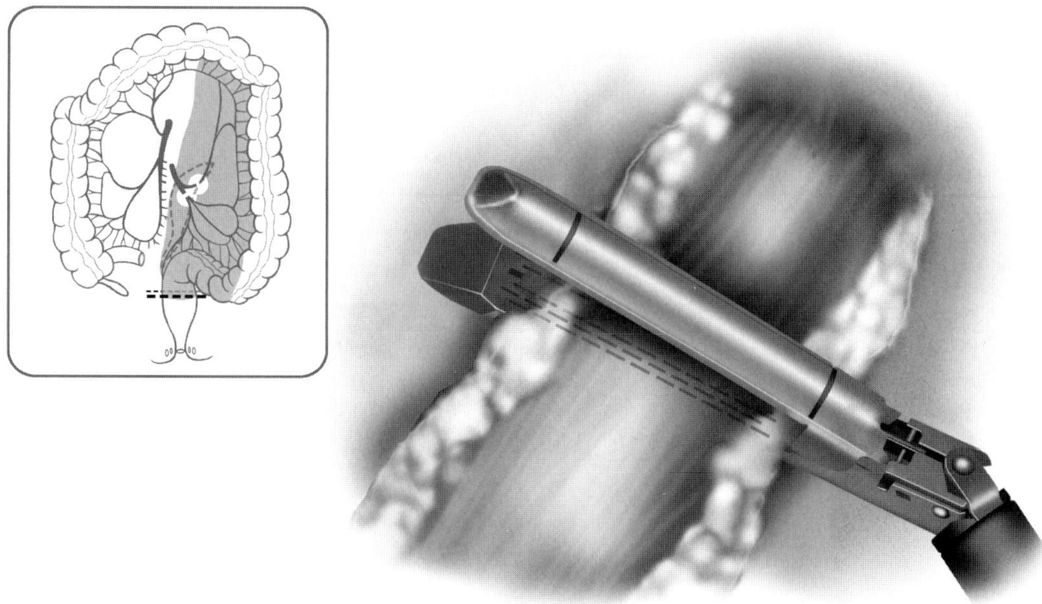

Figure 8.7.9. The rectum is next divided from the right side using one or two applications of an endoscopic stapler.

Phase II: Mobilization of the Left Colon and the Splenic Flexure, Dissection of the Omentum

As soon as the rectosigmoid junction is divided, the surgical team repositions itself for the second phase of the operation, splenic flexure and left colon mobilization. The surgeon works through the suprapubic and the left-lower-quadrant cannulae, whereas the first assistant works through the right-upper-quadrant and the right-lower-quadrant cannulae.

First, the colon is pulled laterally by the assistant or the surgeon. All medial mesenteric attachments should be divided as far cephalad as possible, in a line parallel to and just to the left of the inferior mesenteric vein. Occasionally, there is a left colon or a splenic flexure venous branch that must be isolated and divided during this process. As the posterior surface of the left mesocolon has already been dissected cephalad as far as possible, the colon is now pulled medially and caudally by the assistant using a Babcock and a bowel grasper. This way, the lateral attachments of the left colon are placed under tension and may be divided by the surgeon more easily. This process moves proximally up the colon as the dissection proceeds cephalad. This sequence of retraction and dissection will greatly expedite the splenic flexure takedown (Figure 8.7.10). During this dissection, the surgeon must remain in the proper planes – generally close to the bowel edge laterally, and between Gerota's fascia and the colonic mesentery (Toldt's fascia overlying the Gerota's fascia is swept posteriorly with it).

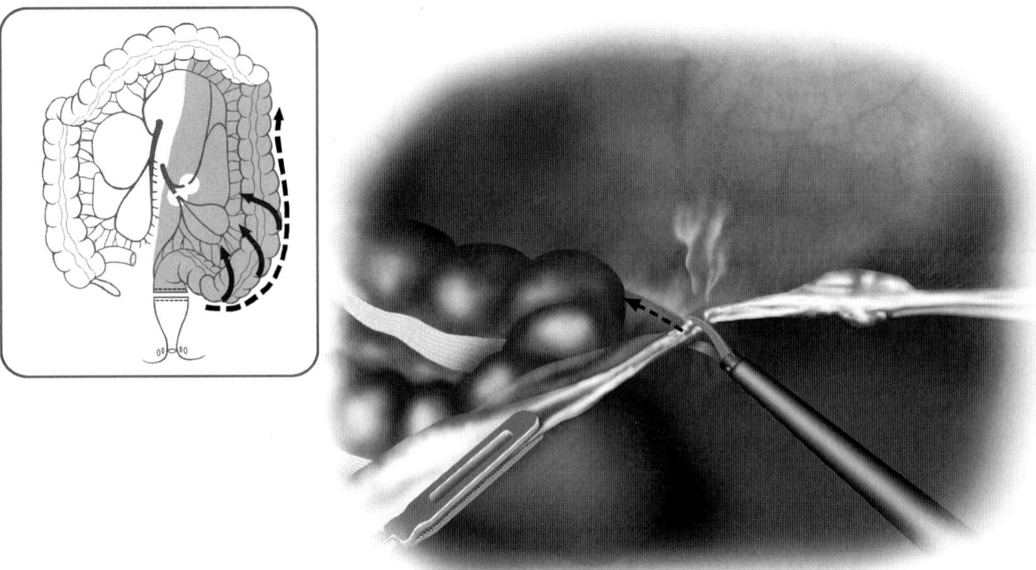

Figure 8.7.10. The colon is reflected medially and dissection of the lateral attachments of the left colon proceed up to the splenic flexure.

In the region of the splenic flexure, the greater omentum gradually appears and is distinguishable from the epiploic appendices by its finer lobulated fatty texture. Separation of the omentum from the colon and these appendices is essential for accurate mobilization of the flexure (Figure 8.7.11). The surgeon may need to switch cannula positions to comfortably reach the splenic flexure, moving from the suprapubic and the left-lower-quadrant cannulae to the left-upper-quadrant and the left-lower-quadrant cannulae.

If the splenic flexure proves difficult to dissect, the dissection can be continued right to left from the distal transverse colon toward the splenic flexure, detaching the omentum from this area as in conventional surgery and gaining entry into the lesser sac (Figure 8.7.12). In our experience, it is important to mobilize the left colon and the left mesocolon as far cephalad as possible in the dorsal mesenteric plane adjacent to Gerota's fascia. This greatly simplifies the mobilization of the splenic flexure, and may simplify dissection of the greater omentum and the lateral adhesions close to the colonic wall. With complete mobilization of the splenic flexure, the surgical team dissects the omentum from the distal transverse colon as far to the right as is possible and practical. This ends the second phase.

Phase III: Transection of the Ileocolic and Middle Colic Vessels, Medial and Lateral Mobilization of the Right Colon and the Hepatic Flexure

At this point, the surgical team repositions itself for the third phase of the procedure, the mobilization of the terminal ileum, right colon, and

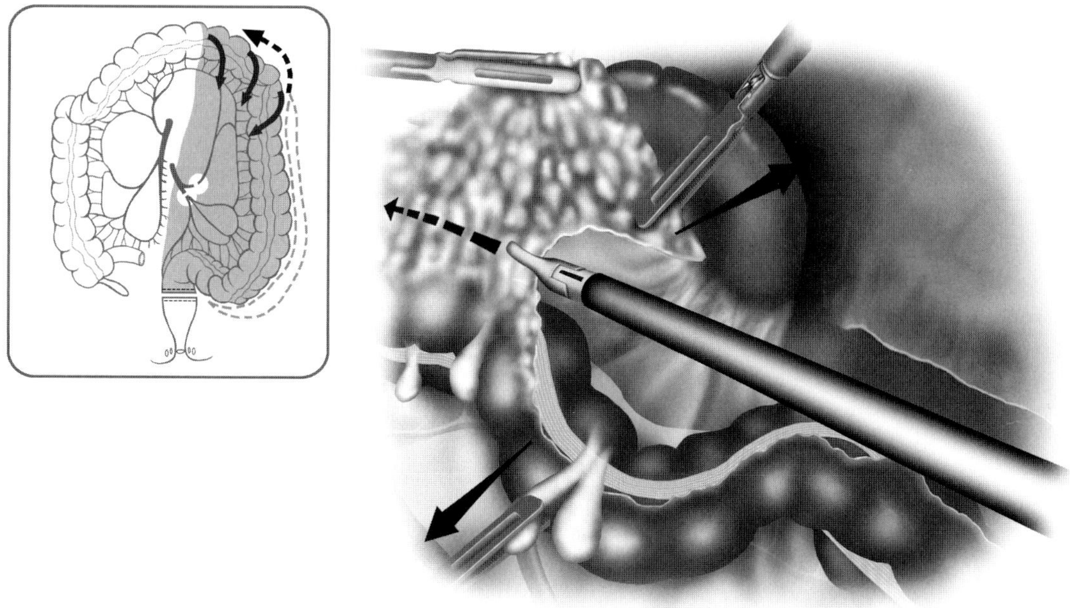

Figure 8.7.11. Separation of the omentum from the colon is required for accurate mobilization of the splenic flexure.

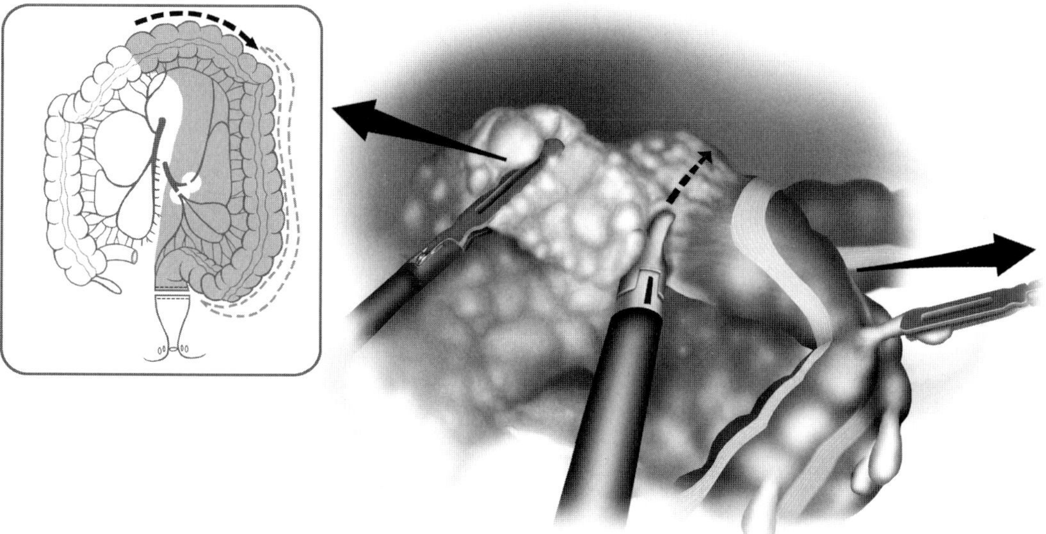

Figure 8.7.12. Splenic flexure mobilization may be expedited with the dissection proceeding from medial to lateral on the transverse colon.

right transverse colon. The patient is tilted left side down and in the Trendelenburg position so the small intestine falls toward the left upper quadrant. The first assistant places the mesentery of ileum and colon laterally close to the ileocecal junction under tension with graspers in the left-upper-quadrant and the left-lower-quadrant cannula sites. Thus, the ileocolic vascular pedicle may be identified more easily. The surgeon begins dissection through the suprapubic and the right-lower-quadrant cannulae, incising the peritoneum below the ileocolic vascular bundle (Figure 8.7.13). This incision is enlarged toward both sides. The ileocolic artery and vein are identified on their dorsal aspects in the front area of the mesentery and are traced to their origin from the superior mesenteric artery and vein. All vessels are carefully dissected at a safe distance from the superior mesenteric artery and vein, and a window through the mesentery is made on either side of the two vessels. The ileocolic pedicle is traced distally to the cecum before division to correctly distinguish it from the superior mesenteric artery and vein. This requires examining the vessels from their ventral aspect also. The pedicles are clipped and then divided, or stapled and transected with an endoscopic vascular stapler or coagulated using a bipolar device (Figure 8.7.14). Again, both ends of the vessels are grasped by surgeon and assistant to be able to control any unexpected bleeding.

Now the ileal and right colonic mesentery are completely freed retroperitoneally by bluntly dissecting a tunnel beginning dorsal to

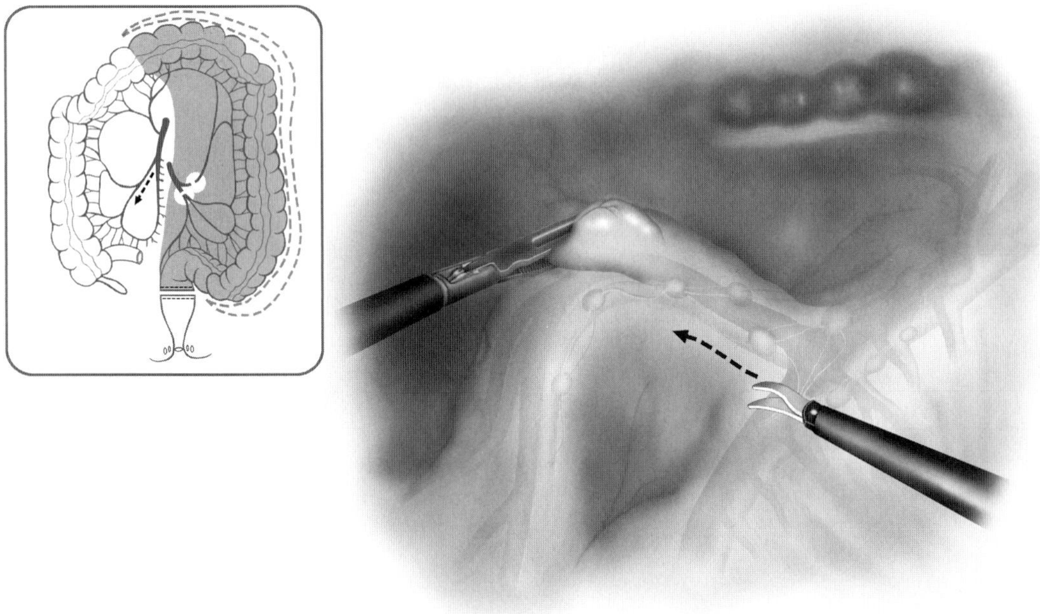

Figure 8.7.13. Phase III begins with an incision just below the ileocolic pedicle.

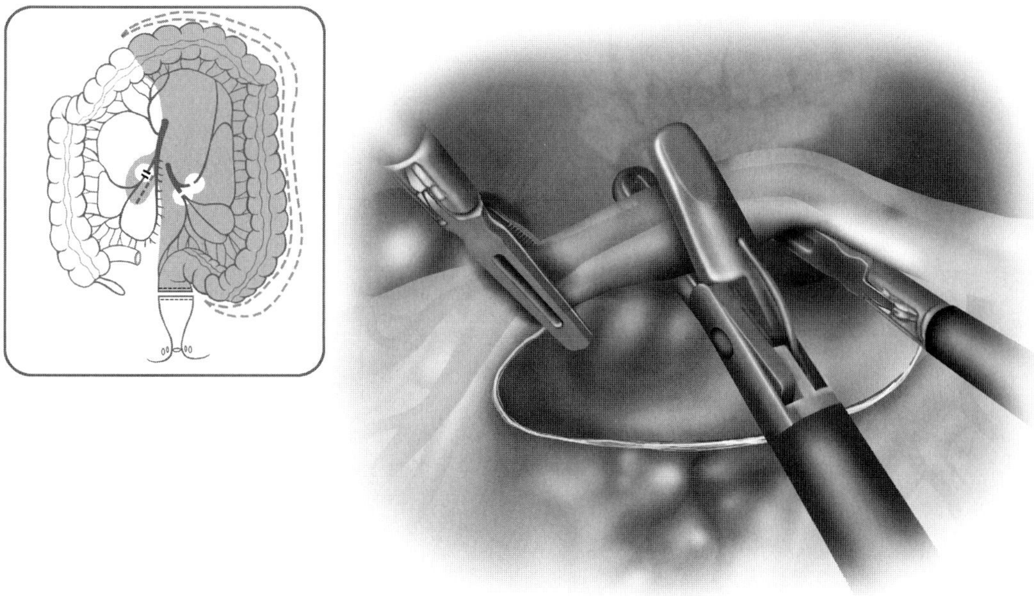

Figure 8.7.14. After mobilizing the pedicle, it is ligated well away from its origin using a bipolar coagulation device.

the ileal mesentery. For this maneuver, the endoscopic paddle is a very useful instrument. The duodenum, the right ureter, the gonadal vessels, and Gerota's fascia become clearly visible. All these anatomic structures are swept down carefully to avoid any injury to them (Figure 8.7.15).

Dissection of the right mesocolon is continued cephalad from the ventral aspect of the right mesenteric root, continuing superiorly and medially until the peritoneal reflection of the right branch or the trunk of the middle colic vessels is seen (Figure 8.7.16). This reflection is divided sharply and blunt dissection is used to isolate the roots of the middle colic vessels. The middle colic vessels are next separated from the retroperitoneal structures and the structures of the lesser omental sac; particular care is needed near the superior aspect of these vessels. Depending on the individual anatomic situation and other factors such as obesity, the middle colic vessels may be separated further centrally close to their roots or further distally in the area of their branches. After circumferential dissection (Figure 8.7.17), the vessels are either coagulated using a bipolar device or ligated with large clips and cut or separated by applying a 30-mm endoscopic vascular stapler. Just to the left of the middle colic pedicle, the mesenteric edge of the transverse colon is grasped, and the peritoneum is incised as far to the left as possible until the region of previous left colonic dissection (phase II of the operation) is reached and connected. Additional vessels of the transverse mesocolon are divided as needed. At this point, the remaining greater

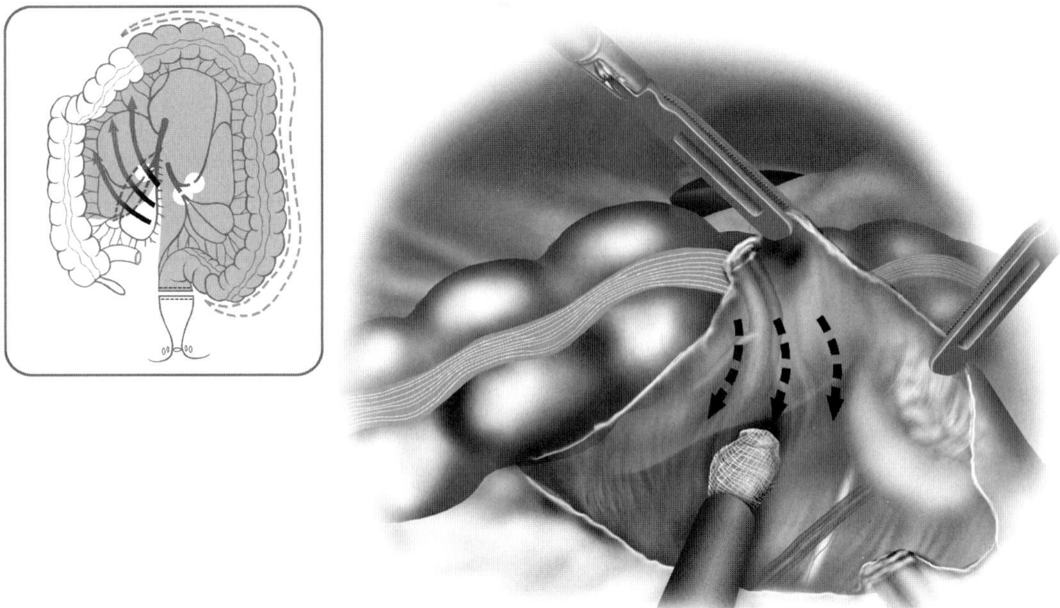

Figure 8.7.15. The ileal and right colonic mesenteric attachments are completely freed retroperitoneally, bluntly dissecting a tunnel dorsal to the ileal mesentery.

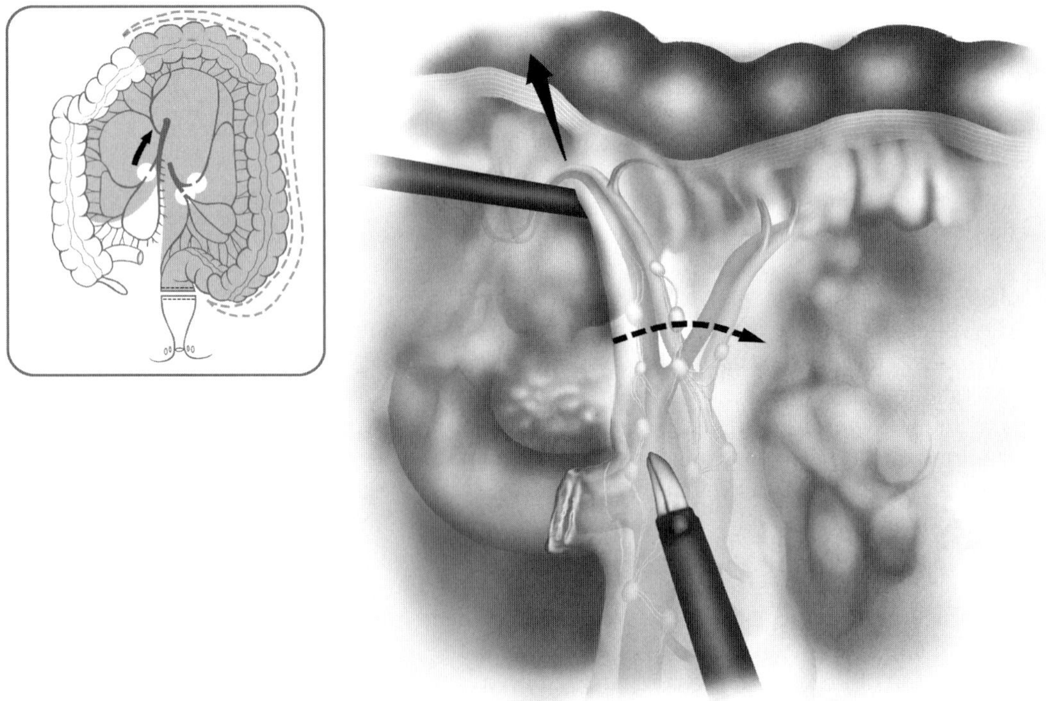

Figure 8.7.16. Just cephalad to the ligated ileocolic pedicle, the middle colic pedicle is identified.

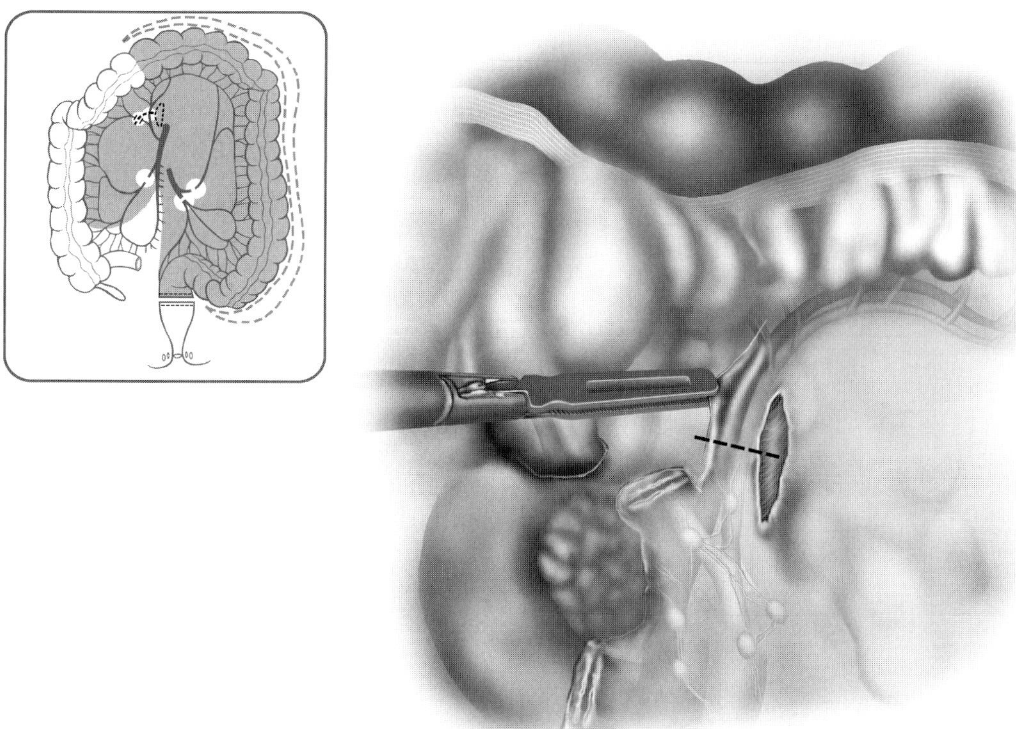

Figure 8.7.17. The ligation of the middle colic vessels may be safer if performed on the right and left branches, rather than on the main trunk.

omental attachments to the right transverse colon are dissected from the colon, thus completely freeing the omentum from the bowel. Vessels of the omentum are sealed using electrocautery, the harmonic scalpel or clipped and divided as necessary.

The terminal ileum is next grasped and the proximal resection line is identified near the ileocecal junction. The mesentery of the terminal ileum and the ileum itself may be divided either laparoscopically inside (e.g., in case of malignancy) or after extraction of the bowel outside of the abdominal cavity which in many cases is faster and does not require a longer incision line. In the rare case of laparoscopic division, the ileal mesentery is completely dissected starting from the left side of the ileocolic pedicle. All mesenteric vessels are clipped, and divided or coagulated. The ileum may be transected using a 45-mm endoscopic stapler.

In the next step, complete mobilization of ileum and right colon is accomplished. The assistant is carefully pulling the terminal ileum and the cecum cephalad and medially. The attachments of the ileum just medial to the base of the appendix are incised, carrying the incision cephalad toward the root of the mesentery and to the inferior edge of the duodenum (Figure 8.7.18). Next, starting at the cecum next to the

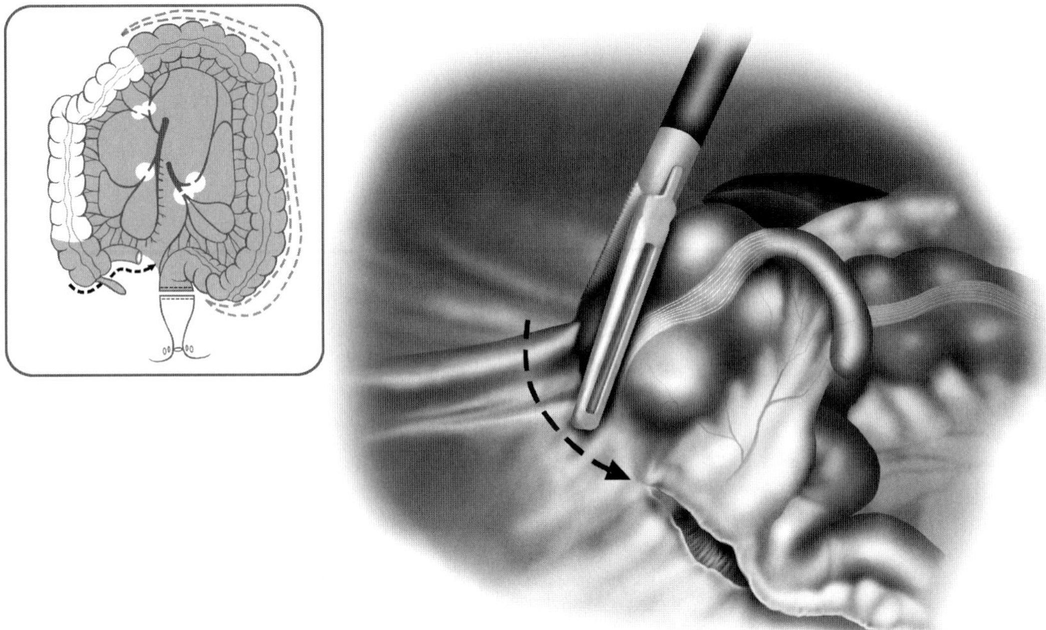

Figure 8.7.18. Attachments of the ileum just medial to the base of the appendix are incised, carrying the incision cephalad toward the root of the mesentery.

root of the appendix, the right colon and the hepatic flexure are completely detached from remaining retroperitoneal structures. The patient's Trendelenburg position should be reversed as the hepatic flexure is reached. Because most of the mobilization of the colon has been performed dorsally, only minor adhesions with the lateral and posterior abdominal wall have to be transected up to and just beyond the hepatic flexure. Then, the last lateral adhesions of the right transverse mesocolon have to be dissected (Figure 8.7.19). Finally, the remaining attachments of the omentum to the proximal transverse colon, then the hepatocolic ligament, are divided (Figure 8.7.20). At this point, the colon should be completely free from surrounding structures. This is checked by running the colon at its entire length from the distal sigmoid orally toward the cecum using Babcock and bowel graspers. At the same time, the colon is moved on top of the small bowel loops to make extraction easily possible. To start this maneuver, especially in obese patients, it may be necessary to tilt the patient left side up again.

Minilaparotomy, Bowel Transection, and Ileorectal Anastomosis

The patient is reversed to a regular position. The distal sigmoid colon is grasped through the right-lower-quadrant cannula, then the suprapubic cannula site is enlarged using a muscle-splitting (small Pfannenstiel) incision and the wound protected using a plastic sleeve device.

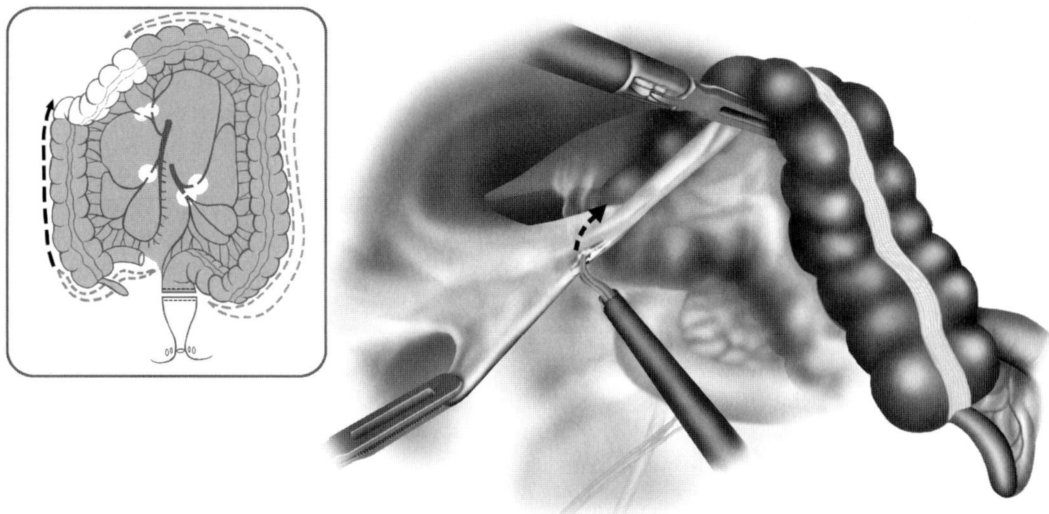

Figure 8.7.19. The last lateral adhesions of the right colon are incised up to the hepatic flexure.

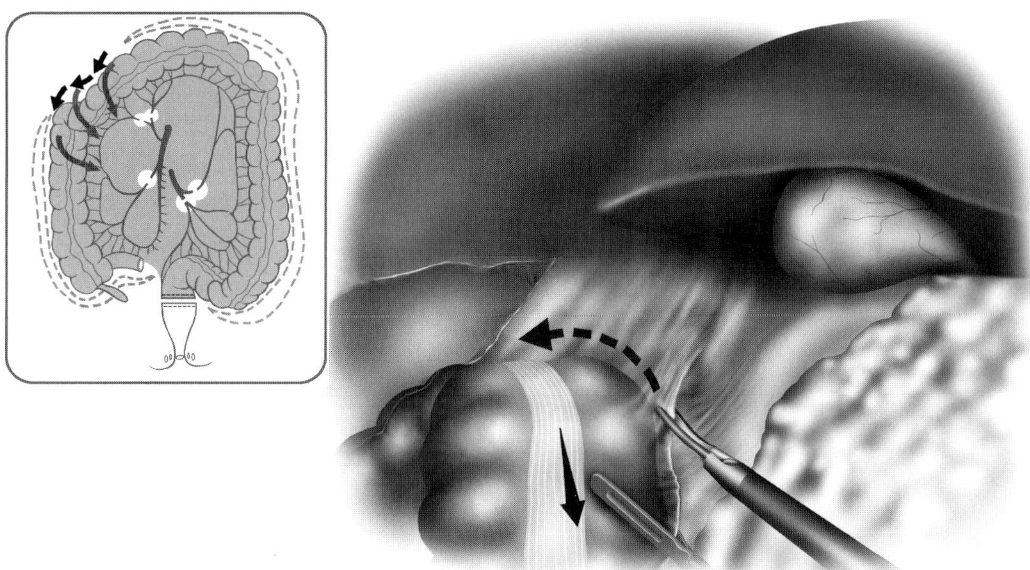

Figure 8.7.20. The hepatocolic ligament is divided from medial to lateral, completely freeing up the right colon.

Pneumoperitoneum is released and the CO_2 insufflator is shut off temporarily. The sigmoid colon is exposed toward the incision and grasped with Allis clamps. The entire colon is pulled out through this wound (Figure 8.7.21). The mesentery of the terminal ileum is now divided extracorporeally toward the considered transection line of the ileum. The terminal ileum is grasped with a purse-string-suture clamp, the straight needles are applied, and the bowel is transected. The specimen is removed. The anvil and the center rod assembly of a 28 circular stapler are placed into the bowel lumen and the purse-string suture is tied in the conventional manner (Figure 8.7.22). The ileum is returned to the peritoneal cavity, and the cavity is copiously irrigated by flushing warm saline in through the suprapubic incision line and suctioning the fluid again through the same incision using a conventional sump suction system. The abdominal wall thereafter is closed with conventional running sutures in two layers (peritoneum and fascia). Pneumoperitoneum is reestablished and the patient is positioned head and right side down again. The shaft of the circular stapler is passed transanally under laparoscopic guidance. The modified plastic spike of the stapler is retracted into the instrument head until the instrument is carefully and completely brought up to the rectal staple line. Then the spike is pushed through the rectal wall just adjacent to the staple line

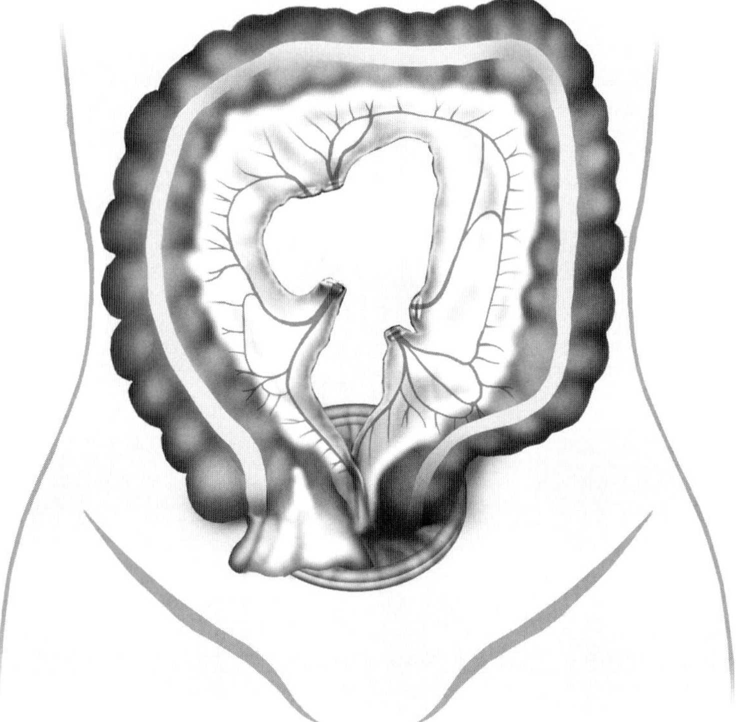

Figure 8.7.21. The entire colon may then be pulled out through the suprapubic incision.

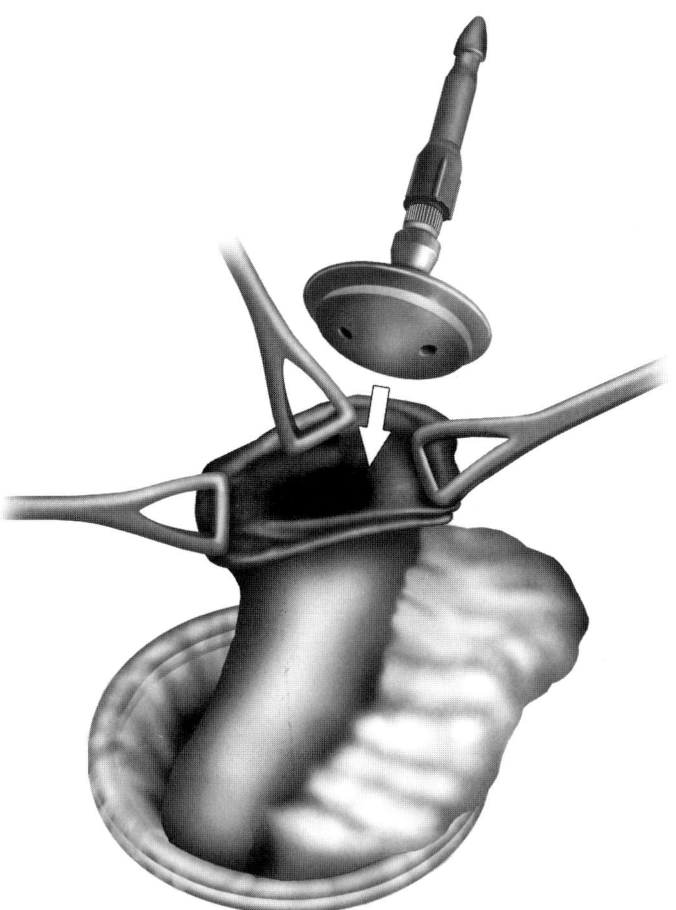

Figure 8.7.22. After removing the entire colon, the center rod and anvil is inserted into the end of the ileum and secured using a purse-string suture.

by turning the wing nut on the stapler handle counterclockwise (Figure 8.7.23).

A standard double-stapling technique is used to form the ileorectal anastomosis. The center rod of the staple protruding from the ileum is grasped with a right-lower-quadrant endoscopic Babcock instrument and is locked into the circular stapler protruding from the rectal stump (Figure 8.7.24). This locking action is easily performed without substantial force as long as the axis of the center rod and the axis of the center post are in a perfect line. Because the center rod is grasped with the Babcock instrument through the right lower quadrant, the tip of the center rod will tend to be directed to the right side of the pelvis. The center post protruding from the rectum should be directed to the left side of the pelvis and the center rod should enter the pelvis from the left side. This maneuver will facilitate locking the center rod into the center post. Before anastomotic formation, the ileal mesentery must be carefully scrutinized along its cut edge to be sure it is not twisted. Excellent visualization of the anastomosis before firing the stapler is

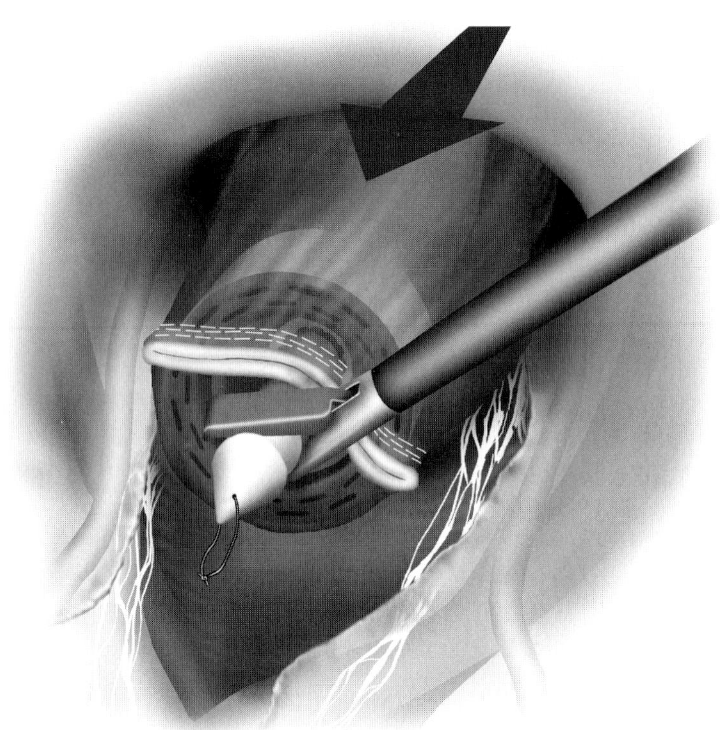

Figure 8.7.23. After passing the circular stapler up to the top of the rectum, the spike is protruded through the rectal wall adjacent to the rectal staple line.

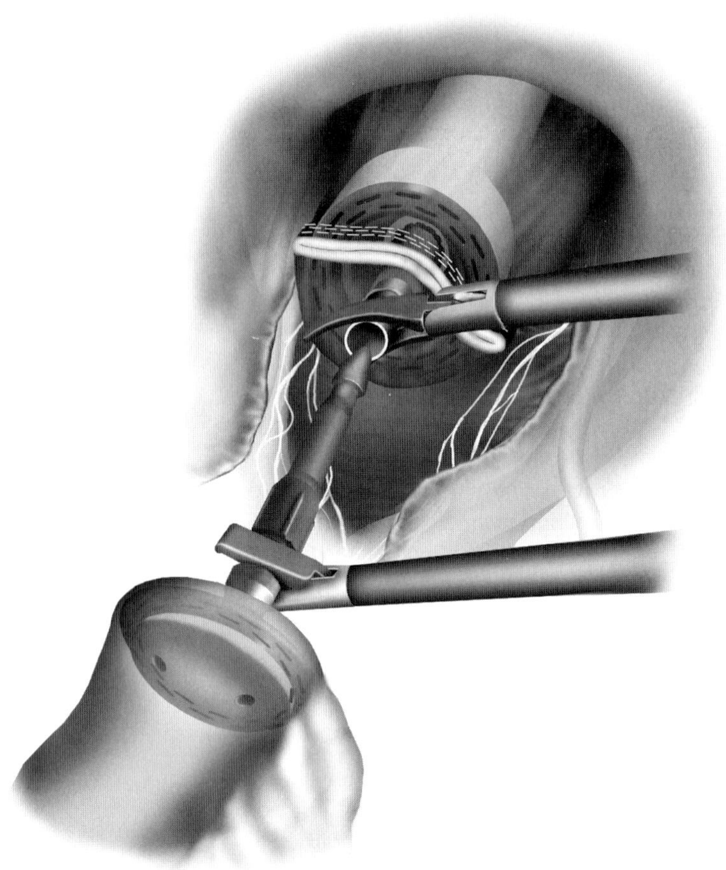

Figure 8.7.24. A standard double-stapled technique is used for the anastomosis of ileum to rectum.

also necessary. The tissue donuts created with the circular staplers are carefully inspected for completeness and are sent for routine pathologic evaluation if the surgeon deems it necessary.

The anastomosis is checked for leaks by filling the pelvis with saline solution, occluding the small bowel lumen several centimeters above the anastomosis applying a bowel clamp and then using a proctoscope to insufflate air into the rectum. No air bubbles should appear.

Special Considerations

Drainage of the abdomen after the conclusion of each case is possible, however, not absolutely necessary. After the pelvis has been carefully irrigated, an atraumatic closed suction drain may be placed in the pelvis through the right- or left-lower-quadrant cannula site. Usually, the drain can easily be passed through the 5-mm cannula and a grasper from the opposite quadrant cannula is used to place the drain into the pelvis. The cannula is then removed.

The vascular anatomy within the mesentery of the transverse colon to the left of the middle colic vessels and in the region of the splenic flexure needs special attention here. Because this area may be difficult to expose, a fundamental understanding of the vessels that may be encountered here is extremely important. Connections between the left colic and middle colic artery are common, with two arcades in the splenic flexure mesentery seen most commonly (33%), followed in frequency by tertiary or primary ones (25% each); arcades with 4, 5, or 6 branches are exceptional (Figure 8.7.25).[20] In 14.5% of specimens, an accessory left colic will arise from the superior mesenteric artery. Also, it is not unusual to find a separate unnamed vein draining from the distal transverse colon directly into the inferior mesenteric vein, or even following a separate course underneath the pancreas to the splenic vein.

When the transverse mesocolon is transected along with the middle colic vessels, entry into the lesser sac is often confusing because of congenital adhesions between the greater omentum, the stomach, and the transverse mesocolon. The omentum may usually be recognized by its fine, fatty lobulations in comparison with the smooth texture of the fat in the transverse mesocolon. The omentum may be quickly encountered superiorly after transection of the transverse mesocolon. Generally, by patiently separating the plane and lysing any congenital adhesions just behind and superior to the middle colic vessels, the lesser sac can be found.

Normally, for cancer located in the transverse colon or close to the hepatic or splenic flexures, extended right hemicolectomies or subtotal colectomies are indicated, including lymph node dissection extending to the root of the middle colic artery and vein. The following points highlight certain techniques that should be used in the rare instance that laparoscopic total abdominal colectomy is performed for cancer (e.g., two synchronous cancers in the proximal and distal colon or one cancer and synchronous large sessile adenoma):

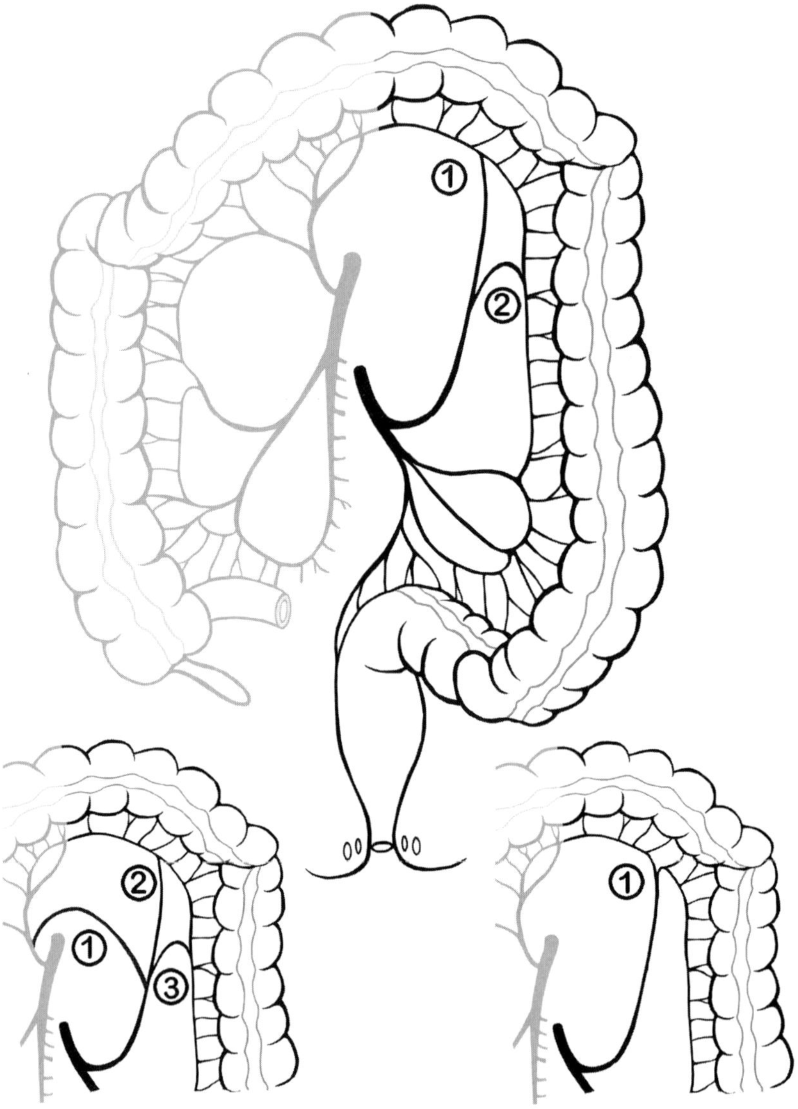

Figure 8.7.25. Mesenteric vascular connections between the left colic and middle colic arteries. Most commonly, there are two (33% of specimens); three arcades and one arcade are less common (25% each). More than three arcades are exceptional.

- All major vessels are ligated proximally with dissection of each of the artery's root at the superior mesenteric artery or aorta and wide mesenteric resection (we use proximal mesenteric vascular division as the routine procedure).
- The transection of the ileum and its mesentery should also be performed laparoscopically. As soon as the bowel is dissected completely free, an endoscopic bowel bag should be passed into the

abdominal cavity through the suprapubic cannula site, and the specimen should be immediately put into the fully opened bag that has been positioned in the pelvis.

- The specimen should be carefully removed and sealed inside the bowel bag after the suprapubic cannula site has been enlarged. This way, the abdominal wall will be protected from any contamination by cancer cells.

The most difficult and also time-consuming part of the procedure is the mobilization of the transverse colon. During medial dissection, it is highly recommended to identify the branches of the middle colic artery and vein very carefully and thoroughly to avoid any unexpected vessel injury in this area of the mesocolon. Surgeon and assistant have to move their instruments very precisely; the mesocolon has to be exposed clearly but carefully. Bleeding from one of these vessels is difficult to stop and may lead to early conversion.

During the completion of the medial dissection coming up orally from the IMA area beyond the splenic flexure one always has to be prepared for another branch of the middle colic vessels to be hidden in the fatty tissue of the mesentery. Also, "tissue triangulation" of the omentum and the transverse colon (see Chapter 6) is crucial during lateral mobilization in this area to facilitate fast orientation and accelerate surgery.

When using cutting devices such as electrocautery or the harmonic scalpel, very high temperatures may be generated in the surrounding tissue leading to the destruction of proteins even several millimeters away from the spot of operation. This is why we avoid using these instruments in the immediate neighborhood of structures carrying mucosa and restrict their application to short-term use of only a few seconds without interruption.

The most important complication in the postoperative course after total abdominal colectomy is anastomotic leakage. The rate of leakage, however, may be kept low by thoroughly testing the anastomosis at the end of surgery (endoscopic and air-leak check). If it still occurs and no conservative treatment by drainage is possible, (laparoscopic) protective ileostomy formation or disconnection of the anastomosis may become necessary. Another complication is anastomotic stricture after double-stapling technique. Such a stricture may be avoided if the anastomosis is checked by rectoscopy in a time range of 4 weeks after the operation. When narrowing is present, the tissue is still soft enough to be widened by carefully pushing the blunt tip of the obturator of the rectoscope beyond the anastomosis. If a stenosis occurs later, stepwise endoscopic dilatation or incision of the scar tissue using electrocautery may be indicated. Bleeding from the anastomosis should be rare if it is checked at the end of surgery. Other complications dealing with the loss of large bowel function are chronic diarrhea, electrolyte disturbances, and dehydration. Conservative treatment replacing liquids and antidiarrheal medication are recommended. In cases of total colectomy for chronic constipation, symptoms may reoccur in the long term. Also in these cases, medical therapy is indicated first.

Conclusions

The laparoscopic approach to total abdominal colectomy is especially attractive as there are a variety of benign indications for this procedure and a previously necessary long midline incision for surgery in all four abdominal quadrants is avoided and replaced by a short suprapubic incision of a few centimeters in length with all the favorable postoperative effects of minimally invasive surgery.

Editors' Comments

Indications: We agree with these indications and the caveats expressed by Dr. Kessler.
Patient positioning: We use a similar setup and positioning.
Instrumentation: We utilize the laparoscopic 5-mm LigaSure V™ device for the mesenteric vascular division.
Cannula positioning: We generally agree with his positioning.
Technique: We now begin the procedure on the right side, and end on the left side, with dissection and division of the rectosigmoid. Our techniques are otherwise very similar. The indications for the use of the hand-assisted technique versus the completely laparoscopic approach will be discussed in Chapter 9.2, entitled *Hand-Assisted Laparoscopic Total Abdominal Colectomy*.

References

1. Caravati F, Ceriani F, Moroni M, et al. The learning curve in laparoscopic resections of the colon and rectum: results and considerations. Chir Ital 2003;55:199–206.
2. Senagore AJ, Delaney CP, Madboulay K, et al. Laparoscopic colectomy in obese and nonobese patients. J Gastrointest Surg 2003;7:558–561.
3. Dunker MS, Bemelman WA, Slors JF, et al. Laparoscopic-assisted vs open colectomy for severe acute colitis in patients with inflammatory bowel disease (IBD): a retrospective study in 42 patients. Surg Endosc 2000;14: 911–914.
4. Hamel CT, Hildebrandt U, Weiss EG, et al. Laparoscopic surgery for inflammatory bowel disease. Surg Endosc 2001;15:642–645.
5. Marchesa P, Milsom JW. Laparoscopic techniques for inflammatory bowel disease. Semin Laparosc Surg 1995;2:246–251.
6. Araki Y, Isomoto H, Tsuzi Y, et al. Clinical aspects of total colectomy: laparoscopic versus open technique for familial adenomatous polyposis and ulcerative colitis. Kurume Med J 1998;45:203–207.
7. Ishida H, Hashimoto D, Inokuma S, et al. Gasless laparoscopic surgery for ulcerative colitis and familial adenomatous polyposis: initial experience of 7 cases. Surg Endosc 2003;17:899–902.
8. Kessler H, Hohenberger W. Laparoscopic assisted restorative proctocolectomy in ulcerative colitis and familial polyposis. J Jpn Surg Soc 2003;28: 648–649.
9. Laparoscopic total colectomy for slow transit constipation. Arch Hung Med Assoc Am 2001;9:10.

10. Marcello PW, Milsom JW, Wong SK, et al. Laparoscopic total colectomy for acute colitis: a case-control study. Dis Colon Rectum 2001;44:1441–1445.
11. Iancu C, Bala O, Tantau M, et al. Laparoscopic total colectomy for asymptomatic familial adenomatous polyposis. Rom J Gastroenterol 2002;11: 47–51.
12. Milsom JW, Ludwig KA, Church JM, et al. Laparoscopic total abdominal colectomy with ileorectal anastomosis for familial adenomatous polyposis. Dis Colon Rectum 1997;40:675–678.
13. Kessler H. Laparoskopische Kolonresektion bei benignen Erkrankungen. Viszeralchirurgie 2003;38:99–106.
14. Bonnard A, de Lagausie P, Leclair MD, et al. Definitive treatment of extended Hirschsprung's disease or total colonic form. Surg Endosc 2001;15:1301–1304.
15. Ho YH, Tan M, Eu KW, et al. Laparoscopic-assisted compared with open total colectomy in treating slow transit constipation. Aust N Z J Surg 1997;67:562–565.
16. Inoue Y, Noro H, Komoda H, et al. Completely laparoscopic total colectomy for chronic constipation: report of a case. Surg Today 2002;32:551–554.
17. Kessler H, Hohenberger W. Laparoskopische Colektomie bei chronischer Obstipation. Langenbecks Arch Surg Kongressbd 2002;230–231.
18. Adachi Y, Sato K, Kakisako K, et al. Quality of life after laparoscopic or open colonic resection for cancer. Hepatogastroenterology 2003;50: 1348–1351.
19. Korolija D, Tadic S, Simic D. Extent of oncological resection in laparoscopic vs. open colorectal surgery: meta-analysis. Langenbecks Arch Surg 2003; 387:366–371.
20. VanDamme J-P, Bonte J. Vascular Anatomy in Abdominal Surgery. Stuttgart: Georg Thieme Verlag; 1990.

Chapter 8.8

Laparoscopic Proctocolectomy with Ileal Pouch to Anal Anastomosis (IPAA)

Peter W. Marcello

Indications

The indications for a laparoscopic proctocolectomy with ileoanal pouch construction are the same whether the procedure is performed by a conventional or laparoscopic approach. Nearly all patients will undergo this operation either for ulcerative colitis refractory to medical therapy or familial adenomatous polyposis. Unless the patient has had multiple prior abdominal surgeries, or known intraabdominal adhesions, the procedure can likely be performed laparoscopically. The surgeon must be skilled in laparoscopic segmental resection and should be experienced in performing a laparoscopic total colectomy before attempting this complex procedure. Because of potential friability of the colon in ulcerative colitis, a surgeon should not perform laparoscopic total colectomy for acute colitis until they are quite comfortable with laparoscopic total colectomy in a noninflamed colon. Obesity (body mass index >30 kg/m^2), was previously considered a contraindication to a laparoscopic total colectomy. However, once the surgeon has performed the procedure in thinner patients, it may be attempted in a more obese population. I do not believe obesity is a contraindication to laparoscopy, but rather I believe this should be a preferred approach to the procedure because it minimizes the potential for significant wound complications.

Patient Positioning and Operating Room Setup

A well-defined operative setup and plan can smooth the progress of a laparoscopic colon resection. By developing a routine approach to patient positioning and instrumentation, anesthetic times can be reduced and the efficiency of the operative team improved. For nearly all cases, an electric table is recommended if available. During the procedure, the patient is likely to be in steep (20′ head-down tilt) Trendelenburg position. The patient will then be rotated side to side during cannula insertion and throughout the procedure. The anesthesia team is often much happier and responsive to alterations in patient positioning when using an electric bed.

The patient is placed in the modified lithotomy position. This allows the surgeon or assistant to stand between the legs during the procedure, especially during colon flexure mobilization. The patient should be positioned with the pelvis just above the lower table break to allow access to the perineum for pelvic manipulation and transanal anastomosis. The legs are placed in padded adjustable stirrups (Dan Allen Stirrups, Bedford Heights, OH). The use of pneumatic compression stockings is highly recommended for prevention of deep venous thrombosis and possibly to prevent lateral nerve injury to the lower extremities. The legs are abducted 20′ to 25′ and the thighs should be minimally elevated. Even mild flexure of the thighs (>10′) can interfere with mobilization of the transverse colon, because instruments passed through the lower abdominal cannulae may abut the thighs as the proximal and distal transverse colon are approached.

To stabilize the body on the table, several additional measures are utilized. A moldable "bean bag" is placed under the patient's head and torso and conforms to the patient with both arms tucked in. Initially, we used padded shoulder harnesses to prevent patient slippage during steep Trendelenburg position. However, two heavy patients (from >700 cases) have developed temporary brachial plexopathy from nerve compression despite the use of heavily padded shoulder harnesses. Currently, a large piece of silk tape (3 inches) placed over the upper chest fixates the upper torso and beanbag to the operating table. Such measures may help prevent vertical or lateral patient slippage during exaggerated Trendelenburg and lateral positioning often called for in laparoscopic colorectal procedures.

The position of the operative team and monitors will vary throughout the procedure (Figure 8.8.1A–C). The goal of the laparoscopic team is to maintain an appropriate unidirectional orientation of the body, working cannulae, and instruments to the monitor location. Ideally, the eyes, hands, and instruments can all converge on the monitor in a straight line. For the rectosigmoid dissection, two monitors are placed lateral to each of the patient's feet. For right, transverse, or left colon dissection, the monitors are shifted upward to the patient's shoulders.

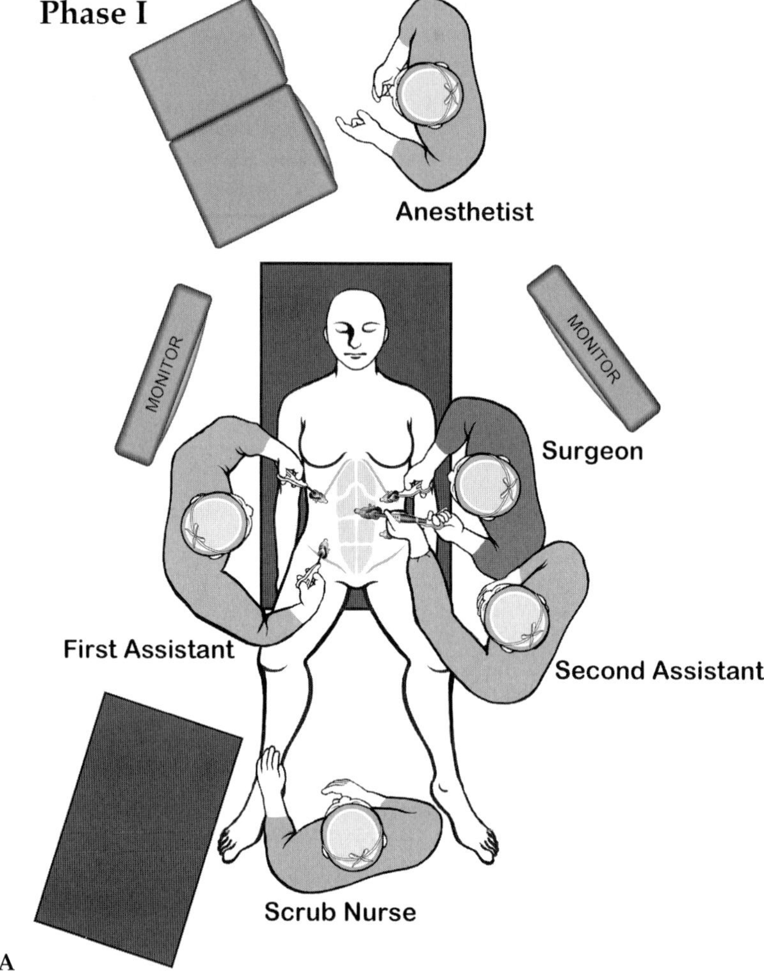

Figure 8.8.1. **A** Positions of the equipment and the surgical team for phase I of the laparoscopic proctocolectomy with ileal pouch procedure.

Phase II

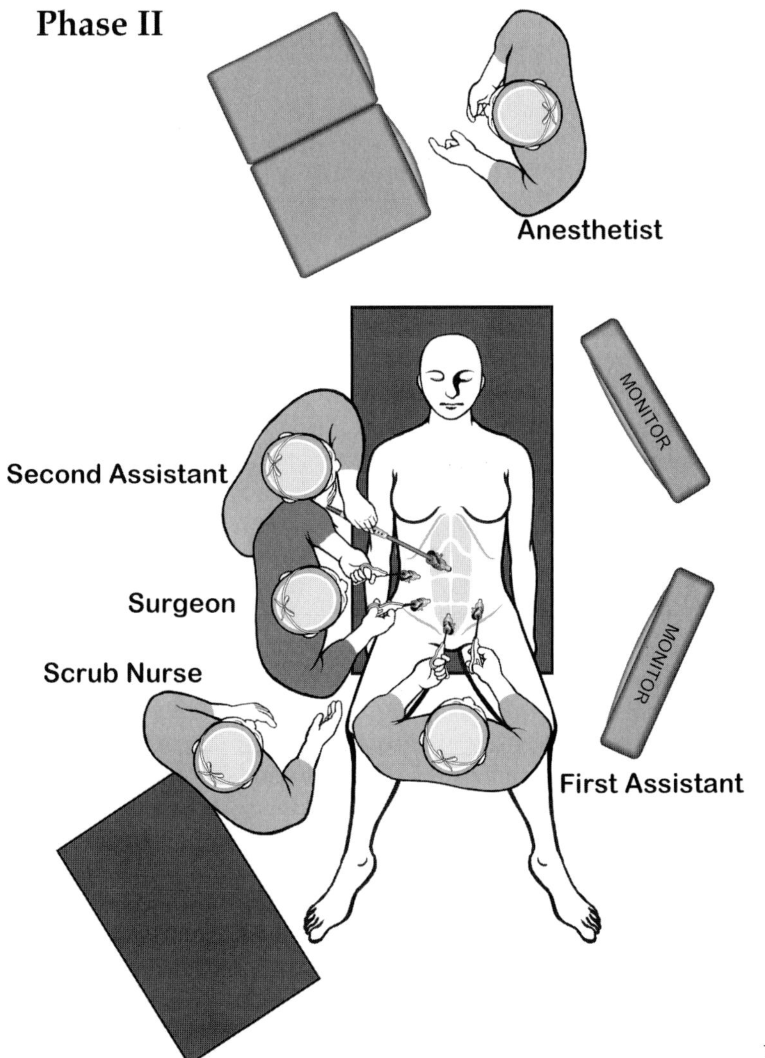

B

Figure 8.8.1. B Positions of the equipment and the surgical team for phase II of the laparoscopic proctocolectomy with ileal pouch procedure.

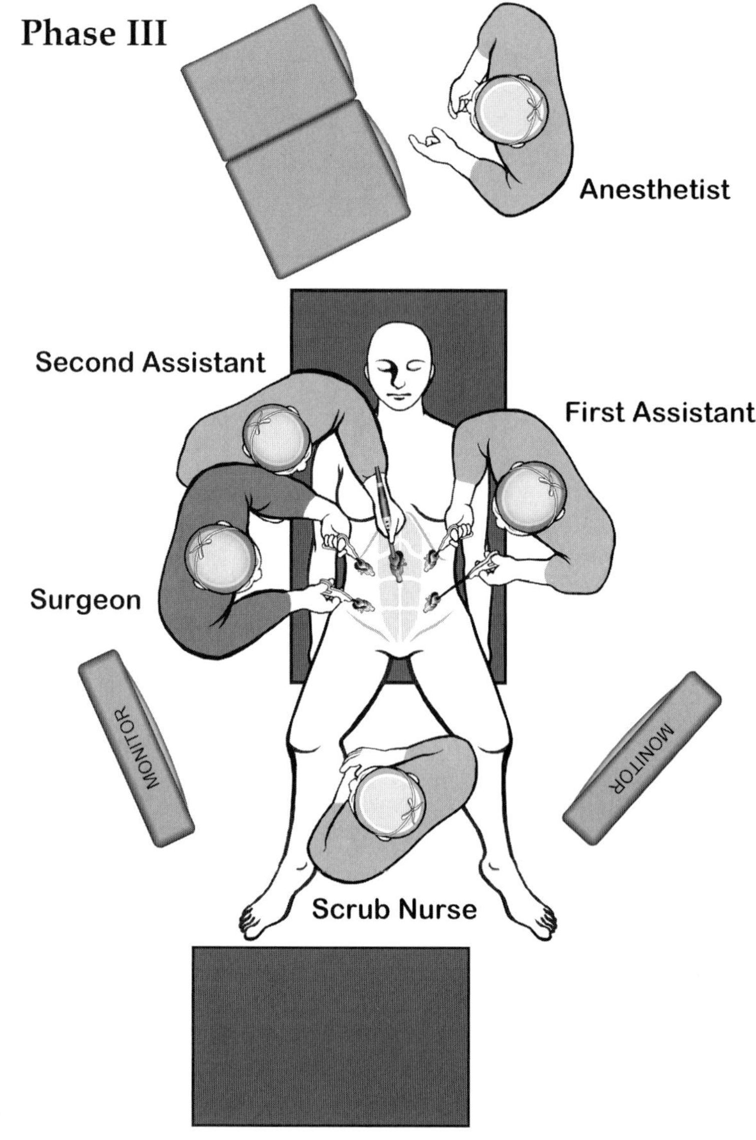

Figure 8.8.1. C Positions of the equipment and the surgical team for phase III of the laparoscopic proctocolectomy with ileal pouch procedure.

Instruments

Specific instruments recommended for laparoscopic total proctocolectomy with ileoanal pouch and diverting loop ileostomy are listed in Table 8.8.1.

Table 8.8.1. Specific instruments recommended for laparoscopic total proctocolectomy with ileoanal pouch and diverting loop ileostomy

5	Cannulae (2 × 12 mm, 1 × 10 mm, 2 × 5 mm)
1	Dissecting device (i.e., LigaSure V™ or Ultrasonic Shears™ or electrosurgery)
1	Laparoscopic scissors
1	Laparoscopic dissector
2	Laparoscopic graspers
1	Long laparoscopic grasper (to reach splenic flexure)
1	Laparoscopic clip applier – large size
4	Endoscopic staplers

Cannula Positioning

A standardized approach to cannula size and placement for all colorectal resections has reduced operative times. Five cannulae are generally required with the camera port placed in the supraumbilical position utilizing an open technique. After a diagnostic laparoscopy to assess feasibility, right-sided cannulae are placed. A 12-mm cannula is placed two fingerbreadths above and medial (2 + 2) to the right anterior superior iliac spine (Figure 8.8.2). This should always be lateral to the rectus sheath to avoid potential injury to the epigastric vessels. The large cannula can accommodate a laparoscopic clip applier, a laparoscopic

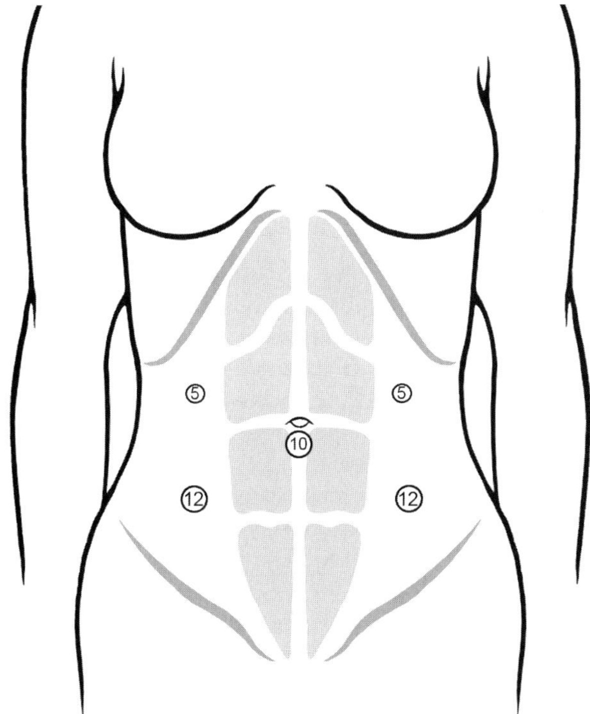

Figure 8.8.2. Positions of the cannulae for the laparoscopic proctocolectomy with ileal pouch procedure.

stapler, or a laparoscopic Babcock clamp. Before placing this cannula, lay a standard laparoscopic instrument from the right lower quadrant site to the left upper quadrant to ensure the instrument can reach the splenic flexure. For taller patients, the cannula will need to be shifted upward. For wider patients, the cannula will need to shift inward. The cannula should still lie outside the rectus sheath. I do not recommend placing the cannula in the site for a right lower quadrant ileostomy in the rectus sheath. This instrument will "sword fight" with the camera and there is potential for an epigastric vessel injury. A 5-mm cannula is placed four fingerbreadths above the lower cannula. One can easily remember this (2 + 2 then 4) measurement. The same approach to cannula placement is performed on the left side. With these five cannulae the entire colon can be devascularized and mobilized.

A 10-mm laparoscope is recommended for the majority of cases. With the advent of high-resolution 5-mm laparoscopes, this may change. I have found using the EndoEYE Deflectable Tip Video Laparoscope by Olympus (Olympus America Inc., Melville, NY), with its flexible tip, has greatly enhanced the performance of laparoscopic colon resection. A 30′ laparoscope is not necessary and may hinder orientation of the field. The camera is often in constant motion during the performance of a laparoscopic colectomy. Overviews and close magnification views are routinely required in vascular pedicle ligation and colon mobilization. The skill of the camera person can enhance or deter the flow of the procedure and may greatly alter the operative times. Because the individual running the camera tends to be the least experienced laparoscopist, I prefer a 0′ laparoscope to limit confusion in orienting the field. The camera person may already be overwhelmed with instructions by the operating surgeon, without the added complexity of a 30′ lens.

Technique

The laparoscopic portion of the procedure is broken into two segments, an extended right colectomy followed by left colectomy. Once the colon is fully mobilized and devascularized, it is brought over the small intestine to the right lower quadrant and all the small intestine is brought to the left of the midline in the left upper quadrant. A 6- to 8-cm muscle-splitting Pfannenstiel incision is created to mobilize and transect the distal rectum from the top of the anal canal, create the pouch, and complete the double-stapled anastomosis in a standard manner. For patients with ulcerative colitis, a loop ileostomy is routinely created through the right rectus muscle, separate from the right lower quadrant cannula site.

The operation begins with the isolation and division of the major vascular pedicles before lateral mobilization of the right colon. The patient is tilted left side down and Trendelenburg position so that the small intestine falls to the left side. The surgeon uses the left-sided cannulae, and the assistant, the right-sided cannulae (Figure 8.8.1a). The assistant, through the right-sided cannulae grasps the cecum and terminal ileum and retracts laterally. This is at a reverse angle to the camera and takes time to master. The ileocolic pedicle is identified as the first vessels crossing over the duodenal sweep. The assistant then grasps the pedicle and elevates the vessels and mesentery (Figure 8.8.3). The surgeon using the left-sided cannulae scores the mesentery just inferior and underneath the pedicle near its origin from the superior mesenteric vessels. A plane is developed underneath the ileocolic pedicle until the duodenum is identified and this structure is swept posteriorly. The pedicle is then isolated from surrounding structures. The ileocolic pedicle is traced distally to the cecum before division to correctly distinguish it from the superior mesenteric artery and vein. Once identification is confirmed, the pedicle is ligated and divided either using the Endo GIA stapler or a LigaSure™ device.

Once the pedicle is divided, the assistant grasps the pedicle and the cut edge of the mesocolon, and the surgeon, using a dissector and bowel grasper, begins a medial to lateral mobilization of the right colon mesentery (Figure 8.8.4). The right ureter and gonadal vessels may be seen in the retroperitoneum of a thin patient. The dissection of the mesocolon from the retroperitoneum continues laterally to the right sidewall, under the colon, then cephalad to the hepatic flexure, and medially to free the mesocolon from the duodenum. Most of the dissection is performed bluntly with minimal sharp or electrocautery dissection except over the duodenum. Here, sharp dissection is often needed to break the fine fibrous attachment between the right mesoco-

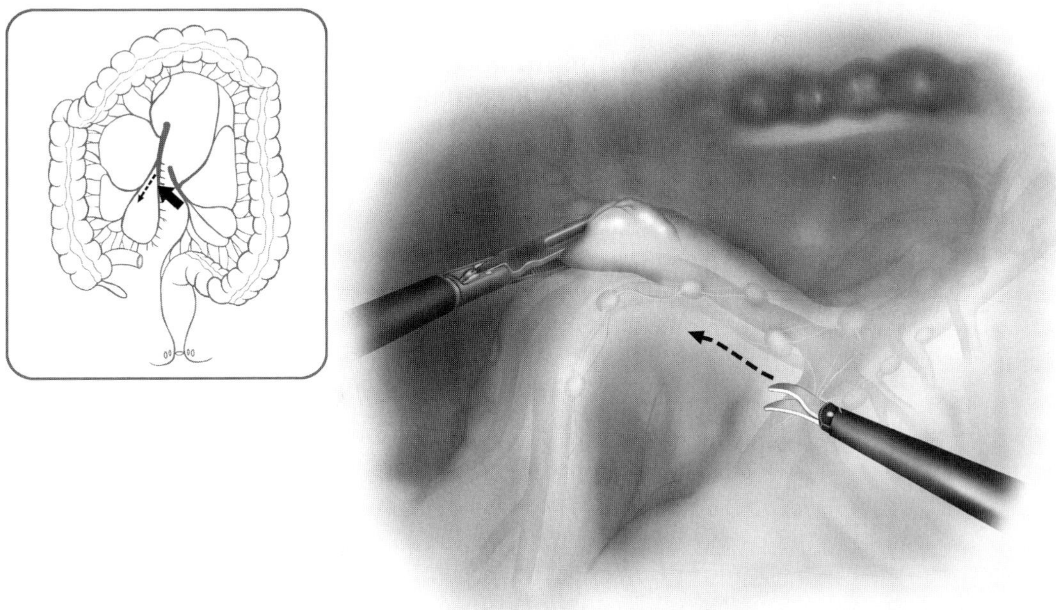

Figure 8.8.3. The initial phase involves an incision just below the ileocolic pedicle, gently placed under tension by the assistant from the right side.

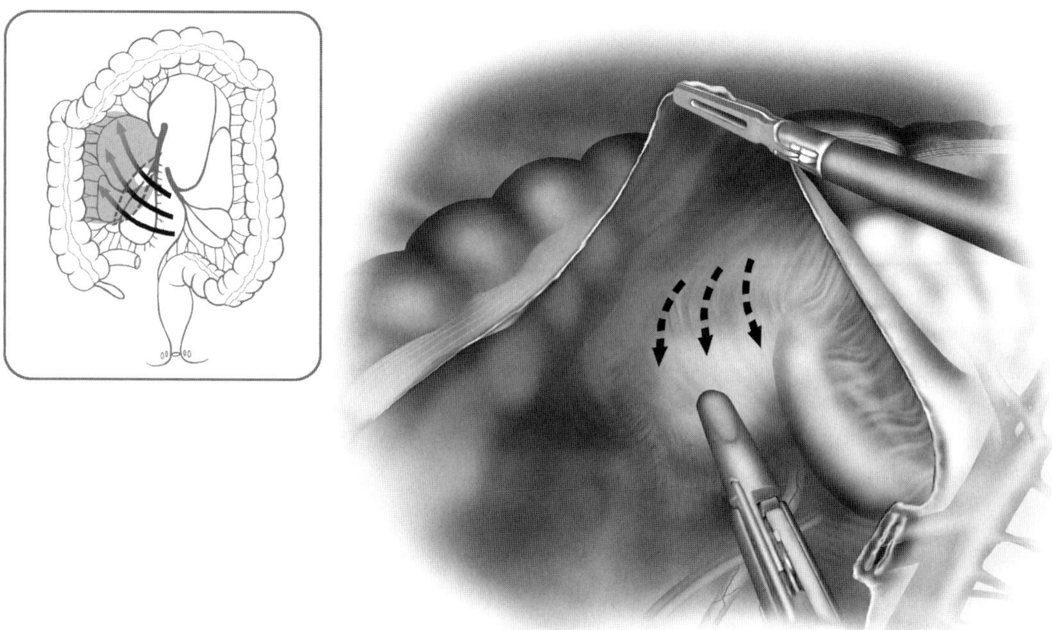

Figure 8.8.4. Once the ileocolic pedicle is divided, a medial to lateral dissection posterior to the right colon mesentery is performed.

lon and duodenum. With this "medial" approach, there is excellent visualization of the dissection from the midline camera port, without the struggle of looking over the colon.

The procedure then shifts to the division of the transverse mesocolon and middle colic vessels. The assistant has an important role in maintaining proper tension and angulation of the transverse mesocolon, to allow the surgeon to correctly identify and ligate the middle colic vessels (Figure 8.8.5). The assistant will elevate the transverse mesocolon in a vertical plane at a 90′ angle to the small bowel mesentery and superior mesenteric artery. This maneuver (called the "Olé maneuver," like the bullfighter's cape) is accomplished by passing a grasper from the right upper quadrant to hold the left side of the transverse mesocolon and another from the right lower quadrant cannula to the right side of the mesocolon. The camera person will often shift to a position between the legs at this time. The surgeon, still on the left side, may then work without the assistant's instruments crossing into the field. The surgeon incises transversely the transverse mesocolon to the left of the middle colic vessels. Here there is usually a well-defined lesser sac opening and the posterior wall of the stomach is visualized (Figure 8.8.6). The surgeon then works across the mesocolon toward the patient's right side and isolates the individual middle colic vessels. Two to three separate branches are identified, isolated, and ligated either with large clips or the LigaSure™ device. The main trunk of the

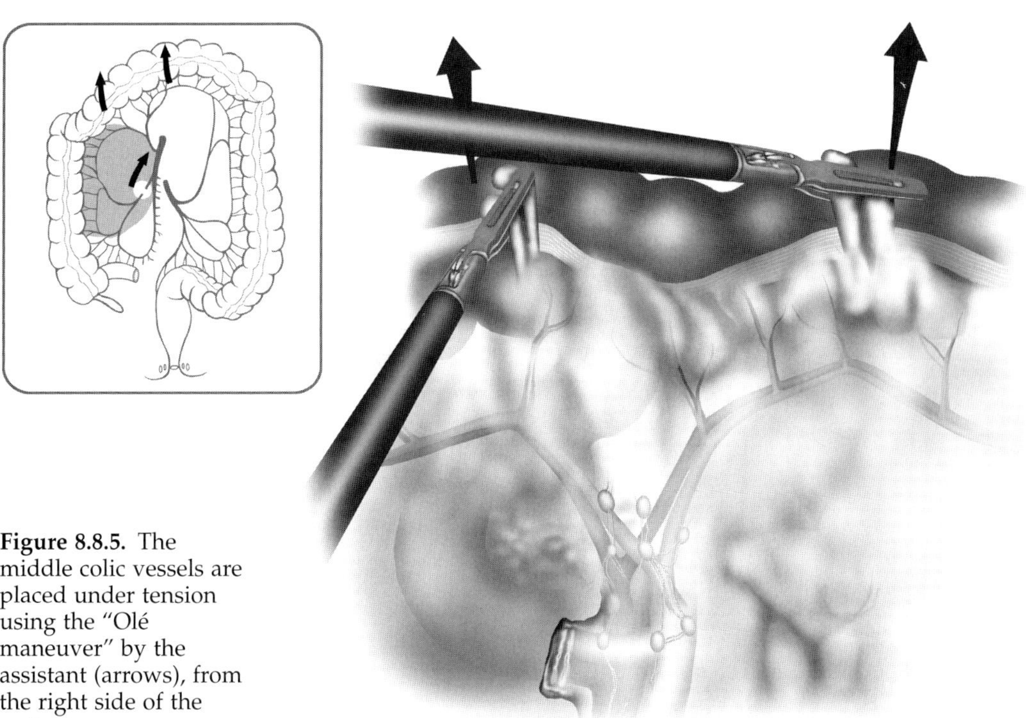

Figure 8.8.5. The middle colic vessels are placed under tension using the "Olé maneuver" by the assistant (arrows), from the right side of the patient.

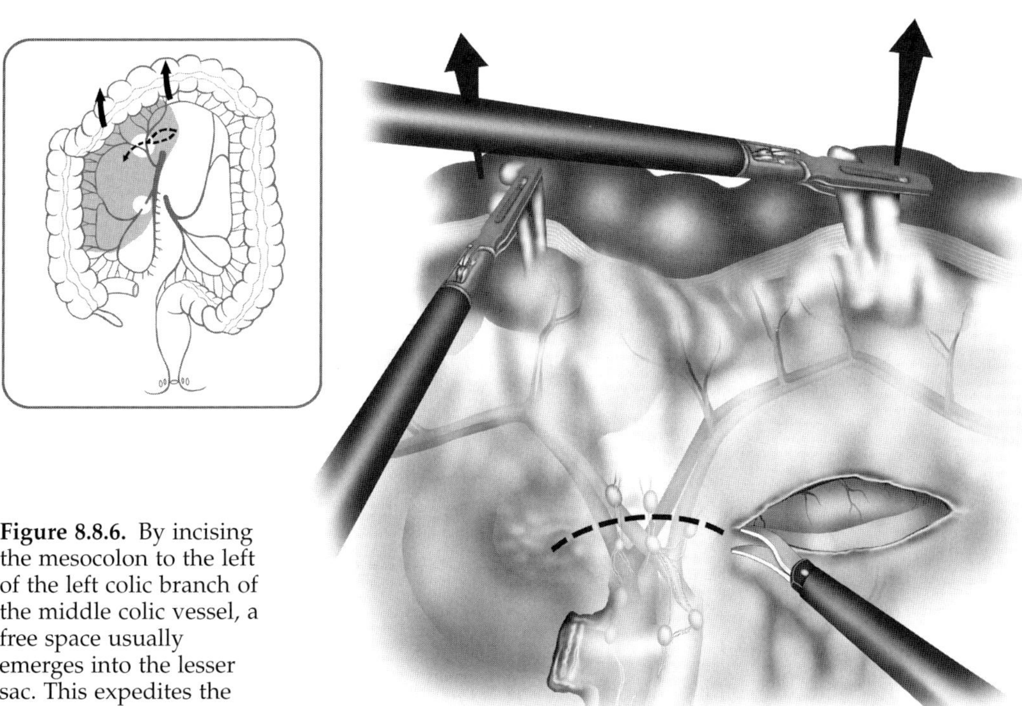

Figure 8.8.6. By incising the mesocolon to the left of the left colic branch of the middle colic vessel, a free space usually emerges into the lesser sac. This expedites the freeing of the pedicle.

middle colic artery is short and rarely visualized either in open or laparoscopic surgery. If the surgeon attempts to divide this main trunk, near the superior mesenteric artery, there is the potential to injure the superior mesenteric artery either directly or indirectly and, therefore, the branches of the middle colic artery should be the target, not the main trunk. Once the middle colic branches are divided, the surgeon continues to work toward the patient's right side, freeing any filmy adhesions between the mesocolon and dorsal side of the omentum. The surgeon may then encounter a right colic pedicle or potentially a large venous trunk called the "gastrocolic trunk." This area over the first portion of the duodenum can often be confusing. It is possible to identify from this approach the gastroepiploic vessels and omental vessels after the mesocolon has been divided.

The surgeon needs to maintain proper orientation of the field. If unsure of the origin of a vessel in this area, the surgeon should proceed with lateral mobilization and return to this once the omentum has been separated from the colon edge. At this junction, the entire right and proximal transverse mesocolon has been divided. One can now visualize the major pedicles, duodenum, and pancreatic head (Figure 8.8.7).

The procedure then turns to the lateral mobilization of the right colon. The appendix and cecum are elevated and the peritoneum is incised to free these structures (Figure 8.8.8). This continues until the point of medial mobilization of the right mesocolon is met. Here the

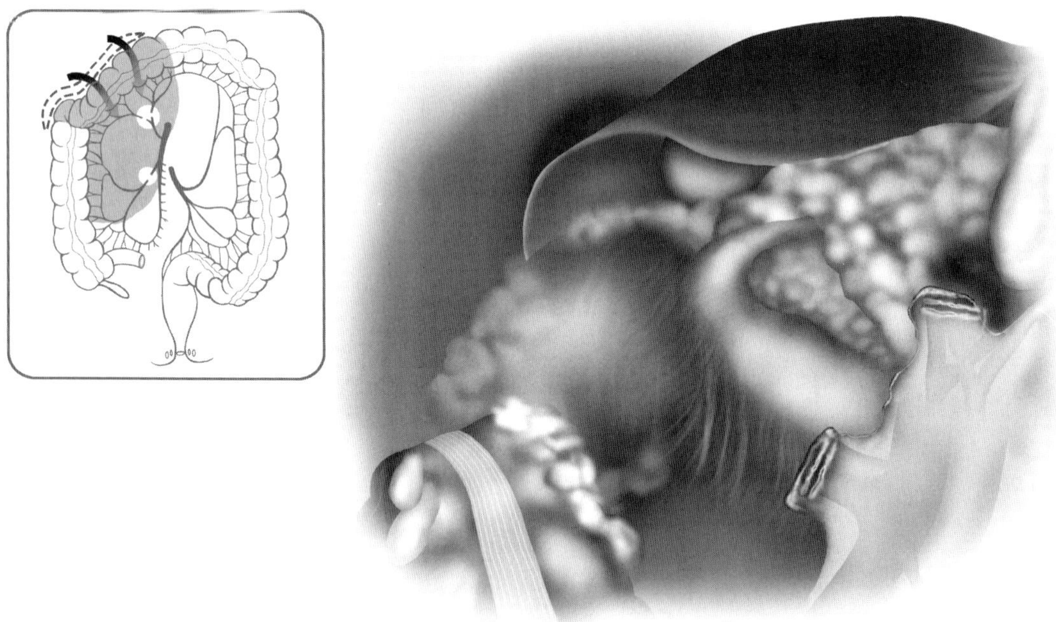

Figure 8.8.7. View after the complete right colon mobilization permits clear view of the head of the pancreas and duodenum.

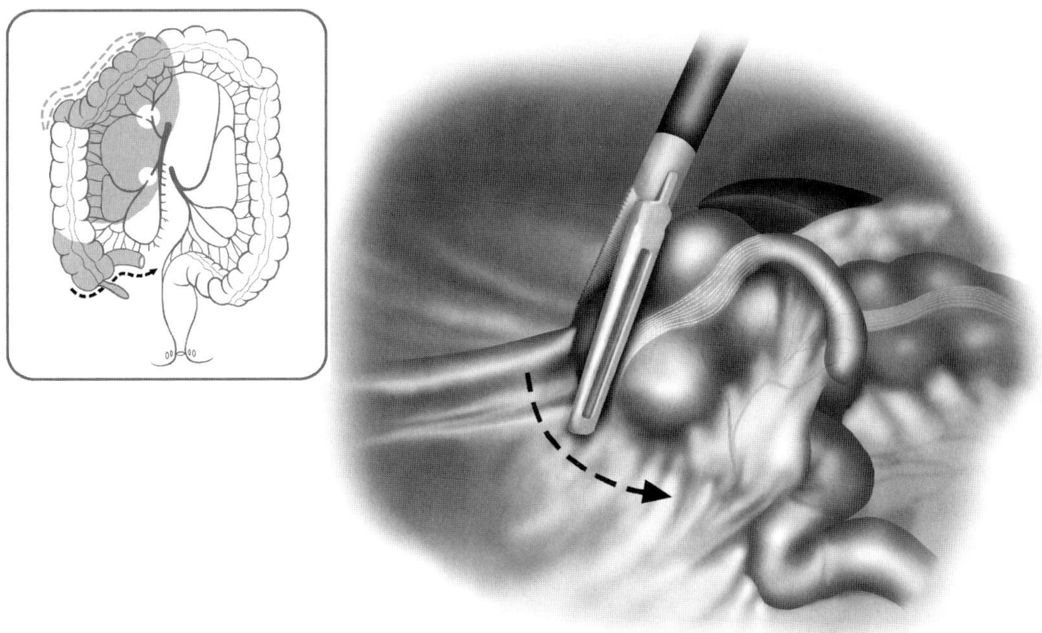

Figure 8.8.8. Lateral mobilization of the right colon starts by incising peritoneum at the base of appendix and cecum.

surgeon will enter an open space, which had been dissected previously during the medial mobilization of the right colon mesentery. The attachments of the terminal ileal mesentery are then divided up to the duodenum. If an ileoanal pouch is to be constructed, the terminal ileal mesentery is further mobilized over the duodenum. This is done with the assistant elevating the ileal mesentery and the surgeon still on the left side freeing the attachments (Figure 8.8.9). The camera is almost vertical during this portion of the procedure, which can be quite disorienting.

The dissection then continues laterally up the right colic gutter where now there remains only a fine line of attachment of the colon to the lateral side wall. The surgeon switches to two graspers to reflect the colon medially as the assistant, through the right lower quadrant cannula, uses a hook cautery to divide the lateral attachments (Figure 8.8.10). At the hepatic flexure, the surgeon separates the omentum from the colon and the assistant, again with the hook cautery, divides the planes. This reproduces the same technique as open surgery with the surgeon providing traction and countertraction and the assistant using the cautery. Once the omentum is freed from the colon edge, it is then separated from the cephalad side of the mesentery until the lesser sac is entered. This can be a very tedious portion of the procedure depending on how fused the mesocolon and omentum are to each other. I will often separate the omentum and colon to the left of midline where the

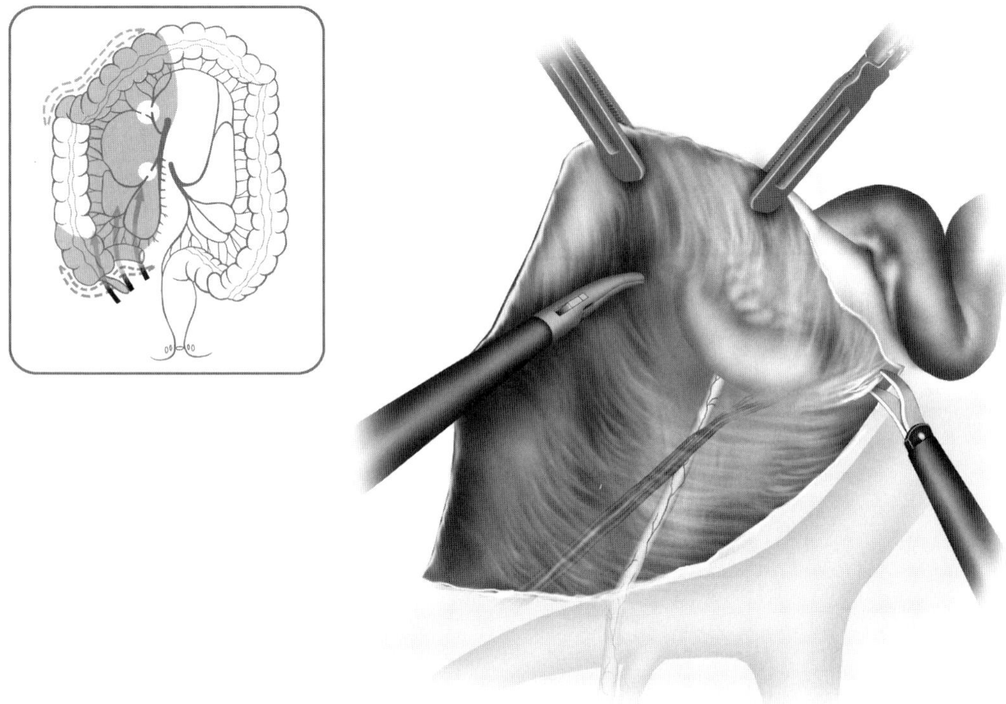

Figure 8.8.9. Attachments of the ileal mesentery are freed up to the duodenum.

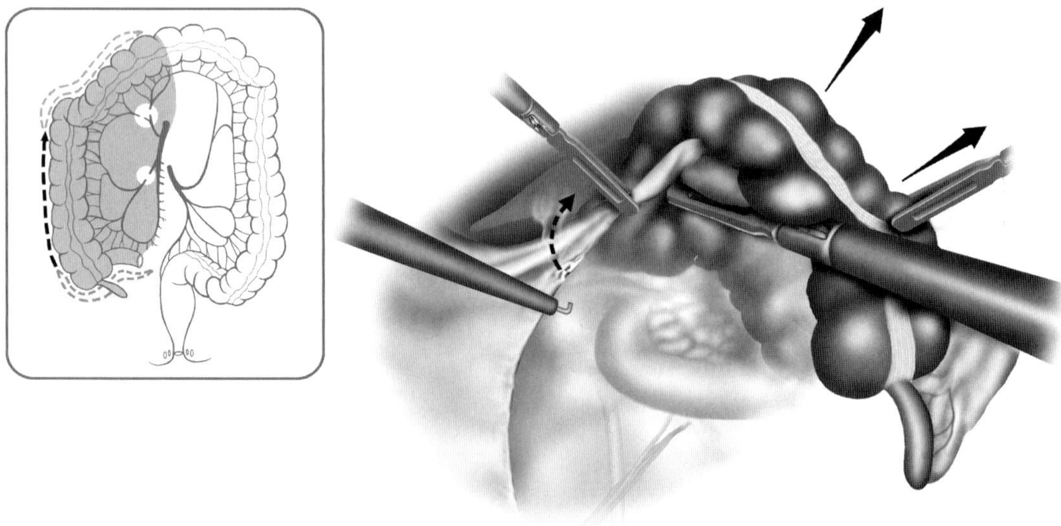

Figure 8.8.10. The lateral attachments of the right colon are divided using a hook cautery instrument.

lesser sac is usually well developed and work back to the hepatic flexure. The entire right colon and terminal ileum are now fully mobilized to a point beyond the midline, completing this portion of the procedure. The colon and terminal ileum should be placed back in anatomic position before beginning the next step to prevent the ileal mesentery from twisting.

The procedure then shifts to the left colon. Monitors and the surgical team are repositioned (Figure 8.8.1B). The patient is placed in steep Trendelenburg and is tilted right side down so the small intestine falls into the right upper quadrant. If the small bowel will not stay out of the pelvis, a sponge can be passed through the 12-mm cannula to help hold the small bowel away. The assistant elevates the inferior mesenteric pedicle and the surgeon makes an incision along the right peritoneal fold of the rectosigmoid mesentery beginning at the sacral promontory (Figure 8.8.11). The incision parallels the course of the inferior mesenteric pedicle and should be opened widely. Using blunt dissection, the inferior mesenteric artery and vein are swept ventrally away from the preaortic hypogastric nerve plexus. Small nerve fibers, which directly enter the mesocolon, are sacrificed and the main nerve plexus is swept dorsally. As dissection is continued medially beneath the inferior mesenteric artery and vein, the left ureter and gonadal vessels are identified and swept posteriorly (Figure 8.8.12). The assistant should grasp the inferior mesenteric artery and mesentery to facilitate exposure underneath the pedicle. If the ureter cannot be readily and easily identified at this point in the dissection, the lateral attach-

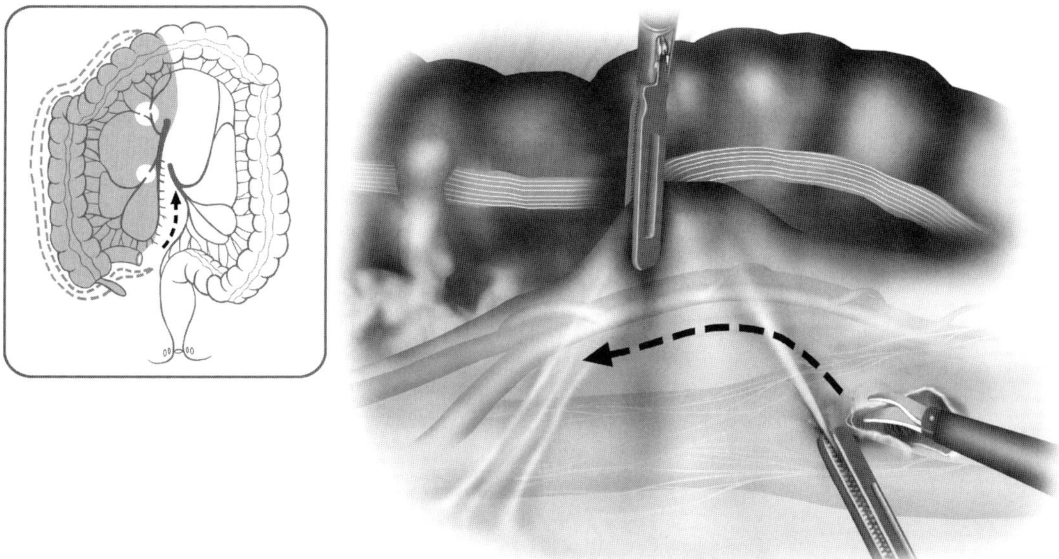

Figure 8.8.11. Dissection of the left colon begins with dissection of the inferior mesenteric artery at the sacral promontory.

ments of the sigmoid colon are incised, the sigmoid colon is mobilized left to right, and the gonadal vessels and left ureter are identified laterally and dissected free of the mesentery.

Once the origin of the inferior mesenteric artery is identified, the peritoneum is incised anteriorly over this pedicle and across the inferior mesenteric vein. The surgeon then uses blunt dissection under the pedicle to create a window lateral to the inferior mesenteric artery and vein below the left colic vessels. A high ligation of the pedicle is not necessary for benign disease. The inferior mesenteric pedicle is ligated and divided either using the Endo GIA stapler or LigaSure™ device. Before firing the stapler or LigaSure™ device, the tips should be clearly visible and the location of the left ureter confirmed (Figure 8.8.13). The proximal and distal sides of the pedicle are grasped so any bleeding can be easily controlled. We prefer to leave the pedicle 1.5–2.0 cm long so if any bleeding occurs, an additional clip or LigaSure™ application can be applied to the pedicle. Once the pedicle is divided, the left colon mesentery then opens and the left colon mesentery is mobilized form medial to lateral in a similar manner as was done for the right colon. The assistant holds the divided distal end of the inferior mesenteric pedicle through the lower port and the cut edge of the left colon mesentery above the pedicle and the surgeon uses blunt dissection with appropriate traction and countertraction to dissect the left colon mes-

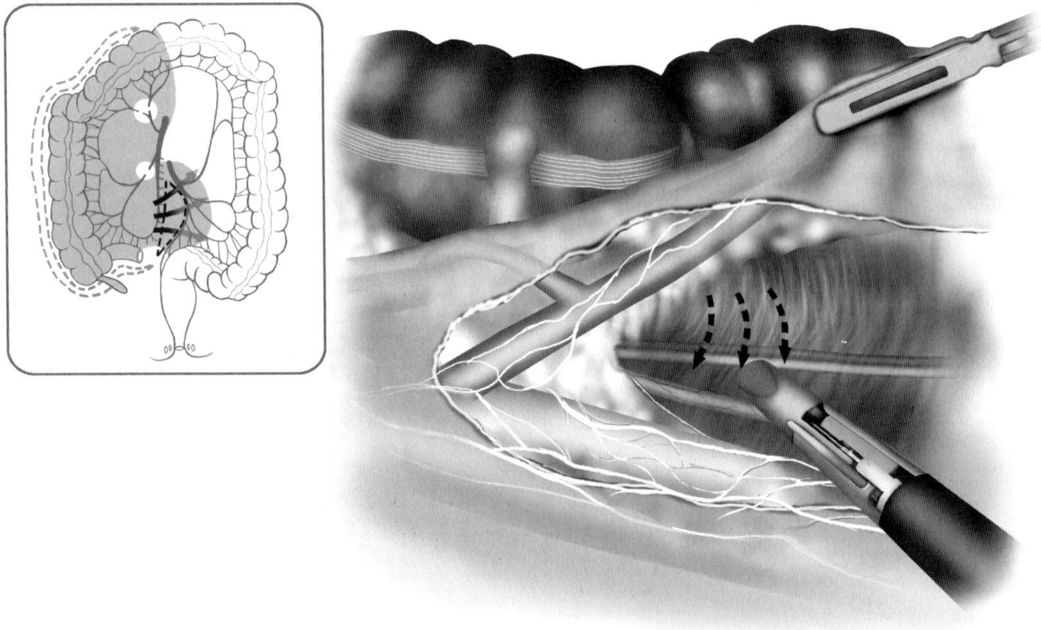

Figure 8.8.12. With dissection of the inferior mesenteric artery, the retroperitoneal attachments are swept posteriorly, and the ureter and gonadal vessels are clearly identified.

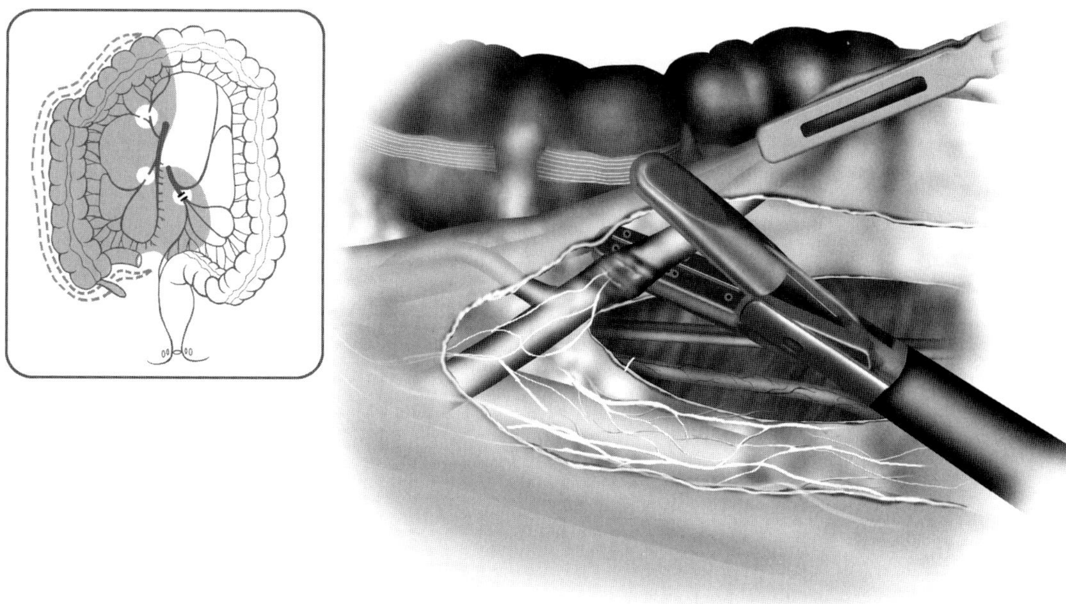

Figure 8.8.13. Once the hypogastric vessels are identified and dissected away from the inferior mesenteric artery, the vessel is ligated with a bipolar device below the left colic artery.

entery from the retroperitoneum. This remains a relatively avascular plane with the exception of a few small vessels on the surface of Gerota's fascia.

The dissection from medial to lateral proceeds out under the sigmoid colon to the lateral side wall, inferiorly into the upper retrorectal space, and superiorly under the splenic flexure. The left-sided monitor is moved from the left foot to the left shoulder. The surgeon then continues dissecting in a cephalad manner, sweeping Gerota's fascia away from the posterior surface of the colonic mesentery. All medial mesenteric attachments should be divided as far cephalad, in a line parallel to and just lateral to the inferior mesenteric vein. The left colic pedicle is identified, isolated, ligated, and divided (Figure 8.8.14). As the dissection continues cephalad, the small bowel will tend to obscure the view. To handle this, the table is repositioned with a slight reverse Trendelenburg and steep left side upward position. If the head is elevated too much above the feet, the transverse colon may hinder the exposure. Once the left colon mesentery is mobilized medially up to the transverse colon, the dissection continues laterally.

The team repositions for the final phase of the colectomy (Figure 8.8.1C). The senior surgeon remains on the patient's right side and will provide medial traction on the colon as the lateral attachments are divided by the assistant standing between the legs. The white line of Toldt is incised with the hook cautery and the point of medial mobiliza-

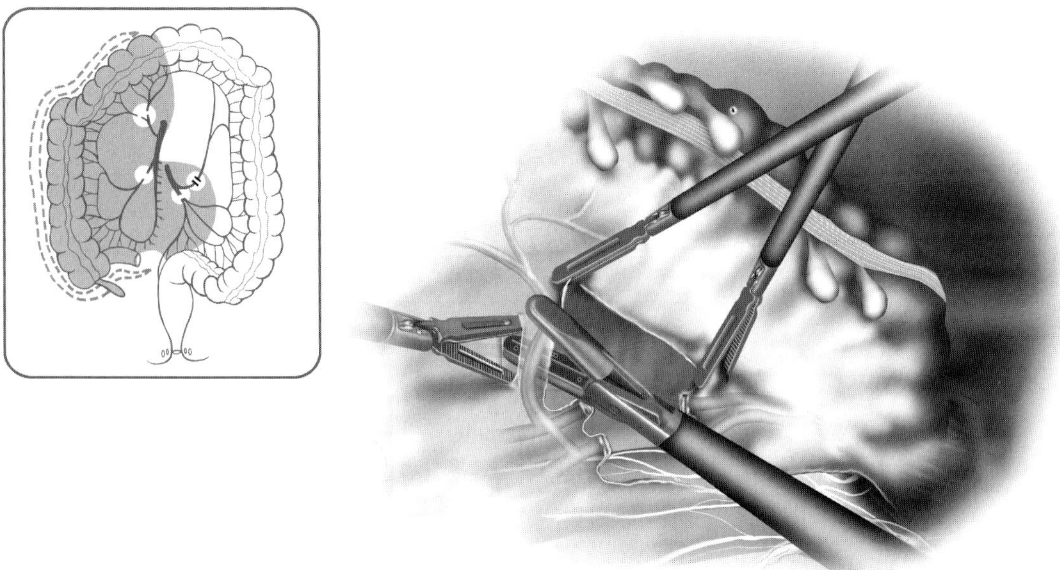

Figure 8.8.14. The left colic pedicle is isolated and divided just after the main vessel ligation.

tion is quickly reached. The colon is retracted medially as the dissection continues cephalad toward the splenic flexure. If the colon has been adequately mobilized from the medial approach, there should only be one or two layers of thin attachments laterally. During this dissection, the surgeon constantly must remain in the proper planes (Figure 8.8.15) – generally close to the bowel edge laterally, between Gerota's fascia and the bowel mesentery.

In the region of the splenic flexure, the greater omentum gradually appears and is distinguishable from the epiploic appendices by its finer lobulated fatty texture. Separation of the omentum from the colon and these appendices is essential for accurate mobilization of the flexure (Figure 8.8.16). Once the first layer of omental attachments is freed (Figure 8.8.17), there is often a secondary attachment of the omentum to the ventral aspect of the distal transverse mesocolon that must be divided. If the splenic flexure proves to be difficult to dissect, the dissection can be continued right to left from the distal transverse colon toward the splenic flexure. The remaining omental attachments can be divided beginning in the mid-transverse colon where they had been previously divided during the right colon mobilization. In our experience, it is important to mobilize the left colon and left mesocolon as far cephalad as possible in the dorsal mesenteric plane adjacent to Gerota's fascia. This greatly simplifies the mobilization of the splenic flexure, and may simplify dissection of the greater omentum and the lateral adhesions close to the colonic wall. Once the splenic flexure is mobilized, the only remaining attachment of the colon is a small segment of

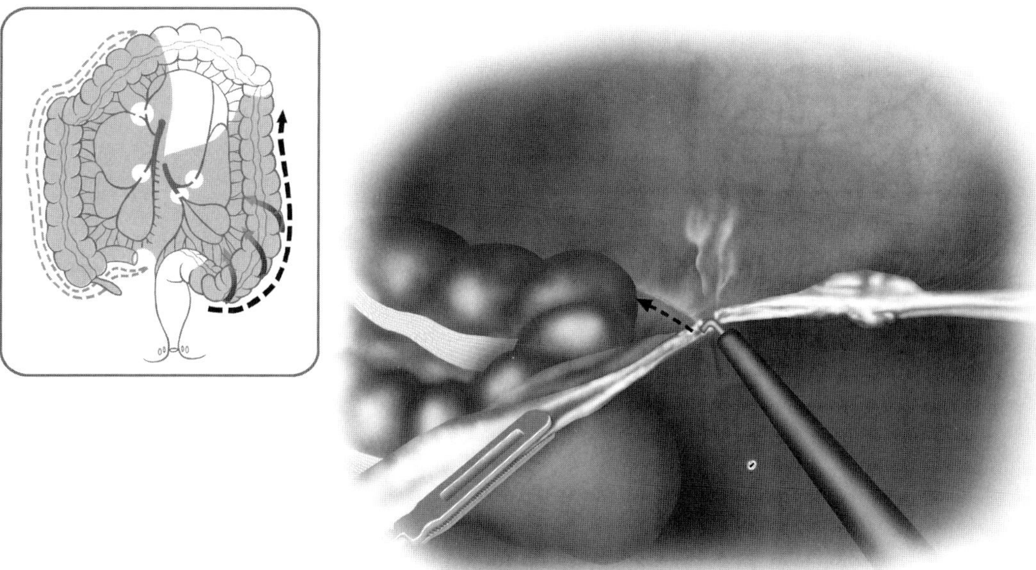

Figure 8.8.15. After medial to lateral dissection of the left mesocolon, the lateral colonic attachments are divided with the hook cautery instrument.

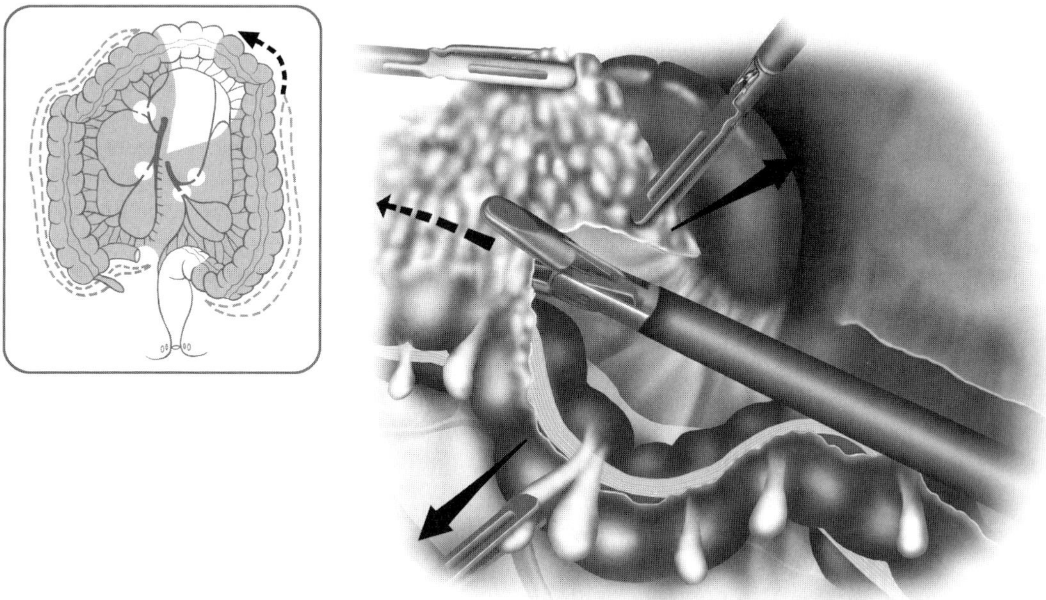

Figure 8.8.16. The omentum is freed from the splenic flexure attachments using a bipolar device.

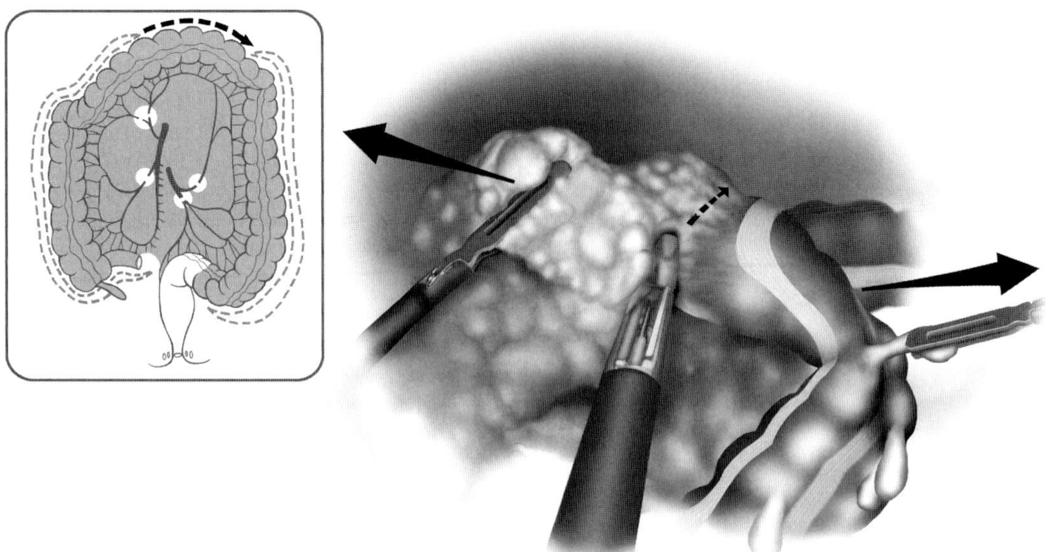

Figure 8.8.17. If dissection is difficult from the lateral side, splenic flexure takedown may be expedited using a medial to lateral approach starting in the middle portion of the transverse colon.

the distal transverse mesocolon. There may be a large venous branch to the inferior mesenteric vein in this segment, which requires ligation and division if identified.

Once these final attachments have been dissected, the entire colon is free and must be placed over the small intestine to prepare for extraction. The patient is typically in a slight reverse Trendelenburg position with the left side upward. To facilitate placement of the colon over the small intestine, the table will be gently shifted to a Trendelenburg and right side upward position. The surgeon, who is now standing between the patient's legs, coordinates the change in table positioning. The surgeon uses the two left-sided cannulae and elevates the splenic flexure and starts to bring this over the small intestine to the right lower quadrant. As this is done, the table is shifted and the small intestine should pass under the colon to the left upper quadrant (Figure 8.8.18). The surgeon continues to pass the colon over the small intestine and follows the mesenteric edge of the colon proximally. Eventually all of the small intestine will lie in the left upper quadrant and the surgeon can trace the mesenteric edge of the small intestine up and over the duodenum (Figure 8.8.19). If this is not performed correctly, the mesentery to the small intestine may twist and not allow the colon to be extracted through the Pfannenstiel incision.

With the colon now in the right lower quadrant, the surgeon has two options. One option is to begin and complete the rectal mobilization laparoscopically and then create the Pfannenstiel incision for rectal transection and pouch construction. If the surgeon has extensive laparoscopic experience, or the patient is moderately obese, this may be the

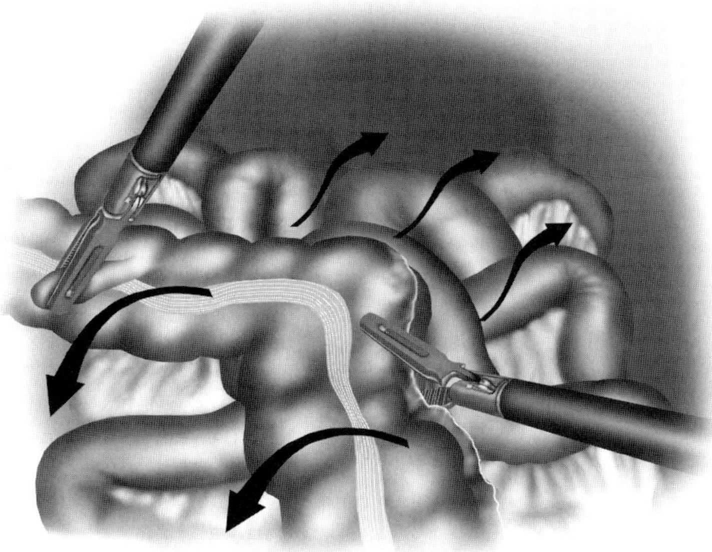

Figure 8.8.18. Once the colon is completely freed, the colon is passed over the small intestines and placed into the right lower quadrant.

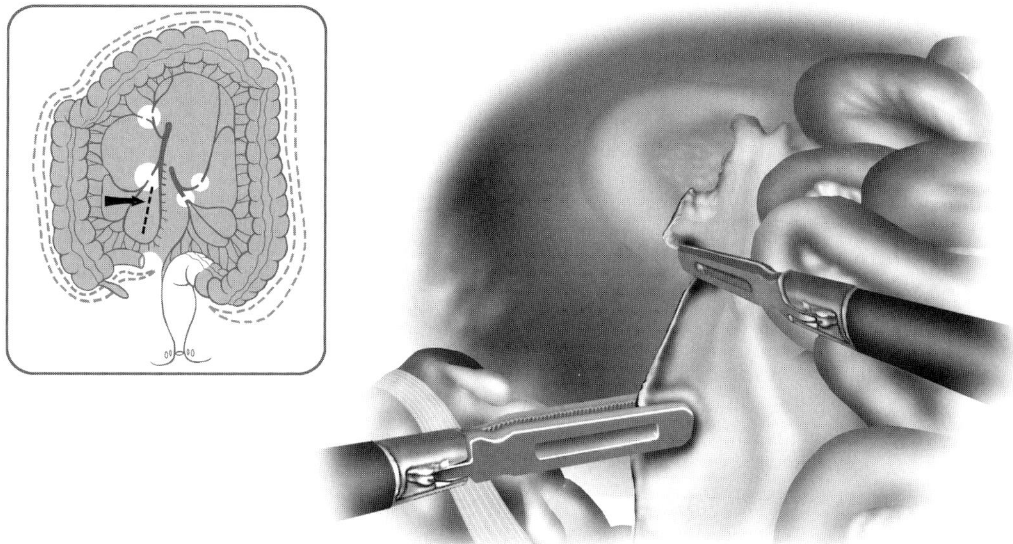

Figure 8.8.19. The surgeon must trace the cut edge of the small intestine mesentery on the right side to be sure that there is no twisting.

preferred approach. The other option is to create the Pfannenstiel incision now and proceed with open rectal mobilization, transection, and pouch construction. This is my preferred approach. Because an incision is needed eventually for pouch construction, one can more easily accomplish rectal mobilization through the open wound. This reduces both the operative time and the technical complexity of the procedure because most surgeons are not skilled in laparoscopic rectal mobilization. If the rectal mobilization is to be performed open, the three 12-mm cannula sites are closed in a transcorporeal manner with absorbable suture before discontinuation of pneumoperitoneum.

An 8-cm Pfannenstiel incision is made two fingerbreadths above the pubic symphysis. The anterior rectus sheath is incised transversely and curved upward at the lateral edges to remain out of the inguinal canal. Superior and inferior flaps are created over the rectus muscle and the peritoneum is incised vertically between the rectus muscles. The peritoneum is incised either to the left or right of the midline inferiorly with care to avoid injury to the bladder wall. A wound protector is placed and a Balfour retractor is used to facilitate the view into the pelvis.

If a loop ileostomy is planned, the incision both in the skin and the anterior rectus sheath for the ileostomy should be made before the Pfannenstiel incision. This is required to prevent a shutter effect at the fascial level of the ileostomy. This can occur if the opening for the ileostomy is made after the Pfannenstiel incision is created and the fascia of the ileostomy is pulled caudally when the fascia of the Pfannenstiel incision is closed transversely (Figure 8.8.20). This may lead to early intestinal obstruction. To avoid this potential complication, the skin and fascial opening for the ileostomy should be made before Pfannenstiel incision. If the ileostomy is created after the Pfannenstiel incision, the fascia of the Pfannenstiel should be pulled caudally as the ileostomy aperture is created. The fascia of the ileostomy should be opened more widely than usual to prevent this complication. If the patient develops evidence of an early bowel obstruction after surgery, narrowing of the ileostomy at the fascial level may be the cause. This can be readily diagnosed by retrograde ileostomy injection or by simply passing a red rubber tube through the ileostomy several inches, which will alleviate the relative obstruction.

Before rectal mobilization, the colon is extracted and divided from the terminal ileum. It is important to maintain proper orientation of the small bowel mesentery during colon extraction. The patient is placed in Trendelenburg position with the right side up to keep the small intestine to the left of midline. A lighted Deaver retractor is used to illuminate the field as the colon is extracted. If performed correctly, one can follow the cut edge of the mesentery up and over the duodenum with all the small bowel remaining to the left of midline. This orientation is maintained for eventual ileoanal pouch construction and anastomosis. The terminal ileum and its mesentery are divided in the usual manner. A tagging suture is placed beneath the staple line of the terminal ileum, and the small bowel is protected with moist laparotomy sponges, in preparation for the rectal dissection.

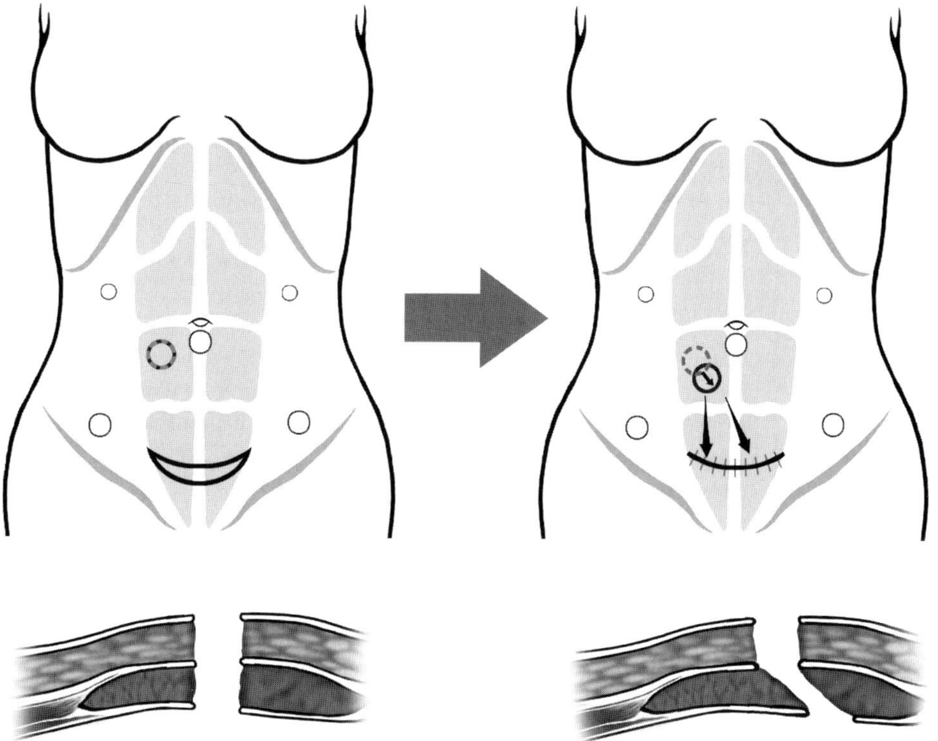

Figure 8.8.20. The incision in the skin and the fascia (both anterior and posterior sheaths) must be carefully aligned so that a "shutter" effect (arrow) does not occur after fascial closure of the suprapubic incision. This could cause an ileostomy obstruction in the postoperative period.

Rectal mobilization through the Pfannenstiel incision can be quite challenging especially in the male pelvis. We use a lighted pelvic retractor and long instruments because often the hand cannot fit through the wound. If necessary, the skin incision can be enlarged to complete the dissection. The rate-limiting factor in viewing the pelvis through the Pfannenstiel is often the skin and not the rectus muscle. Once the rectum is completely mobilized from the abdomen, it may be either divided with a linear stapler or a rectal mucosectomy from the perineal approach may be performed depending on surgeon's preference and patient diagnosis.

Once the colon and rectum are removed, the small intestine is brought through the Pfannenstiel incision and pouch construction and anastomosis is performed according to the surgeon's preference. Before completing the anastomosis, the surgeon should check the orientation of the small bowel mesentery one last time through the Pfannenstiel incision using the lighted retractors. Once the anastomosis is completed, the abdomen is lavaged and a drain may be placed through the left lower cannula site. A loop ileostomy is created in the majority of cases with special care to the opening in the anterior sheath as mentioned above. It is our preference to wrap the ileostomy with Seprafilm (Genzyme Corporation, Cambridge, MA) to facilitate eventual ileostomy closure. The peritoneum of the Pfannenstiel incision is closed vertically and the rectus muscle is loosely reapproximated in the midline with several interrupted sutures to prevent diastases of the rectus. The anterior rectus sheath is closed transversely with two sutures, one coming from each corner to prevent the possible development of a lateral hernia near the internal inguinal ring. The skin incisions are closed and the ileostomy is matured.

Special Considerations

Intraoperative

The most common intraoperative complication associated with laparoscopic total colectomy is bleeding from the vascular pedicles during intracorporeal ligation. Whether vascular clips, laparoscopic vascular staplers, or sealing devices such as LigaSure™ are used, all have the potential to cause minor or significant bleeding. The surgeon must be prepared for this. On the Mayo stand should be several laparoscopic grasping forceps which can be easily reached by the operating surgeon should bleeding occur. Also, maintaining proximal and distal control of the major vascular pedicles is mandatory, so they may be more easily controlled if bleeding is encountered. If bleeding occurs after application of the vascular stapler, it is usually not possible to reapply a second stapler load. The vessel, however, can be controlled by use of an Endoloop (Ethicon Endo-Surgery, Cincinnati, OH) or by clips. The surgeon should be familiar with the use of an Endoloop. Its first application by the surgeon should not be after a major bleeding event. We routinely use Endoloops to ligate the appendiceal stump during laparoscopic appendectomy, to allow our residents to gain experience with this device. If bleeding occurs with the application of clips, it may be controlled with further clip application or with an Endoloop. Finally, I will add a word of caution with the use of the LigaSure™ device. The product works extremely well in most circumstances, but may not be as effective on heavily calcified vessels. If a heavily calcified vessel is encountered, I prefer to control this with a stapler or clips. This would be unusual during laparoscopic restorative proctocolectomy, because the procedure is typically performed in a younger patient population. If bleeding occurs after application of the LigaSure™ device, it may be reapplied to control the bleeding or controlled by use of clips or an Endoloop. Although intraoperative pedicle bleeding is rare, it requires a quick and effective management approach to avoid significant blood loss.

Another complication specific to the laparoscopic portion of this procedure is difficulty in mobilizing the flexures. This is a long operation, which can be made even longer if visualization is inadequate. The vast majority of patients in whom we perform this procedure are young, thin patients. Although this may seem to be the ideal group in whom to perform a laparoscopic procedure, the fact that they are young and thin generally means that they have strong abdominal musculature which does not relax adequately under anesthesia. These taut muscles also do not allow the abdominal wall to distend well after pneumoperitoneum, which can limit visualization, because there is only a small working field between the bowel and parietal peritoneum. This is most noteworthy at the flexures. Also, with a chronically inflamed colon, the omentum may be wrapped tightly over the colon. This is usually seen at the splenic flexure. To manage these issues, it is important to maintain a proper visual field. A 30′ lens or a flexible tip laparoscope such as the EndoEYE™ Deflectable Tip Video Laparoscope by Olympus (Olympus America Inc.) may improve the view at the flexures. Performing as much of the dissection from the posterior plane before attempting mobilization laterally or anteriorly, will elevate the colon from the retroperitoneum which may facilitate the dissection. The table may need to be positioned in a slight reverse Trendelenburg position to keep the small bowel out of the field. If the patient is placed in too steep a reverse Trendelenburg position, the omentum will drift over the colon, impairing visualization. Finally, if the flexure cannot be separated by straight laparoscopic means, a hand-assisted approach should be used to facilitate the procedure. The device can be placed through the Pfannenstiel incision. The use of the hand can greatly enhance dissection of the colon from the omentum and can also assist with blunt mobilization of the colon and mesocolon from the retroperitoneum. A hand-assisted approach to laparoscopic restorative proctocolectomy has now become my personal procedure of choice based on our early results with a hand-assisted technique.[1]

Early Postoperative Concerns

The most common early postoperative complication after laparoscopic restorative proctocolectomy is partial small bowel obstruction or ileus. The treatment of this is generally conservative with intravenous hydration, nasogastric tube decompression, and observation of the patient. The only detail specific to this procedure is swelling or obstruction of the ileostomy. If the ileostomy is manipulated excessively during maturation of the ileostomy, stomal edema may develop within 2–3 days of the procedure. One will then note the swelling of the ileostomy with either diminished stomal output, or thin watery output of low or high quantity. If this is encountered, the patient should not be fed and the swelling allowed to subside before enteral feeding is attempted. This can be a frustrating complication, because the patient is otherwise well and could be discharged were it not for the inability to tolerate a diet. This complication will often delay discharge for 3–4 days, but cannot be rushed. Another type of obstruction specific to this procedure, as mentioned above, is obstruction of the ileostomy at the level of the anterior rectus sheath (Figure 8.8.20). This typically does not present until 2–3 days after surgery, but in this case, there is no swelling of the ileostomy. The patient will develop abdominal distention and emesis, requiring nasogastric decompression. The diagnosis can be made by a retrograde ileostomy injection which will demonstrate dilatation of the distal small bowel up to the fascial level of the stoma. The diagnosis can also be confirmed by passing a red rubber catheter through the ileostomy a distance of 3–4 inches. There will typically be a gush of effluent. This is our preferred initial management approach to this complication. The catheter may be left in place or intermittently passed into the ileostomy for several days to a week until the obstruction resolves. In most circumstances, surgical intervention is not required. If the obstruction does not resolve spontaneously, then a local revision of the ileostomy, to enlarge the fascial aperture, is recommended. This specific complication can be avoided by creating the ileostomy aperture before the Pfannenstiel incision, or by creating a larger opening in the anterior rectus sheath if the ileostomy is created after the Pfannenstiel incision.

Conclusions

Laparoscopic proctocolectomy with ileoanal pouch construction is the most extensive laparoscopic colorectal procedure to perform. However, if broken into its separate components, right and transverse colon mobilization, left colon mobilization, proctectomy, and ileoanal pouch construction, each component is feasible once adequate laparoscopic experience has been achieved with segmental laparoscopic colectomy. The procedure provides significant advantages over a conventional approach for the patient requiring surgery. With an experienced team, the operation can be performed safely and in a reasonable operative time, usually within 5 hours. With the expansion of laparoscopic colectomy, laparoscopic proctocolectomy with ileoanal pouch construction will likely replace the conventional approach in the majority of cases.

Editors' Comments

Indications: We agree with the author regarding his indications.

Patient positioning: Our positioning is very similar. We use a gel pad underneath the patient and do not use any taping or bracing of the patient otherwise.

Instrumentation: We use similar instruments.

Cannula positioning: We generally agree with their positioning.

Technique: We have no major differences to the technique described by Dr. Marcello. We do not use the Seprafilm on a routine basis around the ileostomy site. If the 5-mm LigaSure™ device is used, then one may use 5-mm cannula sites except for the umbilical cannula, because bowel division and stapling is done outside the abdomen through the Pfannenstiel incision. We also agree that this procedure has great potential and the advantages it may offer need to be studied in a prospective manner in the future.

Reference

1. Rivadeneira DE, Marcello PW, Roberts PL, et al. Benefits of hand-assisted laparoscopic restorative proctocolectomy: a comparative study. Dis Colon Rectum 2004;47:1371–1376.

Chapter 9.1

Hand-Assisted Laparoscopic Anterior Resection

Joseph Carter and Richard L. Whelan

Although the safety and feasibility of laparoscopic-assisted segmental colectomy have been demonstrated in a number of studies, there are far less data available concerning sphincter-saving anterior rectal resections. Laparoscopic rectal mobilization and resection at the level of the mid or distal rectum is considerably more difficult than segmental colectomy and provides numerous technical challenges. Anatomic characteristics that conspire to make pelvic dissection difficult include a narrow and deep pelvis, a large uterus, or obesity. There are also reasonable, yet undocumented, concerns regarding inadvertent traumatization of the tumor by the shafts or tips of laparoscopic instruments reaching past and around the lesion. Despite the difficulties, given a surgeon with adequate colorectal and laparoscopic expertise and, importantly, a laparoscopically skilled second assistant to retract and expose, it is possible, in many cases, to perform a laparoscopic total mesorectal excision (TME) of the rectum. Having accomplished this, however, it can be very difficult, especially in a deep pelvis, to transversely divide the rectum with a linear stapler, even with roticulating devices. Thus, in a sizable proportion of cases, in the end, it is necessary to make a larger than anticipated incision in order to complete the distal mobilization and to divide the mesorectum and rectum distally.

Recognizing these difficulties and the high conversion rate, the authors developed and introduced the "hybrid" laparoscopic and open approach.[1] In the hybrid procedure, by design, a portion of the case is done laparoscopically whereas the remainder of the operation is performed via open methods through an infraumbilical incision. Typically, the splenic flexure mobilization, the division of the inferior mesenteric artery (IMA) or main sigmoidal vessels, the colonic division proximally, and the proximal rectal mobilization are accomplished via minimally invasive methods. The remainder of the case, including full rectal mobilization, rectal transection, and the anastomosis, is done through an open incision (in our series, about 11 cm in length).

Indications

The indication for hand-assisted laparoscopic (HAL) anterior resection does not differ from the conventional or purely laparoscopic approach.

Patient Positioning and Operating Room Setup

After placement of an arterial and two intravenous lines as well as venous compression stockings on the legs, the patient is secured in the modified lithotomy position using adjustable stirrups. The thighs should be parallel to the abdomen. The use of a "bean bag" underneath the patient is advised. Both arms are tucked at the patient's side and

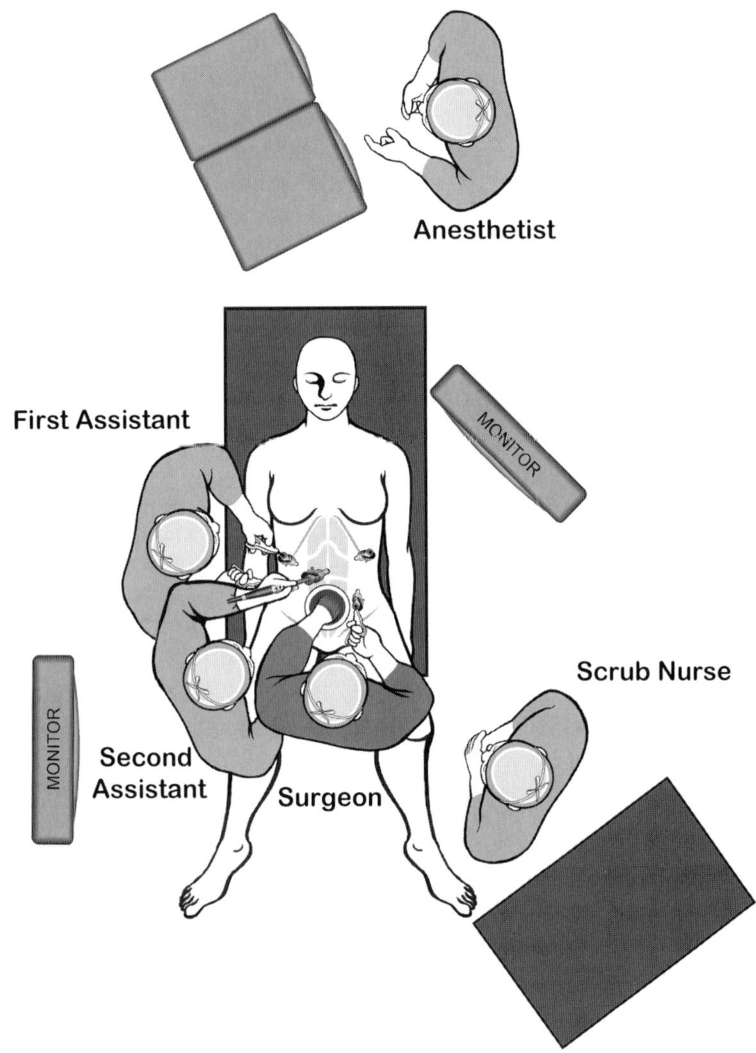

A

Figure 9.1.1. **A** Position of the equipment and the surgical team for the first phase of the HAL anterior resection. **B** Position of the equipment and the surgical team for the second phase (pelvic dissection) of the HAL anterior resection.

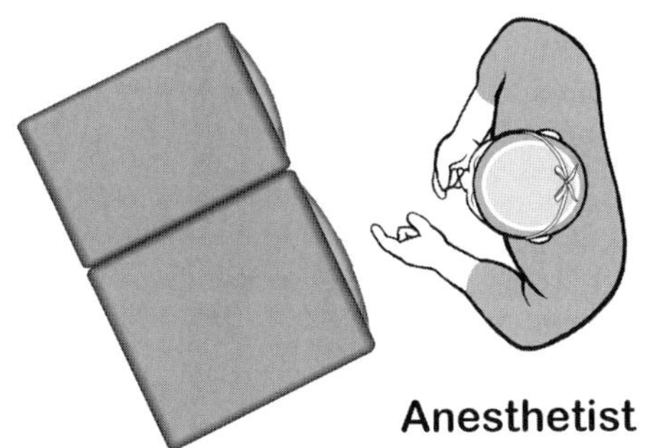

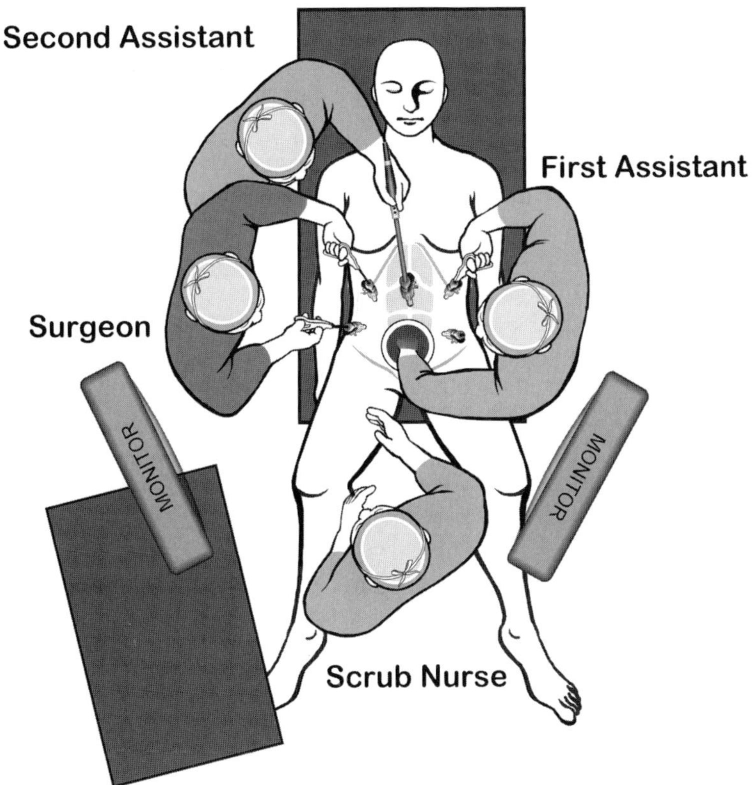

B

Figure 9.1.1. *Continued*

suction is applied to the bean bag. Tape is placed over a pad across the chest to the table at the level of the manubrium to further secure the patient. The monitor on the right side of the patient remains off the right foot throughout the laparoscopic portion of the case. The laparoscopic monitor on the left side is placed off the patient's left shoulder (Figure 9.1.1A). The surgeon stands between the patient's legs with left hand in the abdomen and right hand working via the cannula on the left side. The first assistant stands, with the camera person, on the patient's right side and utilizes the two right-sided cannulae.

Regardless of which specific hand-assisted approach is used, once the main vessels have been divided and the splenic flexure takedown

Table 9.1.1. Specific instruments recommended for HAL anterior rectal resection

5	Cannulae (1 × 12 mm, 1 × 10 mm, 2–3 × 5 mm)
1	Hand-assisted device
1	Dissecting device (i.e., LigaSure V™ or Ultrasonic Shears™ or electrosurgery)
1	Laparoscopic scissors
1	Laparoscopic dissector
2	Laparoscopic graspers
1	Endoscopic stapler

completed, the proximal bowel and remaining mesentery are divided at the chosen level. At this point, if desired, the rectal dissection can be initiated laparoscopically or the minimally invasive part of the operation can be terminated and the open portion of the case begun. In the case of the former, the left-sided monitor must be moved to a position off the left leg or foot. The surgeon moves to the patient's right side whereas the first assistant moves to the left side. The camera person now stands cephalad to the surgeon on the right side (Figure 9.1.1B).

Once the decision has been made to terminate the minimally invasive portion of the operation, fascial sutures are placed to close the 10- and 12-mm cannula wounds and the cannulae are removed. The hand device is removed and a Bookwalter or similar retractor is used to expose the lower abdomen and pelvis. In the majority of cases, it is necessary to extend the skin incision several centimeters to allow open completion of the case. The Allen stirrups can be adjusted for the open part of the case so as to flex the hips and provide better access from below for transanal stapling.

Instruments

Specific instruments recommended for HAL anterior resection are listed in Table 9.1.1.

Cannula and Hand-Device Positioning

It is logical and expedient to place the hand device first, before establishing pneumoperitoneum and placing cannulae. The hand device is placed centrally in the suprapubic region via either a low transverse Pfannenstiel incision or a vertical midline incision (Figure 9.1.2). The latter is advised in situations in which conversion is deemed more likely (obesity, multiple prior operations, etc.). The length of the hand-device incision will vary depending on the surgeon's hand size. Transverse incisions should be made at least 2 cm cephalad to the pubic symphysis to minimize device leakage and to provide access to the left upper quadrant. Once the incision has been completed, the hand device is placed and a hand is inserted into the abdomen after which the cannulae are placed.

It is important to take into account the "footprint" of the hand device when choosing cannula positions. If the cannula and hand are placed too closely together, the intracorporeal hand is more likely to block the path of instruments inserted through the cannula. A four-cannula arrangement with an optional fifth cannula is recommended. A 10-mm cannula, usually placed just above the umbilicus, is the first to be inserted. The hand is used to protect the abdominal viscera as the first cannula is placed in the absence of pneumoperitoneum; the latter is established once this first cannula is fully inserted. A 12-mm cannula is inserted in the right lower quadrant, lateral to the rectus muscle, about at the level of the anterior superior iliac spine (more cephalad in those with long and broad abdominal walls). This cannula should either be placed at the site chosen for a diverting loop ileostomy (marked in the holding area preoperatively) or, at least, 3–4 cm away from the stoma site. Utilizing the stoma location usually requires that the cannula be placed through the rectus muscle. A 5-mm cannula is inserted approximately 4 fingerbreadths above the 12-mm cannula, also lateral to the rectus muscle. Finally, a 5- or 10-mm cannula is placed in the left lower quadrant lateral to the rectus muscle and below the level of the umbilicus (10 mm is needed if a 10-mm tissue ligating and dividing device is to be used from this location). The optional fifth cannula is best placed in the left upper quadrant lateral to the rectus

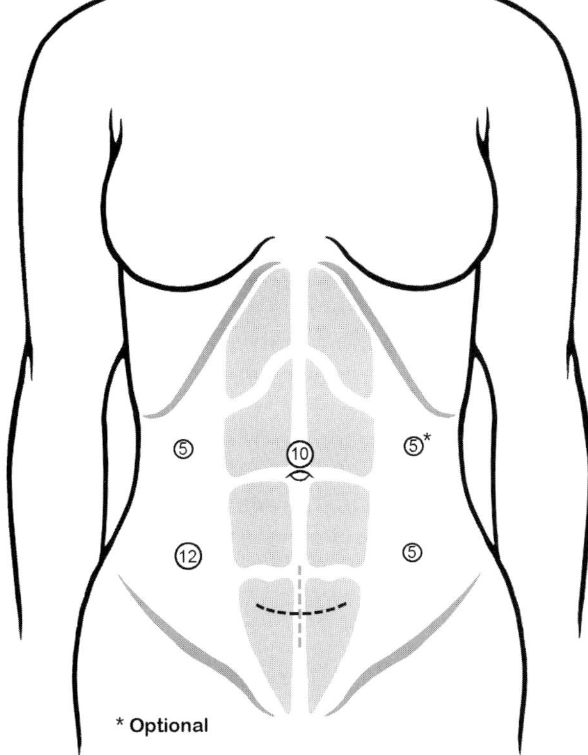

Figure 9.1.2. Positions of the cannulae and the hand-assist device for the HAL anterior resection.

border. It is advised that some type of cannula anchor be used (threaded cannula or grip, or skin suture tethers that are wrapped around the insufflation arm of the cannula).

Technique

There are two basic approaches to mobilize the left colon and ligate the vessel, medial to lateral and lateral to medial. The medial to lateral approaches allow prompt mobilization and division of the main vessels proximally which is recommended by many experts in the cancer setting. There are two ways to do the medial to lateral mobilization: The first initiates dissection at the level of the sacral promontory whereas the second starts at the level of the inferior mesenteric vein (IMV). A brief description of each method follows.

Medial to Lateral Approach Starting at the Sacral Promontory

In the first method, the dissection is begun at the sacral promontory at the right base of the rectosigmoid colon. The surgeon stands between the legs with left hand in abdomen and right hand holding a bowel grasper through the left-sided cannula; the first assistant and camera person are on the patient's right side. The table is placed in the Trendelenburg position with the right side tilted down so that the small bowel will shift into the right upper quadrant. The surgeon may place a towel in the peritoneal cavity via the hand-assist device to pack the small bowel out of the way. The omentum is then swept cranially above the transverse colon to expose the mesentery.

The surgeon uses his hand to grasp the sigmoid mesentery and elevate it ventrally and to the left (Figure 9.1.3). This maneuver exposes the groove between the inferior mesenteric vascular pedicle and the retroperitoneum. The first assistant uses both right-sided cannulae; a grasper in one hand to facilitate exposure and a cutting device in the other. Using the endoscopic scissors, the first assistant incises the peritoneum immediately to the right and below the vascular pedicle. The incision starts at the sacral promontory and is continued a short distance both into the pelvis and toward the head to provide some working space. The surgeon then places his fingers underneath the vascular pedicle, and uses blunt dissection in order to lift the pedicle ventrally as well as to sweep the preaortic hypogastric plexus dorsally. The first assistant places the graspers underneath the cut edge of the incised peritoneum to help elevate the vascular pedicle and expose the retroperitoneum. Blunt dissection is performed laterally until the left ureter and the gonadal vessels are visualized through this mesenteric window (Figure 9.1.4).

The peritoneum is further scored cephalad, just dorsal to the sigmoidal vessels on the medial aspect of the mesentery to the IMA level. The surgeon carefully grasps the artery with his hand, and continues blunt dissection posteriorly and laterally to reach the IMV. As the surgeon controls both of these vessels, the assistant incises the peritoneum across the pedicle to create a peritoneal window lateral to the vein. Both

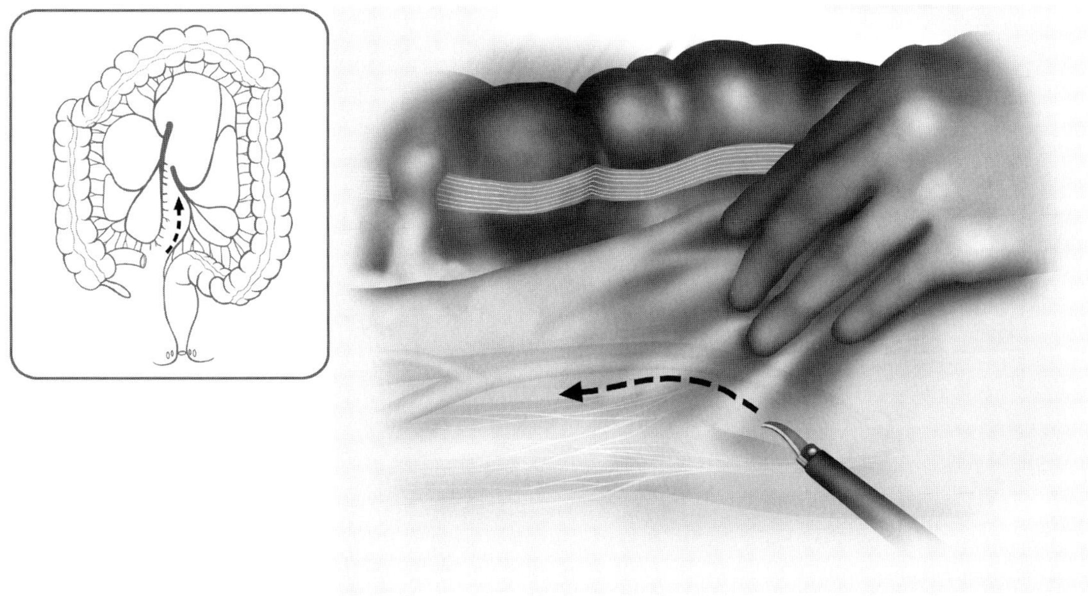

Figure 9.1.3. In initiating the dissection of the IMA and IMV, the surgeon grasps the pedicle with the left hand and elevates it ventrally and to the left.

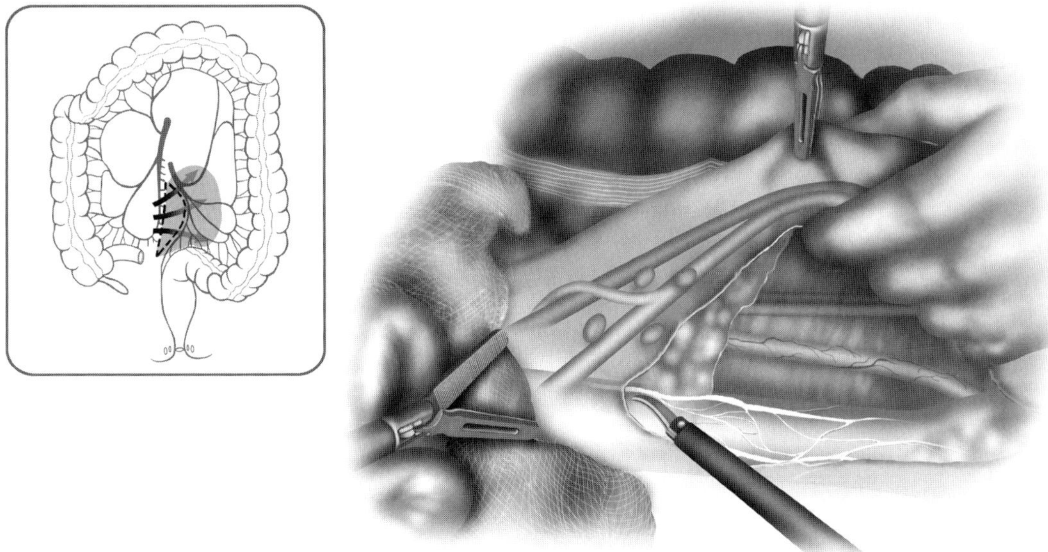

Figure 9.1.4. Blunt dissection is performed beneath the IMA to expose the left ureter and the gonadal vessels.

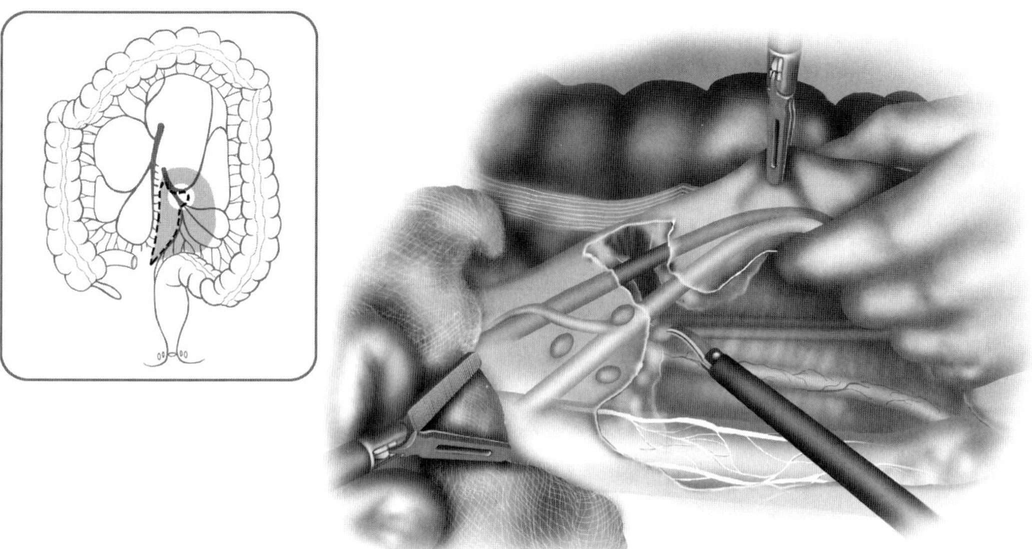

Figure 9.1.5. Both the IMA and IMV are prepared for ligation by dissection away from the retroperitoneal structures and creating a window in the mesentery lateral to the IMV.

vessels should now be clearly exposed and retracted away from the retroperitoneal structures, making them ready for ligation (Figure 9.1.5). The artery and vein are then divided either proximal to or just distal to the left colic artery, depending on the preference of the surgeon. We prefer to ligate the vessels with an endoscopic coagulation device instead of with an endoscopic stapler or surgical clips (Figure 9.1.6). Blunt dissection continues posterior to the left colon mesentery, with the first assistant elevating the mesentery, and the surgeon's fingers sweeping, dorsally, the retroperitoneal fat and the anterior aspect of Gerota's fascia (Figure 9.1.7). Dissection should continue until the lateral attachments of the left colon are encountered at the splenic flexure. The correct dissection plane is avascular.

The next step in flexure takedown is separation of the greater omentum from the transverse colon. The surgeon initially grasps the transverse colon and retracts it caudally with the intracorporeal left hand while holding up the reflected omentum with a grasper held with the right hand, thus exposing the avascular attachments between these two structures (Figure 9.1.8). Starting at the mid-transverse colon, the assistant uses a grasper to improve exposure and a scissors to divide the avascular attachments and enter the lesser sac; once entered, the surgeon can place his fingers into the lesser sac in order to palpate, bluntly dissect, and expose the remaining attachments. After the omentum is separated, the colon should only be attached by the lieno-colic ligament and lateral attachments. The surgeon places his hand posterior to the colon mesentery and retracts the colon medially. Using

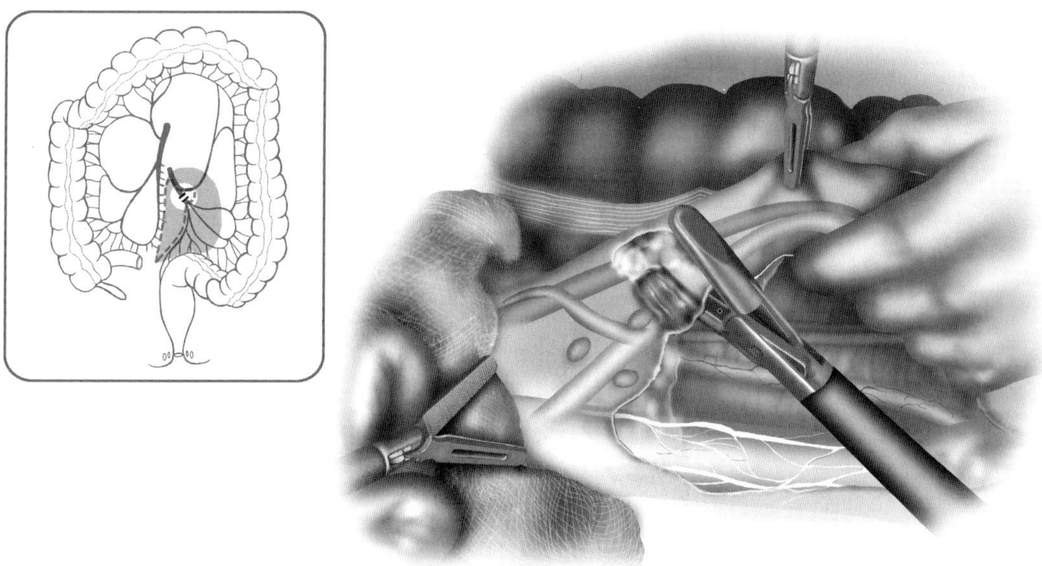

Figure 9.1.6. An endoscopic coagulation device is used to simultaneously ligate and divide the inferior mesenteric pedicle.

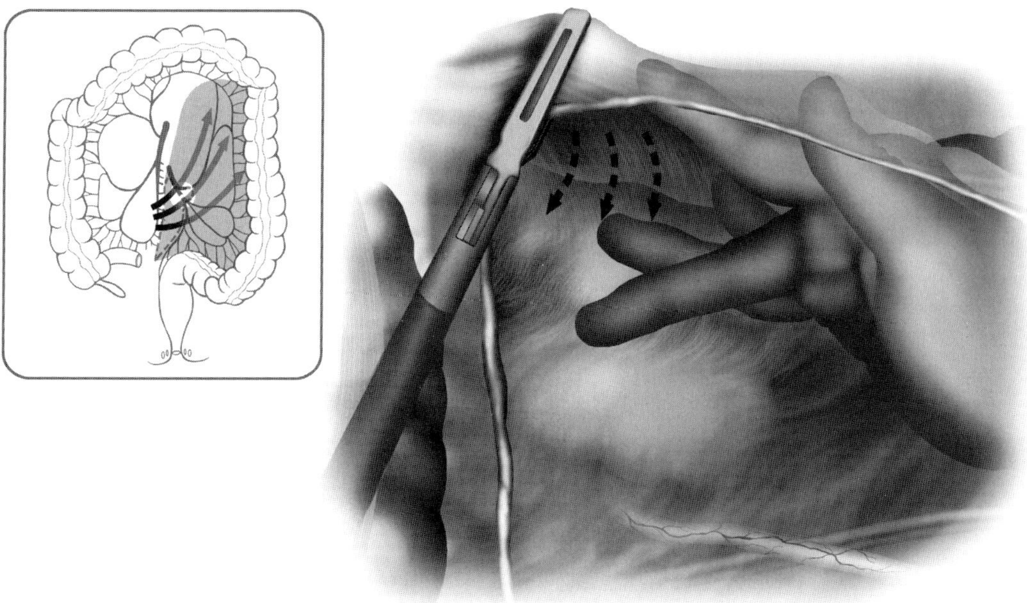

Figure 9.1.7. The medial to lateral dissection continues by sweeping Gerota's fascia away from the left colonic mesentery.

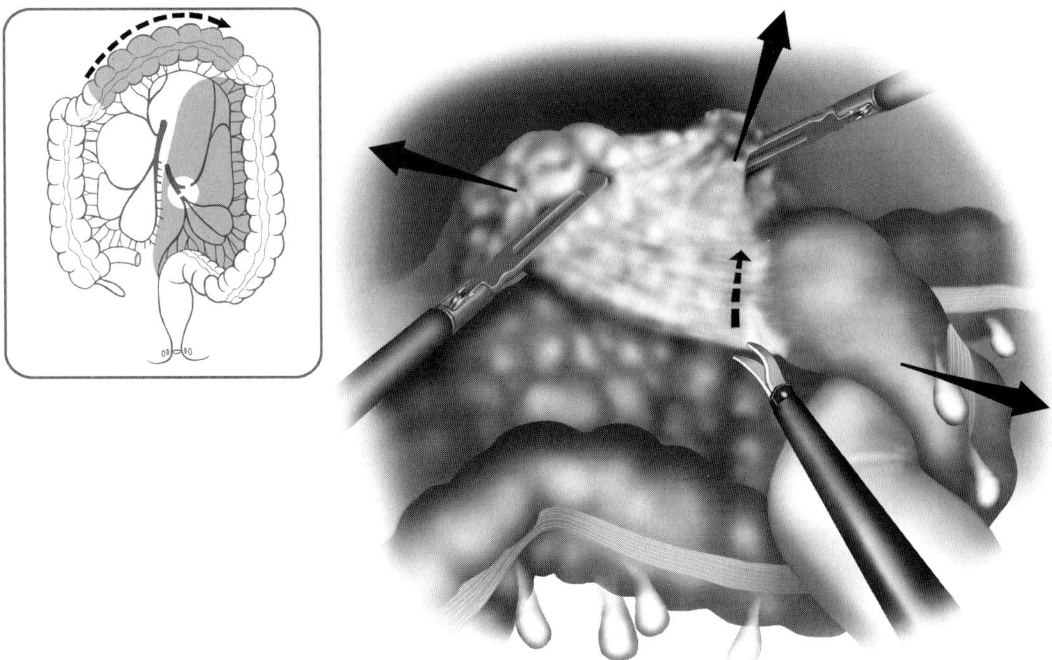

Figure 9.1.8. Takedown of the splenic flexure involves separation of the greater omentum from the distal transverse colon, using the left hand to advantage in retracting the colon caudally.

the endoscopic scissors in his right hand, the surgeon then divides the lateral attachments starting at the distal descending colon and proceeding cephalad. Division of the lienocolic ligament completes mobilization of the splenic flexure (Figure 9.1.9).

Medial to Lateral Approach Starting at the IMV

The alternate medial to lateral approach commences at the level of the IMV. Using this technique, the dissection is initiated cephalad to the IMA takeoff. The room and equipment setup as well as the position of the surgeon and assistants are the same as for the method just described. The table is placed in slight reverse Trendelenburg with the right side down. The back of the surgeon's intracorporeal hand is used to hold back the proximal ileum and the small bowel from the base of the descending colon mesentery, thus exposing the IMV and the ligament of Treitz. The surgeon's right hand grasps and elevates the descending colon which puts the mesentery on stretch. The first assistant grasps the left transverse mesocolon just beneath the bowel and retracts it upward with one hand, while using a scissors or other device in the other hand to score the peritoneum parallel to and a short distance from the IMV (Figure 9.1.10). This starting point is either just medial or lateral to the IMV depending on whether the vein is to be sacrificed or preserved. This opening is enlarged and a window created through

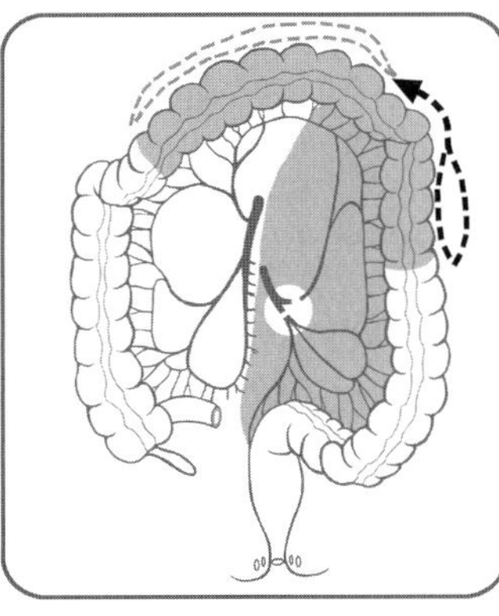

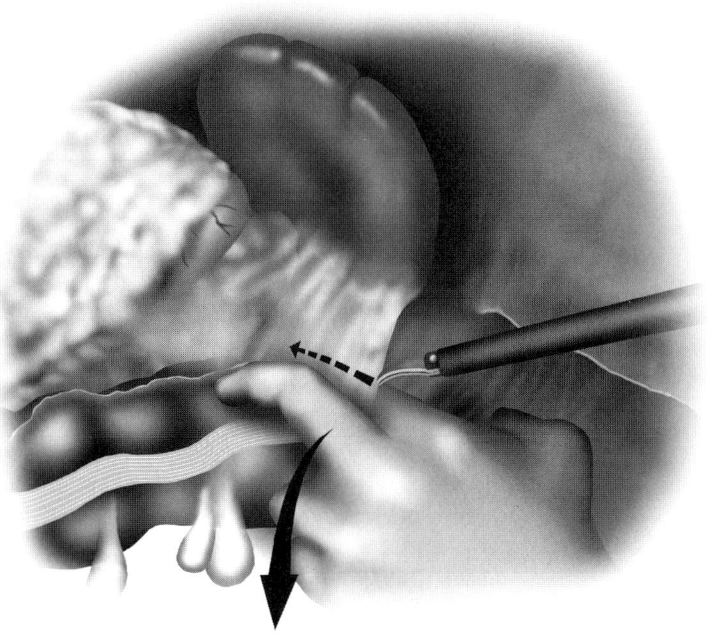

Figure 9.1.9. The lienocolic ligament is finally taken down using endoscopic scissors with the surgeon's right hand through the left-sided cannula.

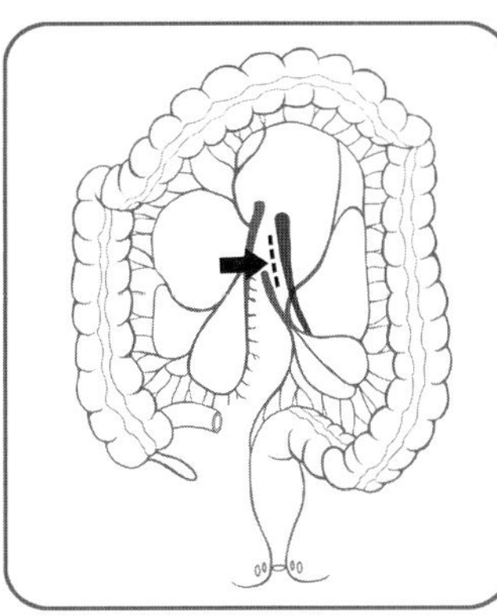

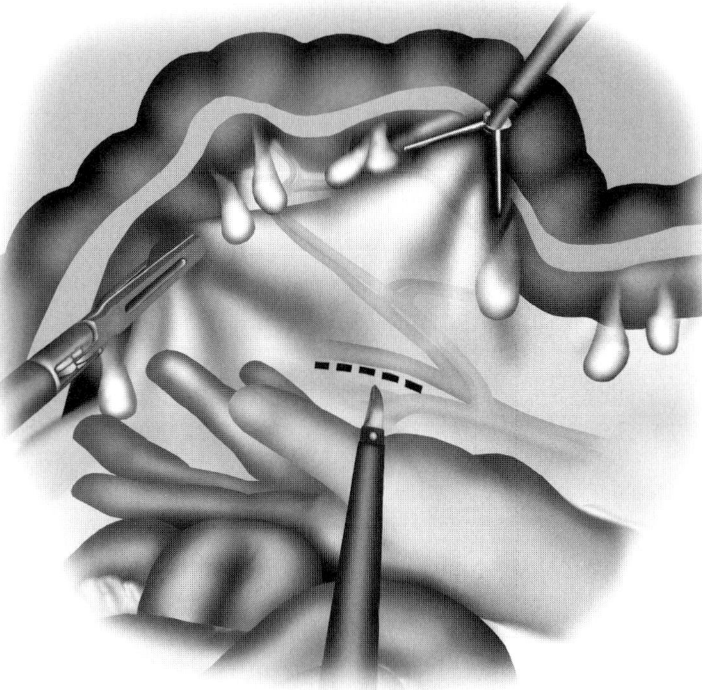

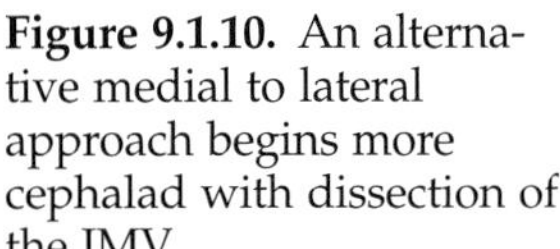

Figure 9.1.10. An alternative medial to lateral approach begins more cephalad with dissection of the IMV.

which the dissection can be initiated. Next, the plane between the posterior aspect of the mesentery and the anterior surface of Gerota's fascia is established through this window and continued laterally.

The hand and the laparoscopic instruments are alternately used to lift the mesentery upward, thus exposing the dissection plane, or to do the actual dissection. The cephalad extent of this mobilization is the inferior edge of the pancreas; the caudal limit is the left colic vessels. To continue the mobilization caudally, either the IMA (or the left colic vessels) must be divided or a new window created between the left colic vessels and the first sigmoid branch off the main sigmoidal vessel. The left ureter and gonadal vessels are then bluntly dissected down and away from the underside of the colonic mesentery as the dissection continues caudally toward the left iliac fossa (Figure 9.1.11). Next, the omentum is dissected away from the left half of the transverse colon. Then, as described earlier, the lesser sac is entered and the remaining flexure attachments are taken down. To complete the mobilization of the left transverse colon, the base of its mesocolon must be divided ventral to its insertion along the inferior border of the pancreas (Figure 9.1.12). Care must be taken to preserve the marginal vessels when performing this step. The final step is the division of the thin lateral peritoneal attachments of the descending colon.

Lateral to Medial Approach

The room setup and staff positioning are the same; the table is placed in mild reverse Trendelenburg with the right side tilted down and the omentum reflected cephalad. The surgeon, standing between the legs, grasps the descending colon with his left hand and retracts it medially

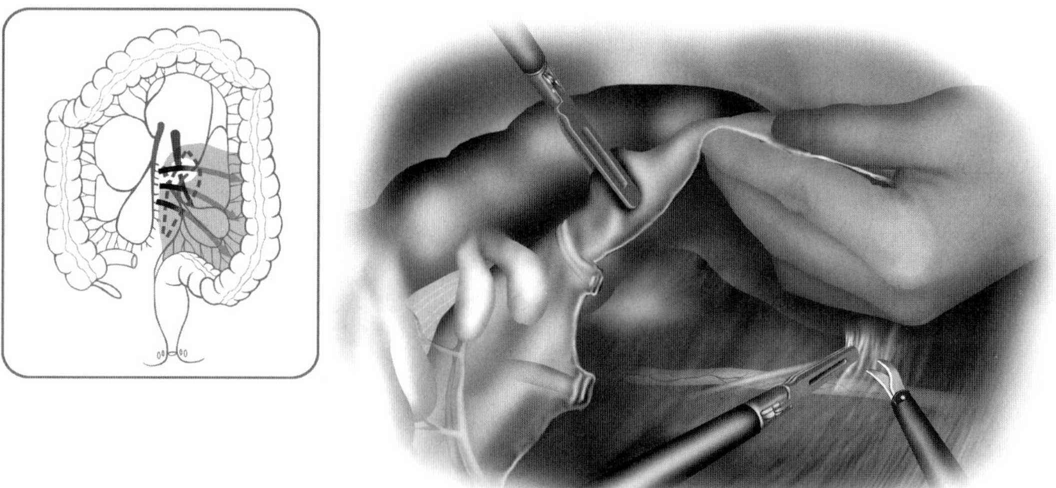

Figure 9.1.11. Dissection of the gonadal vessels and ureter from the mesocolon.

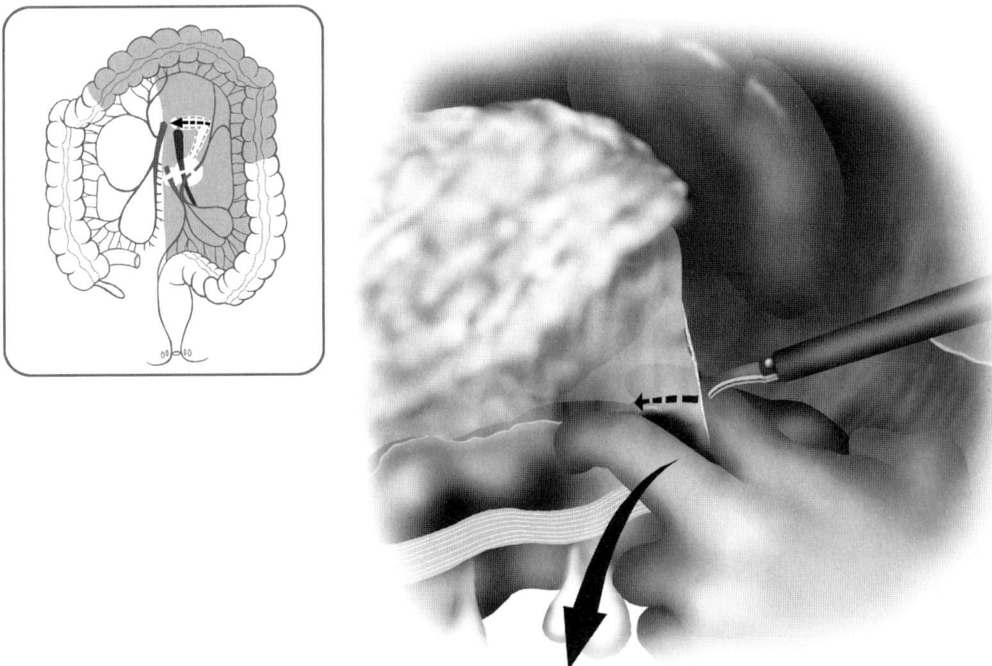

Figure 9.1.12. Dissection of the mesocolon of the left transverse colon from the inferior border of the pancreas.

while using his right hand to initiate dissection by dividing the line of Toldt via the left-sided cannula (Figure 9.1.13). The first assistant uses two graspers to retract the proximal left colon and keep the small bowel and omentum out of the way. As the colon is detached, medial and upward traction by the hand must be increased. The proper dissection plane between the anterior aspect of Gerota's fascia and the underside of the mesocolon must be found; it is usually not evident at the start. Once the mobilization is well underway, the hand can be repositioned lateral to the colon; the back of the hand is used to retract the mesocolon (draped over it) medially and upward which exposes the proper (purple colored) dissection plane. The assistant holds the left colon out of the way. It is important to fully mobilize the descending mesocolon to a point medial to the IMV. Dissection proceeds toward the flexure and, if possible, the lienocolic attachments are divided.

Next, the omentum is separated from the left transverse colon as previously described (Figure 9.1.8). The intracorporeal hand, either left or right, is then used to identify the IMA and IMV. The mesentery can be displayed broadly by draping the colon over the surgeon's hand. The assistant then uses scissors to create windows in the mesentery between the vessels after which the artery and vein are ligated proximally at the desired location. The bowel and remaining mesentery are next divided at the chosen level.

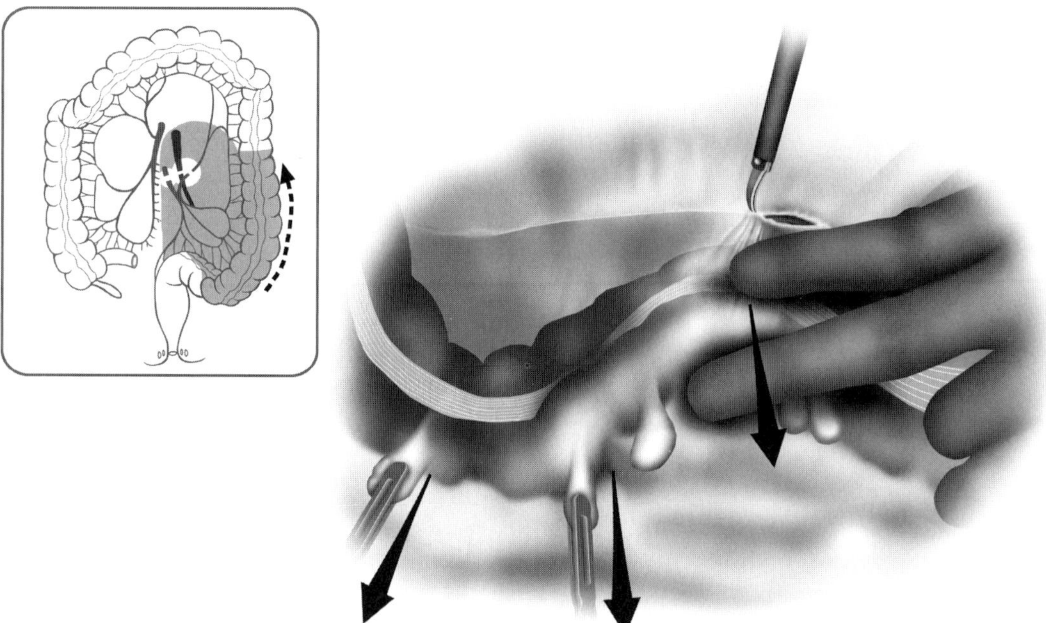

Figure 9.1.13. Lateral mobilization of the left colon along the line of Toldt.

Rectosigmoid and Rectal Mobilization, Distal Rectal Division, and Anastomosis

After completing the steps of: 1) The flexure takedown, 2) proximal devascularization, and 3) bowel division, there are two options. The first is to laparoscopically initiate the pelvic portion of the operation, whereas the second possibility is to commence the open part of the operation. It is the authors' impression that the open dissection, via a limited laparotomy incision, is facilitated by having fully scored the pelvic peritoneum laterally and anteriorly and also by establishing the presacral plane before ending the minimally invasive portion of the operation. Additionally, although unproven, it is again our impression that it is easier to identify and preserve the hypogastric presacral nerves laparoscopically.

Minimally Invasive Rectal Dissection

The left monitor is repositioned lateral to the left foot or leg; the surgeon moves to the patient's right side and the first assistant to the left (Figure 9.1.1B). The patient is placed in Trendelenburg position and tilted right side down. This part of the case can be accomplished with the hand in or out of the abdomen. Provided the pelvis is sufficiently large, the assistant can grasp and retract the rectosigmoid upward with either the right or left hand. The remaining hand is used to provide and improve exposure. The surgeon using a grasper and a scissors then performs the dissection. The rectum and the surrounding structures and sidewalls must be retracted and placed on tension in order to reveal the proper planes. Care is taken to identify and preserve the hypogastric nerves while establishing the proper plane that will permit full resection of the mesorectum (Figure 9.1.14). The initial lateral and anterior dissection can often be initiated laparoscopically without difficulty. Once the dissection has been fully commenced and the planes have been established, the open portion of the case should be initiated.

Open Portion of the Operation

A variety of retractors are used to provide exposure through the limited incision including a Bookwalter or other table-affixed retractor and long hand held St. Marks or Deaver retractors. A final incision length of 9–12 cm is usually required and will vary depending on the surgeons' hand size and the body habitus of the patient. If not already done, the mobilized left colon is exteriorized and divided proximally with a linear stapler. Because the open rectal resection technique has been well described elsewhere, it will not be reviewed in detail here. Suffice it to say that a TME type mobilization is performed. Confirmation of lesion location and rectal washout with a tumoricidal solution

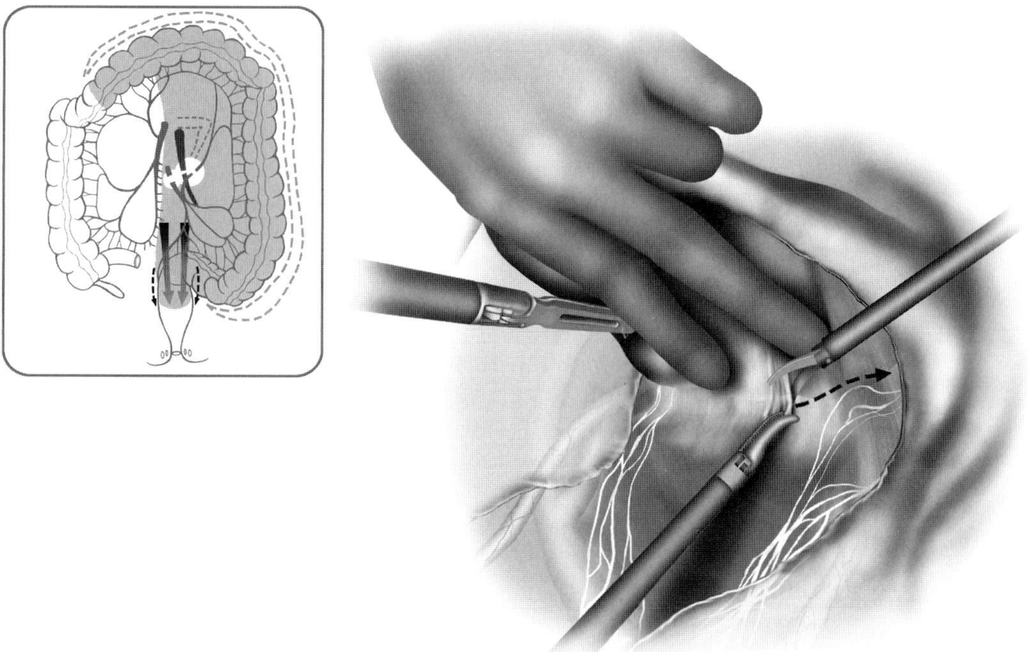

Figure 9.1.14. "Hand-assisted" laparoscopic mobilization of the rectum.

(9:1 dilution of standard 10% povidone solution with saline to obtain a final concentration of 1%) should be standard procedure before stapling and transecting the rectum. Full rectal mobilization as well as ligation and division of the mesorectum and the distal rectum are performed after which a double-stapled anastomosis via a transanally placed circular EEA device is accomplished. For distal rectal lesions, instead of stapling across the rectum, a rectal mucosectomy followed by a hand-sewn coloanal anastomosis may be necessary. Proximal diversion via a loop ileostomy may be warranted depending on the height of the anastomosis, a history of pelvic radiation, a positive leak test, and individual surgeon's judgment.

Special Considerations

A preliminary report that compared hybrid results to those of a group of fully open patients demonstrated that there was no difference at all in the pathologic resection parameters (margins, lymph node harvest, etc.) between the groups while also revealing a significantly shorter length of stay and return of bowel function for the hybrid group. Because the small laparotomy incision was, in the end, required, it was logical to make the infraumbilical incision early in the case and to place a hand device into it so as to take advantage of the benefits of hand-assisted (HAL) techniques throughout the laparoscopic portion of the case.

HAL methods offer several advantages over purely laparoscopic approaches, including tactile feedback and the ability to manually palpate, retract, and bluntly dissect. The latest generation of devices also allows the surgeon to work laparoscopically with the hand outside the abdomen or to insert a laparoscopic cannula through the device itself, thus adding a traditional cannula. A growing number of experts believe that hand-assisted methods decrease operative times, reduce conversion rates, and facilitate the teaching of advanced laparoscopic techniques.[2,3] It is far easier for a well-trained open surgeon to learn how to work with one hand in the abdomen. The length of the hand-assist wound largely depends on the hand size of the surgeon and, thus, will vary. In regard to hybrid low anterior resections, in the end, an incision large enough to permit open completion of the case is needed; this usually requires enlarging the hand incision.

There are currently limited reports in the literature describing the results of hybrid low anterior resection for rectal neoplasms. We previously reported our results of 31 patients who underwent a hybrid resection for rectal cancer. Compared with 25 open patients, the laparoscopic patients had significantly shorter incision lengths, time to first bowel movements, and mean length of stay.[2] Importantly, there were no differences between the groups with regard to any of the pathologic parameters such as lymph node harvest or proximal and distal margins. Two other pilot studies, involving 16 and 10 patients undergoing HAL anterior resection, confirmed that the procedure could be performed safely with a low complication rate.[4]

Conclusions

It is clear that TME type methods are associated with a superior outcome compared with less radical or stringent techniques. Furthermore, it has also been well demonstrated that the experience and the training of the surgeon are critical variables in determining outcome in this setting. Laparoscopic and hand-assisted hybrid operations must conform to the same oncologic standards. It is also critical that surgeons embarking on these operations have sufficient minimally invasive experience obtained by performing resections for benign disease and for colon cancers.

Presently, in the majority of patients, it is not possible to perform a laparoscopic distal sphincter-saving rectal resection without making an incision large enough to get a hand inside. Regardless, it seems that the use of hybrid methods and the avoidance of a full laparotomy are associated with, at least, some short-term benefits. The use of hand-assisted methods in this setting is logical. It is the impression of a growing number of surgeons that the hand-assisted method is easier to learn and is a bit quicker than the standard laparoscopic/open hybrid operation. Confirmation of these impressions awaits the performance of a large prospective randomized trial.

Editors' Comments

Indications: We believe that patients with rectal lesions below the peritoneal reflection requiring circumferential mobilization completely down to the pelvic floor are potentially not good indications for even a HAL resection. This relates to the need for complex dissection deep in the pelvis and the need for a distal rectal washout. Otherwise, we agree that the indications are not different from open surgery.

Patient positioning: We do not use a bean bag as described in this chapter. A gel-like pad beneath the patient, which adheres on its own to the operating table, is all we use.

Instrumentation: We use similar instruments.

Cannula positioning: We use only 5-mm cannulae in addition to the hand device at the standard sites.

Technique: We would emphasize the initial aspect of this procedure is a thorough evaluation of the entire abdomen, including the liver in cancer patients. We generally begin the dissection medially starting at the sacral promontory. Once we complete lymphovascular pedicle isolation, then we perform left colon mobilization and splenic flexure takedown. Peripheral mesenteric dissection and bowel diversion at the proximal resection line may be done using open technique through the hand port.

The laparoscopic approach to rectal mobilization is our preferred method. We sometimes use the hand port and draw the rectosigmoid up through this for strong countertraction (Figure 9.1.15, with inset). Once the rectum is fully dissected, we then perform distal rectal washout, bowel transection, and low anastomosis through the hand port incision.

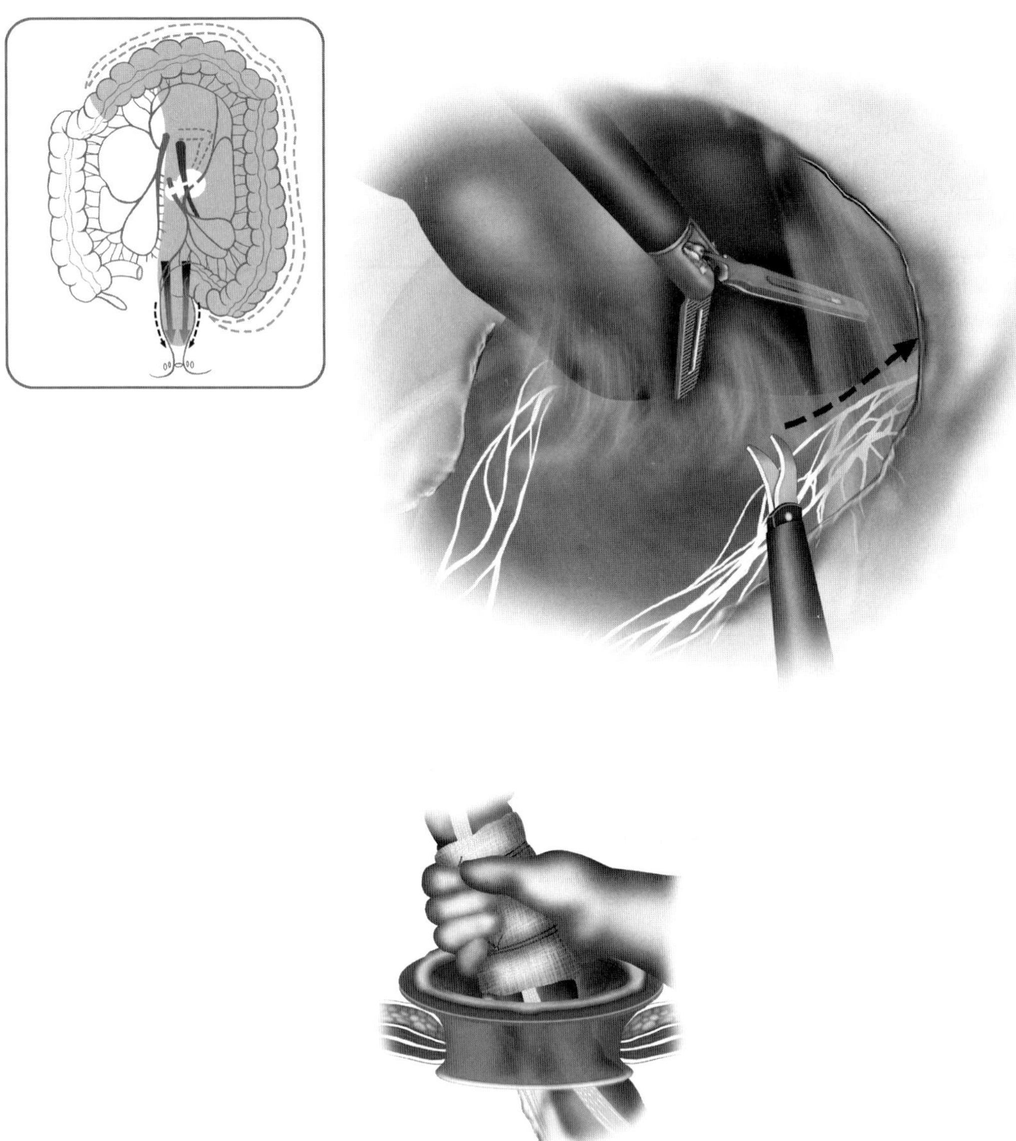

Figure 9.1.15. Mobilization of the rectum by pulling the rectum through the hand port (inset).

We have found that using a disposable plastic wound retracting device (Alexis retractor, Applied Medical) is valuable.

References

1. Vithiananthan S, Cooper Z, Betten K, et al. Hybrid laparoscopic flexure takedown and open procedure for rectal resection is associated with significantly

shorter length of stay than equivalent open resection. Dis Colon Rectum 2001;44:927–935.
2. Romanelli JR, Kelly JJ, Litwin DE. Hand-assisted laparoscopic surgery in the United States: an overview. Semin Laparosc Surg 2001;8:96–103.
3. Nakajima K, Lee SW, Cocilovo C, et al. Hand-assisted laparoscopic colorectal surgery using GelPort. Surg Endosc 2004;18:102–105.
4. Nakajima K, Lee SW, Cocilovo C, et al. Laparoscopic total colectomy: hand-assisted vs standard technique. Surg Endosc 2004;18:582–586.

Chapter 9.2

Hand-Assisted Laparoscopic Total Abdominal Colectomy

Toyooki Sonoda

Indications

The mobilization of the entire abdominal colon and transection of the bowel at the rectosigmoid junction remains one of the more challenging of the laparoscopic operations. An ileorectal anastomosis is created for most noninflammatory conditions, but a total abdominal colectomy and end ileostomy may be necessary in cases of severe colitis. The following are the main indications for this procedure: Fulminant colitis (ulcerative colitis, Crohn's, infectious), colonic inertia, familial adenomatous polyposis with rectal sparing, or hereditary nonpolyposis colorectal cancer.

The use of hand-assisted surgery adds tactile feedback and allows for safe handling of the colon, and has been shown to decrease operative times compared with conventional laparoscopic surgery when used in the setting of a total colectomy.[1] The operation is divided into four key components: 1) Dissection of the right colon, 2) transverse colon, 3) descending and sigmoid colon, and 4) splenic flexure.

Patient Positioning and Operating Room Setup

After induction of general anesthesia, an orogastric tube and Foley catheter are inserted. The patient is placed in a modified lithotomy position using adjustable stirrups, with both arms tucked at the sides. Venous compression stockings are used in all cases. The patient is placed in Trendelenburg position (20° head-down tilt), and a hand-assist port is placed in the suprapubic position. For the first phase of the operation (right colon mobilization), the surgeon and first assistant stand on the patient's left side, and the second assistant stands between the legs (Figure 9.2.1A). This position is maintained for the second phase of the operation, or the transverse colon mobilization.

Then, for the third portion of the operation (descending and sigmoid colon mobilization), the surgeon and the first assistant move to the right side of the patient. The second assistant stands between the legs of the patient, only helping as needed (Figure 9.2.1B). For the splenic flexure takedown, the surgeon stands between the legs, with the first and second assistants on the right side of the patient (Figure 9.2.1C).

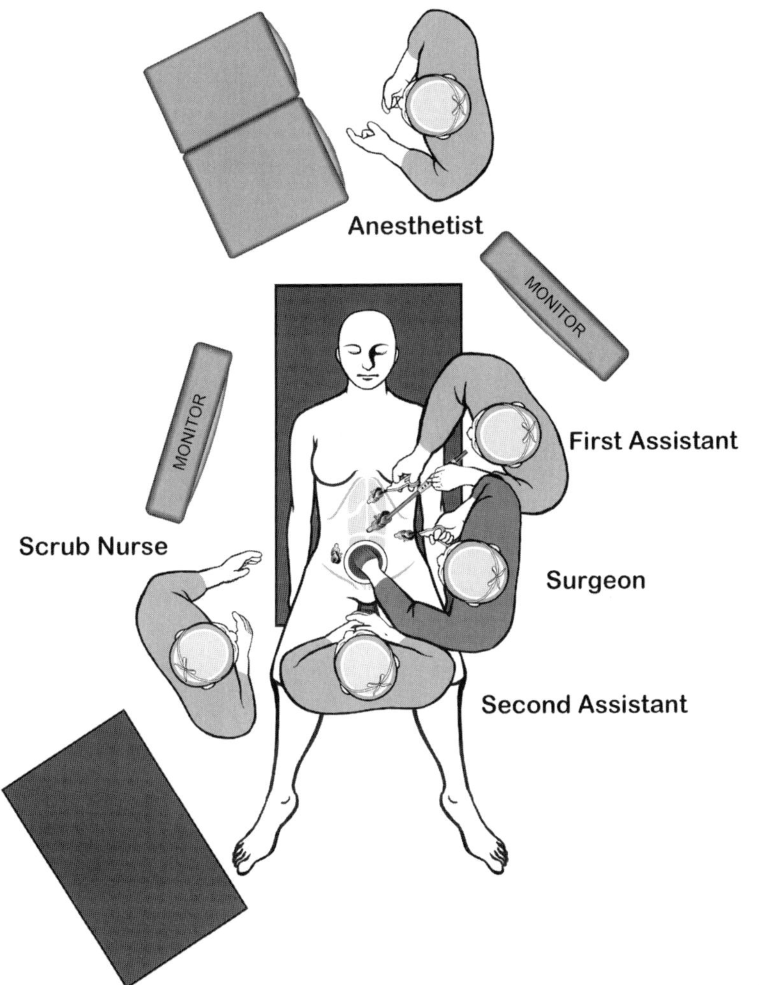

Figure 9.2.1. A Position of the equipment and the surgical team for the HAL total abdominal colectomy during the first and second phases of the procedure.

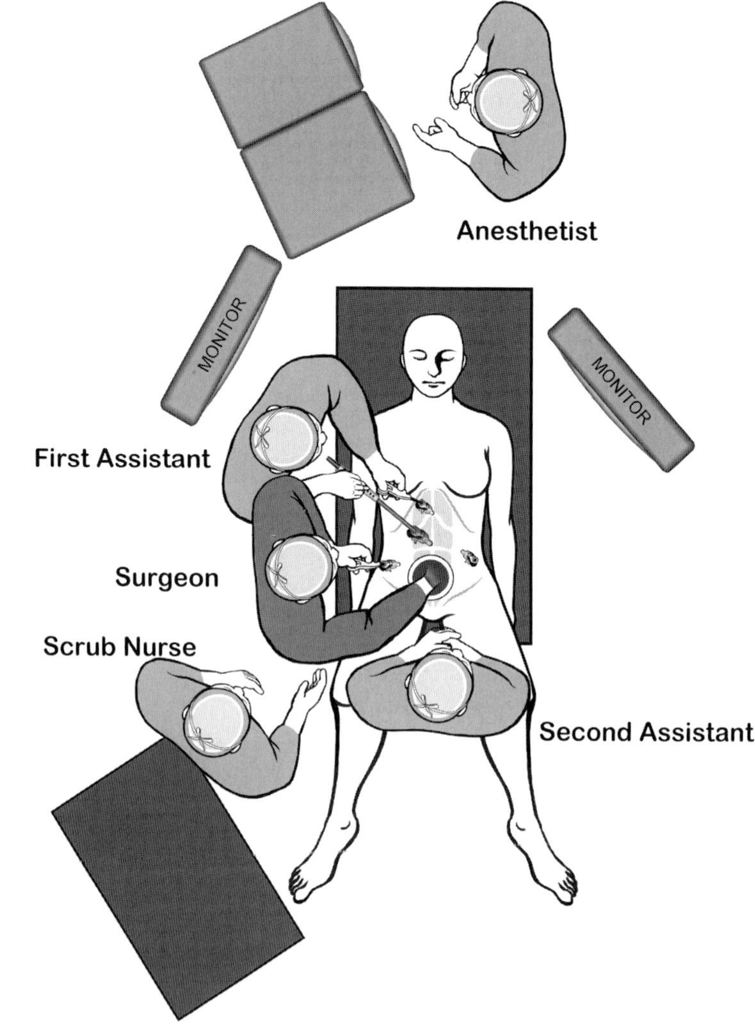

B

Figure 9.2.1. B Position of the equipment and the surgical team for the HAL total abdominal colectomy during the third phase of the procedure.

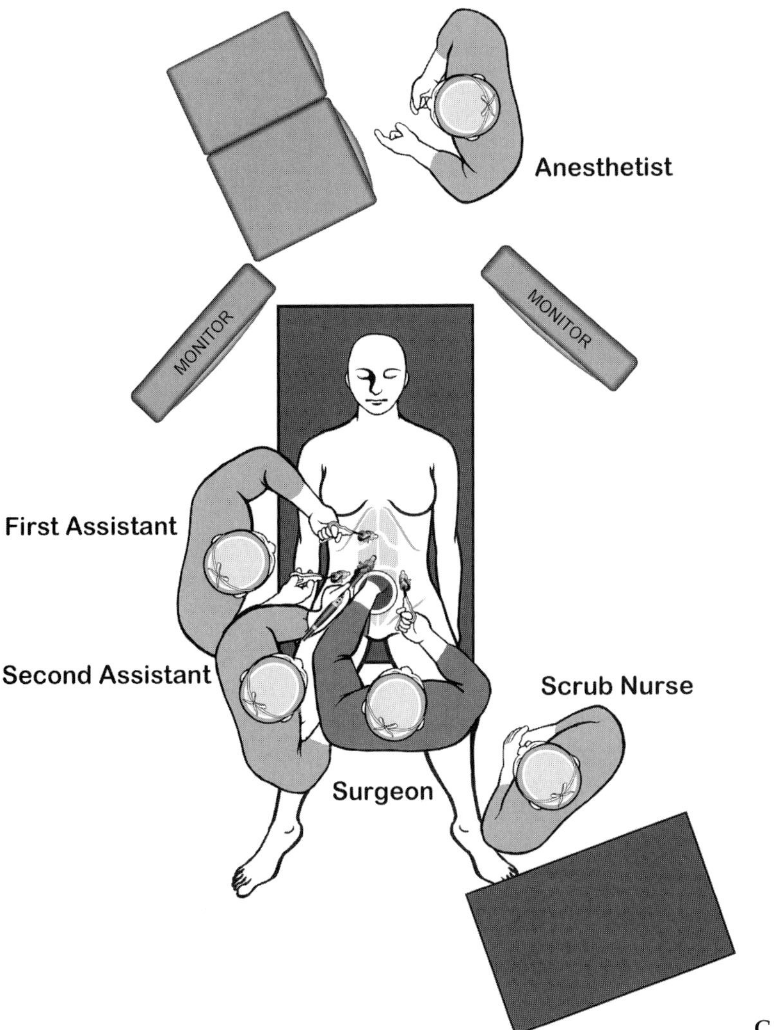

Figure 9.2.1. C Position of the equipment and the surgical team for the HAL total abdominal colectomy during splenic flexure takedown.

Table 9.2.1. Specific instruments recommended for HAL total abdominal colectomy with ileorectal anastomosis

5	Cannulae (2 × 10 mm, 2 × 5 mm)
1	Hand-assisted device
1	Dissecting device (i.e., LigaSure V™ or Ultrasonic Shears™ or electrosurgery)
1	Laparoscopic scissors
1	Laparoscopic dissector
2	Laparoscopic graspers
1	Endoscopic stapler

Instruments

Specific instruments recommended for hand-assisted laparoscopic (HAL) total abdominal colectomy with ileorectal anastomosis are listed in Table 9.2.1.

Cannula Positioning

The preferred location for the hand-assist device is in the suprapubic region through a Pfannenstiel incision, about 2 fingerbreadths above the upper border of the symphysis pubis. This results in good cosmesis and probably lessens pain compared with a vertical incision. However, a vertical midline suprapubic incision may be used if conversion to open surgery is a realistic possibility (anticipated adhesions, or early on in a surgeon's experience). By placing the hand port in the suprapubic position, the division of the bowel and anastomosis can be performed using open techniques.

The cannulae are placed as shown in Figure 9.2.2. If an end ileostomy is planned, this site must be marked before the induction of anesthesia, while the patient is awake and sitting up. The right abdominal stoma site can be used to place a cannula through it.

Technique

Medial to Lateral Dissection

The procedure begins with the patient in Trendelenburg position. A Pfannenstiel (or vertical suprapubic) incision is created, usually 6–9 cm in size, just large enough to insert one's gloved hand. The general rule is to make the incision as large as the surgeon's glove size (for example, size 7 glove = 7-cm incision). Superior and inferior flaps are created of the anterior rectus fascia, and the rectus abdominus is split in the midline and the peritoneum opened. Before inserting the hand-assist device, a hand is placed into the abdomen to confirm that the umbilical area is free of adhesions (for the optical cannula insertion), and a 10-mm supraumbilical port is inserted while the hand lifts the abdominal wall and shields the underlying bowel loops from injury. A suprapubic incision is preferred to one below the umbilicus, because the size of the hand port device may cause collisions with the infraumbilical

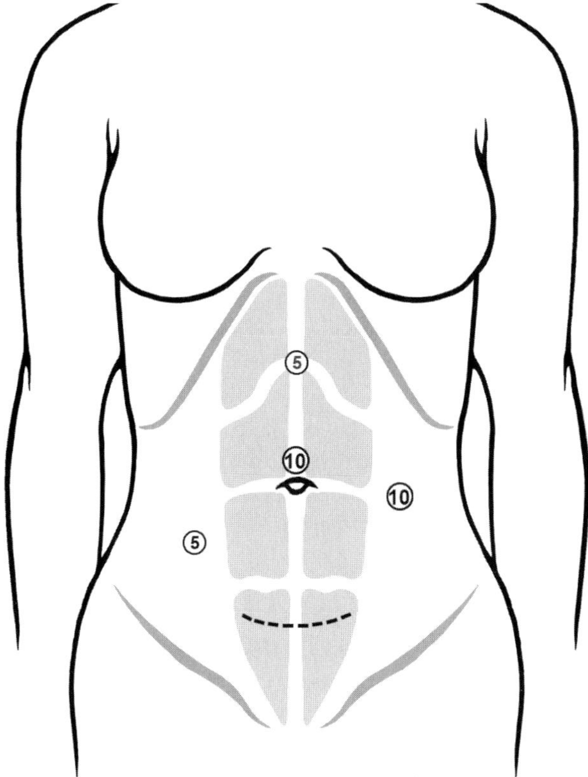

Figure 9.2.2. Position of the cannulae for the HAL total abdominal colectomy.

port. The hand port is fashioned to the suprapubic incision, and carbon dioxide pneumoperitoneum is established. Additional ports are placed, as in Figure 9.2.2. The laparoscope is placed through the supraumbilical cannula and the abdomen explored.

The surgeon and assistants set up for the right colon mobilization, as illustrated in Figure 9.2.1. The patient is placed in steep Trendelenburg with the right side up. The surgeon inserts his/her left hand into the hand port, and with a bowel grasper in the right hand through the left abdominal port, the transverse colon is retracted cephalad and the omentum is lifted above the transverse colon. The proximal small bowel is swept to the left of the patient and the terminal ileum is swept inferiorly, exposing the duodenum and the anterior aspect of the right colonic mesentery. The ileocecal region of the bowel is placed on anterolateral traction to identify the ileocolic artery and vein, which bowstring through the mesentery when placed on traction; this pedicle is usually easily identified. The proximal segment of the ileocolic artery and vein normally courses just inferior to the duodenum, and the duodenum is an important initial landmark. The first assistant helps by both holding the camera and by retracting the transverse colon cephalad using a bowel grasper placed through the epigastric port. The thumb and index finger of the surgeon's left hand are used to grasp the ileocolic artery and vein through the mesentery to retract it anteriorly. A monopolar scissors is used to incise the mesentery just inferior and superior to the ileocolic vessels, isolating them (Figure 9.2.3). These vessels are then divided at their appropriate level; in the case of benign disease, they are divided comfortably away from the origin. The vessels can be divided using a vessel-sealing device such as the LigaSure™ device, or the artery and vein can be isolated separately using an endoscopic dissector and clipped (Figure 9.2.4). In nearly 87% of cases, the right colic artery arises as a tributary of the ileocolic artery and not from the superior mesenteric artery,[2] and the ileocolic artery is usually divided proximal to the take-off of the right colic artery.

The left hand is then used to retract the distal edge of the divided ileocolic vessels, exposing the posterior aspect of the right colonic mesentery. The assistant helps by lifting up the thin mesenteric edge above the duodenum. A medial to lateral retromesenteric dissection is performed, first by bluntly sweeping down the second portion of the duodenum, separating it from the posterior aspect of the transverse mesocolon (Figure 9.2.5). The head of the pancreas is exposed carefully, as this dissection can result in a considerable amount of venous bleeding if performed too vigorously. This plane is maintained and dissected laterally, staying in the plane anterior to the retroperitoneal fascia as the fascia is bluntly swept down. The hand is inserted further and further underneath the mesentery, as Gerota's fascia is further swept away laterally, until this dissection is carried underneath the right

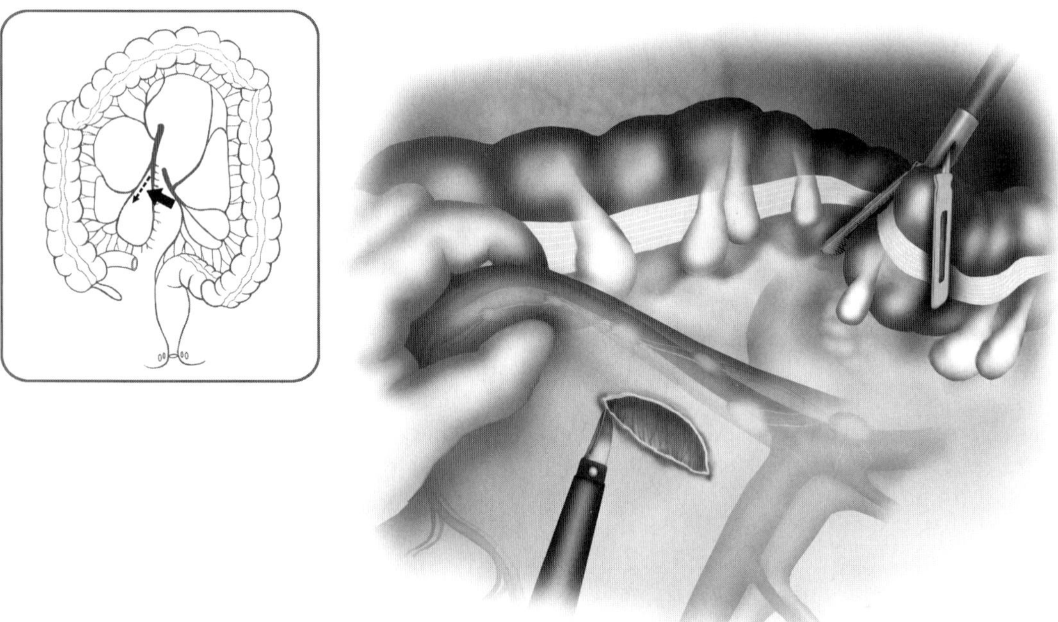

Figure 9.2.3. Isolation of the ileocolic pedicle begins with an incision just below it.

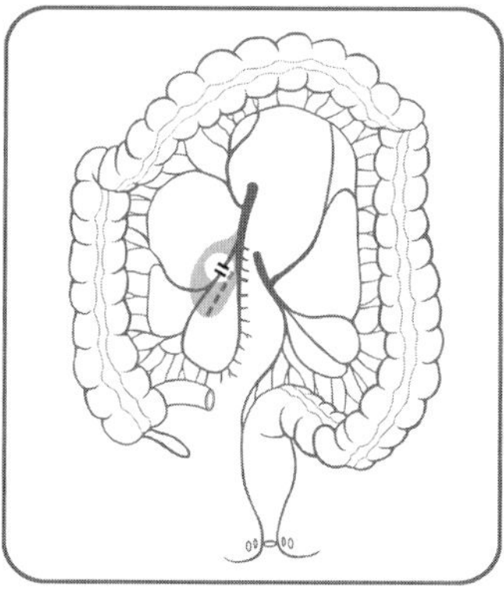

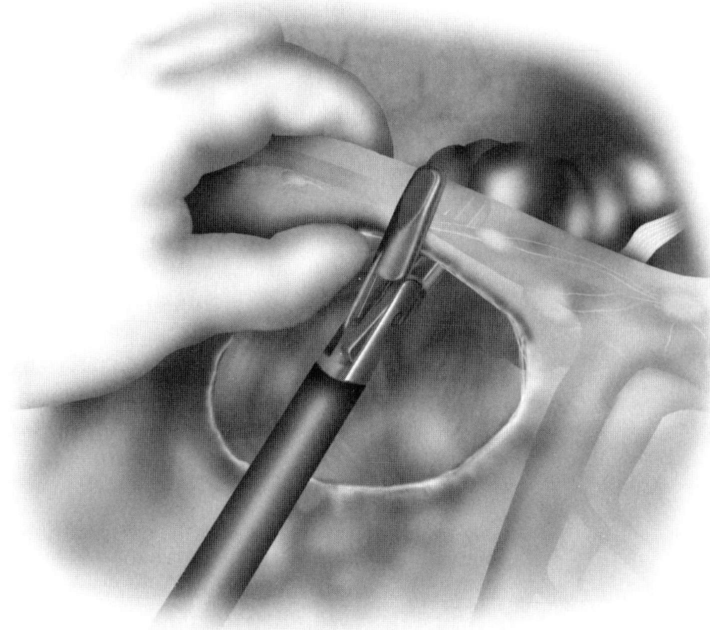

Figure 9.2.4. The vessels can be divided using a vessel sealing device such as the LigaSure™.

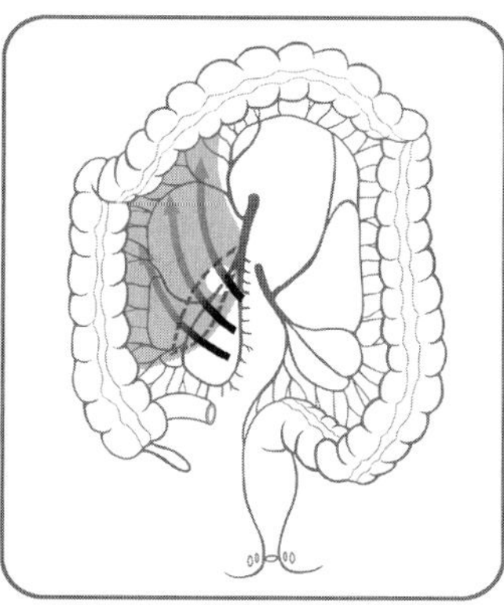

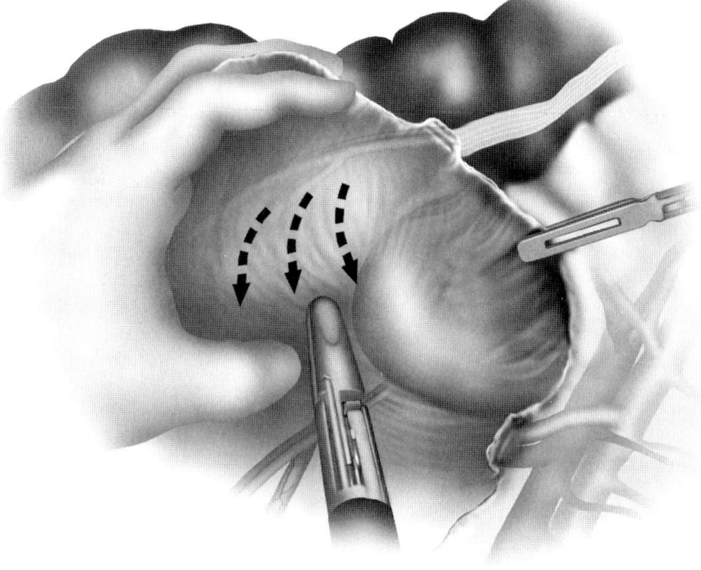

Figure 9.2.5. A medial to lateral approach to the mobilization of the right colon is used, beginning with sweeping the second portion of the duodenum carefully away from the mesocolon.

colon to the lateral abdominal wall, as well as underneath the hepatic flexure. Within the ileal mesentery, the ileal branch of the ileocolic vessel must not be torn by aggressive dissection underneath the cecum.

Next, the terminal ileum is grasped with the left hand and retracted cephalad, and electrosurgery is used to detach the ileum from the retroperitoneal structures. Occasionally, the hand can become an obstruction to the dissecting instrument, and in this case, the hand is removed and the monopolar shears inserted directly through the hand port and manipulated with the left hand. The dissection is taken around the appendix and cecum, sweeping away the residual retroperitoneal attachments to the cecum. With the left hand retracting the right colon medially, the monopolar scissors is inserted into the right abdominal port and used by the first assistant to divide the lateral attachments of the right colon (Figure 9.2.6). If the medial dissection was taken to the lateral abdominal wall, this attachment should be a thin sheet of peritoneum. This dissection is taken in a cephalad direction, eventually mobilizing the hepatic flexure. Depending on the case, the monopolar shears may need to be used from the epigastric port closer to the hepatic flexure. Placing the patient in reverse Trendelenburg position may help with hepatic flexure takedown.

At this point in time, again in Trendelenburg position with the right side up, the dissecting instrument is placed through the left abdominal port, and the omental dissection is begun. The assistant, still standing at the left of the patient, grasps the omentum, placing anterior traction

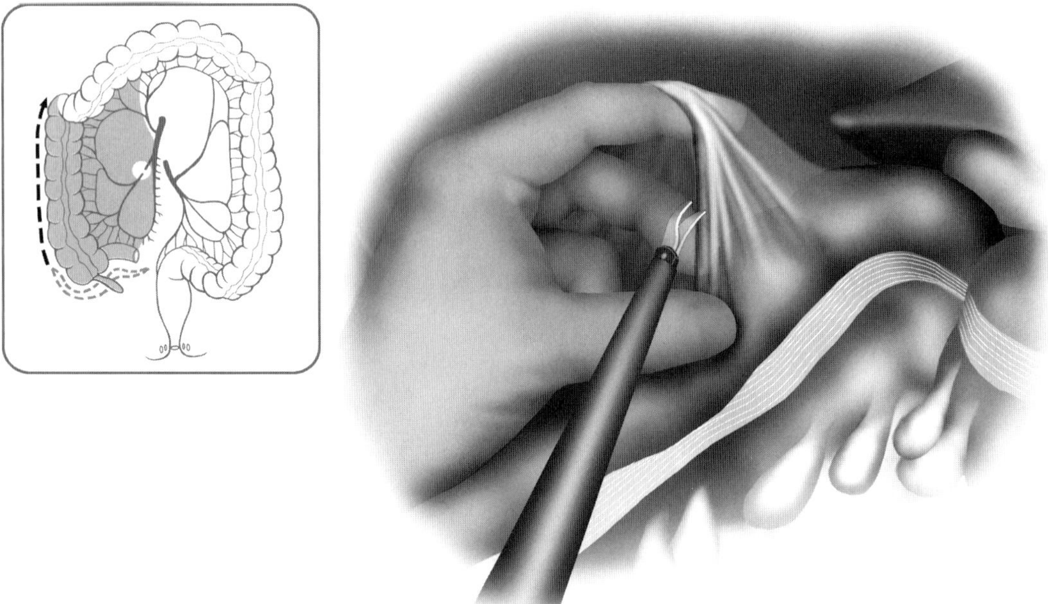

Figure 9.2.6. The lateral attachments are divided using monopolar electrosurgery, with the left hand providing medial retraction on the colon.

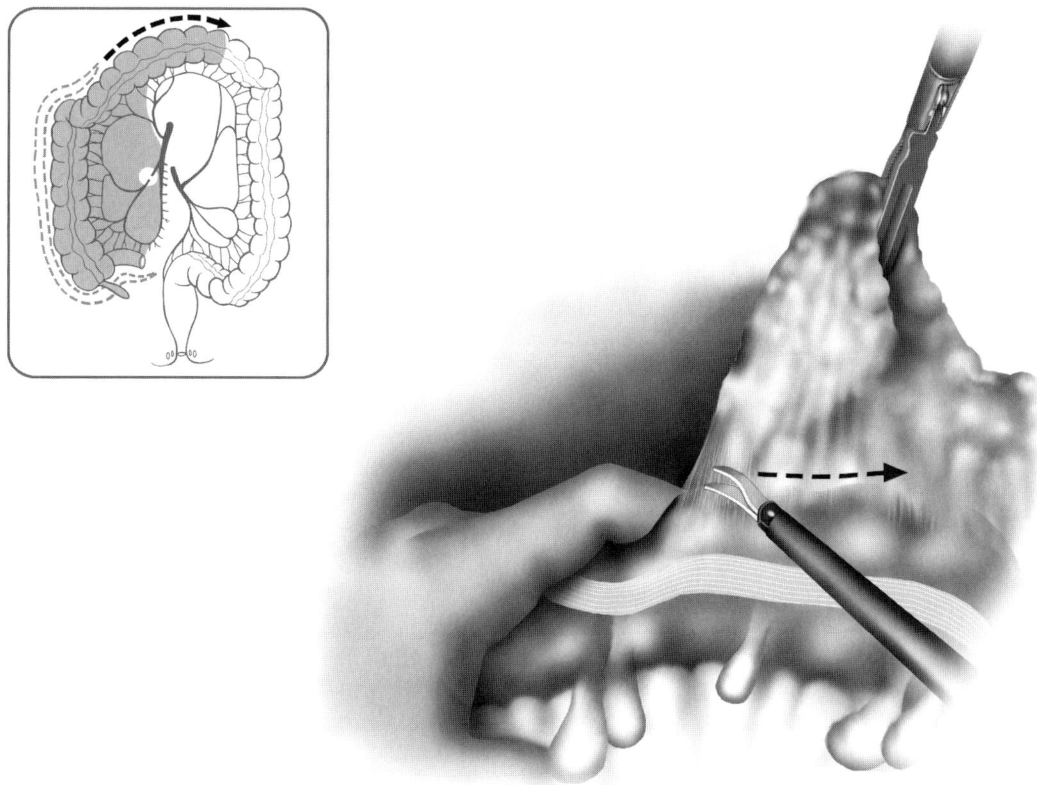

Figure 9.2.7. Omental dissection is performed from right to left.

on it, as the transverse colon is held by the left hand of the surgeon. Initially starting this dissection in the midtransverse colon and working back toward the hepatic flexure seems to allow for the easiest dissection. Larger omental vessels are divided using the LigaSure™, and care is taken to stay close to the colonic wall. After the omentum is freed from the hepatic flexure, the omental dissection is performed from right to left, mobilizing the omentum off of the transverse colon as one would in conventional surgery (Figure 9.2.7). With the surgeon positioned on the left side of the patient, dissection should be limited to the middle colic vessels and the transverse mesocolon to the right of the midline. Dissection to the left side of these areas becomes very difficult and should be reserved for later phases of the operation.

The assistant, from the left side of the patient, retracts the transverse mesocolon anteriorly, displaying the middle colic vessels (which can be visualized behind the peritoneum with traction) to the surgeon. In nearly one-third of the cases, an arterial branch will be present to the right colic angle. A finger is passed underneath the cut mesenteric edge, and is hooked around this branch, isolating it. This vessel is divided using the LigaSure™, or clipped and divided. The head of the pancreas is further swept down gently, and a finger is passed behind the middle colic vessels. It is important to remember that the vascular anatomy of the middle colic system is extremely variable, and there can be up to five different vessels behaving as arteries and branches. The pattern of the "true middle colic artery," or a single stem branching into a right and left branch may be present in only 46% of cases. Especially in more obese patients in whom the middle colic vessels may be "hidden" in a thickened mesentery, the hand-assisted approach allows the surgeon to feel pulsations within the mesentery. The right branch of the middle colic artery is identified and a finger is hooked around it, as a mesenteric window is created between the right and left branches (Figure 9.2.8). This vessel is divided. Then, a finger is passed around the left middle colic branch, and a window made to the left of this branch. This branch is then divided in the same way. When the dissection is completed to the left of the middle colic vessels, attention is turned to the left colon.

The operating room setup is changed as in Figure 9.2.1B. Still in steep Trendelenburg position, the patient is airplaned with the left side up. The small bowel loops are swept to the right of the patient. Near the ligament of Treitz, a left colic artery is usually seen branching from the inferior mesenteric artery (88% of cases). This vessel bowstrings and becomes visible through the mesentery when anterolateral traction is placed on the left colon. The surgeon's right hand is inserted through the hand port, and this vessel is grasped and retracted anteriorly. The assistant helps with retraction of the left colon with a bowel grasper inserted from the left abdominal port. With the monopolar shears inserted through the right abdominal port (manipulated with the left hand), mesenteric windows are created on both sides of this vessel, and the vessel is isolated and divided with the LigaSure™ device (Figure

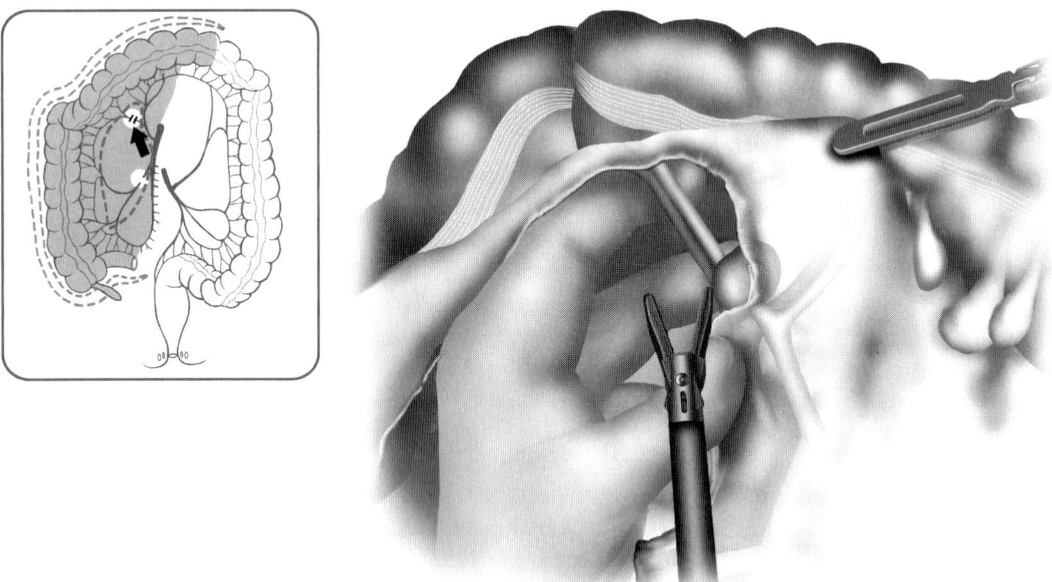

Figure 9.2.8. The right branch of the middle colic vessel is dissected as a finger is hooked around it.

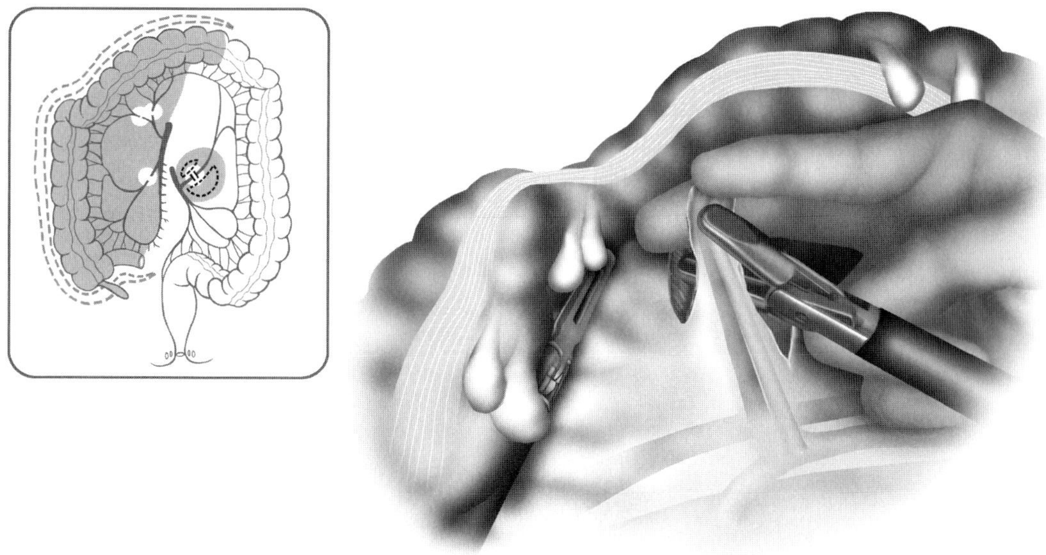

Figure 9.2.9. The left colic artery is isolated using finger retraction, and divided with a LigaSure™ device.

9.2.9). Adjacent to the ligament of Treitz (superior to the inferior mesenteric artery) is probably the easiest place to enter the correct retromesenteric plane to start a medial to lateral mobilization, and in benign disease this approach is preferred. With the right hand lifting the cut edge of the mesentery and exposing the mesenteric window, the retroperitoneal fascia including Gerota's fascia is bluntly swept down from the posterior aspect of the mesentery (Figure 9.2.10). The assistant helps in exposing this window. The hand is inserted further into this window and dissection is continued to the lateral abdominal wall. Initially, this plane is dissected inferiorly as far as possible, behind the first sigmoidal branch. Then, the same plane is developed in a cephalad direction, continuing to sweep down the retroperitoneal fascia until near the top of the kidney. Here, the mesentery of the colon attaches to the inferior border of the pancreas, and attention must be given so that the dissection does not carelessly continue posterior to the pancreas and injure the splenic vein.

At this point in time, the right hand is removed from the hand port, and the monopolar scissors is inserted through the hand port itself for lateral mobilization of the sigmoid colon. It is helpful for the assistant to move to the right side of the patient to assist through the epigastric port. Medial traction is placed on the sigmoid colon using bowel graspers, and the lateral attachments of the sigmoid colon are taken down with the monopolar scissors (Figure 9.2.11). Sharp and blunt dissection is used to carefully "peel" the sigmoid colon and mesosigmoid away from the retroperitoneal structures. The left ureter and gonadal vein

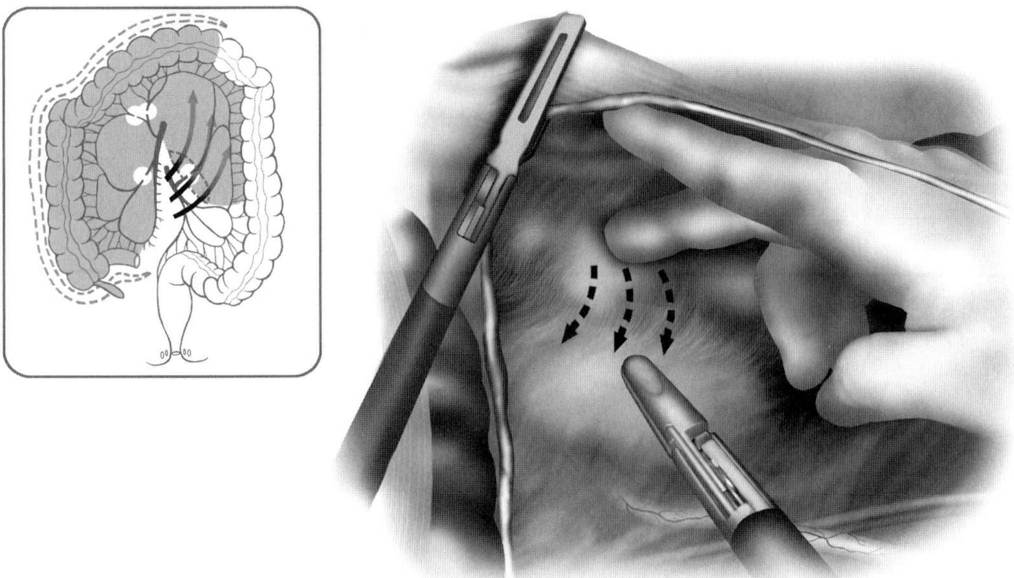

Figure 9.2.10. The surgeon's right hand is used to elevate the left colonic mesentery and Gerota's fascia is bluntly swept down using one or two fingers.

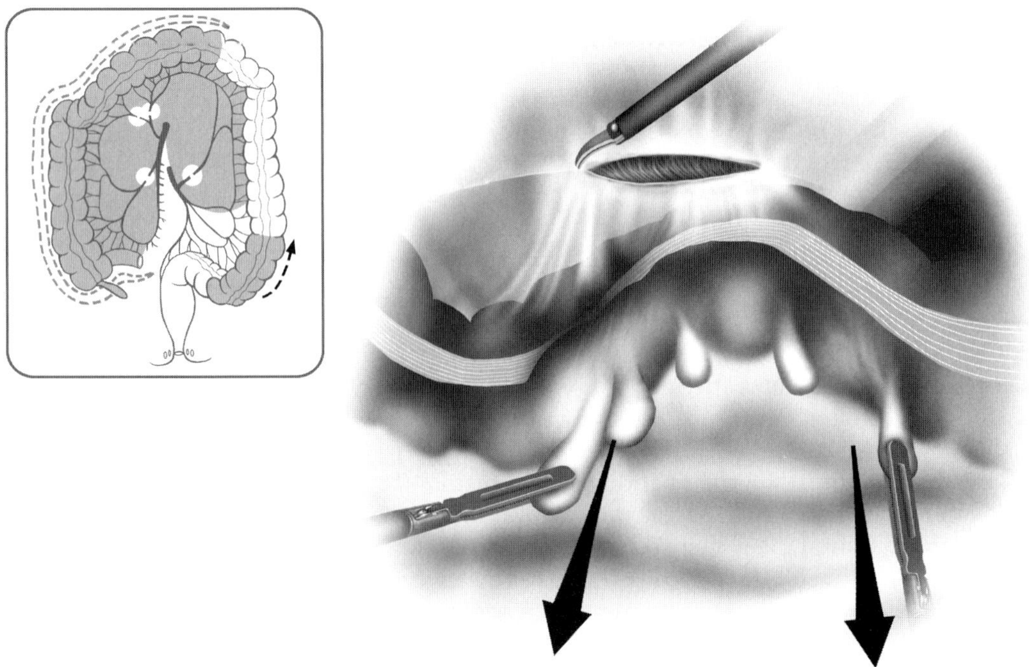

Figure 9.2.11. Medial traction is placed on the sigmoid colon, and the "white line" of Toldt is incised using monopolar scissors.

should be identified underneath the preserved retroperitoneal fascia. The dissection using this approach is taken in a superior direction until difficult. The left hand is placed back into the hand-assist device, and the monopolar shears inserted into the left abdominal port. The sigmoid colon is grasped and placed on medial traction, and the lateral attachment of the descending colon is further divided, heading toward the splenic flexure (Figure 9.2.12). This attachment should be a thin sheet of peritoneum if the medial to lateral retromesenteric dissection was taken to the lateral abdominal wall. Near the splenic flexure, the dissection becomes easier with the surgeon standing between the legs and, therefore, this lateral dissection is paused. The mobilization of the left and sigmoid colon is completed and, with this surgical method, the inferior mesenteric artery and sigmoidal branches remain intact. The sigmoidal branches may be isolated and divided intracorporeally before moving on to the splenic flexure dissection, or they can be left for later division using open surgery through the Pfannenstiel incision.

For the splenic flexure takedown, the surgeon moves between the patient's legs, as in Figure 9.2.4. The left hand is placed through the hand port, and the LigaSure™ 5 or 10 mm through the left abdominal port. The first assistant moves to the right of the patient and inserts bowel graspers into the right abdominal and epigastric ports. The patient is placed in a reverse Trendelenburg position.

The splenic flexure has several attachments, including the splenocolic ligament and the greater omentum. It is also held in place posteriorly by its retroperitoneal attachment, and the dissociation of Gerota's fascia from the posterior aspect of the mesentery in the previous

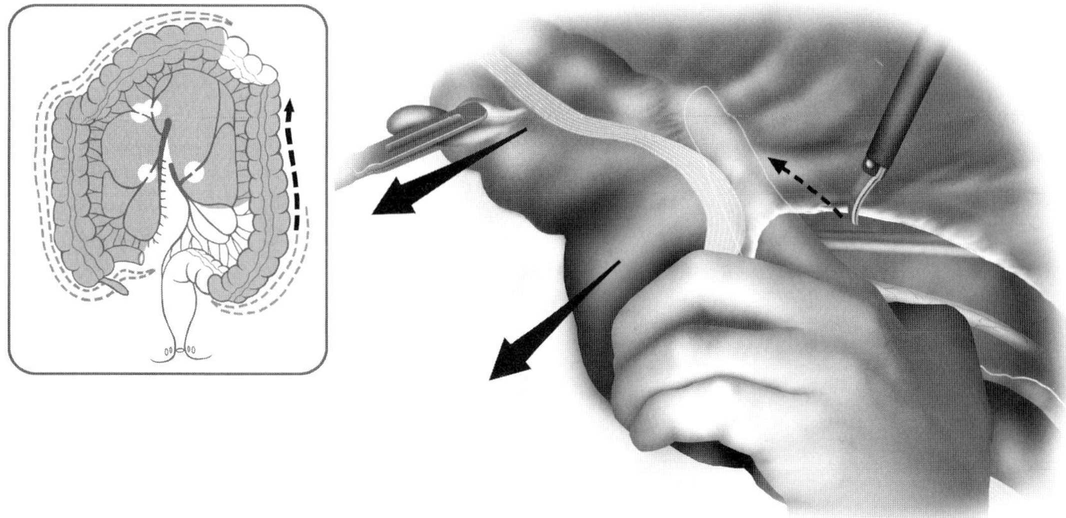

Figure 9.2.12. Using strong medial traction with a hand inserted in the port, lateral attachments of the left colon are incised.

surgical step allows for the splenic flexure to "drop down" toward the surgeon, distancing itself from the spleen and allowing for a safe dissection. The left hand grasps the proximal descending colon and retracts this inferiorly and medially. The assistant retracts the omentum as this is dissected off the wall of the splenic flexure using the LigaSure™ (Figure 9.2.13). Then, the splenocolic ligament is carefully dissected from laterally, staying as close to the colon as possible. This left to right dissection is continued, entering the lesser sac, and the omentum is further mobilized from the distal transverse colon. Here, the remaining omental attachments may be dissected from right to left, back toward the splenic flexure to meet the previous dissection. This should liberate the entire splenic flexure, and the remaining colonic attachment becomes the mesentery to the splenic flexure and distal transverse colon. By retracting the transverse colon toward the pelvis, the dorsal aspect of this mesenteric attachment is exposed. This mesentery is dissected with the LigaSure™ from lateral to medial until the pancreas is visualized and, at this level, the dissection is continued inferior to the pancreas (Figure 9.2.14). An intermesenteric vessel may be present between the middle and left colic arteries, and mesenteric vessels within this mesentery are divided. By dynamically retracting the transverse colon inferiorly from several directions, the final peritoneal attachments of the transverse colon are visualized and divided. Now,

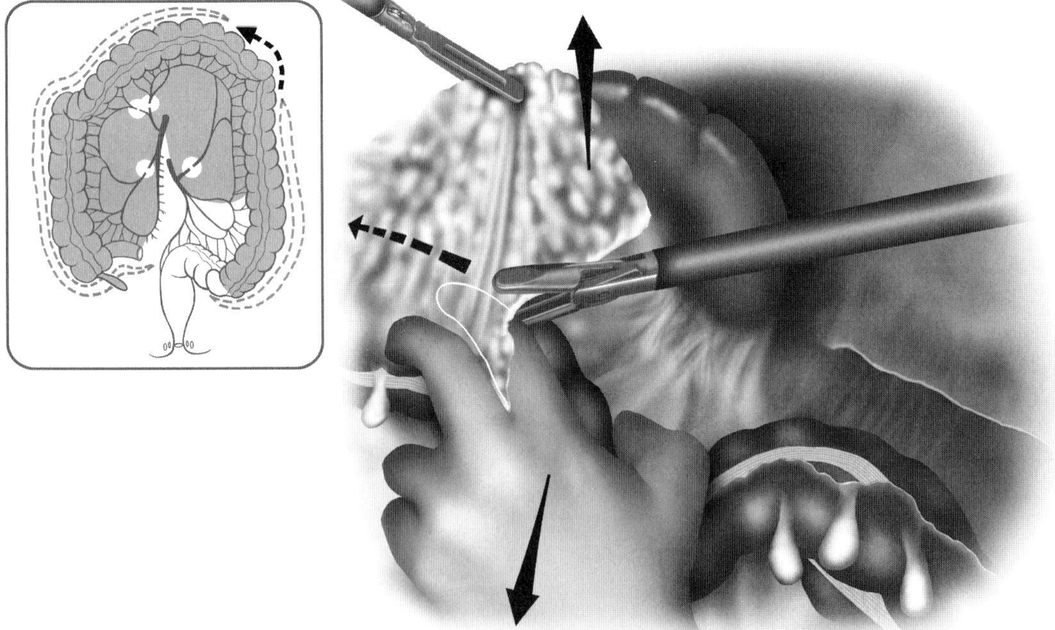

Figure 9.2.13. As an assistant retracts the omentum cephalad, the splenic flexure of the colon is freed with a LigaSure™ device.

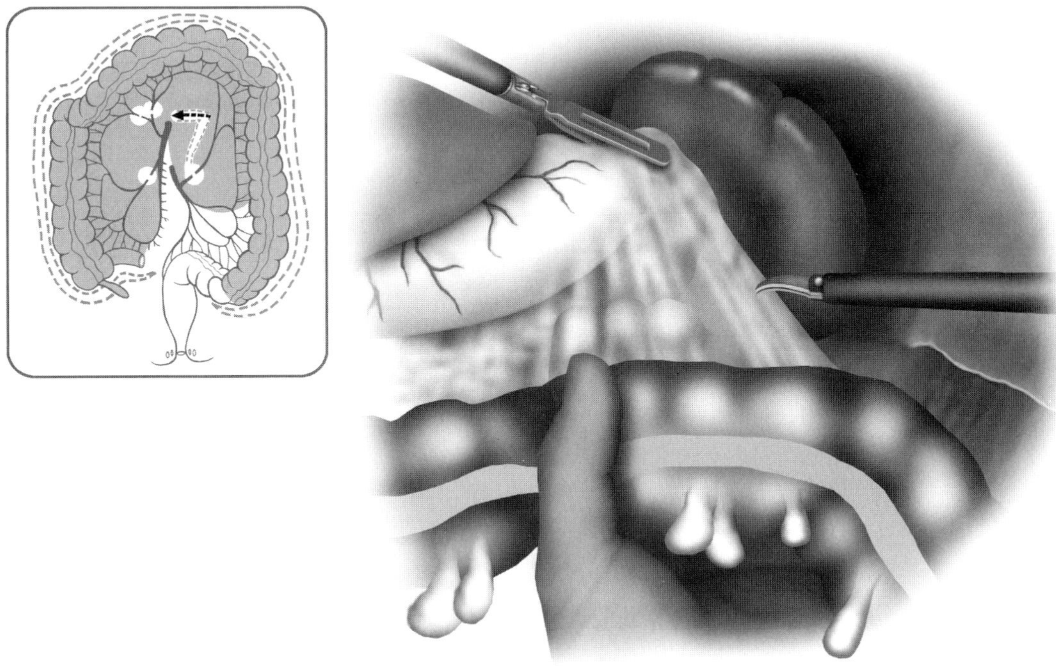

Figure 9.2.14. The last remnants of the transverse colon mesentery are freed from lateral to medial just inferior to the pancreas.

the entire abdominal portion of the colon should be free. The colon is placed above the small bowel loops, ready for extraction, as the patient is placed back in a Trendelenburg position.

Through the hand-assist device, the transverse colon is grasped, and the entire colon is exteriorized (Figure 9.2.15). The remaining portions of the operation will utilize conventional "open" surgical techniques. Staying inferior to the cut edge of the ileocolic vessels, the ileal mesentery is divided toward the ileocecal junction, dividing the ileal and accessory ileal branches. The terminal ileal wall is cleaned off and divided. If a stapled ileorectal anastomosis is planned, a purse-string is placed into the cut edge of the ileum and the center rod and anvil of a circular stapler are inserted into it. If an end ileostomy is planned, a linear cutting stapler is used to transect the distal terminal ileum. As the ileum can easily twist around its mesentery inside the abdomen, two seromuscular stay sutures are placed into the wall of the terminal ileum, and the sutures are left outside the body to prevent twisting as the ileum is placed back into the abdomen.

The specimen is now free proximally, and attention is given to the sigmoid colon. Any attachments of the sigmoid colon that were not adequately divided intracorporeally are dissected at this time through the Pfannenstiel incision using open techniques. The colon is retracted caudally, and the remaining sigmoidal arteries are isolated and divided (preserving the inferior mesenteric artery), until the top of the rectum is reached (Figure 9.2.16). The preservation of the inferior mesenteric

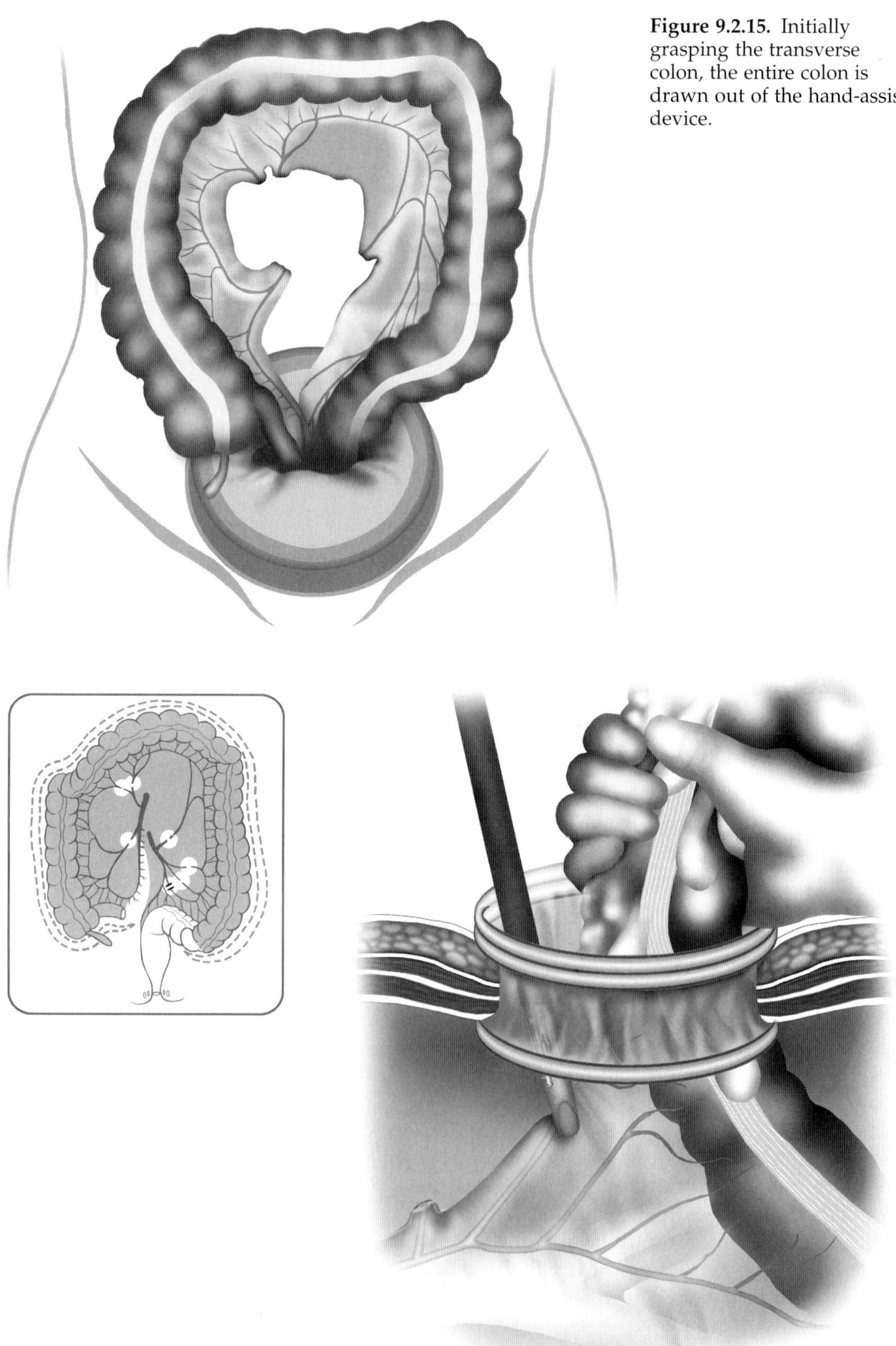

Figure 9.2.15. Initially grasping the transverse colon, the entire colon is drawn out of the hand-assist device.

Figure 9.2.16. Remaining sigmoid branches of the inferior mesenteric vessels are divided through the hand port site using open techniques until the top of the rectum is reached.

artery will assure good blood supply to the rectal stump (especially if the distal sigmoid colon is left intact), and the hypogastric nerves will remain completely untouched. The top of the rectum is stapled using a 30- or 45-mm linear stapler as in conventional surgery, liberating the total colectomy specimen. The end of the ileum is located, and a stapled ileorectal anastomosis created by inserting an end-to-end stapler into the rectum (CEEA 28 or 31 mm). Both donuts are checked for integrity, and a leak test is routinely performed by immersing the anastomosis in saline and injecting air under pressure into the rectum. The hand-assisted approach allows the surgeon to place reinforcing sutures if necessary, and for surgeons that prefer a single-stapled anastomosis (instead of a double-stapled one), a Proline purse-string can easily be placed into the mouth of the rectal stump. If an end ileostomy is planned, a stoma aperture is created in the right lower quadrant just as in open surgery, splitting the rectus abdominus muscles.

Approach if Cancer of the Rectum Is an Issue

If there is concern about malignancy, the inferior mesenteric artery should be divided laparoscopically very proximally as part of a complete lymphadenectomy. In this case, the surgical approach dealing with the left and sigmoid colon will change. The setup for this portion of the operation will be as in Figure 9.2.2. With the patient in Trendelenburg position with the left side up, the surgeon stands on the right side of the patient, with the first assistant between the legs. The first assistant places a hand through the hand-assist device and retracts the sigmoid colon anterolaterally, out of the pelvis. Starting at the sacral promontory using monopolar scissors, the surgeon creates a wide incision in the mesosigmoid, staying just posterior to the inferior mesenteric artery. An avascular plane is present here, and this is bluntly developed, sweeping the right and left hypogastric nerves away from the posterior aspect of the inferior mesenteric artery. The mesentery is opened in a superior direction toward the origin of the inferior mesenteric artery, further developing this plane (Figure 9.2.17). Using the hand to retract the inferior mesenteric pedicle anteriorly, the retroperitoneal fascia is swept down, developing the retromesenteric plane from medially to laterally. The left ureter and gonadal vein are visualized and protected. After identification of these structures, the inferior mesenteric artery and vein are isolated proximally and divided (Figure 9.2.18). The surgeon then inserts the right hand into the hand port, lifting the cut edge of the mesentery, and blunt dissection is continued laterally to the abdominal wall, staying anterior to the retroperitoneal fascia as the fascia is swept down. The dissection is initially taken inferiorly underneath the sigmoid colon, and then cephalad, sweeping Gerota's fascia down from the posterior aspect of the left colonic mesentery, heading toward the top of the left kidney. At this point, the lateral attachments of the sigmoid and left colon are taken down as in the previous description.

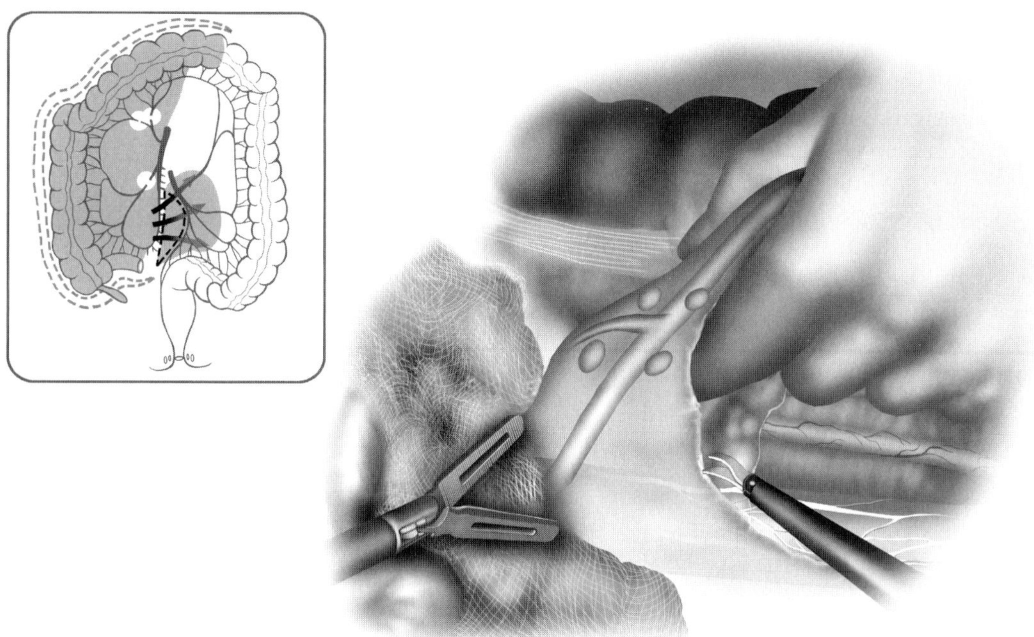

Figure 9.2.17. For an oncologic dissection of the inferior mesenteric vessels, dissection is begun at the region of the sacral promontory, dissecting between the posterior aspect of the inferior mesenteric artery and the hypogastric nerves.

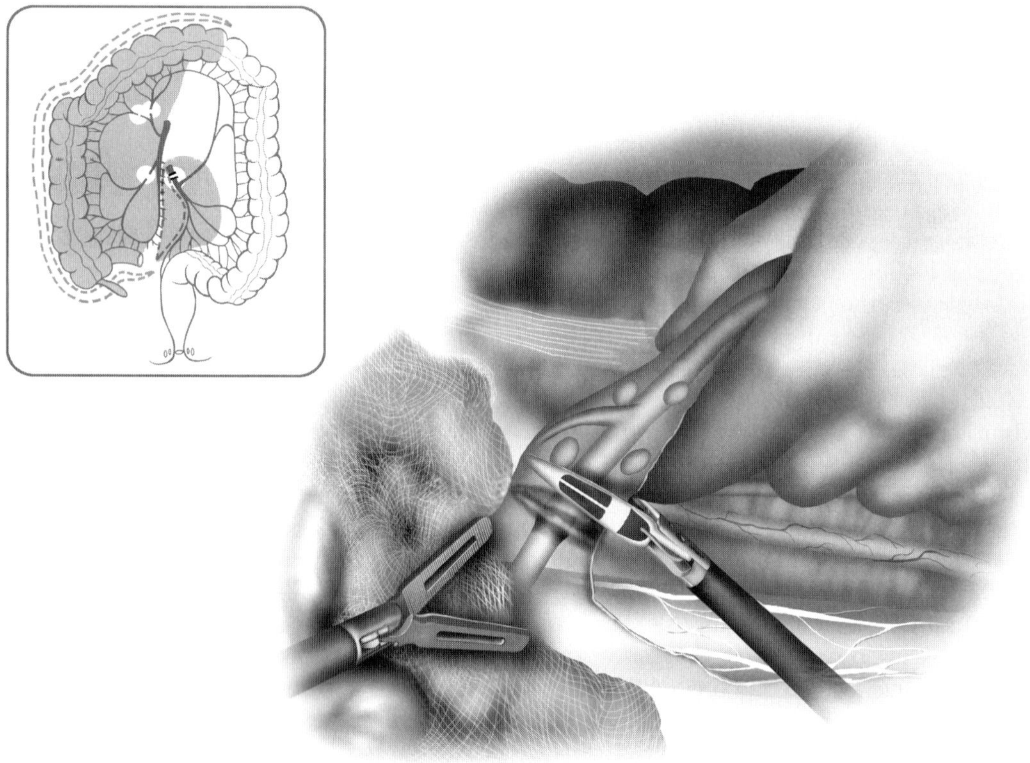

Figure 9.2.18. The inferior mesenteric artery and vein are divided proximally after identifying the left ureter and gonadal vessels.

Special Considerations

A profound understanding of mesenteric anatomy should help limit unnecessary surgical bleeding. During medial to lateral mobilization of the left colon, the surgeon should be careful to stay anterior to the retroperitoneal fascia and to clearly identify the left ureter before transaction of the inferior mesenteric artery.

One potential complication unique to the total colectomy is dehiscence of the staple line of the rectal stump in the case of severe colitis. This complication is difficult to prevent if the patient has severe inflammation and is malnourished. To prevent a pelvic abscess in this situation, we implant the closed end of the mucus fistula into the subcutaneous space of the suprapubic wound (see Figure 9.2.5); if a stump dehiscence were to occur, this would result in a wound infection rather than a pelvic abscess. To implant the rectal stump into the wound, it will need to be left slightly longer (transected at the distal sigmoid colon), and tacked to the lower aspect of the peritoneal opening before closure of the peritoneum. The fascia is not closed entirely, but closed around the colon laterally, which protrudes through the fascia centrally.

Conclusions

The laparoscopic mobilization of the total abdominal colon is a difficult and time-consuming procedure, but the use of hand-assisted surgery has improved operative times. The utilization of a hand port may allow less-experienced laparoscopic surgeons to tackle this daunting procedure. Furthermore, in cases of fulminant colitis, the surgeon may feel more comfortable dissecting the fragile colon using a hand rather than small laparoscopic graspers. In our practice, the hand-assisted approach has become the preferred method for performing a total colectomy.

Editors' Comments

Indications: We agree with these indications.

Patient positioning: We generally have the surgeon stand between the legs for both the right and left colon mobilization and mesenteric dissection, using the right hand for the right colon and the left hand for the left colon. The first assistant stands on the left side by the patient for the right colon and on the right side of the patient for the left colonic parts.

Cannula positioning: We use the same sites, but avoid using the stoma site for a cannula, as it is usually too close to the umbilicus, and thus any instrument crowds the laparoscope.

Technique: Our technique is similar to those described, and we believe it is a valuable method for the total colectomy using laparoscopic techniques.

References

1. Nakajima K, Lee SW, Cocilovo C, et al. Laparoscopic total colectomy: hand-assisted vs standard technique. Surg Endosc 2004;18:582–586.
2. VanDamme J-P, Bonte J. Vascular Anatomy in Abdominal Surgery. Stuttgart: Georg Thieme Verlag; 1990.

Chapter 10.1

Diagnostic Laparoscopy

Martin R. Weiser and Alessandro Fichera

Evaluation of the visceral organs, peritoneum, retroperitoneum, and pelvis is an integral component of abdominal surgery, and the ability to appraise the abdomen laparoscopically has been well established. The magnified view offered by current videoscopes and the maneuverability within the abdomen allows for a thorough and complete evaluation.

Indications

The efficacy of diagnostic laparoscopy has been well studied in solid organ malignancy. Conlon et al.[1] described 115 patients with radiographically resectable peripancreatic tumors that underwent extended diagnostic laparoscopy before planned curative resection. In 41 patients, additional disease previously not appreciated on preoperative imaging was noted at laparoscopy. These patients with metastatic disease avoided unnecessary laparotomy. The addition of staging laparoscopy in the entire cohort raised the overall resectability rate from 35% to 76% in patients undergoing laparotomy.

The efficacy of diagnostic laparoscopy has also been proven in high-risk colorectal cancer patients.[2] In 14 patients with near obstructing rectal cancers, diagnostic laparoscopy was performed before initiation of neoadjuvant chemoradiation. All patients were thought to have locally advanced, but resectable, disease based on radiographic imaging. At laparoscopy, four patients (29%) had diffuse peritoneal disease which significantly altered their treatment strategy resulting in avoidance of unnecessary laparotomy. Thus, in colorectal cancer patients in whom there is a significant question regarding primary staging or diagnosis that could alter the treatment strategy, diagnostic laparoscopy may be indicated.

Patient Positioning and Operating Room Setup

We often use epidural anesthesia if colorectal resection is anticipated at the same time as diagnostic laparoscopy. The patient is usually placed in modified lithotomy position and sequential pneumatic devices on the lower extremities are routinely used. The arms are placed at the patient's sides and the patient is secured in position with either a bean bag or Plexiglas sleighs because steep rotation and tilting of the operating table is often necessary. Monitors are placed on the right and left sides of the table and the exact position is dictated by any additional procedures to be performed (Figure 10.1.1).

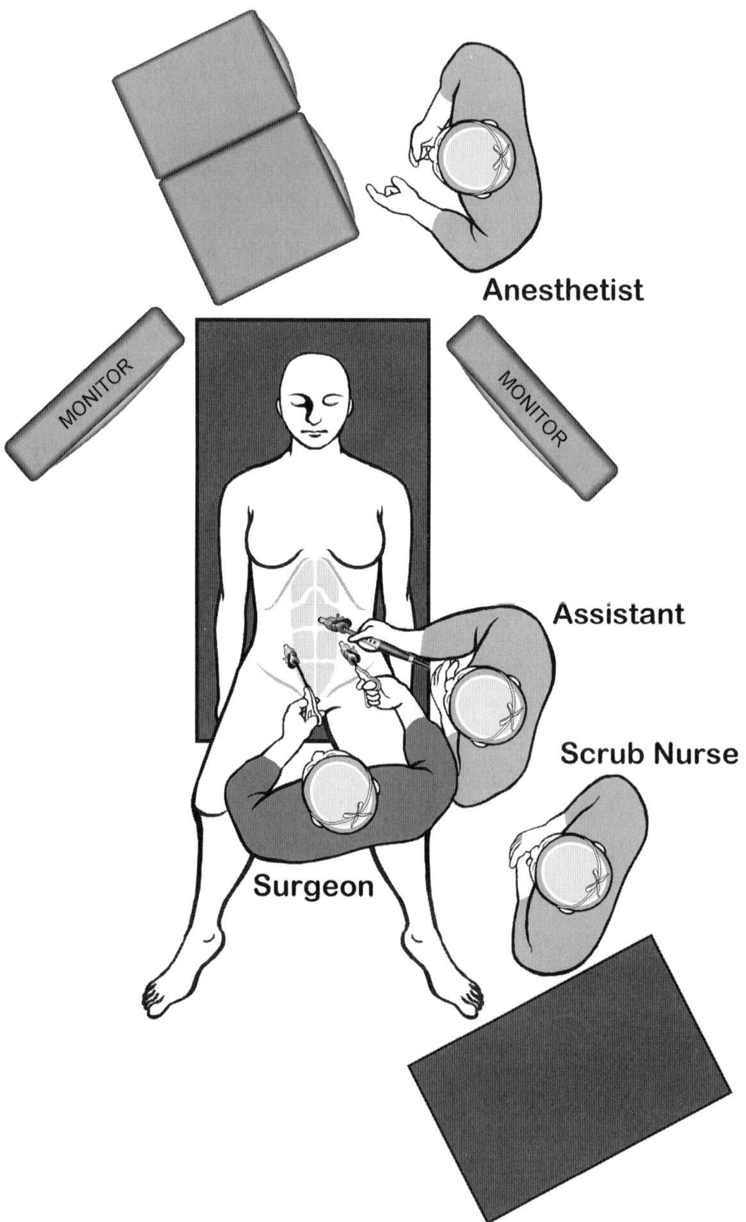

Figure 10.1.1. Positions of the surgical team and equipment for the diagnostic laparoscopy at the beginning of the procedure.

Table 10.1.1. Specific instruments recommended for diagnostic laparoscopy

3–5	Cannulae (1 × 10 mm, 2–4 × 5 mm; only 5-mm cannulae may be used if a 5-mm videoscope is available)
2	Laparoscopic bowel graspers
1	Laparoscopic ultrasound

Instruments

Specific instruments recommended for diagnostic laparoscopy are listed in Table 10.1.1.

Cannula Positioning

Although cannula placement is modified by additional procedures that may be performed, at least three cannulae are usually required for a thorough examination of the peritoneum, visceral organs, and retroperitoneum (Figure 10.1.2). With improved optics, 5-mm videoscopes can be used for many procedures. If ultrasound is needed, at least one 10-mm additional cannula will be required, likely on the right side, because this will allow liver ultrasonography most easily. When diag-

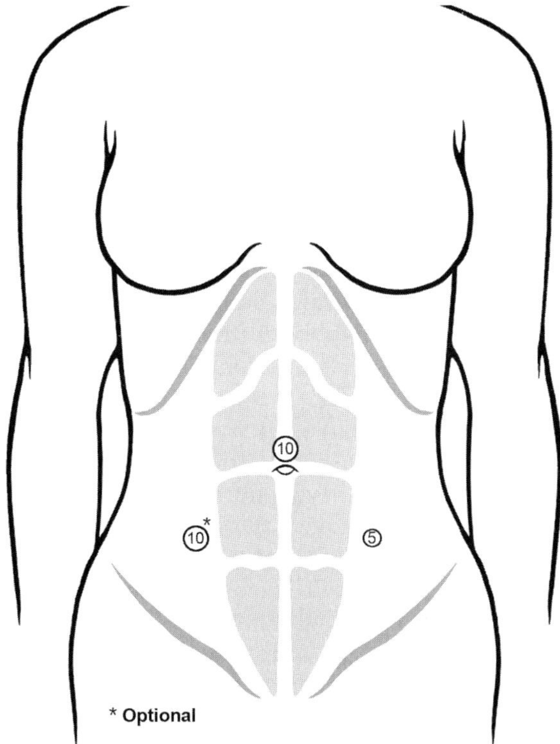

Figure 10.1.2. Cannula positions for the diagnostic laparoscopy. If liver ultrasound is used, the right cannula should be a 10-mm size (asterisk).

nostic laparoscopy with or without biopsy is solely performed, we use a three-cannula technique (one cannula for a 5-mm 30° videoscope, a second for a 10-mm laparoscopic ultrasound, and a third for a 5-mm instrument). A 10-mm cannula is placed at the umbilicus and two additional 5-mm cannulae are placed in the right and left mid abdomen lateral to the rectus abdominus muscle. If a colectomy is anticipated, the cannula setup is altered according to the procedure to be performed. For example, if the colon is to be resected, we use a five-cannula technique with a 10-mm flexible videoscope. A 10-mm cannula is placed at the umbilicus, a 12-mm cannula in the lower quadrant opposite the segment of colon to be resected for the endoscopic stapler, and three additional 5-mm working cannulae in the other remaining abdominal quadrants.

Technique

The extent of exploration is somewhat dictated by the disease process. For example, in inflammatory bowel disease, it is critical to fully evaluate the entire intestine to confirm diagnosis and determine the extent of disease. Only after the small bowel has been thoroughly examined and cleared of disease can Crohn's disease be excluded and an ileal pouch fashioned for patients with presumed ulcerative colitis. Furthermore, in patients with Crohn's disease in whom skip lesions are not uncommon, the small bowel must be fully evaluated so all areas are adequately addressed. In cases of colorectal cancer, careful evaluation for peritoneal, retroperitoneal, and liver metastases is critical, and intraoperative findings can change the surgical plan.

Once all cannulae are placed, the abdomen is systematically evaluated. The upper abdomen is first explored with the patient in reverse Trendelenburg position, which allows the abdominal viscera to move downward with gravity. The flexible tip or 30° videoscope allows full evaluation of the dome of the liver and diaphragms. The lesser sac and retroperitoneum can be easily evaluated by opening the gastrohepatic ligament either with electrosurgery, ultrasonic scalpel, or LigaSure™ device. A fan retractor can be used to lift up on the left liver to allow visualization and evaluation of the retroperitoneum. Evaluation of the pancreas, celiac axis, and periportal adenopathy can be evaluated with the aid of the laparoscopic ultrasound. After visual inspection, the liver parenchyma is fully evaluated with ultrasound (Figure 10.1.3). Segments II–VIII can be well visualized by placing the ultrasound probes on the surface of the liver. Evaluation of segment I (caudate lobe) requires placing the probe beneath liver segments II and III and adjacent to the vena cava. Small visible lesions can easily be biopsied with a cupped forceps or excised with ultrasonic scalpel or cautery. Hemostasis is easily controlled with a 5-mm argon beam coagulator or electrosurgery. Deeper intraparenchymal lesions that are visualized on ultrasound can be biopsied using a trajectory guided TRU-cut needle under ultrasound guidance. The current laparoscopic ultrasound probe (Bruel & Kjaer, Naerum, Denmark) has an attachable needle guide that allows for ultrasound guided biopsy.

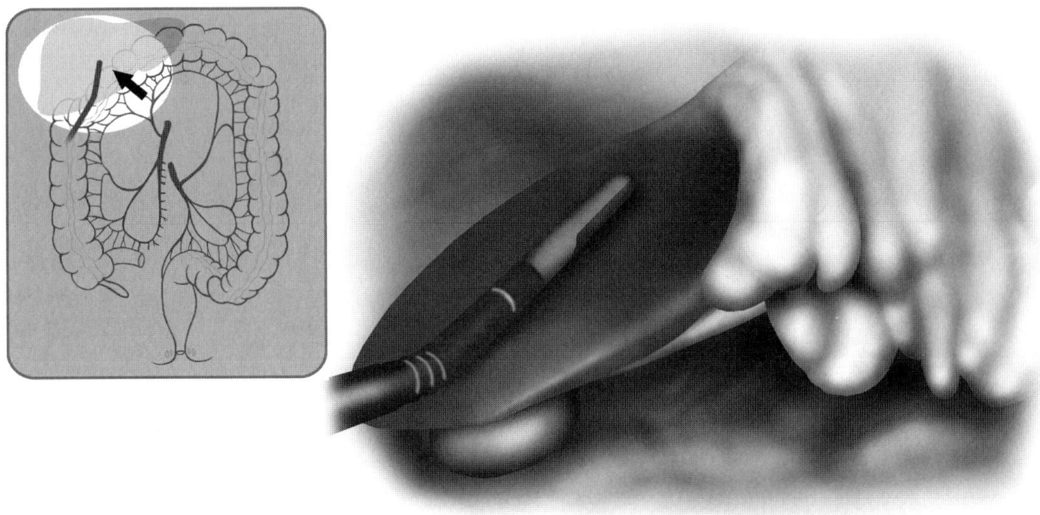

Figure 10.1.3. A laparoscopic ultrasound probe can be readily used to assess the liver and retroperitoneal structures during diagnostic laparoscopy.

The mid abdomen is well visualized with the patient in the Trendelenburg position. The omentum is visualized and then placed over the liver, which brings the transverse colon superiorly for full evaluation. With the transverse colon in the upper abdomen, the small bowel and mid-abdominal retroperitoneum is easily visualized and evaluated. The patient is then tilted with the right side down, the small intestine is placed in the right abdomen, and the ligament of Treitz identified under the left transverse colon (Figure 10.1.4, with inset). The inferior mesenteric vein located adjacent to the ligament of Treitz and the left colon and its mesentery are easily identified including the origin of the inferior mesenteric artery. In this position, periaortic adenopathy can be evaluated and biopsied if necessary. Laparoscopic ultrasound with Doppler can be useful when evaluating retroperitoneal adenopathy. The origin of the inferior mesenteric artery and sigmoid mesentery are also well visualized. While keeping the patient in this position, the sigmoid colon and its mesentery are evaluated in the lower abdomen.

Attention is then placed back at the ligament of Treitz to begin evaluation of the small intestine. Using either a hand-over-hand or hand-to-hand technique (see Chapter 8.1), all surfaces of the small bowel are visualized as it is passed from one bowel grasper to the other (Figure 10.1.5). Once the distal jejunum/proximal ileum are reached, it is necessary to tilt the patient with the left side down – then the loops of intestine can be easily placed into the left side of the abdomen. This permits easy completion of the small bowel examination to the cecum. In cases of inflammatory bowel disease, sites of stricture can be marked with suture for later resection or stricturoplasty. In the left side down position, the second and third portions of duodenum are visualized as are

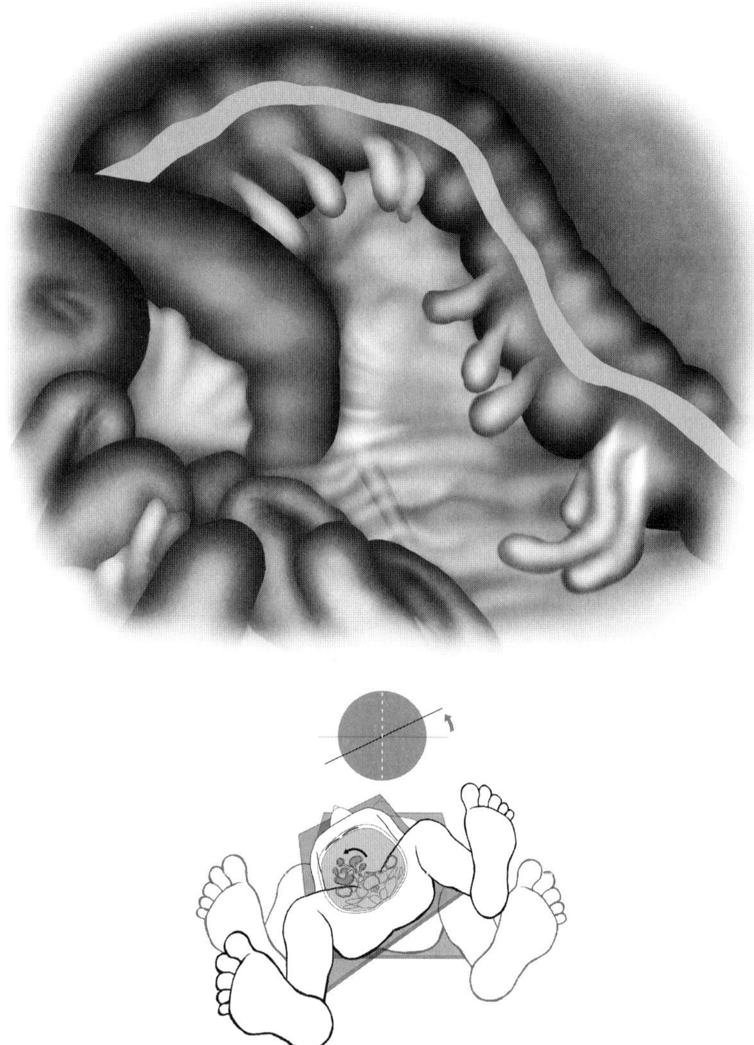

Figure 10.1.4. "Running" of the small bowel begins with appropriate positioning of the patient (inset: patient in left side up with intestines retracted to the right) and starting the evaluation at the ligament of Treitz. Note that the inferior mesenteric vein is readily seen even in moderately obese patients.

the ileocolic and middle colic pedicles. The appendix, cecum, right colon, and hepatic flexure are identified and evaluated with bowel graspers.

By next placing the patient in deep Trendelenburg position, the pelvic organs can be well visualized. The small bowel is placed in the mid and upper abdomen. The lower sigmoid colon and rectum can be inspected with bowel graspers and the peritoneal reflections including the cul-de-sac between rectum and the anterior organs are well visualized. In females, the ovaries, fallopian tubes, and uterus are inspected (Figure 10.1.6).

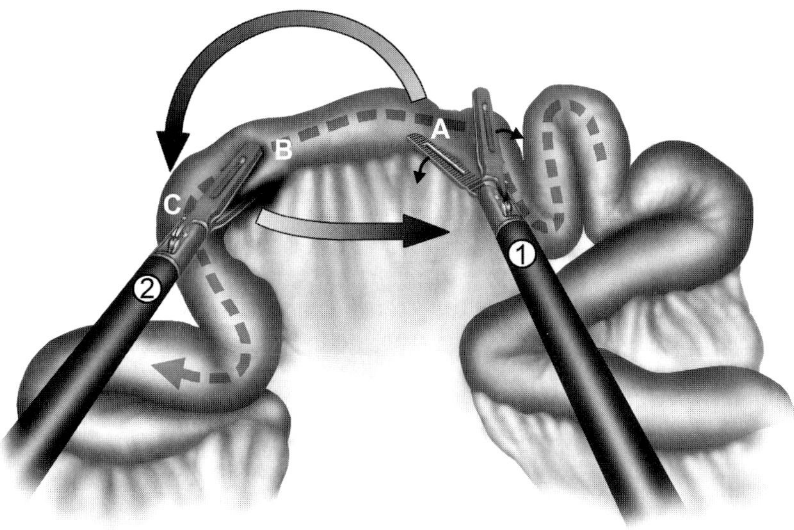

Figure 10.1.5. Running the bowel using the "hand-over-hand" technique: The right-handed grasper (1) releases the bowel and prepares to move from point A on the bowel to point C, whereas the left-handed grasper (2), at point B, prepares to slide underneath the other grasper.

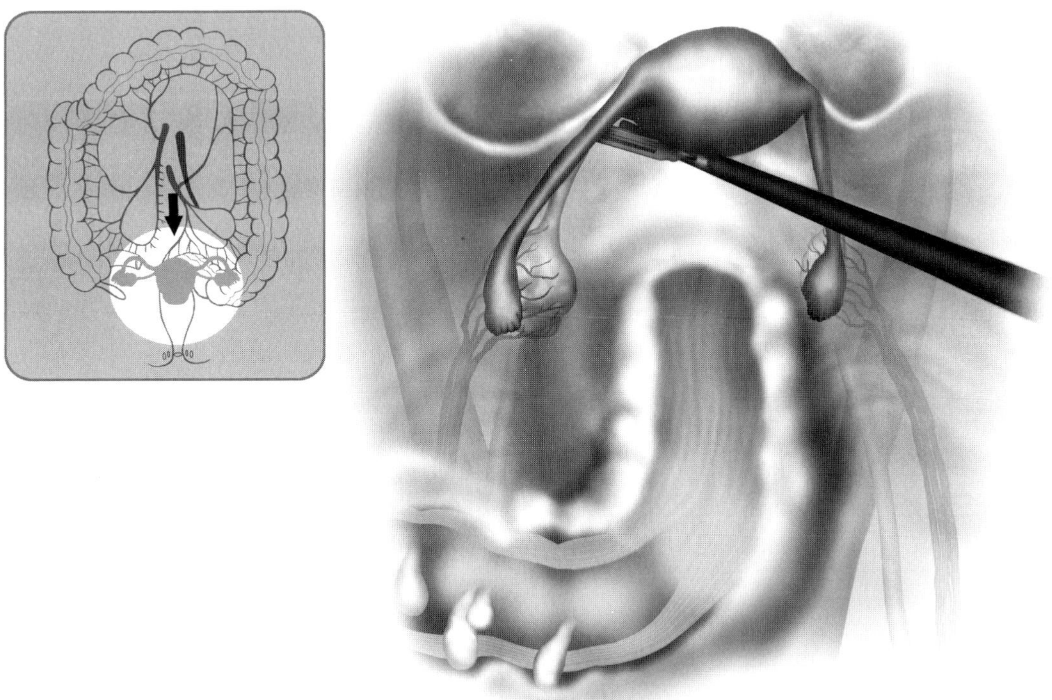

Figure 10.1.6. Diagnostic laparoscopy nearly always affords an excellent view of the uterus, Fallopian tubes, and ovaries.

Special Considerations

The limitations of laparoscopy including loss of direct tactile sensation are overcome by enhanced visualization and increased reliance on visual cues, the use of ultrasound, and indirect palpation with laparoscopic instruments. Current videoscopes permit 15–20× magnification and the diagnostic scope of the examination can be further enhanced with laparoscopic ultrasound. Although direct palpation is not possible, the operating surgeon can indirectly palpate abnormal areas by maneuvering an instrument over the suspected region.

Colonic abnormalities can be evaluated with intraoperative colonoscopy. The use of carbon dioxide as the inflating gas for colonoscopy allows for rapid reabsorption and resolution of bowel distension so this is never an inhibitory factor during laparoscopic surgery.[3]

Recent technologic advances in laparoscopic ultrasound probes with four-way steerable scanning head, integrated biopsy system, and color flow mapping allow for full evaluation of intra-abdominal organs such as the liver and the retroperitoneum. Integrated biopsy systems, such as the one provided by Bruel & Kjaer, allow for real-time ultrasound targeted TRU-Cut biopsies. Intraoperative liver ultrasound is a proven diagnostic modality. This has been clearly demonstrated in patients with known liver metastases where liver ultrasound at the time of liver metastasectomy often identifies additional lesions that alter the surgical plan.[4,5] However, the use of routine liver ultrasound in nonmetastatic disease is less established. In a study of 63 patients undergoing diagnostic laparoscopy before curative colorectal resection, two patients were noted to have hepatic lesions not previously picked up on computed tomography scan.[6] In another study of 33 patients that underwent preoperative laparoscopy and liver ultrasound, one patient was found to have liver metastases missed by preoperative computed tomography scan.[7] Although not conclusively proven, it is reasonable to perform liver ultrasound in high-risk patients to assess for metastatic disease because the procedure is noninvasive and relatively quick.

Conclusion

Full evaluation of the abdomen and pelvis are an integral component of any abdominal surgery, and this is easily performed laparoscopically. The limitations related to lack of direct tactile sensation are more than compensated by the advances in technology including magnified videoscopes which allow for enhanced visualization, ability to maneuver throughout the abdomen and pelvis, and laparoscopic ultrasound.

Editors' Comments

Indications: We would add that certain rare patients with Crohn's disease may require diagnostic laparoscopy to rule out another etiology, e.g., ileitis with unusual clinical course or massively enlarged mesenteric lymph nodes to rule out lymphoma.

Patient positioning: We place the patients in similar positions.

Instrumentation: If intraoperative endoscopy becomes necessary, a colonoscope with CO_2 insufflation may be preferable.

Cannula positioning: The cannula positioning always depends on the individual case and situation.

Technique: We generally follow a pattern of clockwise exploration starting in the right upper quadrant.

References

1. Conlon KC, Dougherty E, Klimstra DS, et al. The value of minimal access surgery in the staging of patients with potentially resectable peripancreatic malignancy. Ann Surg 1996;223:134–140.
2. Koea JB, Guillem JG, Conlon KC, et al. Role of laparoscopy in the initial multimodality management of patients with near-obstructing rectal cancer. J Gastrointest Surg 2000;4:105–108.
3. Nakajima K, Lee SW, Sonoda T, et al. Intraoperative carbon dioxide colonoscopy: a safe insufflation alternative for locating colonic lesions during laparoscopic surgery. Surg Endosc 2005;19(3):321–325.
4. Foroutani A, Garland AM, Berber E, et al. Laparoscopic ultrasound vs triphasic computed tomography for detecting liver tumors. Arch Surg 2000;135:933–938.
5. Tsioulias GJ, Wood TF, Chung MH, et al. Diagnostic laparoscopy and laparoscopic ultrasonography optimize the staging and resectability of intraabdominal neoplasms. Surg Endosc 2001;15:1016–1019.
6. Milsom JW, Jerby BL, Kessler H, et al. Prospective, blinded comparison of laparoscopic ultrasonography vs. contrast-enhanced computerized tomography for liver assessment in patients undergoing colorectal carcinoma surgery. Dis Colon Rectum 2000;43:44–49.
7. Goletti O, Celona G, Galatioto C, et al. Is laparoscopic sonography a reliable and sensitive procedure for staging colorectal cancer? A comparative study. Surg Endosc 1998;12:1236–1241.

Chapter 10.2

Laparoscopic Stoma Formation

Sang Lee

Stoma formation is well suited for a laparoscopic approach. It is technically simple to perform and requires a limited number of cannula sites. Unlike the Trephine (open) method of stoma formation, a thorough intraabdominal exploration with the laparoscope can be performed without making additional incisions. Although the benefits of laparoscopic surgery can be expected after laparoscopic stoma formation, to date, there is no prospective randomized trial comparing outcomes of open and laparoscopic stoma formation. There are some retrospective studies, which suggest a low complication rate, shorter hospitalization, and less pain after laparoscopic stoma formation.[1–4]

Indications

Indications for laparoscopic stoma formation do not differ from those of open surgery. Laparoscopic stoma formation can be performed independently for a variety of indications or as a part of more complex gastrointestinal surgery. A variety of intestinal sites can be chosen for stoma formation; the terminal ileum, transverse colon, and sigmoid colon are the most common sites chosen for stoma formation. The choice for different sites depends on indications and subsequent procedures planned. A loop ileostomy is preferred as a temporary stoma site especially when further colon and rectal surgery is planned in the future. For a permanent ostomy site, end sigmoid colostomy with less output is favored. For either, it is essential to carefully select the site of the stoma preoperatively in concert with a stoma nurse.

Patient Positioning and Operating Room Setup

General anesthesia is used, and we place an orogastric tube and a Foley catheter in order to minimize the chances of damaging the stomach or the bladder during cannula insertion. Pneumatic compression stockings are used in all patients. Two video monitors are placed angling toward the patient at shoulder level. Some surgeons recommend performing the procedure with the patient in the supine position but we prefer the modified lithotomy position using padded stirrups. This position allows the surgeon or assistant to stand between the patient's legs, while the other surgeon stands on the left side of the patient (for ileostomy formation) and facilitates complete inspection of the small intestines (Figure 10.2.1). A mirror image of this setup is used for the sigmoid colostomy formation. The hips and knees are gently flexed to an angle no greater than 15° to avoid laparoscopic instruments colliding with the patient's thighs.

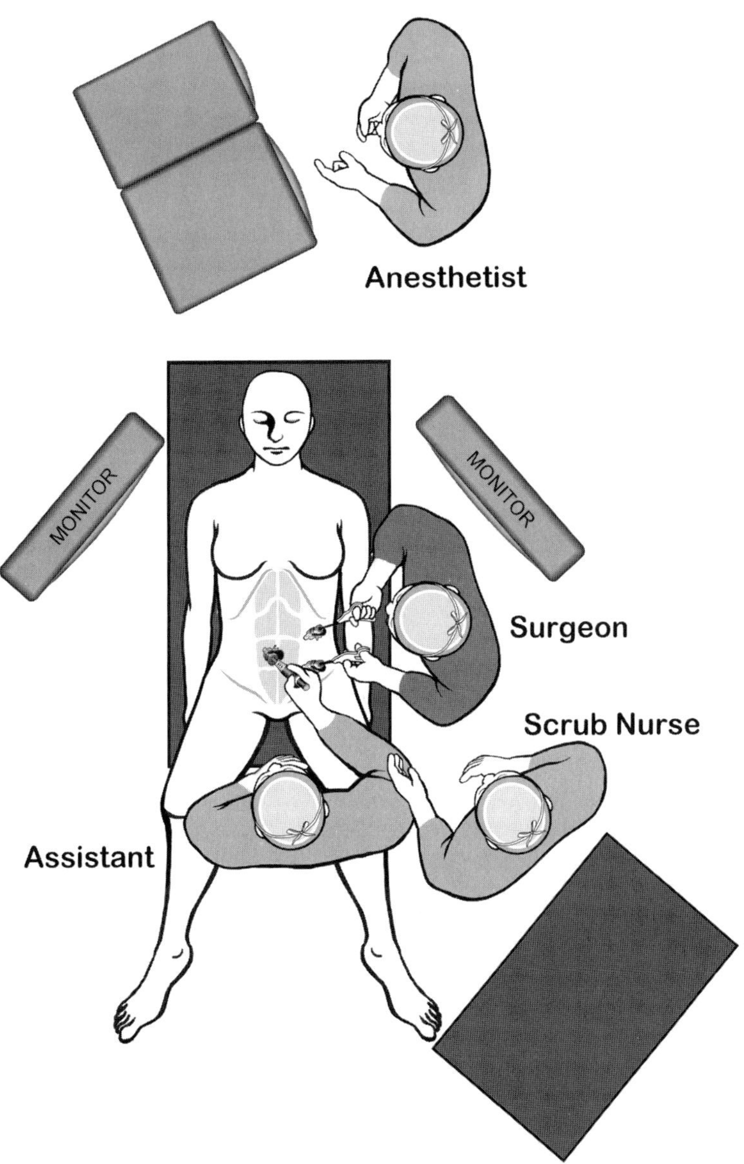

Figure 10.2.1. Positions of the surgical team and the equipment for the laparoscopic stoma formation procedure.

Table 10.2.1. Specific instruments recommended for laparoscopic stoma creation

2–4	Cannulae (1 × 12 mm, 1–3 × 5 mm)
2	Laparoscopic graspers
1	Laparoscopic needle holder

Instruments

Specific instruments recommended for laparoscopic stoma creation are listed in Table 10.2.1.

Cannula Positioning

Positioning and number of cannulae placed (Figure 10.2.2, for the ileostomy formation) largely depend on the extent of intraabdominal manipulations expected. Most patients with "virgin" abdomens, not requiring extensive adhesiolysis, can be performed using a more limited number of cannulae, whereas a thorough inspection of the entire small

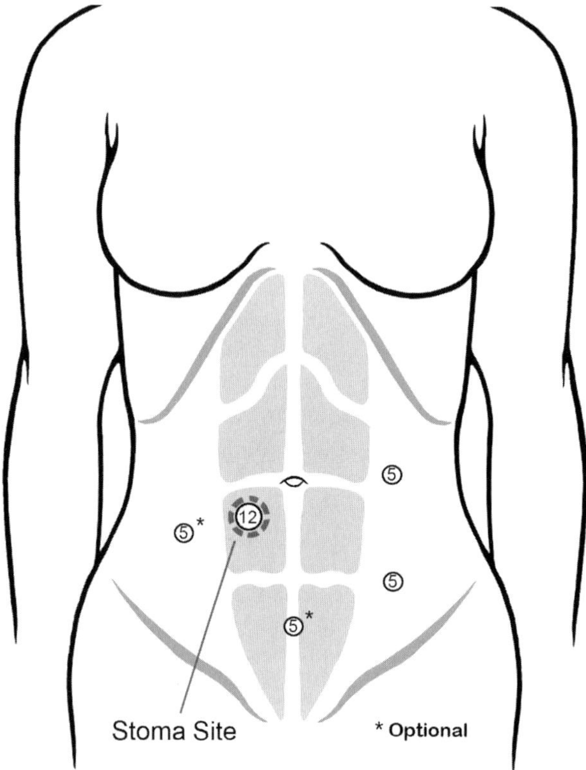

Figure 10.2.2. Positions of the cannulae for the laparoscopic ileostomy formation. Use of optional cannulae (*) should be used with a low threshold if this makes the procedure easier, especially when adhesions are present.

intestines may require at least four cannulae. Although it is tempting to minimize the number of cannulae, there should be no hesitation in inserting one or two additional 5-mm cannulae, if this will allow better exposure and easier manipulations of the tissues.

Technique

Loop Ileostomy

The peritoneal access is achieved through the preoperatively chosen ostomy site, nearly always planned inside the rectus sheath (Figure 10.2.2). For loop ileostomy formation, the right lower quadrant site is generally preferred. A 3-cm disk of skin is excised at the site. Subcutaneous tissue is divided longitudinally onto the abdominal fascia. The anterior leaf of the rectus sheath is divided longitudinally using a Bovie and the rectus muscle is spread in the direction of the muscle exposing the posterior rectus sheath. The peritoneum is entered using the open technique by dividing the posterior rectus sheath and peritoneum between the two Allis clamps. Posterior sheath is then divided to a length of 3 cm, large enough to accommodate insertion of two fingers. Three Allis clamps are then used to grasp the edges of the posterior rectus sheath equidistant from each other (Figure 10.2.3A). Three full-thickness bites of the posterior fascia are taken just underneath each Allis clamp, forming a "stay" purse-string suture (Figure 10.2.3B). The two ends of the purse-string suture are then drawn through a precut 2-inch-length 18-French red rubber catheter using a Rummel tourniquet (Figure 10.2.3C). A 12-mm cannula is inserted and the purse-string suture (Rummel tourniquet) is tightened around the cannula and secured using a hemostat clamp (Figure 10.2.4). A 12-mm cannula is best suited in terms of preventing leakage of pneumoperitoneum, and also allows any instrument to be inserted through it. It is not necessary to keep the size of this cannula small because it will be enlarged to accommodate the bowel at the end of the procedure anyway. An additional 5- to 10-mm cannula is inserted in the left lower quadrant of the abdomen lateral to the rectus sheath and above the level of pelvic brim under direct vision. An angled camera is inserted through the left lower quadrant cannula and a segment of ileum approximately 10–20 cm proximal to the ileocecal valve is gently grasped using a bowel grasper.

Identification of the terminal ileum is facilitated by retracting the small intestines in the cephalad direction out the pelvis and by gently grasping the cecum in the anterior-lateral direction. Visualization of the ligament of Treves, located on the antimesenteric border of the terminal ileum just proximal to the ileocecal valve is also helpful in identifying the anatomy. If extensive adhesiolysis is required, an additional 5-mm cannula should be placed in the left side of the abdomen approximately 4 fingerbreadths above the left lower quadrant cannula.

Once the suitable segment of the ileum is identified, it is then gently brought up to the abdominal wall and exteriorized through the ostomy site. The proximal and distal limbs of the intestine are then marked

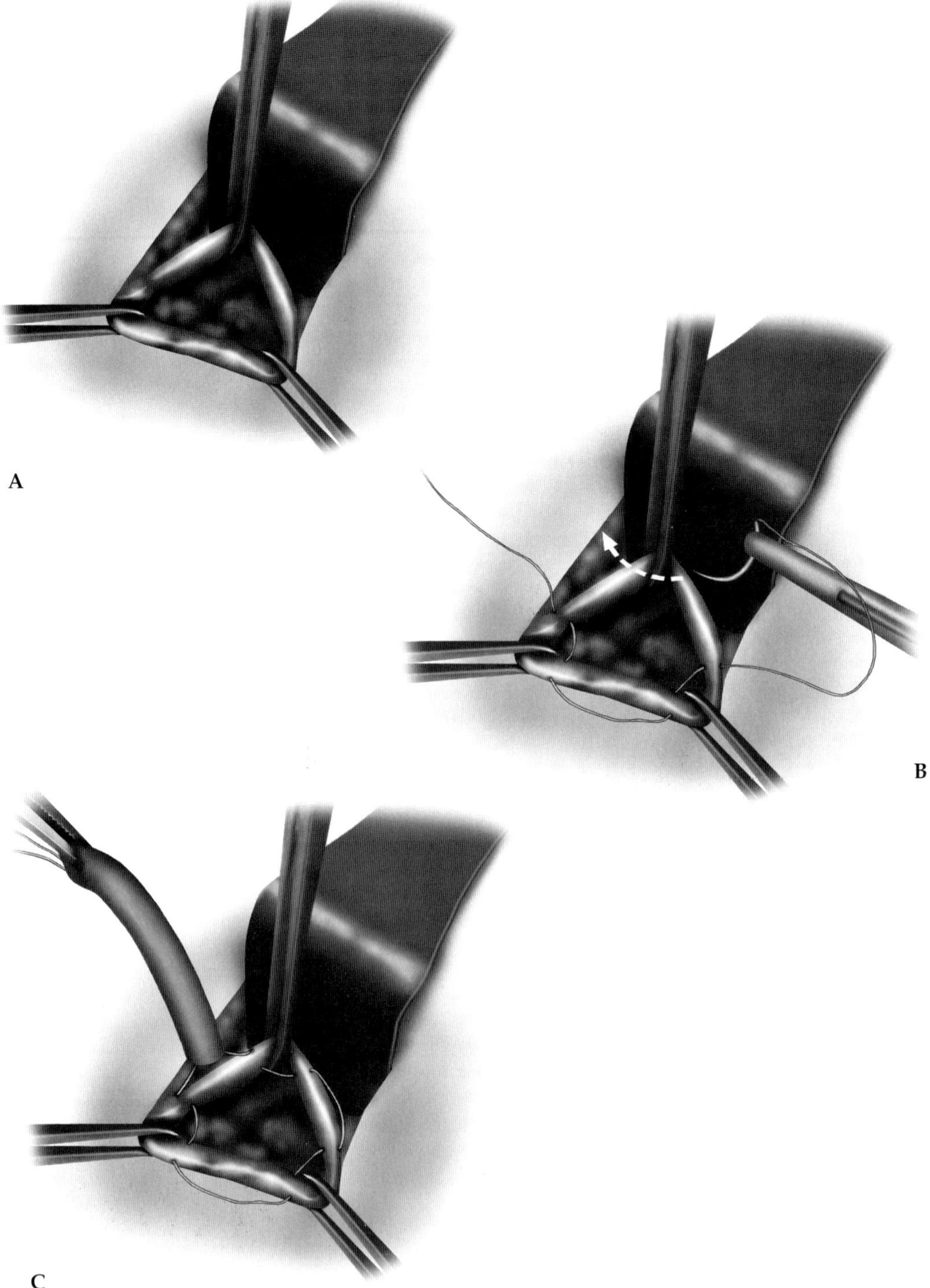

Figure 10.2.3. Insertion of the cannula at the stoma site. **A** Three Allis clamps are used to grasp the posterior sheath in performing the initial cannula insertion using an "open" technique at the stoma site. **B** Three "bites" of the posterior sheath are taken in preparation for making a "stay" suture for placement of an occluding Rummel tourniquet at the stoma site. **C** Placement of the Rummel tourniquet permits minimal leakage after cannula placement.

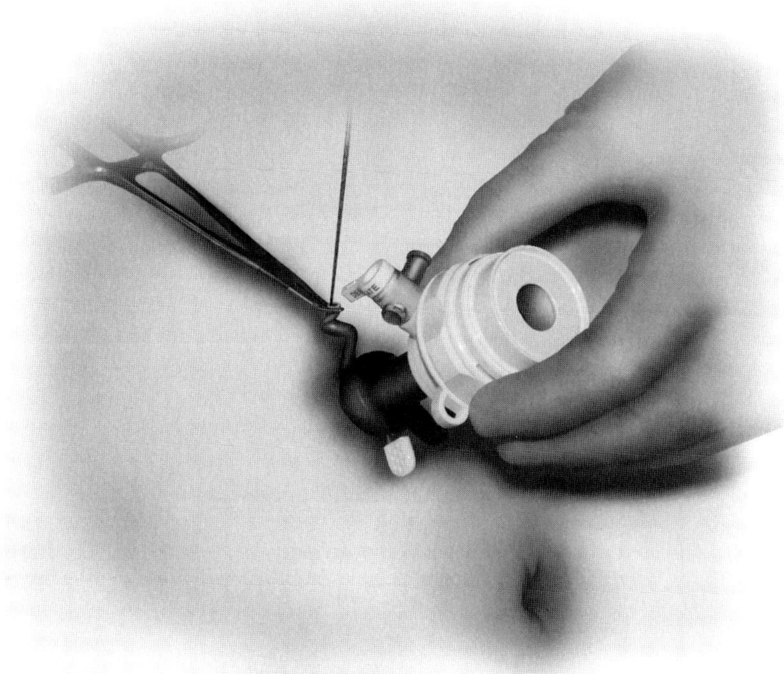

Figure 10.2.4. A 12-mm cannula is inserted and the Rummel tourniquet is tightened.

extracorporeally with different colored sutures for orientation. The marked intestinal loop is then replaced into the abdomen and a cannula is reinserted into the ostomy site and secured with the Rummel tourniquet. The proper orientation of the marking sutures is confirmed under pneumoperitoneum. Alternatively, the sutures may be placed laparoscopically (Figure 10.2.5). The left lower quadrant cannula site is closed and the stay suture at the ostomy site is removed. The ileum is exteriorized using an instrument placed through the stoma site, taking care to keep it oriented with the sutures placed properly. We use a purple or blue ("sky is up") colored suture material placed proximally, and a darker (chromic, "brown-is-down") colored one placed distally (Figure 10.2.6). Once a stoma bridge is placed under the loop, we dilate the fascia to 2 fingerbreadths, then exteriorize the loop onto the anterior abdominal wall. The ileostomy is then matured after placing sterile dressings over the other cannula sites (Figure 10.2.7).

In more complex cases such as in Crohn's disease, a thorough exploration of the small intestines, in addition to stoma formation is required. In this situation, more cannulae may be required to adequately inspect the entire length of the small intestines. The patients in this situation should be placed in the modified lithotomy position. Pneumoperitoneum is first established through the right lower quadrant ostomy site as described above. Two additional cannulae are placed in the left side

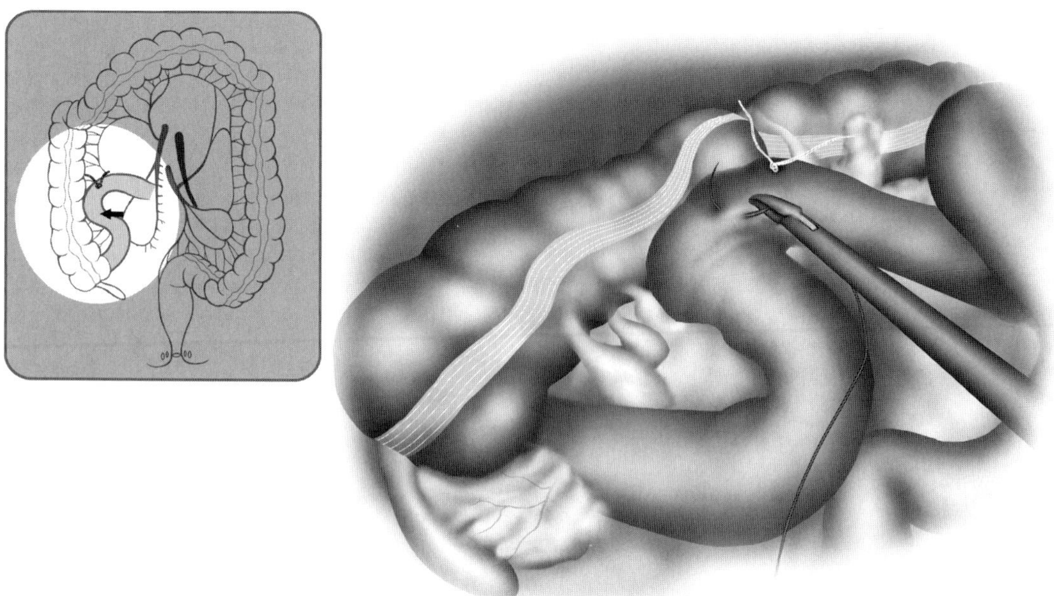

Figure 10.2.5. Marking sutures are placed in order that the bowel is properly oriented when it is drawn out through the stoma site cannula. The proximal suture is purple or blue, and the distal suture is brown (chromic, "brown is down").

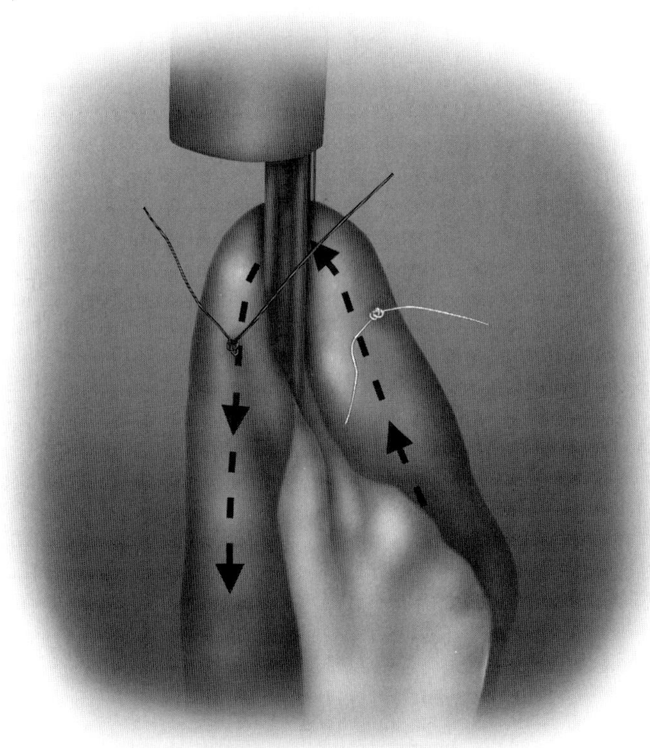

Figure 10.2.6. Careful orientation of the proximal and distal limbs of the intestine is necessary to be sure that the stoma is matured properly.

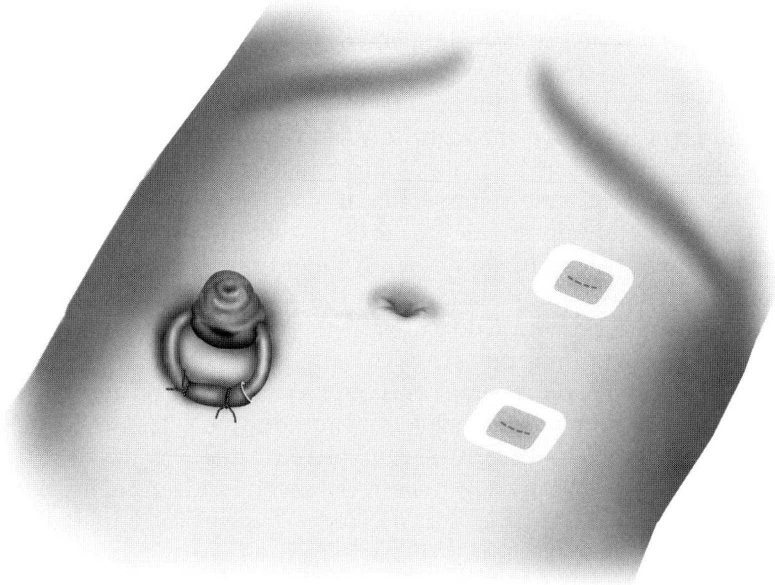

Figure 10.2.7. The stoma is matured after placing the occlusive dressings over the cannula site wounds.

of the abdomen, lateral to the rectus sheath. The inferior cannula is placed above the pelvic brim and the superior cannula is placed approximately 4 fingerbreadths above the inferior cannula. Placement of a 10-mm cannula in the left lower quadrant is useful if intracorporeal marking of the intestines is planned.

The patient is initially placed in the Trendelenburg position with the right side up to facilitate retraction of the small intestines into the left upper quadrant of the abdomen. The surgeon stands between the patient's legs and uses instruments placed through the two lower quadrant ports in order to run the bowel. For this, the patient is placed with the left side up and in a slight reverse Trendelenburg position (see Chapter 8.1). The ligament of Treitz is identified by placing the small intestinal loops over to the right upper quadrant of the abdomen. To best approach the terminal ileum, the surgeon operates through the two cannulae in the left side of the abdomen. Once the exploration of the small intestines is completed, a segment of the ileum can be exteriorized and the ostomy matured as described previously.

Sigmoid Colostomy

The technique for laparoscopic sigmoid colostomy formation is similar to that described for diverting loop ileostomy. The patient is placed in the modified lithotomy position. Two video monitors are placed at an angle near the patient's knees. A 12-mm cannula is inserted through the premarked left lower quadrant colostomy site as described earlier. After establishing pneumoperitoneum, a camera is inserted and a cannula is placed in the right lower quadrant lateral to the rectus muscle above the pelvic brim. In patients with a less mobile sigmoid colon, an additional cannula is inserted approximately 4 fingerbreadths above the right lower quadrant port. Using a pair of laparoscopic scissors, the lateral attachments of the sigmoid colon are mobilized. If the descending colon needs to be mobilized, addition of a cannula in the suprapubic area is useful. In this case, the surgeon can operate while standing between the patient's legs. The assistant facilitates the dissection by standing on the right side of the patient and retracting the sigmoid colon toward the right side of the patient. In obese patients, it may be necessary to divide the mesentery and colon in order to perform an end colostomy. Intracorporeal division of the intestines can be accomplished by introducing a laparoscopic GIA stapler through the 12-mm cannula placed usually in the right lower quadrant of the abdomen. Alternatively, a mobilized loop of the sigmoid colon can be exteriorized and divided extracorporeally using a GIA stapler. The procedure is then completed as is usual with an open procedure.

Special Considerations

The laparoscopic approach to create a stoma is a straightforward procedure that combines a good intraabdominal inspection with a minimally invasive procedure.

Although there is no large prospective randomized controlled trial comparing laparoscopic versus open stoma formation to date, many studies report the laparoscopic method to be safe and effective. Hollyoak et al.[5] compared the outcomes of 55 patients who underwent either laparoscopic (40) or open (15) stoma formations in their institution. They reported significantly shorter operative time (54 versus 72 minutes), shorter time to return of bowel function (1.6 versus 2.2 days), and shorter length of stay (7.4 versus 12.6 days) for laparoscopic stoma formation. They also reported lower morbidity and mortality associated with the laparoscopic technique. In this series, 5% of the laparoscopic patients were converted to open technique because of extensive adhesions from previous surgery. Other studies also report extensive adhesions as the most common reason for conversion.[1–4] Most studies report extremely low conversion rates for patients with no history of previous abdominal surgeries.

Conclusion

A laparoscopic technique should be considered for all patients who are undergoing stoma formation because it is usually a simple and straightforward procedure. Laparoscopic techniques appear to be safe and effective. They allow a thorough evaluation of associated intraabdominal pathology without causing extensive surgical trauma.

Editors' Comments

Indications: We generally agree with the indications, and also prefer a loop ileostomy for temporary stoma. In an emergent situation with left-sided colon obstruction, it may be practical to consider transverse colostomy. In the absence of bowel distension, laparoscopy affords the opportunity to look around the abdomen.

Patient positioning: A nasogastric tube or Foley catheter is not always necessary, especially if the indication for stoma creation is not obstruction. A simple supine position can also be used in straightforward cases.

Instrumentation: In most cases, only two cannulae are needed to create a loop ileostomy.

Cannula positioning: We always start to dissect the stoma site and decide then where to place the other cannulae needed.

Technique: It is not always necessary to excise the skin for temporary stomas. A simple incision is sufficient. Some surgeons also prefer to incise the fascia horizontally. A rod may not be needed unless there is a lot of tension on the stoma. For a transverse colostomy, the initial incision is made more cephalad in the rectus sheath. Otherwise, the procedure is similar.

References

1. Fuhrman GM, Ota DM. Laparoscopic intestinal stomas. Dis Colon Rectum 1994;37:444–449.
2. Jess P, Christiansen J. Laparoscopic loop ileostomy for fecal diversion. Dis Colon Rectum 1994;37:721–722.
3. Ludwig KA, Milsom JW, Garcia-Ruiz A, et al. Laparoscopic techniques for fecal diversion. Dis Colon Rectum 1996;39:285–288.
4. Oliveira L, Reissman P, Nogueras J, et al. Laparoscopic creation of stomas. Surg Endosc 1997;11:19–23.
5. Hollyoak MA, Lumley J, Stitz RW. Laparoscopic stoma formation for faecal diversion. Br J Surg 1998;85:226–228.

Chapter 10.3

Laparoscopic Adhesiolysis

Yoshifumi Inoue

Intraabdominal adhesions are the inevitable result of abdominal operations.[1] Postoperative adhesions are not always symptomatic, but a small percentage do become symptomatic as an acute or chronic small bowel obstruction. An adhesive small bowel obstruction is estimated to develop in 3% of all patients who have undergone laparotomy.[2] Beck et al.[3] reviewed 18,912 patients with open abdominal surgery and found 14.3% had obstruction within 2 years, with 2.6% requiring adhesiolysis. Moreover, the incidence increases significantly after major abdominal operations and reoperation causes more adhesions.[4]

The goal of surgical treatment of acute small bowel obstruction should focus on avoiding operative delay and reducing the morbidity associated with bowel strangulation.[5] In the early era of laparoscopy, prior abdominal surgery was a relative contraindication to treat acute small bowel obstruction. According to this concept, laparotomy has been used in the treatment of small bowel obstruction caused by postoperative adhesions. But today, with the development of improved laparoscopic operative techniques and devices, laparoscopic lysis of adhesions for acute and chronic small bowel obstruction does have a role in some instances.[6,7]

Because laparoscopic approaches have some advantages with less pain, early recovery of bowel movement, less problems about abdominal wall cicatrization, a shorter hospital stay and incapacitation of patient activity, and an improved aesthetic effect,[8] there remains some hope that some of these benefits would be realized in laparoscopic adhesiolysis. Especially important is the theoretical advantage that the development of fewer postoperative adhesions compared with open laparotomy and fewer wound complications would result in a lower risk of subsequent obstructions.[9]

Indications

The indications for laparoscopic adhesiolysis for small bowel obstruction are identical to those for open surgery. Patients should be excluded from the indications of laparoscopic adhesiolysis when there are signs of bowel perforation or necrosis. Indications for lysis of adhesions must be individualized to the patient, and immediate operation and resection by laparotomy are indicated in cases of acute abdomen secondary to intestinal obstruction or perforation.

In patients with a radiologic diagnosis of small bowel obstruction, diagnosis should be achieved through a combination of clinical and radiologic parameters. Plain X-ray films, ultrasound images, or computed tomography scans may show small bowel dilatation, wall thickening, and abnormal distribution of intraluminal gas and air-fluid levels. In many of these cases, a point of partial or complete obstruction will be detected by contrast imaging through a nasal long intestinal tube.

Initially, many of the patients may be carefully observed during a period of conservative treatment that consists of measures such as fasting, placement of long intestinal tubes, and the administration of peripheral or central intravenous fluids, electrolytes, and nutrition. Observation includes serial abdominal radiographs, physical examination, volume and characteristics of drainage fluids, and appropriate laboratory tests. Patients in whom the bowel obstruction resolves within 1 week and who fulfilled the following criteria are considered candidates for laparoscopic adhesiolysis: 1) At least two prior episodes of small bowel obstruction, 2) confirmed improvement in physical signs of peritoneal inflammation, and 3) disappearance of air-fluid levels on plain abdominal X-ray films. The patients with elevated white blood count, temperature elevation, massively dilated bowel, and exquisite abdominal tenderness could be considered for laparoscopic exploration, but then should be converted rapidly to an open procedure if necrotic bowel is suspected or severe extensive adhesions or distension are present.

Finally, in laparotomy, to determine the site of obstruction, a large incision is usually required, and there may be significant manipulations of the bowel. However, in the case of a band-like adhesion, the obstruction is usually relieved speedily laparoscopically with relative ease.[10] These types of patients are best suited for laparoscopic lysis of adhesion for small bowel obstruction.

Patient Positioning and Operating Room Setup

The patient is placed in the supine position with abducted arms and supports mounted to the sites of the table which allow safe tilting and lateral rotation of the operating table. A nasogastric tube and urinary catheter are placed. If a long intestinal tube is placed in the preoperative period, we do not place a nasogastric tube. Preoperative antibiotics are administered with gram-negative and anaerobic coverage to prevent surgical site infection. Two video monitors are used: Principally, the video monitor to the patient's right is positioned inferiorly at the level of hip and the monitor to the left positioned superiorly at the level of the shoulder. This positioning forms a plane parallel to the root of the superior mesenteric artery and allows the operating surgeon to look and work in the same direction as the camera orientation. But the configuration of the operating room arrangement should be flexible to permit modifications during the operation. For instance, for right-sided adhesions, the surgeon should operate from the left, with the monitor placed on the patient's right (Figure 10.3.1A). The inverse positions should be arranged for left-sided adhesions (Figure 10.3.1B). The surgeon can stand at the patient's right for midline adhesions or those on both sides.

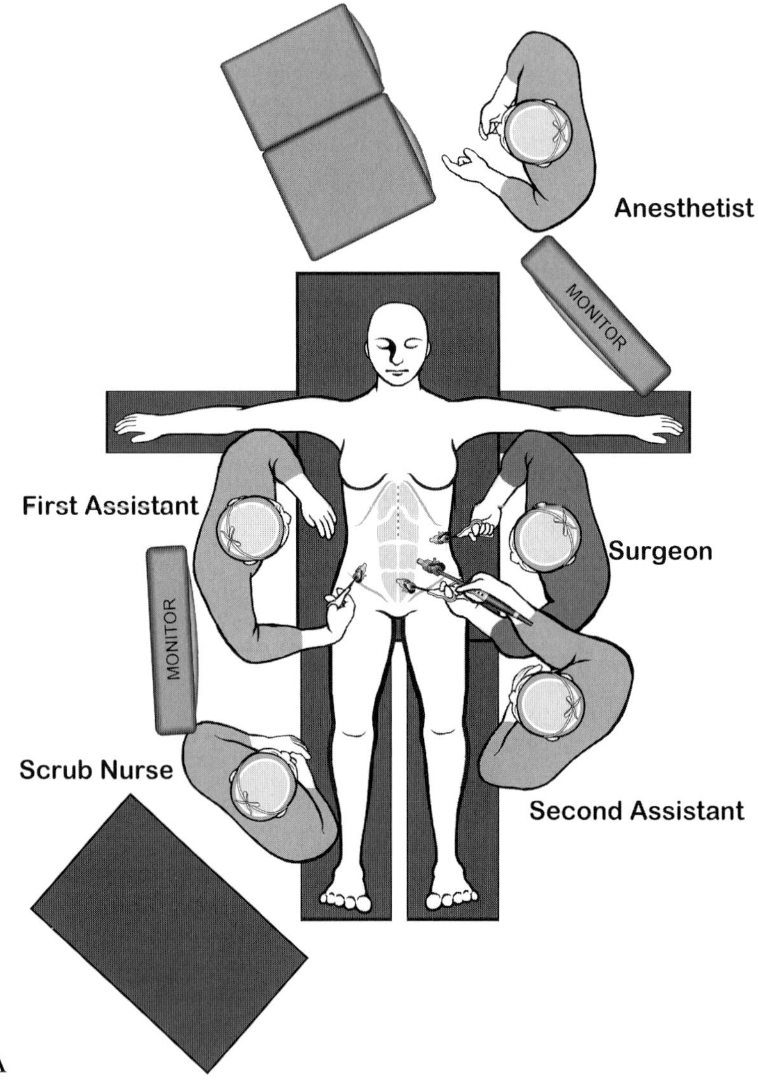

Figure 10.3.1. Positions of the surgical team and equipment for laparoscopic adhesiolysis. **A** Setup for the situation in which adhesions are primarily on the right side. **B** Setup for the situation in which adhesions are primarily of the left side.

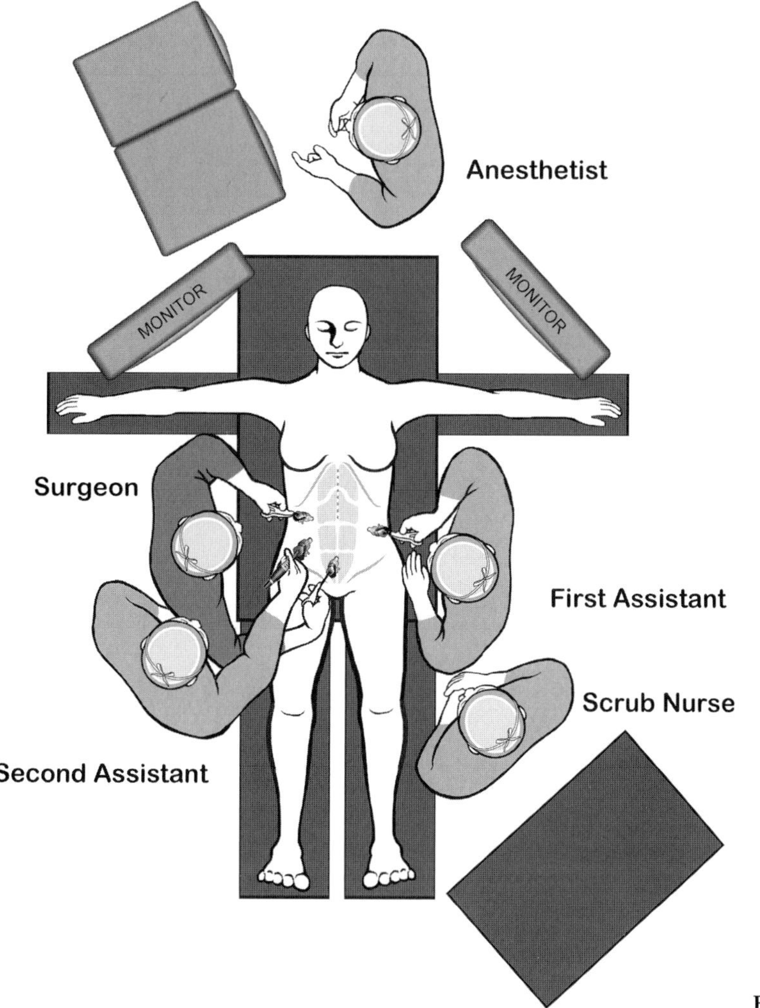

Figure 10.3.1. *Continued*

Patients should be prepared and draped in a way that allows rapid conversion to an open procedure when necessary.

Instruments

Specific instruments recommended for laparoscopic adhesiolysis are listed in Table 10.3.1.

Table 10.3.1. Specific instruments recommended for laparoscopic adhesiolysis

3–5	Cannulae (1 × 10 mm, 2–4 × 5 mm)
1	Dissecting device (i.e., LigaSure V™ or Ultrasonic Shears™ or electrosurgery)
1	Laparoscopic dissector
2	Laparoscopic graspers

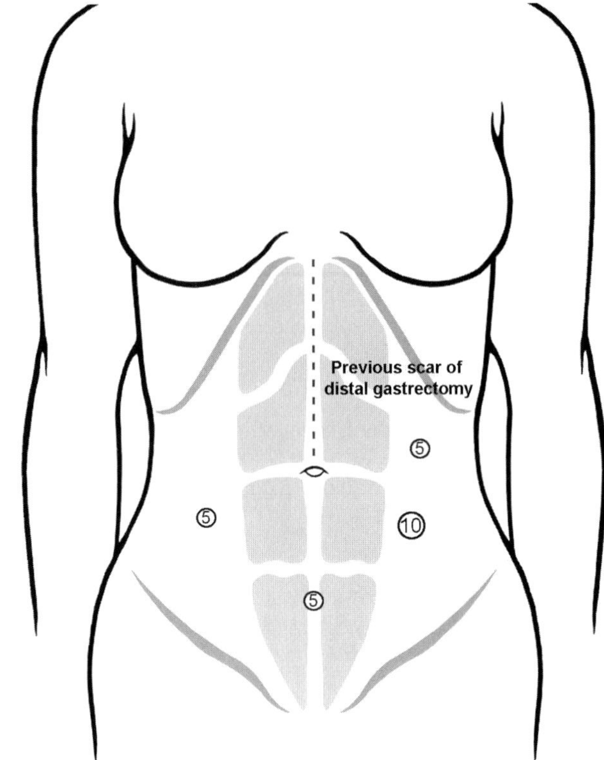

Figure 10.3.2. Positions of the cannulae for laparoscopic adhesiolysis when adhesions are primarily on the left side. The 10-mm cannula is for insertion of the laparoscope.

Cannula Positioning

Because virtually all patients have undergone previous surgery, special care must be taken in establishing the pneumoperitoneum and inserting the initial trocar. According to the size and position of scars and the kind of previous operations, the first trocar site is placed at a site away from the previous incisions. This is frequently in a virgin part of the abdomen 5–10 cm away from any previous scars. When there is a scar in the infraumbilical part, the first port of entry will be in the epigastrium or the right or left upper abdominal quadrants. When there is a scar in the upper median abdomen, the first port will be inserted in the right or left lower abdominal quadrants (Figure 10.3.2).

We now routinely use the open method of entering the abdominal cavity by performing a cut-down procedure for trocar insertion. Using an open technique for trocar insertion safely allows entry into the peritoneum even in the face of mechanical bowel obstruction with dilated loops of bowel.

Technique

A minimum of three cannulae are used: 10 mm for the camera and two additional (usually 5-mm) cannulae to obtain good triangulation between the instruments. After inserting the initial 10-mm cannula, the peritoneal cavity is insufflated with CO_2 to the level of 8–10 mm Hg of pressure. After the camera is introduced through this cannula, two 5-mm cannulae for manipulation will be inserted into the peritoneal cavity under direct visualization. When there is not enough space to insert another 5-mm cannula, lysis of adhesions to abdominal wall is performed before the additional 5-mm cannula is inserted.

The actual dissection is usually started by adhesiolysis between small intestine or omentum to the parietal abdominal wall (Figure 10.3.3). A proper pressure of pneumoperitoneum, such as 12–14 mm Hg, helps to put the point or line for lysis under tension. The use of scissors without electrosurgery during this procedure has been proven to be advantageous in the dissection of the mostly nonvascularized fields of adhesions. Using a monopolar or bipolar electrode often causes the contraction of adhesional strands, leading to the risk of injuring adherent loops of bowel. Meticulous attention should be given so as not to injure the serosa of bowel. If the distance between bowels and abdominal wall is enough to apply a harmonic scalpel, this instrument is extremely useful because the temperature at the lateral side of the blade is not so high as to cause thermal injury to the intestinal wall (Figure 10.3.4).

After all adhesions to parietal abdominal wall are lysed, the small intestine is followed in a retrograde manner with atraumatic bowel graspers, beginning at the terminal ileum when possible. Care is taken to avoid bowel injury by grabbing the mesentery and avoiding direct handling of

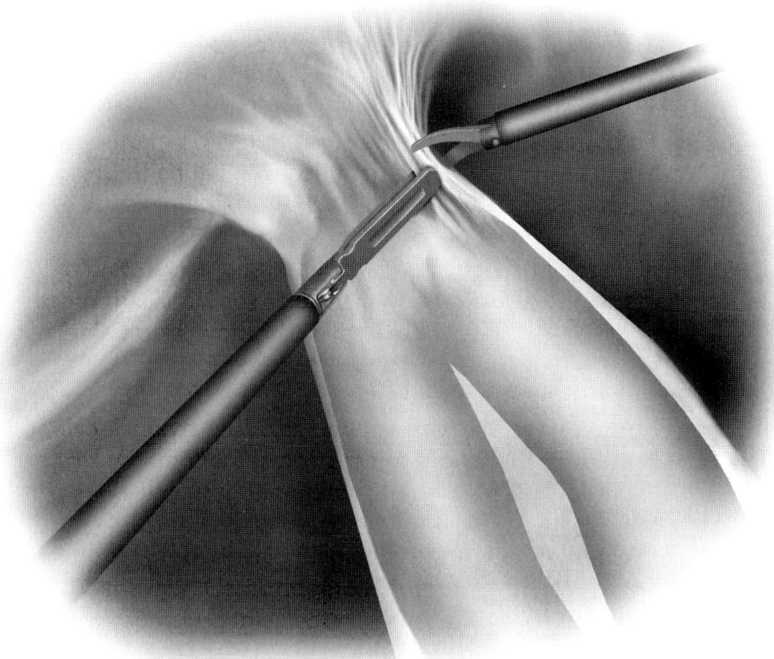

Figure 10.3.3. Dissection is usually initiated by lysing adhesions between small bowel loops and the anterior abdominal wall.

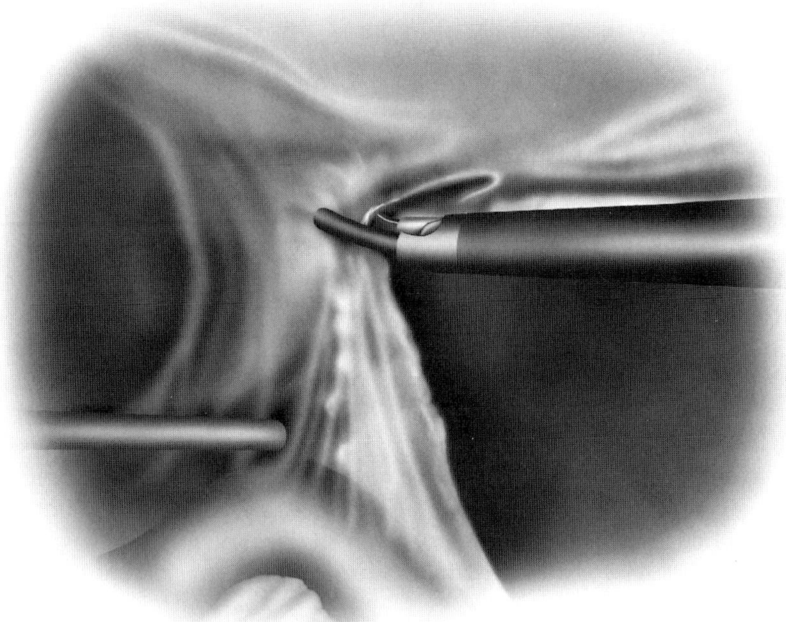

Figure 10.3.4. If the length of adhesion between the abdominal wall and intestine is greater than 4–5 mm, use of an ultrasonic dissecting device may be considered.

the dilated intestinal serosa. Placing the patient in the steep Trendelenburg position and tilting the patient with the left side down permits the surgeon to visualize the cecum properly and enhances running of the small bowel. This process should continue until a transition point between dilated and decompressed intestine is found and the responsible adhesion is identified. The point of transition is usually identified between a proximal dilated loop of small intestine and a distal decompressed loop. Gentle manipulation of the bowel loops using the graspers should be performed to identify the obstructing adhesive band.

If the cause of obstruction of small intestine is an adhesive band, it is usually easy to resolve. A grasping instrument is then passed beneath this band, thus isolating it over the mesentery. Again, it is worth emphasizing that using a monopolar or bipolar electrode often causes the contraction of adhesional strands, leading to risk of injuring adherent loops of bowel. Vascularized strands with a sufficient length are dissected after prior ligation using clips, or ligatures administered either by the intra- or extracorporeal knotting technique. It is possible that large hemoclips can be used to clip the band on both sides of the grasper. A hooked electrosurgery tip is then used to divide the band.

When a point of obstruction is not clearly identified, lysis continues until all suspicious adhesions or bands responsible for the symptoms are dissected as with the approach for small bowel obstruction by laparotomy. We also evaluate the entire small intestine even if a convincing obstruction at one point is found.

After small bowel obstruction is resolved by manipulation, the entire bowel is then examined again for signs of intestinal injury during the exploration. If dense adhesions are encountered, laparotomy should be performed. But we try to make the incision as short as possible. Additionally, if nonviable intestine is encountered, the abdomen should be opened through an incision that is long enough to safely manage the problem. Assuming that laparoscopic adhesiolysis to resolve the small bowel obstruction is successful, the abdominal cavity should be irrigated with saline solution, and the omentum placed between the intestine and ventral wall of the abdomen as much as possible.

After final thorough control with complete hemostasis, the inserted ports are retracted under visual control with the camera. In case of extensive adhesiolysis, we position a silicone drain in that area to allow for an early detection of postoperative bleeding and perforation of intestine.

Special Considerations

Conversion to laparotomy should not be considered a complication of the laparoscopic approach and in fact laparoscopic adhesiolysis has one of the highest risks of conversion to an open method.

The main reasons for conversion to laparotomy include dense adhesions, nonviable intestine, suspected tumor, or iatrogenic perforation during laparoscopy. The presence of dense adhesions is the most common cause of conversion to laparotomy.[11–13]

Laparoscopic adhesiolysis with scissors may be inconvenient because of bleeding. Electrodissection causes tissue damage and delayed intestinal perforations because of its excessive heat production. Bipolar scissors has the advantage of reducing the electrosurgical complications but still has potential for delayed thermal injury. The ultrasonically activated scalpel causes less heat production compared with electrosurgery, thereby theoretically lowering the risk of delayed perforations.

Because of dilated and fragile thin-walled bowel, the risk of traumatic iatrogenic enterotomies is increased during bowel manipulation. In addition, when exploring the bowel between two manipulating bowel graspers, both instruments should remain in view at all times. When one clamp leaves the visual field, it is difficult to appreciate the amount of traction being applied. Also, if an enterotomy should occur, it may not be appreciated. At the time of dissection, countertraction is necessary.[14] The left hand of the surgeon can be applied over the workplace on the abdominal wall, avoiding the need of accomplishing excessive traction of the bowel with the grasper, which could result in danger of intestinal laceration. What is of great concern is the proper handling of the dilated, and often fragile, loops of intestine. We believe that the use of nontraumatic bowel clamps minimizes this complication, and they are strongly recommended, as smaller sharp dissectors and graspers could result in injury and tearing of the bowel.

The most important early postoperative complication is delayed intestinal perforation resulting in panperitonitis. Electrodissection may cause tissue damage and this is sometimes manifested as intestinal perforations after one to three postoperative days. If there is not a drain placed, discovery of panperitonitis could be delayed. Therefore, if adhesiolysis is performed extensively, we recommend routine placement of a silicone drain.

The most important late postoperative complication is recurrent small bowel obstruction. The cause of the recurrent episodes of obstruction could be attributed to incomplete adhesiolysis at the previous operation. The adhesions should be completely lysed, but we sometimes hesitate to explore entire intestine when there are multiple adhesions and when the main portion of obstruction is resolved.

Finally, newly developed adhesions originating from adhesiolysis operation may cause recurrent bowel obstruction. Although it has been reported by several investigators that laparoscopic surgery leads to fewer adhesions compared with laparotomy,[15,16] there still may be a possibility of recurrent bowel obstruction.

Conclusion

Laparoscopic adhesiolysis is a relatively new procedure, and it must be scrutinized to determine which patients are best suited to undergo a trial of laparoscopic adhesiolysis. Emergency situations in acute small bowel obstruction combine several circumstances unfavorable for laparoscopy: A limited work area and a distended and fragile small bowel.[17] Laparoscopic adhesiolysis in the nonemergency situation may produce better results. Laparoscopic adhesiolysis seems to be appropriate in patients without signs of bowel perforation or other factors outlined earlier that may predispose patients to either an intraoperative complication or unsuccessful laparoscopic adhesiolysis.

Laparoscopic treatment of small bowel obstruction is effective when done properly, leads to a speedy convalescence and shorter hospital stay, and has good long-term results.[18] The potential advantages of laparoscopic surgery are clear and may include less intraabdominal adhesion formation and fewer wound complications, as well as less postoperative pain. This makes laparoscopic adhesiolysis for small bowel obstruction an attractive procedure. But rapid conversion to laparotomy should always be considered in patients with dense adhesions in order to accomplish the operation for small bowel obstruction safely.

Editors' Comments

Indications: We all agree that the concept of considering laparoscopic methods for intestinal obstruction is increasing. However, there are obvious patients with a prior history of extensive surgeries, peritonitis, or known dense adhesions for which a laparoscopic approach should never be considered.

Patient positioning: We always use the modified lithotomy position, so there is the possibility that the surgeon or assistant may stand between the legs or have access to pelvic structures (rectum or vagina) as needed during the operation. The use of gravity should also be considered, i.e., tilting of the patient in various positions so that bowel loops can be displaced to the surgeon's advantage.

Instrumentation: Our instrumentation does not differ markedly, but we try to have a 5-mm laparoscope available, because this allows the surgeon to place this scope into any cannula during the operation in case of extensive adhesions. We use microscissors, with avoidance of electrosurgery whenever possible, to prevent the inadvertent thermal injury to bowel. Safe and atraumatic bowel graspers are also key tools, and there are now such graspers with short jaws, which permit working in close spaces as may be found in the abdominal cavity of patients with adhesions. We do not use a long intestinal tube in the preoperative treatment of small bowel obstruction.

Cannula positioning: We try to use the upper quadrants for the initial cannula site, because just below the ribs is often the least adhesion-prone area in the abdominal cavity. This is a judgment call that the surgeon must make at the time of the operation. Once the initial cannula is placed, we often will sound out the abdominal wall for the other cannulae by first piercing the additional cannula sites with a long 21-gauge needle, which then confirms that the proposed site is clear of adhesions. Once the camera is placed and two additional cannulae are in place (all three lined up for dissection in the region of interest), then the surgeon really has a chance to work with great precision.

Technique: We perform a procedure very much as Dr. Inoue describes. We avoid electrosurgery on the bowel loops, and accept some bleeding from the filmy adhesions. This is not likely to be of any consequence. We also would use the LigaSure V™ (ValleyLab, Boulder, CO) to dissect off omentum from the abdominal wall. Although a harmonic scalpel may be helpful, we prefer the 5-mm LigaSure V™, and also believe that the lateral thermal spread is minimal. In instances where there is not a major blood vessel in the tissue being divided, we only use LigaSure™'s electrical energy for 1–2 seconds. This usually is effective for minor bleeding points.

Regarding antiadhesion agents, one of us has used Seprafilm sheets (Genzyme, Cambridge, MA), ground up into a powder in the operation room, and injected this through a cannula at the conclusion of the operation around the sites of greatest adhesions. However, whether this may prevent further adhesions is not proven. We do not place any drain at the conclusion of the operation.

Finally, the entire adhesiolysis may not be possible using the laparoscopic approach, but it may permit a directed approach which may save the need for a huge incision. For example, the laparoscopy may demonstrate that the adhesion or obstruction is in the pelvis, thereby permitting either a limited lower midline or a Pfannenstiel incision.

Laparoscopic methods will not replace laparotomy in the treatment of adhesive small bowel obstruction, but there are patients in whom a laparoscopic method should be considered. Our final advice is that the surgeon should be prepared to "convert" early in the assessment of this technique, with safety and effectiveness far out weighing whether laparoscopy was successful.

References

1. Weibel MA, Majno G. Peritoneal adhesions and their relation to abdominal surgery. A postmortem study. Am J Surg 1973;126:345–353.
2. Francois Y, Mouret P, Tomaoglu K, et al. Postoperative adhesive peritoneal disease. Laparoscopic treatment. Surg Endosc 1994;8:781–783.
3. Beck DE, Opelka FG, Bailey HR, et al. Incidence of small-bowel obstruction and adhesiolysis after open colorectal and general surgery. Dis Colon Rectum 1999;42:241–248.
4. Becker JM, Dayton MT, Fazio VW, et al. Prevention of postoperative abdominal adhesions by a sodium hyaluronate-based bioresorbable membrane: a prospective, randomized, double-blind multicenter study. J Am Coll Surg 1996;183:297–306.
5. Mucha P Jr. Small intestinal obstruction. Surg Clin North Am 1987; 67:597–620.
6. Freys SM, Fuchs KH, Heimbucher J, et al. Laparoscopic adhesiolysis. Surg Endosc 1994;8:1202–1207.
7. Franklin ME, Dorman JP, Pharand D. Laparoscopic surgery in acute small bowel obstruction. Surg Laparosc Endosc 1994;4:289–296.
8. Vierra M. Minimally invasive surgery. Annu Rev Med 1995;46:147–158.
9. Kavic SM, Kavic SM. Adhesions and adhesiolysis: the role of laparoscopy. JSLS 2002;6:99–109.
10. Bastug DF, Trammell SW, Boland JP, et al. Laparoscopic adhesiolysis for small bowel obstruction. Surg Laparosc Endosc 1991;1:259–262.
11. Ibrahim IM, Wolodiger F, Sussman B, et al. Laparoscopic management of acute small-bowel obstruction. Surg Endosc 1996;10:1012–1014.
12. Strickland P, Lourie DJ, Suddleson EA, et al. Is laparoscopy safe and effective for treatment of acute small-bowel obstruction? Surg Endosc 1999; 13:695–698.
13. Navez B, Arimont JM, Guiot P. Laparoscopic approach in acute small bowel obstruction. A review of 68 patients. Hepatogastroenterology 1998; 45:2146–2150.
14. Carbajo Caballero MA, Martin del Olmo JC, Blanco JI, et al. Therapeutic value of laparoscopic adhesiolysis. Surg Endosc 2001;15:102–103.
15. Moore RG, Partin AW, Adams JB, et al. Adhesion formation after transperitoneal nephrectomy: laparoscopic v open approach. J Endourol 1995;9:277–280.
16. Bulletti C, Polli V, Negrini V, et al. Adhesion formation after laparoscopic myomectomy. J Am Assoc Gynecol Laparosc 1996;3:533–536.
17. Chosidow D, Johanet H, Montariol T, et al. Laparoscopy for acute small-bowel obstruction secondary to adhesions. J Laparoendosc Adv Surg Tech A 2000;10:155–159.
18. Sato Y, Ido K, Kumagai M, et al. Laparoscopic adhesiolysis for recurrent small bowel obstruction: long-term follow-up. Gastrointest Endosc 2001;54:476–479.

Chapter 10.4

Rectopexy with and Without Sigmoid Resection

Alessandro Fichera and Martin R. Weiser

Indications

Management of rectal prolapse has evolved over many centuries, but it is still generating interest and controversies involving its etiology, functional aspects, and surgical management.[1–4] A surgical approach should be carefully chosen after a thorough functional evaluation and should not be based on the surgeon's familiarity and preference for a particular technique but rather on the fitness of the patient and the functional disorders so often associated with rectal prolapse, among them incontinence or constipation.[5,6] The use of laparoscopic methods does not broaden or modify the indications.

We prefer a laparoscopic rectopexy with sigmoid resection in the young and fit patient with a significant history of constipation. A simple laparoscopic suture rectopexy is reserved for patients predominantly incontinent but without significant constipation.

Laparoscopy has shown to have several attractive features in the surgical treatment of rectal prolapse. Laparoscopic mobilization of the rectum is feasible and safe. Magnified visualization is afforded by new-generation videoscopes that facilitate precise dissection, preservation of the autonomic nerves, and avoidance of severe presacral bleeding. Even with the availability of advanced laparoscopic techniques, selection of the appropriate operation continues to be problematic for surgeons.

Perineal procedures, although less invasive, have a relatively high recurrence rate with overall acceptable short-term results and they should be offered exclusively to the high-risk elderly patients. For the younger and healthier patient population, an abdominal approach is preferred because of a lower recurrence rate. In this group, a complete evaluation of the associated symptoms is mandatory to achieve the best long-term functional results. For patients with significant constipation, a sigmoid resection should be considered in combination with rectopexy in order to provide significant improvement of their symptoms. However, in patients with severe incontinence, a suture rectopexy alone is sufficient and a resection may worsen their continence issues.[5,6]

Patient Positioning and Operating Room Setup

After an epidural catheter is activated and general anesthesia attained, a Foley catheter and a nasogastric tube are inserted. Venous compression devices in the lower extremities are routinely used. The patient is placed in modified low lithotomy position, which allows an assistant to stand between the patient's legs for transanal insertion of a stapling

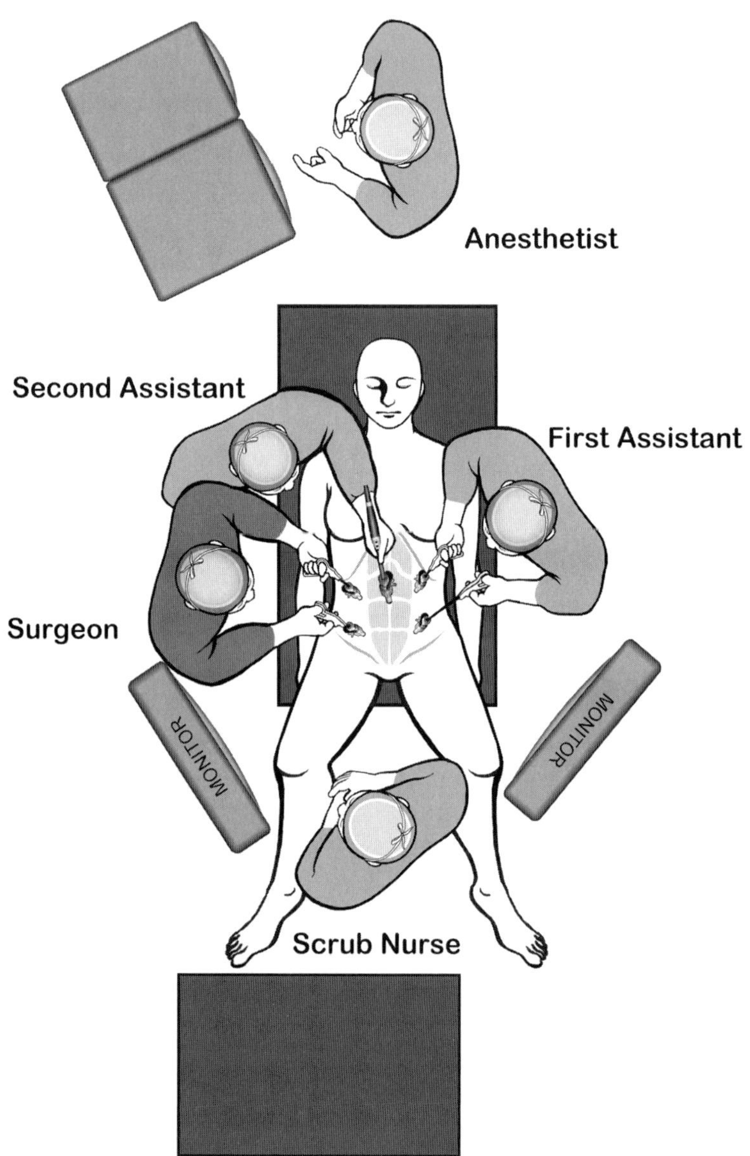

Figure 10.4.1. Positions of the equipment and the surgical team for laparoscopic rectopexy.

device when a sigmoid resection is performed. Early epidural activation is advantageous because it affords sympathetic blockade, which preserves intestinal peristalsis, prevents distension, and facilitates small bowel retraction and pelvic visualization. When a rectal resection and anastomosis is planned, the rectum and colon are irrigated with at least 1000 cc of warm saline or water until clear before draping the patient. Some surgeons also use diluted Betadine irrigation to theoretically prevent local septic complications if microscopic spillage occurs during the construction of the anastomosis.

After adequate venous access has been established, both upper extremities are secured at the patient's side, the abdomen is prepped and draped in the usual sterile manner, and the patient is then placed in slight Trendelenburg position. At least two monitors are necessary for laparoscopic rectal dissection, resection, and/or anastomosis and they should be placed at the foot of the table, so that both the surgeon and the assistants can maintain online visualization. Also, suction and electrosurgical devices are placed at the foot of the table (Figure 10.4.1).

Instruments

Specific instruments recommended for laparoscopic rectopexy with resection are listed in Table 10.4.1.

Cannula Positioning

A 5- or 10-mm cannula is initially inserted using the open technique just below the umbilicus. Additional 5-mm cannulae are inserted just lateral to the rectus abdominis muscles in the left upper and right upper quadrants. A 12-mm cannula is placed in the right lower quadrant just lateral to the rectus abdominis muscles over McBurney's line for the endoscopic stapler to be used for bowel resection. A 5- or 10-mm cannula is placed in the left lower quadrant depending on instrumentation. The left lower cannula or umbilical site can be used for specimen extraction by enlarging it to 3–4 cm (Figure 10.4.2).

Table 10.4.1. Specific instruments recommended for laparoscopic rectopexy with resection

5	Cannulae (1 × 12 mm, 1 × 10 mm, 3 × 5 mm)
1	Dissecting device (i.e., Ligasure V™ or Ultrasonic Shears™ or electrosurgery)
1	Laparoscopic scissors
1	Laparoscopic dissector
2	Laparoscopic graspers
1	Laparoscopic needle holder
1	Laparoscopic knot pusher
1	Endoscopic paddle
1	Endoscopic stapler

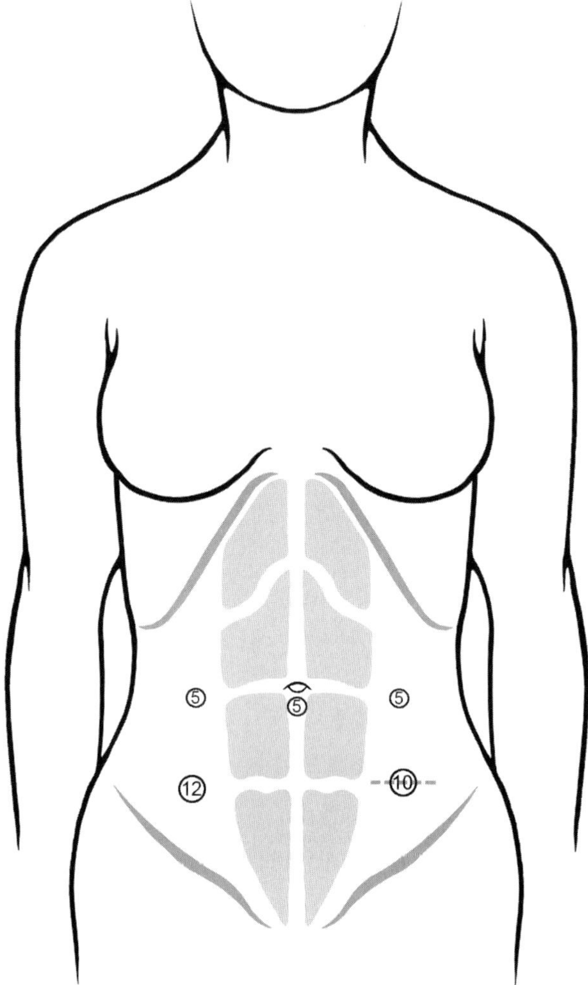

Figure 10.4.2. Positions of the cannulae for laparoscopic rectopexy.

Technique

When the pneumoperitoneum is established at 15 mm Hg and ports are placed, full evaluation of the abdominal cavity is performed, as the majority of these patients are elderly. The patient is placed in Trendelenburg position with the left side tilted up. The small bowel is gently retracted out of the operating field using atraumatic bowel graspers. The combination of sympathetic blockade afforded by the epidural administration of local anesthetics, gravity from the Trendelenburg position, and gentle manipulation of the small bowel allows visualization of the sigmoid mesentery and pelvis. The rectum, sigmoid, and descending colon are evaluated. Typically, there is a significant redundancy of the rectosigmoid with a very low peritoneal cul-de-sac.

Rectopexy Without Sigmoid Resection

Using a bowel grasper, the rectum and colon are gently retracted up and out of the pelvis to allow for visualization of the sacral promontory and the vascular anatomy of the rectosigmoid area. Dissecting from the right side, the peritoneum over the sacral promontory is incised (Figure 10.4.3) and the superior hemorrhoidal pedicle is identified and retracted superiorly. The left ureter must be clearly visualized through the submesenteric window to avoid injuring it (Figure 10.4.4). When these two important structures are clearly visualized, the peritoneal incision is extended, first cephalad to the aortic bifurcation and the hypogastric nerves are swept dorsally away from the superior hemorrhoidal artery and vein, then caudally in the pelvis for several centimeters. The assistant at this time with the atraumatic bowel grasper is grasping the cut edge of the peritoneum and retracting the rectum anteriorly and to the left to allow safe mobilization of the rectum in the presacral space. This plane is avascular allowing for a bloodless dissection down to Waldeyer's fascia at the third sacral vertebra. This fascia is sharply incised and the dissection is continued distally down to the pelvic floor (Figure 10.4.5).

Next, the left lateral sigmoid attachments are incised and the rectum and sigmoid colon are retracted by the assistant to the patient's right side. The peritoneum to the left of the rectum is incised to allow complete mobilization of the rectosigmoid (Figure 10.4.6). The dissection is extended posteriorly to join the plane previously dissected on the right

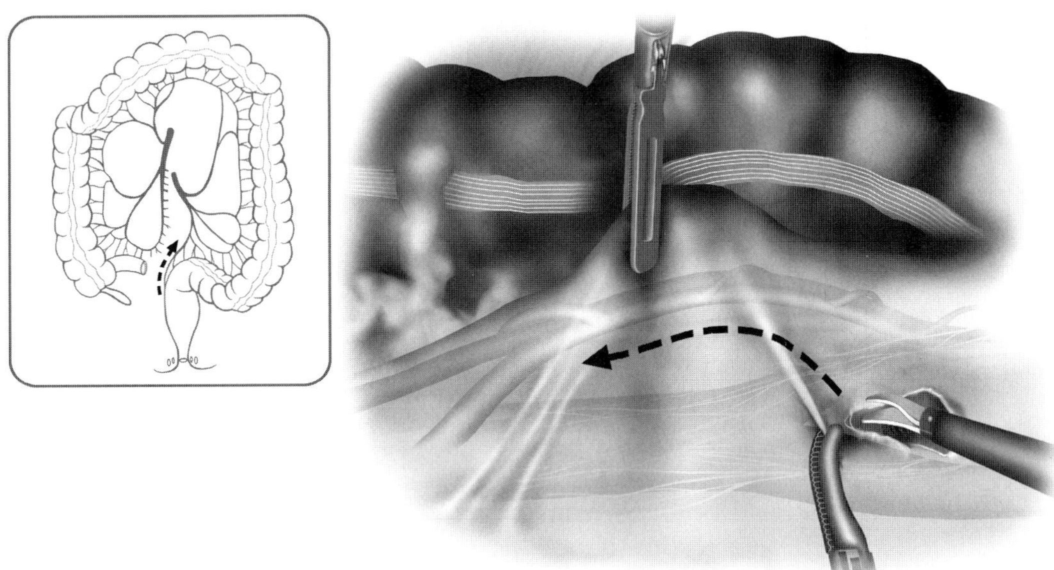

Figure 10.4.3. From the patient's right side, the peritoneum over the sacral promontory is incised.

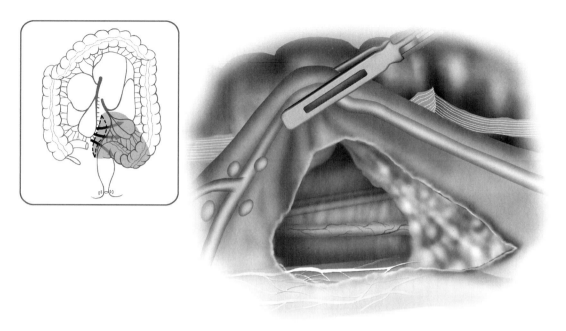

Figure 10.4.4. The left ureter is clearly visualized through the submesenteric window.

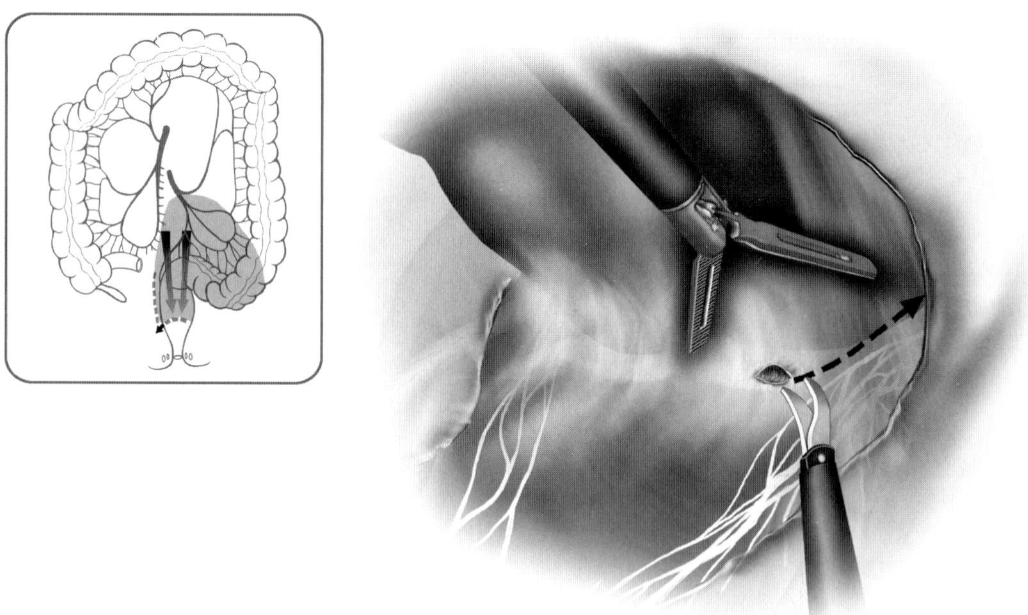

Figure 10.4.5. After division of Waldeyer's fascia, the dissection is continued to the pelvic floor posteriorly.

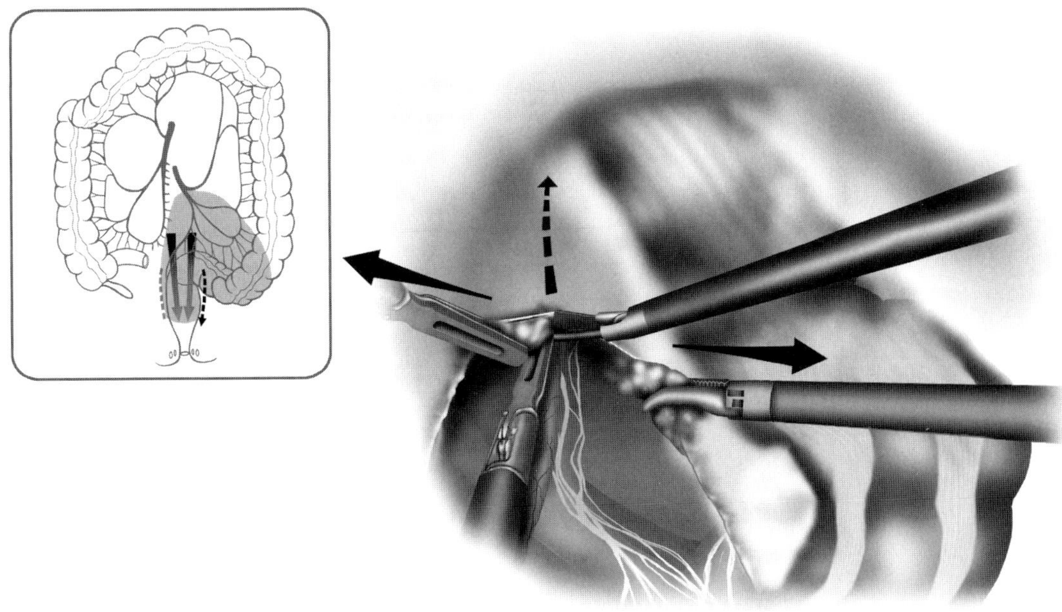

Figure 10.4.6. The left lateral sigmoid attachments are incised while the assistant to the patient's right side retracts the rectum and sigmoid colon.

side. The peritoneal reflexion is incised; however, the true lateral rectal stalks are exposed but left undisturbed.[7] The completeness of dissection is determined visually or with the aid of a double-gloved finger in the rectum (Figure 10.4.7). Using a laparoscopic instrument, the surgeon's finger should be palpable just above the pelvic floor. Further mobilization of the peritoneal reflection is continued anteriorly at the level of the cul-de-sac if necessary. It is important again to preserve the lateral rectal stalks.[7] At this point, if only a rectopexy is planned, the rectum is placed under moderate tension by the assistant through the left lower quadrant port sites.

A 0 nonabsorbable suture is passed through the right lower quadrant cannula into the peritoneal cavity. The needle is grasped by the needle holder in the right lower quadrant cannula and is driven through the presacral fascia, about 1 cm below the sacral promontory and about 1 cm to the right of the midline (Figure 10.4.8). The needle is then passed through the lateral rectal stalks in a location so that the rectum will be under mild tension (Figure 10.4.9). Intra- or extracorporeal knot-tying is performed. Often, we will use extracorporeal tying in which the suture is pulled out of the abdomen and a Roeder knot is performed and slit with a knot pusher to tighten the suture. At this point, a second rectopexy suture is placed in the same manner 1 cm cephalad from the previous one on the patient's right side.

The surgeon at this time places tension on the rectum toward the right presacrum. If this maneuver does not cause excessive angulation

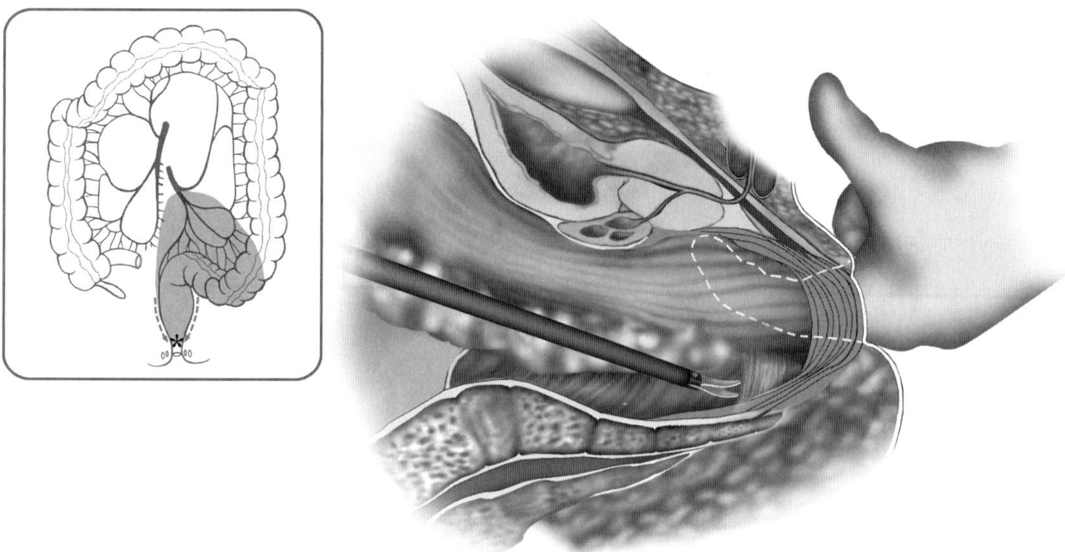

Figure 10.4.7. Insertion of a double-gloved finger into the rectum may aid in determining the completeness of dissection of the rectum.

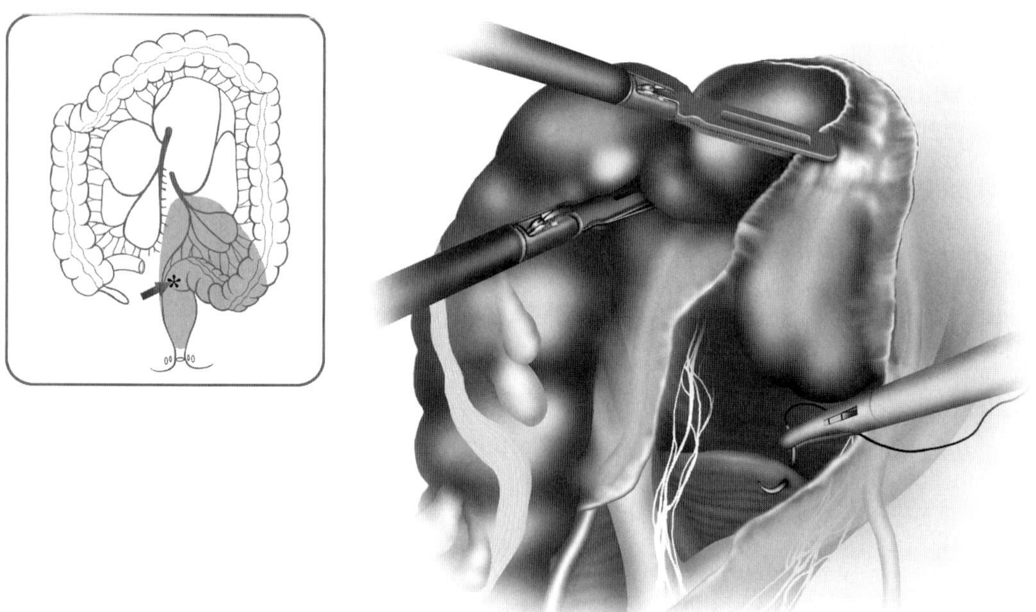

Figure 10.4.8. The first rectopexy suture is driven through the presacral fascia, about 1 cm below the sacral promontory and about 1 cm to the right of the midline.

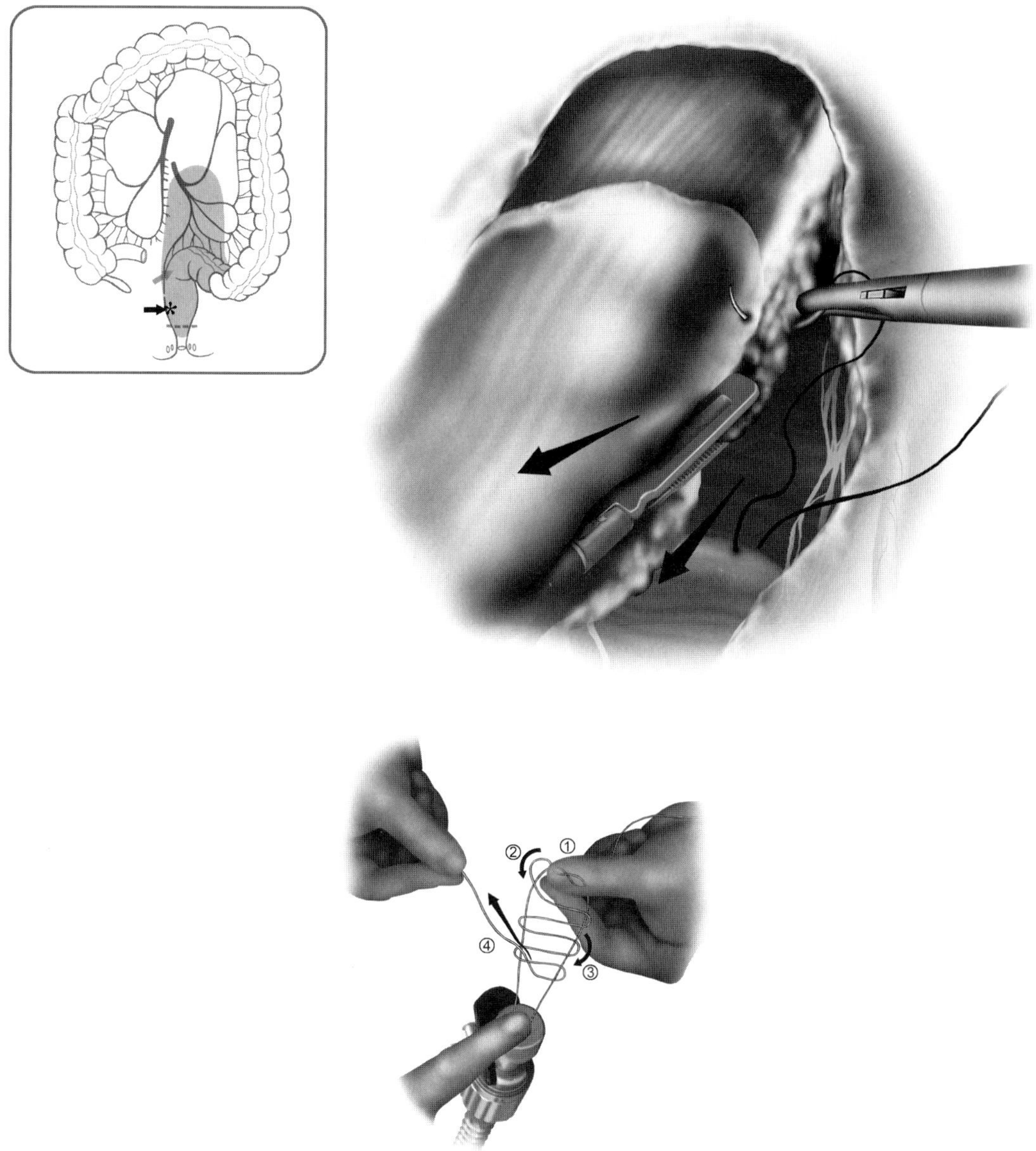

Figure 10.4.9. The needle is then passed through the lateral rectal stalks in a location so that the rectum will be under mild tension (inset: Use of the externally tied Roeder now is used, allowing for rapid tying of the rectopexy sutures).

or tension, rectopexy sutures can be placed on the patient's left side. This is indeed a controversial point and some authors would not place rectopexy sutures bilaterally in order to avoid possible rectosigmoid angulation especially when a resection is not planned. At the completion of the rectopexy, an intraoperative proctoscopy is performed past the rectopexy site to make sure that no angulation or constriction of the lumen has occurred.

Resection Rectopexy

After performing the complete mobilization, the sigmoid colon is then retracted toward the left side of the pelvis by the assistant. It is important to have a clear understanding at this point of the vascular anatomy of the rectosigmoid as well as the location of the left ureter, which was initially identified through the window underneath the superior hemorrhoidal vessels on the left side. This procedure preserves the left colic artery, dividing only the sigmoid branches of the inferior mesenteric artery.[8] Viability of the distal bowel in this way presents no problem and is supplied by the middle and superior hemorrhoidal vessels. The proximal blood supply is usually adequate through the left colic artery, which is also preserved. The sigmoid branches are dissected at their takeoff from the superior hemorrhoidal artery and are sealed and divided with the LigaSure™ device. Mobilization of the mesentery leading to the proximal and distal transection points is also completed from the patient's right side. The assistant on the left side is retracting the sigmoid to the left side of the pelvis.

It is important to remember that when this operation is performed for prolapse, the rectum should be mobilized to the pelvic floor and laterally to the level of the lateral stalks, but the anastomosis should be performed at or just below the sacral promontory. At the distal resection point, the mesorectum is divided with the LigaSure™ device. The assistant retracts the rectum up and out of the pelvis and toward the left side with the surgeon completing the distal dissection from the right side.

Once this is accomplished, an endoscopic stapler is inserted through the right lower quadrant port site, placed across the upper rectum, and deployed. Because of the high level of transsection, the stapler may need to be fired twice to completely divide the rectum at this point. When this is accomplished, the left lower quadrant or umbilical cannula site is enlarged to 3–4 cm to allow exteriorization and proximal transection of the specimen.

When the abdominal cavity is entered and the pneumoperitoneum is evacuated, a wound protector is inserted. The divided sigmoid colon is then delivered through the incision. Proximal division of the mesentery can be completed extracorporeally and the proximal limit of the resection is identified, circumferentially freed from the mesentery and divided between clamps. At this point, a pursestring is applied over the distal stump and the center rod and anvil of a circular stapler 31 mm is inserted and secured in place.

Tension over the mesentery of the sigmoid and descending colon is evaluated at this time and further mobilization is achieved if needed. The distal stump is inserted back into the abdominal cavity. Interrupted fascial stitches are placed to close the extraction site around a port and pneumoperitoneum is reestablished.

When that is achieved, the assistant holds the distal sigmoid colon to allow proper orientation of the mesentery and avoid torsion. The second assistant between the legs of the patient inserts the shaft of the circular 31-mm stapler. A suture is placed in the spike of the stapler to facilitate laparoscopic removal. The stapler is passed transanally and guided to the rectal staple line. The spike of the circular stapler is then advanced adjacent to the rectal staple line and removed by grasping the suture. The spike is removed through the right lower quadrant port site.

The surgeon then grasps the center rod of the circular stapler anvil and inserts it into the shaft of the stapler. Proper orientation of the mesentery is further checked. The assistant allows for retraction of the sigmoid colon for adequate visualization of the mesentery. The stapler is then closed and deployed. The stapler is released and extracted transanally. The two rings are checked. A leak test is performed by insufflating the rectum transanally while the pelvis is filled with fluid and the descending colon is occluded to detect air leaks from the anastomosis. The pelvis is then copiously irrigated with warm sterile saline solution using a laparoscopic suction irrigator.

The rectopexy is then performed distal to the anastomosis as previously described. Proctoscopy is performed to ensure that there is no angulation or constriction. The cannulae are removed in a routine manner and the cannula sites are closed.

Special Considerations

As described in the previous section, a clear understanding and definition of the anatomy of the pelvis at the time of dissection and exposure are mandatory to avoid intraoperative complications.

Two major structures ought to be identified and avoided intraoperatively: The left ureter and the presacral veins. As in any sigmoid and rectal resection, the left ureter is at risk for injury if not properly visualized and retracted out of the operating field. The left ureter should be immediately visualized upon opening the right peritoneum and creating a window underneath the superior hemorrhoidal vessels. When the left ureter is identified, it should be dissected downward away from the operating field together with the gonadal vessels. Another area where the ureter could be injured is at the level of the left pelvic rim if the incision at the peritoneal reflexion on the left is taken too laterally. It is mandatory when incising the peritoneum on the left side of the pelvis that the surgeon retracts the rectum to the right and the first assistant incises the peritoneum medially. At that level, the ureter is usually lateral and it is critical to dissect in the correct plane.

It is our practice in any laparoscopic procedure that if the anatomy of the ureter is not clearly visualized, laparoscopy is aborted and a laparotomy is performed. Similarly, in situations of inadvertent ureteral injury, conversion to open laparotomy is essential to assess the extent of damage. Resection of damaged tissue and repair over a stent is usually possible. Because there is no retroperitoneal inflammation in these patients, routine use of ureteral stents is not indicated.

When performing the rectopexy over the sacral promontory, it is important to place the sutures at least 1 cm off the midline to avoid the presacral veins. In case of a presacral bleed, an attempt to direct pressure should be performed and it is often indicated to tie the suture that has been placed over the injured vein and eventually add additional stitches. If the bleeding cannot be controlled with laparoscopic methods, clearly a conversion is indicated.

A specific complication in patients that have had only a suture rectopexy is the angulation of the redundant sigmoid colon after placement of the sutures. This problem should be detected and avoided by intraoperative inspection of the lumen with a rigid proctoscope before evacuating pneumoperitoneum. If this condition is not noted intraoperatively, the patient will present with difficulty evacuating and worsening constipation in the months after surgery. This is indeed a difficult problem to manage at that point and will require takedown of the previous rectopexy and possibly a sigmoid resection. Usually, these are patients with redundant sigmoid colon at the time of the initial rectopexy.

In patients who have had a resection rectopexy, anastomotic leak is always a concern. Similar to any other intestinal anastomosis, tension over the anastomosis ought to be avoided. Viability and vascularization of the stumps should be left intact by preserving the left colic artery and the superior hemorrhoidal artery as previously described. In case of a clinically evident anastomotic leak, oral intake should be immediately discontinued; the patient should be started on intravenous fluids and antibiotics, and evaluated with a Gastrografin enema to assess the extent of the leak. Management can vary from observation to having to perform a diverting loop ileostomy and drainage of the pelvic sepsis. If a leak is noted at the completion of the anastomosis, careful evaluation should be performed. This should be done before completing the rectopexy so that a 360° view of the anastomosis is possible. If the area of leakage is identified, it should be reinforced with intracorporeal sutures. If the leak is not controlled by this measure, treatment options include temporary diversion, takedown and re-creation of the anastomosis, and conversion to an open procedure for further evaluation.

Frequent early postoperative sequelae that are not specific to the operations described include urinary retention and postoperative ileus.

A Foley catheter is kept in place until the epidural infusion has been discontinued. This is to prevent postoperative urinary retention, especially in the older male patient population. A clear visualization of the hypogastric and the sacral nerves helps in avoiding long-term urinary and sexual dysfunction.

Return of bowel function can also be delayed especially in patients with a history of chronic constipation. Our practice is to allow the patient to have a clear liquid diet the day immediately after surgery. We watch for progression of recovery of intestinal function. When passage of gas has been documented, at that time the patients are allowed to be advanced to a low residue diet and discharged home.

Other laparoscopic techniques for repair of complete rectal prolapse have been described. Specifically, tacking of the rectum to the sacrum using either polypropylene mesh or a sling has been described. We believe that a rectopexy or a resection rectopexy are much simpler procedures and as effective as those that include mesh insertion.[9,10] Further details on the long-term results of this procedure will be provided in Chapter 11.6.

Conclusions

To achieve adequate long-term functional results in patients with rectal prolapse, either open or laparoscopically, a careful preoperative evaluation and the selection of the appropriate surgical technique based on the physiologic parameters of the specific patient are required. If these principles are applied to laparoscopy, there is no reason to believe that our long-term results will be less optimal than those achieved in the best series of conventional open approach, while the advantages of a less invasive technique will then benefit this patient population.

Editors' Comments

Indications: We would consider sigmoid resection in most young and healthy patients even if not symptomatically constipated because constipation tends to worsen after simple rectopexy.

Patient positioning: We place the monitors near the knees of the patient. Electrosurgical devices are placed lateral to the patient, and the suction device is placed near the head of the patient in our setup.

Instrumentation: We use similar instruments.

Cannula positioning: Our positioning is similar.

Technique: We strongly advocate use of the surgeon's double-gloved hand placed into the rectum to check the level of dissection. We use a size 2–0 nonabsorbable (braided) on a ski-needle (atraumatic) for the rectopexy. We also advocate intraoperative endoscopy to check patency of the lumen after application of the rectopexy sutures. We avoid placing stitches on both sides of the rectum because they may constrict the lumen of the bowel. If conversion is required, we will consider a Pfannenstiel incision, because this heals rapidly and the resultant scar will be hidden in the suprapubic area. If bleeding is the indication for conversion, a midline incision permits entry into the abdomen more quickly.

References

1. Heah SM, Hartley JE, Hurley J, et al. Laparoscopic suture rectopexy without resection is effective treatment for full-thickness rectal prolapse. Dis Colon Rectum 2000;43:638–643.
2. Himpens J, Cadiere GB, Bruyns J, et al. Laparoscopic rectopexy according to Wells. Surg Endosc 1999;13:139–141.
3. van Dalen RM, Modi AK, Hershman MJ. How to do it in surgery: laparoscopic rectopexy. Br J Hosp Med 1997;58:587–588.
4. Xynos E, Chrysos E, Tsiaoussis J, et al. Resection rectopexy for rectal prolapse. The laparoscopic approach. Surg Endosc 1999;13:862–864.

5. Eu KW, Seow-Choen F. Functional problems in adult rectal prolapse and controversies in surgical treatment. Br J Surg 1997;84:904–911.
6. Madbouly KM, Senagore AJ, Delaney CP, et al. Clinically based management of rectal prolapse. Surg Endosc 2003;17:99–103.
7. Kellokumpu IH, Kairaluoma M. Laparoscopic repair of rectal prolapse: surgical technique. Ann Chir Gynaecol 2001;90:66–69.
8. Ignjatovic D, Bergamaschi R. Preserving the superior rectal artery in laparoscopic anterior resection for complete rectal prolapse. Acta Chir Iugosl 2002;49:25–26.
9. Tsugawa K, Sue K, Koyanagi N, et al. Laparoscopic rectopexy for recurrent rectal prolapse: a safe and simple procedure without a mesh prosthesis. Hepatogastroenterology 2002;49:1549–1551.
10. Kessler H, Jerby BL, Milsom JW. Successful treatment of rectal prolapse by laparoscopic suture rectopexy. Surg Endosc 1999;13:858–861.

Chapter 11.1

External Evidence of Laparoscopic Colorectal Surgery

Jeffrey W. Milsom, Bartholomäus Böhm, and Kiyokazu Nakajima

The following chapters are dedicated to the external evidence of laparoscopic colorectal surgery. We believe that 15 years after the first laparoscopic colon resections we should be able to give some reliable and valid statements concerning effectiveness of laparoscopic colorectal surgery. Therefore, we performed, with the help of several coauthors, a systematic review on different topics and attempt to answer the most relevant clinical questions.

The external evidence of therapeutic trials should always be carefully evaluated because the methodological quality of the trials influences the interpretation of the results. The results are the results. But whether we take them seriously to draw firm and solid conclusions depends largely on the confidence we have in them. Thus, the different methodological qualities of the trials yield to different levels of recommendations. We trust the conclusions of well-designed and -performed trials much more than less-well-designed studies, which are more prone to many types of bias.

According to modern epidemiologic standards, a hierarchy in the quality of clinical studies (Table 11.1.1) and the recommendations gained from these studies is well established (Table 11.1.2). It is always very important to critically state the quality of the trials so that the level of recommendation can be clearly seen.

If a difference between conventional and laparoscopic surgery is assumed, it should be described as relative risk reduction (RRR) and absolute risk reduction (ARR) so that the number of patients needed to prevent (NNT) one complication can be calculated (NNT = 1/ARR).

Data extraction from the literature was sometimes difficult because some results were not differentiated between groups and thus we had to include them in the further analysis as missing values. Continuous data in different series are sometimes given as mean and standard deviation and sometimes as median and range. To perform our analysis, therefore, we arbitrarily accepted median values as mean, and the range divided by 6 was taken as standard deviation, using the sometimes questionable assumption of a symmetric distribution of the data. At times, we calculated the missing standard deviation by the

Table 11.1.1. Levels of evidence (a "hierarchy of quality") of clinical therapeutical trials

Level of evidence	Type of study
1a	Systematic review (with homogeneity) of RCTs
1b	Individual RCT with narrow CI
1c	All-or-none decision
2a	Systematic review (with homogeneity) of cohort trials
2b	Individual cohort study (including poor-quality RCT; or <80% of follow-up)
2c	"Outcomes" research
3a	Systematic review (with homogeneity) of case-control studies
3b	Individual case-control study
4	Case series (cohort studies or case-control studies of poor quality)
5	Expert opinion without explicit clinical appraisal, or based on physiology, bench research, or first principles

given *P* value according to the recommendations of the Cochrane Collaboration.

All comparative data were included in the meta-analyses we performed, despite their questionable methodological value. The summary of the possible treatment effects was calculated using a random effects metaanalysis by the review manager software (Revman 4.2) from the Cochrane Collaboration. All data are given in Forrest plots which show the raw data, the risk ratio (RR), or weighted mean difference (WMD) including the 95% confidence interval (CI). The area of the block in our figures indicates the weight assigned to the study.

It could be painful for purist statisticians to read our analysis because we applied excellent statistical tools to data of sometimes questionable statistical value, i.e., clinical studies which were not from randomized controlled trials (RCTs). It is an accepted statistical rule that data should not be included in a review in which the risk of bias is high, even if there is no better evidence. We know how important it is to follow this rule and how misleading a review may be if such data are included. We are well aware that our review may seriously overestimate any treatment effect shown in the analysis, but our final assessment (see conclusion) is tempered by the weakness of the current data. If there is a benefit of the laparoscopic approach, the effect size cannot reliably be estimated from the current data in the surgical literature.

Table 11.1.2. Grades of recommendation

A	Consistent level 1 studies
B	Consistent level 2 or 3 studies or extrapolations from level 1 studies
C	Level 4 studies or extrapolations from level 2 or 3 studies
D	Level 5 evidence or troublingly inconsistent or inconclusive studies of any level

Therefore, although the quality of most of the studies is level 3 or higher – except for colorectal cancer – and strong publication and selection bias are obvious, the evidence presented in these reviews is the best available. But using modern statistical analytical methods, we must surmise that most arguments supporting laparoscopic surgical methods, drawn from these data, need further support by better trials. The major statistical reason to analyze and summarize these data, despite their pitfalls, is to generate hypotheses which may be evaluated in further controlled studies.

Chapter 11.2

Outcomes After Laparoscopic Adhesiolysis

Michael Seifert

Adhesions are a common sequela after abdominal surgery and may also form after intraabdominal inflammatory diseases. Adhesions are an important etiology of acute or chronic intestinal obstruction or even chronic pain, and must be suspected as a leading cause of abdominal pain whenever the patient has undergone previous abdominal surgery. Ray et al.[1] reported an estimated 303,836 hospitalizations for adhesiolysis-related procedures in the United States in 1994. Although this frequency may herald the importance of adhesions leading to hospitalizations or surgery, primary adhesiolysis was required only in 19% of all cases.

The use of laparoscopy to treat adhesions is not new. Adhesiolysis using a laparoscope has been performed by gynecologists decades ago (before videolaparoscopy) to treat chronic pelvic pain or infertility related to fallopian tube obstruction. Currently, complex and extensive adhesiolysis is feasible using laparoscopic techniques, thus surgeons have adopted this minimally invasive approach to treat abdominal pain or bowel obstruction in selected patients. This chapter will review the evidence base related to these two indications.

Methods

Search of Literature

The MEDLINE database via PUBMED was searched for English literature published since 1990. The MeSh terms "adhesiolysis" and "surgery" were used for the search. All abstracts found in the literature were evaluated. Individual case reports and small case series (less than 30) were excluded. Included were all other case series, case-control, cohort, or randomized studies. Studies were separated in two groups: Surgery for chronic pain and surgery for intestinal obstruction. If the pain was caused by intestinal obstruction, the study was included in the obstruction group.

Outcomes

We analyzed the frequency of conversion to a conventional approach, the duration of surgery, the length of postoperative hospital stay, morbidity and mortality, and success of adhesiolysis. In some but not all studies, the previous number of laparotomies was given and the mechanism of obstruction (isolated bands, dense adhesions, or other) were described. If long-term results were available, the length of follow-up and recurrence rate (pain or obstruction) were documented.

Data Analysis

The overall quality of the studies is low, thus all conclusions should be drawn cautiously. Most studies are retrospective[2–8] or prospective[9–11] case series. Because difficult cases would be biased toward conversion to laparotomy (or were primarily operated on using an open method), a valid comparison between the laparoscopic and conventional approach is actually not feasible analyzing the available data. In addition, the studies are so heterogenous that the numeric results are not summarized but all results are expressed as the range of the reported results. One study was found that compared the conventional and laparoscopic approaches using a matched-pair analysis.[12] Only one randomized trial is available that investigated the role of laparoscopic adhesiolysis in patients with chronic pain.[13]

Results

The reasons for laparoscopic adhesiolysis were acute bowel obstruction but more often suspected chronic bowel obstruction with pain.

Laparoscopic Surgery for Acute Small Bowel Obstruction

In surgery for acute bowel obstruction, isolated bands were found in 30%–55%, dense adhesions in 30%–45%, internal hernia or strictures in about 2%. Conversions were reported in 20%–60% (Table 11.2.1). The most common reasons for converting cases to open surgery were inability to identify the origin of obstruction, nonviable intestine, iatrogenic perforation, or suspected malignancy.

The intended laparoscopic procedure was "successful" in 35%–100% depending on the underlying disease. This approach relieved the symptoms in almost all cases with chronic obstruction but in less than half with acute obstruction. If isolated bands were the reason for obstruction, the procedure was highly successful. But the success markedly decreased if dense adhesions caused obstruction.

The operative time ranged from 30 to 240 minutes. Many authors reported about serious intraoperative complications such as enterotomies which were sometimes missed and detected some days later during emergent laparotomy because of peritonitis. In these cases, some small perforations were obviously caused by an instrument or electrosurgery. The risk of perforation was very high, especially in

Table 11.2.1. Indication, morbidity, mortality, conversion to open surgery, duration of surgery (operative time), and mean length of hospital stay (stay)

Author	Year	Indication	n	Morbidity	Mortality	Conversion	Operative time [min]	Stay [days]
Freys et al.	1994	CSBO	58	6	0	0		
Benoist et al.	1996	ASBO	31	6	0	15		
Ibrahim et al.	1996	ASBO/CSBO	33	1	0	11	–	–
							64 (15–180)	
Bailey et al.	1998	ASBO	65	–	–	30	108 (55–160)	2.9 ± 0.7
Leon et al.	1998	ASBO/CSBO	40	6	–	26		
Navez et al.	1998	ASBO	68	14	2	37	77	6.6
Strickland et al.	1999	ASBO	40	16	0	16	68	3.6
							71 (20–230)	
Chosidow et al.	2000	ASBO/CSBO	134	5	0	21		(0–27)
Agresta et al.	2000	ASBO/CSBO	63	1	0	11	45 (20–65)	–
Suter et al.	2000	ASBO	83	26	2	36	–	–
Levard et al.	2001	ASBO/CSBO	308	47	7	140	–	14 (1–56)
Wullstein et al.	2003	ASBO	52	10	0	27	103	11.3
Franklin et al.	2003	ASBO	167	31	4	13	20–180	5 (2–42)
Chopra et al.	2003	ASBO/CSBO	34	18	2	11	150–240	7.3–13.3
							110 (30–230)	
Borzellino et al.	2004	ASBO/CSBO	65	8	0	13		4.4 (1–22)

CSBO, chronic small bowel obstruction; ASBO, acute small bowel obstruction.

prolonged procedures with significant distension of the small bowel to a diameter of more than 4 cm.[14]

Morbidity was low (0%–22%) if the laparoscopic approach could be successfully accomplished. Morbidity was substantially higher, up to 80%, in converted cases and could possibly exceed the expected morbidity after primary conventional surgery. If the case could be solved laparoscopically, the recovery was very smooth and short. Mortality was low in most series but in one study approached almost 43%.[15] The reported hospital stay was 6–8 days after laparoscopy and more than 12 days after laparotomy.

Laparoscopic Surgery for Chronic Bowel Obstruction

If laparoscopic surgery was performed for chronic abdominal or pelvic pain, conversion was rarely reported. Authors also reported, in most cases, a low morbidity (0%–15%) and mortality (0%–2%).[16] For example, in a prospective study from Onders and Mittendorf,[17] 70 patients with abdominal pain underwent laparoscopy. Other pathologies than adhesions were found and laparoscopically treated (13 hernias, 5 abnormal appendices, and 2 abnormal gallbladders). Adhesions were only reported in 45 patients. Fifty (71.4%) patients had long-term pain relief after an average follow-up of 129 weeks.

Swank et al.[18] also reported about 200 patients with adhesions as the cause of pain. Complete adhesiolysis was accomplished in 82%, almost complete adhesiolysis in 10%, and incomplete adhesiolysis in 8%. The postoperative relief of pain was surprisingly independent of the degree of adhesiolysis.

Malik et al.[19] reported very encouraging long-term results of laparoscopic adhesiolysis for chronic abdominal and pelvic pain. They sent a questionnaire to 187 patients from whom 101 answered. The follow-up was 6–18 months. The surgery was uneventful in all patients. The laparoscopic pain score markedly decreased in almost all patients and in about 50% the pain was completely relieved. Similar to Swank's study, the pre- and postoperative reported pain scores did not correlate with the amount or degree of adhesions.

To evaluate the precise role of laparoscopic adhesiolysis in patients with chronic abdominal pain during at least 6 months, Swank et al.[13] accomplished a randomized blinded trial in 100 patients who were assigned to either a thorough diagnostic laparoscopy only or subsequent laparoscopic adhesiolysis. After 6 and 12 months, in more than 50% of all cases, the pain and quality of life were improved. However, there was no difference between groups, i.e., the favorable effect was also seen in the group without adhesiolysis, undergoing only a diagnostic laparoscopy!

Discussion

There is no question that laparoscopic adhesiolysis can safely be accomplished in selected patients. But the literature also supports the idea that serious complications and even death have been reported after such procedures. It should always be performed by well-trained laparoscopic surgeons who are educated both in advanced laparoscopic surgery as well as conventional open intestinal surgery.[4]

A good indication for the laparoscopic approach is partial or a recurrent small bowel obstruction without a significantly dilated bowel. Bands or dense adhesions in a nondilated small bowel can be lysed without major morbidity. If a malignant adhesion is suspected, the case should be converted to open surgery, if this is a curable situation, or biopsies only done from the abdominal cavity if a far-advanced disease state is encountered.

Acute bowel obstruction is not a good indication for laparoscopic surgery based on the current literature, but the laparoscopic approach may be successful in highly selected patients. Borzellino et al.[20] excluded all patients with "generalized or local peritonitis, associated incisional hernia, absence of less than two abdominal quadrants free of adhesions at the echographic mapping, and the presence of massive bowel distension associated with diffuse air-fluid levels on abdominal X-ray." This selection appears clinically wise and only 65 of 135 patients (48.1%) were selected for the laparoscopic approach in his series. Still, 13 of 65 patients had to be converted to a conventional approach even with these criteria.

Sometimes it is crucial to quickly decide whether surgery is needed at all to avoid perforation or gangrene. Even if clinically available, sonographic and radiologic examinations are not conclusive to decide upon the feasibility of the laparoscopic approach, but, in rare situations, laparoscopy may be an excellent option to clarify the situation.

Acute obstruction may be extremely challenging and should be quickly converted to an open method if difficulties are encountered at the beginning of the operation. The distended abdomen and dilated bowel make the working space very small. Inadvertent perforation by a Veress needle or laparoscopic instrument has been frequently reported.[21] Some authors recommend laparoscopic suture repair of small lacerations if there is no gross contamination. Greater injuries or soiling of the peritoneal cavity by intestinal contents is a clear indication for conversion to conventional surgery.

Based on the current evidence, to reduce intraoperative morbidity, especially in patients with a distended abdomen, an open access for the initial cannula insertion seems mandatory because the pattern of adhesions is unpredictable. Surgeons should not risk an inadvertent injury to the intestine by a blind insertion of the Veress needle or trocar. In addition, the friable and distended bowel is easily injured by brisk and ungentle handling or by using traumatic graspers or sharp instruments. Running the bowel has to be done very gently. Grasping the mesentery may reduce the risk of bowel injury but may increase the risk of serious bleeding.

Does the laparoscopic approach offer a really clear advantage in patients with acute bowel obstruction? Because randomized trials or even good cohort studies are not available, the question cannot yet be answered. Currently, there is only level 4 or 5 evidence to support the use of laparoscopy in acute or chronic intestinal obstruction, or in chronic abdominal pain patients. It is obvious that the laparoscopic approach is successful in patients with "minor" adhesions who might have done also very well by a small laparotomy. Thus, it is not fair to compare the laparoscopic procedure with the converted or conventional cases even when a match-pair study suggests advantages (if the laparoscopic approach is successful).

The role of laparoscopy is twofold in patients with suspected adhesions or chronic abdominal pain: It may be diagnostic to rule out other pathologies, or therapeutic to lyse adhesions. In these cases, the laparoscopic approach seems to be a valuable option if surgery is considered.

One reason to advise patients without evidence of clear obstruction, who have already undergone an extensive negative workup, to undergo a diagnostic laparoscopy is that adhesions may decrease the movement and distensibility of the intestine and thus cause pain. In patients with pain in the right lower quadrant, laparoscopic appendectomy is worthwhile if no other definitive cause is found. Most patients have complete relief after appendectomy.

Is laparoscopy justified for chronic abdominal pain not related to bowel obstruction? If diagnostic laparoscopy is performed for chronic pain, a pathology is found in a high percentage of patients in some nonrandomized studies, in which authors suggest that the pain score is markedly reduced after surgery or even completely diminished in almost 50%.[22–24] Patients in these reports are likely a highly selected group. The value of adhesiolysis was questioned by only one randomized trial.[13] In this study, if a patient was thoroughly explored by a diagnostic laparoscopy and a pathology excluded, then additional adhesiolysis did not improve long-term outcome. Thus, it remains controversial whether surgery of any type (laparoscopic or open) should be performed for chronic abdominal pain.

Whether the laparoscopic approach causes less adhesions postoperatively compared with the conventional approach is suspected from animal and some clinical studies[25] but not clearly proven by clinical studies. There is much good experience of "less adhesions" after laparoscopic surgery (level 5 evidence), but solid evidence for this is thus far lacking.

Conclusion

Laparoscopic adhesiolysis may be a worthwhile procedure in selected patients. If adhesiolysis for acute obstruction is intended, some risk factors such as peritonitis, previous malignant disease, or complex conventional adhesiolysis have been reported frequently in the literature, and suggest that the laparoscopic approach must be considered cautiously. Laparoscopic surgery for chronic bowel obstruction or even pain can be accomplished with low morbidity, but the long-term results are good in at most 50% of all patients, and this evidence comes from nonrandomized studies (level 3b and 4 evidence). Important factors for a favorable outcome are good surgical judgment and proper selection of patients.

Final Questions for Consideration

1. Does the laparoscopic approach cause less morbidity?
   This is unknown. If the laparoscopic approach is successful treating acute bowel obstruction, the morbidity may be low in simple cases, but high in converted cases. The overall morbidity in patients with chronic bowel obstruction or pain is low (Recommendation C).
2. Does the laparoscopic approach cause less mortality?
   This is also unknown and unlikely (Recommendation C).
3. Does the laparoscopic approach have any short-term advantages?
   This is unknown because there are no comparative studies (Recommendation D).
4. Does the laparoscopic approach increase the cost of the operation?
   This is unknown because there are no comparative studies (Recommendation D).
5. Are the long-term results in favor of the laparoscopic approach?
   This is unknown because there are no comparative studies (Recommendation D).

References

1. Ray NF, Denton WG, Thamer M, et al. Abdominal adhesiolysis: inpatient care and expenditures in the United States in 1994. J Am Coll Surg 1998;186:1–9.
2. Ibrahim IM, Wolodiger F, Sussman B, et al. Laparoscopic management of acute small-bowel obstruction. Surg Endosc 1996;10:1012–1014.
3. Chopra R, McVay C, Phillips E, et al. Laparoscopic lysis of adhesions. Am Surg 2003;69:966–968.
4. Bailey IS, Rhodes M, O'Rourke N, et al. Laparoscopic management of acute small bowel obstruction. Br J Surg 1998;85:84–87.
5. Leon EL, Metzger A, Tsiotos GG, et al. Laparoscopic management of small bowel obstruction: indications and outcome. J Gastrointest Surg 1998;2:132–140.
6. Agresta F, Piazza A, Michelet I, et al. Small bowel obstruction. Laparoscopic approach. Surg Endosc 2000;14:154–156.
7. Levard H, Boudet MJ, Msika S, et al. Laparoscopic treatment of acute small bowel obstruction: a multicentre retrospective study. ANZ J Surg 2001;71:641–646.
8. Suzuki K, Umehara Y, Kimura T. Elective laparoscopy for small bowel obstruction. Surg Laparosc Endosc Percutan Tech 2003;13:254–256.
9. Al-Mulhim AA. Laparoscopic management of acute small bowel obstruction. Experience from a Saudi teaching hospital. Surg Endosc 2000; 14:157–160.
10. Chosidow D, Johanet H, Montariol T, et al. Laparoscopy for acute small-bowel obstruction secondary to adhesions. J Laparoendosc Adv Surg Tech A 2000;10:155–159.
11. Franklin ME Jr, Gonzalez JJ Jr, Miter DB, et al. Laparoscopic diagnosis and treatment of intestinal obstruction. Surg Endosc 2004;18:26–30.
12. Wullstein C, Gross E. Laparoscopic compared with conventional treatment of acute adhesive small bowel obstruction. Br J Surg 2003;90: 1147–1151.

13. Swank DJ, Swank-Bordewijk SC, Hop WC, et al. Laparoscopic adhesiolysis in patients with chronic abdominal pain: a blinded randomised controlled multi-centre trial. Lancet 2003;361:1247–1251.
14. Suter M, Zermatten P, Halkic N, et al. Laparoscopic management of mechanical small bowel obstruction: are there predictors of success or failure? Surg Endosc 2000;14:478–483.
15. Rosin D, Kuriansky J, Bar ZB, et al. Laparoscopic approach to small-bowel obstruction. J Laparoendosc Adv Surg Tech A 2000;10:253–257.
16. Vrijland WW, Jeekel J, Van Geldorp HJ, et al. Abdominal adhesions: intestinal obstruction, pain, and infertility. Surg Endosc 2003;17:1017–1022.
17. Onders RP, Mittendorf EA. Utility of laparoscopy in chronic abdominal pain. Surgery 2003;134:549–552.
18. Swank DJ, Van Erp WF, Repelaer Van Driel OJ, et al. Complications and feasibility of laparoscopic adhesiolysis in patients with chronic abdominal pain. A retrospective study. Surg Endosc 2002;16:1468–1473.
19. Malik E, Berg C, Meyhofer-Malik A, et al. Subjective evaluation of the therapeutic value of laparoscopic adhesiolysis: a retrospective analysis. Surg Endosc 2000;14:79–81.
20. Borzellino G, Tasselli S, Zerman G, et al. Laparoscopic approach to postoperative adhesive obstruction. Surg Endosc 2004;18:686–690.
21. Navez B, Arimont JM, Guiot P. Laparoscopic approach in acute small bowel obstruction. A review of 68 patients. Hepatogastroenterology 1998; 45:2146–2150.
22. Dunker MS, Bemelman WA, Vijn A, et al. Long-term outcomes and quality of life after laparoscopic adhesiolysis for chronic abdominal pain. J Am Assoc Gynecol Laparosc 2004;11:36–41.
23. Schietroma M, Carlei F, Altilia F, et al. The role of laparoscopic adhesiolysis in chronic abdominal pain. Minerva Chir 2001;56:461–465.
24. Nezhat FR, Crystal RA, Nezhat CH, et al. Laparoscopic adhesiolysis and relief of chronic pelvic pain. JSLS 2000;4:281–285.
25. Swank DJ, Hop WC, Jeekel J. Reduction, regrowth, and de novo formation of abdominal adhesions after laparoscopic adhesiolysis: a prospective analysis. Dig Surg 2004;21:66–71.

Chapter 11.3

Outcomes After Laparoscopic Colectomy for Diverticular Disease

Steffen Minner

The incidence of diverticulosis of the colon increases gradually with age so that by the eighth decade of life almost 80% of the elderly have some diverticula of the colon. Only a minority of these patients complain about acute or chronic diverticulitis and are candidates for surgery.

The indications for emergent surgery are well established: Acute abdomen with perforation and diffuse peritonitis. A more conservative approach may be chosen in patients with acute diverticulitis and local peritonitis or abscess. Most surgeons try to treat the inflammatory process first using antibiotics and computed tomography scan-guided percutaneous drainage of abscess, followed by elective resection with colorectal anastomosis if there is more than one episode, or if the first episode is complicated by abscess. Emergent surgery is indicated only if the clinical situation does not improve under proper treatment with antibiotics and bowel rest either in the hospital or as an outpatient, depending on the clinical judgment of a particular case.

The most common indication for surgical therapy in diverticular disease is chronic sigmoid diverticulitis complicated by recurrent infection, bleeding, stenosis, or fistula to adjacent organs or the skin. These conditions are usually cured by sigmoid resection with colorectal anastomosis. Because all the above-named procedures have been performed conventionally and laparoscopically, the available external evidence should give us a good idea of the value of the laparoscopic approach to treating these patients.

Methods

Search of Literature

The MEDLINE database via PUBMED was searched for English literature published since 1991. The MeSh terms "diverticulitis" and "laparoscopic*" were used for the search. All 240 abstracts of the discovered literature were evaluated. Individual case reports and small case series (less than 20) were excluded as well as mixed studies which included patients with cancer, adenomas, or other inflammatory diseases. Included were 24 observational studies (15 simple case series and 9 comparative cohort studies).

Outcomes

The studies were carefully analyzed and the following items extracted if given: Morbidity, mortality, the proportion of conversion to a conventional approach, the duration of surgery, time to first flatus, time to resumption of a regular diet, and the length of postoperative hospital stay. The same endpoints were looked at in the comparative cohort studies, summarized in an "intent-to-treat" analysis, and compared between laparoscopic and conventional surgery. If long-term results were available, the length of follow-up and recurrence rate were documented.

Data Analysis

The overall quality of the studies is level 3–5. There are no randomized controlled trials (RCTs) that compared both approaches in patients with diverticulitis. This is somewhat surprising because in some countries diverticular disease is the most common indication for laparoscopic sigmoid resection. In theory, it should be easy to set up some RCTs from experienced centers. One small study compared whether the anastomosis should be accomplished after closure of the laparotomy and establishing a pneumoperitoneum or through a small suprapubic incision.[1]

Most of the studies we found were very small retrospective or prospective case series which were excluded from this analysis. Fifteen larger studies with more than 20 patients were evaluated (Table 11.3.1). Nine comparative cohort studies were also included (Table 11.3.2).

Results

The indications for elective resection were mainly acute diverticulitis or chronic diverticulitis with stenosis, with only occasional patients having fistula to the bladder. The conversion rate ranged from 4% to 26%, the operative time 120–240 min, the time to tolerate regular diet 1–21 days, the length of hospital stay 2–55 days, the morbidity 0%–23.7%, and the mortality 0%–3% (Table 11.3.1).

In the comparative cohort studies, the relative risk (RR) of morbidity was 0.37 [confidence interval (CI) 0.25–0.56] (Figure 11.3.1) in the laparoscopic group and the RR of wound infection was only 0.4 (CI 0.17–0.94) (Figure 11.3.2). The weighted mean difference (WMD) of the operative time was 76.9 (CI 15.5–138.3) minutes longer in the laparoscopic group (Figure 11.3.3) and the hospital stay was 4.1 (CI

Table 11.3.1. Results of case series

Author	Year	n	Conversion [%]	Morbidity [%]	Mortality [%]	Operation time [min]	Diet [days]	Stay [days]
Eijsbouts et al.[5]	1997	41	15	17	0	195	–	6.5
Franklin et al.[4]	1997	164	9	15	–	120 (90–240)	–	–
Bouillot et al.[6]	1998	50	8	14	0	195 (150–280)	–	10 (6–22)
Stevenson et al.[7]	1998	100	8	21	0	180 (60–310)	–	4 (2–33)
Köckerling et al.[8]	1999	304	7	16	3	–	–	–
Schlachta et al.[9]	1999	92	7	18	0	150–165	3	5–6
Siriser et al.[10]	1999	65	5	14	0	179 ± 44	2.6 ± 1.3	7.6 ± 3
Smadja et al.[11]	1999	54	9	13	0	298 ± 61	2.3 ± 0.7	6.4 ± 2.7
Berthou et al.[12]	1999	110	8	7	0	167 ± 65	–	8,2–13,5
Martinez et al.[13]	1999	38	7	24	0	215 ± 66	3 ± 1.7	4 ± 1.3
Vargas et al.[14]	2000	69	26	0	0	155 (90–320)	–	–
Trebuchet et al.[15]	2002	170	4	8	0	141 ± 36	3.4 ± 2.1	8.5 ± 3.7
Le Moine et al.[16]	2003	168	14	21	0	240 (210–300)	4.8 (2–21)	–
Schwandner et al.[17]	2004	396	7	17	2	193 (75–400)	6.8 (3–19)	11.8 (4–71)
All		2000	9.9	14.5	0.3			

Table 11.3.2. Method of the comparative cohort studies

Author	Period (months)	n	Rate
Bruce et al.[18] Retrospective chart review. Two independent surgical teams which performed either laparoscopic or conventional resection.	36	42	1.2
Liberman et al.[19] Fourteen laparoscopic resections were compared with matched medical records of 14 open cases.	36	28	0.8
Köhler et al.[20] Laparoscopic resections were performed by a single surgeon and prospectively documented. The laparoscopic group was compared with a historical group of the same institution.	18	29	1.6
Tuech et al.[21] Prospective study. Patients may also be included in the study by Thaler et al. Two separate surgical teams were used to perform either laparoscopic or conventional resection.	72	46	0.6
Faynsod et al.[22] Retrospective chart review. The laparoscopic cases were matched with 20 open resections.	87	43	0.5
Dwivedi et al.[23] Retrospective chart review. Two hundred twenty-three charts were primarily reviewed and 69 excluded. Two surgeons accomplished exclusively all laparoscopic resections.	66	154	2.3
Senagore et al.[3] Retrospective chart review. All laparoscopic resections were performed by a single surgeon.	22	132	6.0
Thaler et al.[2] Laparoscopic and open resection were performed by two institutions from 1992 to 2000. Primary endpoint was recurrence. It was not stated how many patients were followed. Retrospective chart review on all patients operated on because of diverticulitis.	108	148	1.4

The period of surgery and number of resections are given to calculate the resection rate per month and institution (rate).

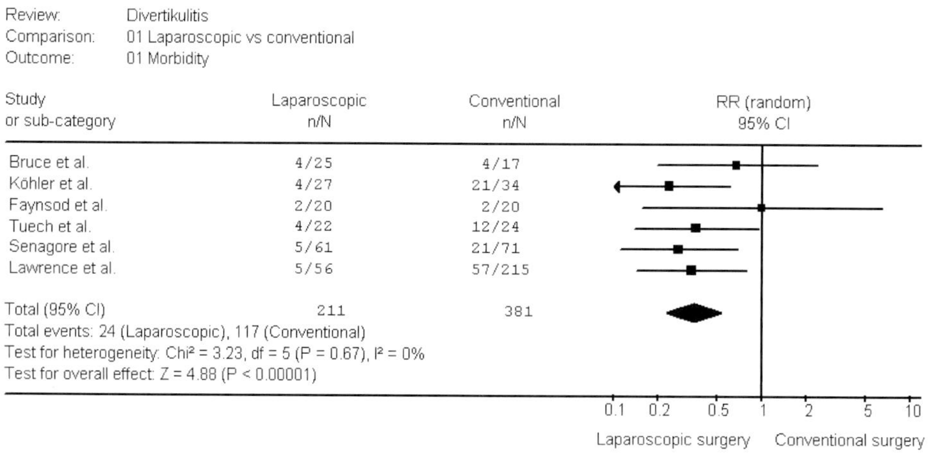

Review: Divertikulitis
Comparison: 01 Laparoscopic vs conventional
Outcome: 01 Morbidity

Study or sub-category	Laparoscopic n/N	Conventional n/N
Bruce et al.	4/25	4/17
Köhler et al.	4/27	21/34
Faynsod et al.	2/20	2/20
Tuech et al.	4/22	12/24
Senagore et al.	5/61	21/71
Lawrence et al.	5/56	57/215
Total (95% CI)	211	381

Total events: 24 (Laparoscopic), 117 (Conventional)
Test for heterogeneity: $Chi^2 = 3.23$, df = 5 (P = 0.67), $I^2 = 0\%$
Test for overall effect: Z = 4.88 (P < 0.00001)

RR (random) 95% CI: 0.1 0.2 0.5 1 2 5 10
Laparoscopic surgery Conventional surgery

Figure 11.3.1. Morbidity [risk ratio (RR) including the 95% CI] after laparoscopic and conventional surgery for diverticulitis.

Review: Divertikulitis
Comparison: 01 Laparoscopic vs conventional
Outcome: 03 Wound infection

Study or sub-category	Laparoscopic n/N	Conventional n/N
Köhler et al.	2/27	7/34
Tuech et al.	1/22	4/24
Dwivedi et al.	1/66	2/88
Senagore et al.	0/61	5/71
Lawrence et al.	0/56	7/215
Total (95% CI)	232	432

Total events: 4 (Laparoscopic), 25 (Conventional)
Test for heterogeneity: $Chi^2 = 1.04$, df = 4 (P = 0.90), $I^2 = 0\%$
Test for overall effect: Z = 2.37 (P = 0.02)

RR (random) 95% CI: 0.01 0.1 1 10 100
Laparoscopic surgery Conventional surgery

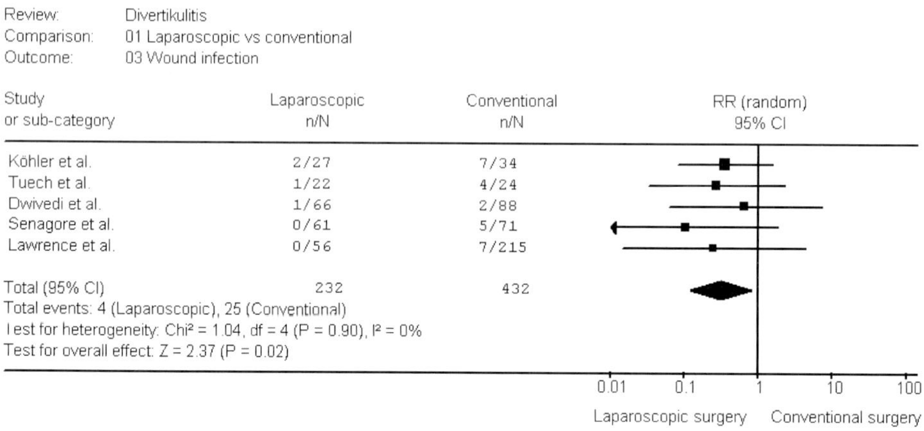

Figure 11.3.2. Wound infections [risk ratio (RR) including the 95% CI] after laparoscopic and conventional surgery for diverticulitis.

Review: Divertikulitis
Comparison: 01 Laparoscopic vs conventional
Outcome: 04 Operative time

Study or sub-category	N	Laparoscopic Mean (SD)	N	Conventional Mean (SD)	WMD (random) 95% CI
Bruce et al.	25	397.00 (9.10)	17	115.00 (5.10)	282.00 [277.69, 286.31]
Köhler et al.	27	165.00 (21.00)	341	121.00 (21.00)	44.00 [35.77, 52.23]
Faynsod et al.	20	251.00 (68.00)	20	243.00 (49.20)	8.00 [−28.78, 44.78]
Dwivedi et al.	66	212.00 (7.20)	88	143.00 (5.70)	69.00 [66.89, 71.11]
Senagore et al.	61	109.00 (7.00)	71	101.00 (7.00)	8.00 [5.60, 10.40]
Lawrence et al.	56	170.00 (45.00)	215	140.00 (49.00)	30.00 [16.52, 43.48]
Total (95% CI)	255		752		73.88 [−8.25, 156.02]

Test for heterogeneity: $Chi^2 = 11938.58$, df = 5 (P < 0.00001), $I^2 = 100.0\%$
Test for overall effect: Z = 1.76 (P = 0.08)

WMD (random) 95% CI: −1000 −500 0 500 1000
Laparoscopic surgery Conventional surgery

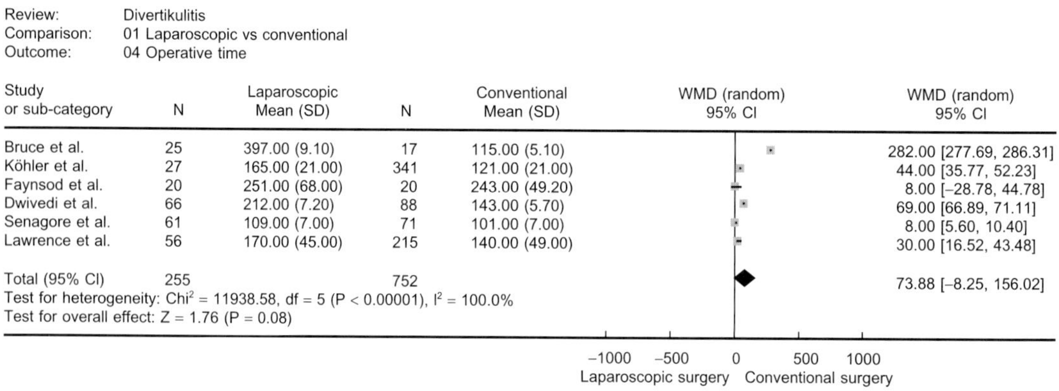

Figure 11.3.3. Operative time (WMD including the 95% CI) after laparoscopic and conventional surgery for diverticulitis.

Review: Divertikulitis
Comparison: 01 Laparoscopic vs conventional
Outcome: 08 Hospital stay

Study or sub-category	N	Laparoscopic Mean (SD)	N	Conventional Mean (SD)
Bruce et al.	25	4.20 (1.10)	17	6.80 (1.10)
Köhler et al.	27	7.90 (1.20)	34	14.30 (2.30)
Faynsod et al.	20	4.80 (2.30)	20	7.80 (1.50)
Dwivedi et al.	66	4.80 (1.20)	88	8.80 (1.50)
Senagore et al.	61	3.10 (0.20)	71	6.80 (0.40)
Total (95% CI)	199		230	

Test for heterogeneity: $Chi^2 = 48.03$, df = 4 ($P < 0.00001$), $I^2 = 91.7\%$
Test for overall effect: Z = 10.01 ($P < 0.00001$)

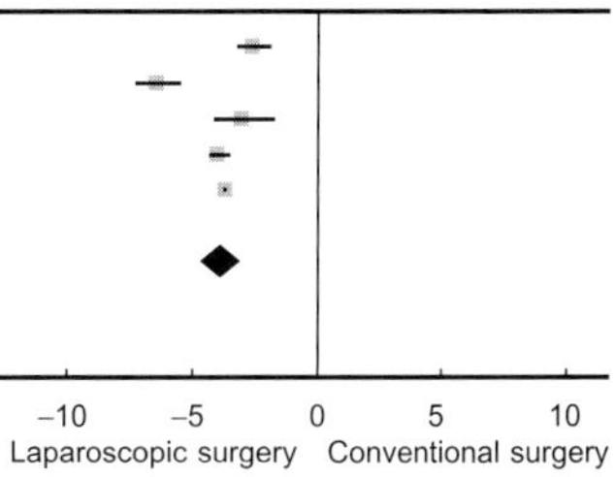

Figure 11.3.4. Hospital stay (WMD including the 95% CI) after laparoscopic and conventional surgery for diverticulitis.

2.4–5.8) days shorter (Figure 11.3.4). Mortality was very low and not different.

Recurrence after resection was investigated in one study (n = 236).[2] The authors described a low recurrence rate of 5% (n = 12) but they did not state how many patients were actually followed. A difference between laparoscopic and conventional surgical groups was not found.

One study (n = 132) analyzed the direct costs for laboratory services, pharmacy, radiology, anesthesia, operating room, and hospitalization.[3] The direct costs per case were $3.458 ± 437 for laparoscopic resections and $4.321 ± 501 for conventional procedures. The length of stay was 3.1 ± 0.2 days in the laparoscopic group and 6.8 ± 0.4 days in the conventional group.

Discussion

Elective laparoscopic colectomy for diverticular disease is at least as safe as conventional surgery because: 1) Morbidity seemed to be lower, and 2) mortality is at least the same. Whether there is a shorter period of postoperative ileus or whether patients experience less pain are also questionable because of a lack of quality of comparative data. The described shorter periods of ileus and postoperative pain in noncomparative case series are not supportive data favoring laparoscopic over conventional surgery and may only suggest that early feeding accelerates postoperative recovery. Some surgeons may point to the results of RCTs on colorectal cancer (see Chapter 11.5) to support their belief about the superiority of the laparoscopic approach. However, surgery for diverticulitis differs in many aspects from oncologic surgery.

Regarding the role of the laparoscopic technique in emergent situations, i.e., in patients with acute diverticulitis with perforation or abscess, some surgeons advocate the laparoscopic approach.[4] They described good results with a relative low proportion of conversions in experienced hands. We advocate caution in adoption of this approach, because proper treatment of perforated diverticular disease with peritonitis is a challenging task even in conventional surgery. Whether it is successfully treated laparoscopically or conventionally is less important than aspiring to achieve a low mortality and morbidity. The appeal of a laparoscopic approach lies in the avoidance of a large abdominal incision, which may become an incredibly morbid feature if infection, dehiscence, or herniation result. However, it should only be considered in highly selected patients without distended bowel and performed by a very experienced team.

Therefore, if enthusiasts of the laparoscopic approach aspire to convince other people that the laparoscopic approach is superior based on sound evidence-based surgical methodology, this must be achieved with convincing data not yet available. Our personal bias favors the laparoscopic colectomy for diverticular disease surgery, but our personal recommendation is based on grade D evidence which, by itself, cannot support that other surgeons must learn laparoscopic surgery.

Conclusions

The available surgical literature provides evidence that laparoscopic colectomy for diverticular disease is a safe procedure and is not associated with higher morbidity or mortality than conventional surgery in experienced hands. Whether it should be applied in the emergency situation in patients with perforated diverticulitis and peritonitis is questionable. The superiority of laparoscopic resections has to be shown in the future through well-designed studies.

Final Questions for Consideration

1. Does the laparoscopic approach lead to less morbidity?
   Not really known because the incidence is low and RCTs are missing (Recommendation C).
2. Does the laparoscopic approach lead to less mortality?
   Not really known because the incidence is very low and RCTs are missing (Recommendation C).
3. Does the laparoscopic approach have any short-term advantages?
   Likely. If RCTs on colorectal cancer surgery are accepted as substitutes, there may be some short-term advantageous (Recommendation C).
4. Are costs increased by the laparoscopic approach?
   Unlikely. The available data are scarce and prospective total costs analysis not accomplished (Recommendation D).
5. Are long-term results in favor of the laparoscopic approach?
   Unlikely. The very few available data showed no difference (Recommendation D).

References

1. Bergamaschi R, Tuech JJ, Cervi C, et al. Re-establish pneumoperitoneum in laparoscopic-assisted sigmoid resection? Randomized trial. Dis Colon Rectum 2000;43:771–774.

2. Thaler K, Weiss EG, Nogueras JJ, et al. Recurrence rates at minimum 5-year follow-up: laparoscopic versus open sigmoid resection for uncomplicated diverticulitis. Surg Laparosc Endosc Percutan Tech 2003;13:325–327.
3. Senagore AJ, Duepree HJ, Delaney CP, et al. Cost structure of laparoscopic and open sigmoid colectomy for diverticular disease: similarities and differences. Dis Colon Rectum 2002;45:485–490.
4. Franklin ME Jr, Dorman JP, Jacobs M, et al. Is laparoscopic surgery applicable to complicated colonic diverticular disease? Surg Endosc 1997;11: 1021–1025.
5. Eijsbouts QA, Cuesta MA, de Brauw LM, et al. Elective laparoscopic-assisted sigmoid resection for diverticular disease. Surg Endosc 1997;11:750–753.
6. Bouillot JL, Aouad K, Badawy A, et al. Elective laparoscopic-assisted colectomy for diverticular disease. A prospective study in 50 patients. Surg Endosc 1998;12:1393–1396.
7. Stevenson AR, Stitz RW, Lumley JW, et al. Laparoscopically assisted anterior resection for diverticular disease: follow-up of 100 consecutive patients. Ann Surg 1998;227:335–342.
8. Köckerling F, Schneider C, Reymond MA, et al. Laparoscopic resection of sigmoid diverticulitis. Results of a multicenter study. Laparoscopic Colorectal Surgery Study Group. Surg Endosc 1999;13:567–571.
9. Schlachta CM, Mamazza J, Poulin EC. Laparoscopic sigmoid resection for acute and chronic diverticulitis. An outcomes comparison with laparoscopic resection for nondiverticular disease. Surg Endosc 1999;13:649–653.
10. Siriser F. Laparoscopic-assisted colectomy for diverticular sigmoiditis. A single-surgeon prospective study of 65 patients. Surg Endosc 1999;13:811–813.
11. Smadja C, Sbai IM, Tahrat M, et al. Elective laparoscopic sigmoid colectomy for diverticulitis. Results of a prospective study. Surg Endosc 1999;13:645–648.
12. Berthou JC, Charbonneau P. Elective laparoscopic management of sigmoid diverticulitis. Results in a series of 110 patients. Surg Endosc 1999;13:457–460.
13. Martinez SA, Cheanvechai V, Alasfar FS, et al. Staged laparoscopic resection for complicated sigmoid diverticulitis. Surg Laparosc Endosc Percutan Tech 1999;9:99–105.
14. Vargas HD, Ramirez RT, Hoffman GC, et al. Defining the role of laparoscopic-assisted sigmoid colectomy for diverticulitis. Dis Colon Rectum 2000;43:1726–1731.
15. Trebuchet G, Lechaux D, Lecalve JL. Laparoscopic left colon resection for diverticular disease. Surg Endosc 2002;16:18–21.
16. Le Moine MC, Fabre JM, Vacher C, et al. Factors and consequences of conversion in laparoscopic sigmoidectomy for diverticular disease. Br J Surg 2003;90:232–236.
17. Schwandner O, Farke S, Fischer F, et al. Laparoscopic colectomy for recurrent and complicated diverticulitis: a prospective study of 396 patients. Langenbecks Arch Surg 2004;389:97–103.
18. Bruce CJ, Coller JA, Murray JJ, et al. Laparoscopic resection for diverticular disease. Dis Colon Rectum 1996;39:S1–S6.
19. Liberman MA, Phillips EH, Carroll BJ, et al. Laparoscopic colectomy vs traditional colectomy for diverticulitis. Outcome and costs. Surg Endosc 1996;10:15–18.
20. Köhler L, Rixen D, Troidl H. Laparoscopic colorectal resection for diverticulitis. Int J Colorectal Dis 1998;13:43–47.

21. Tuech JJ, Pessaux P, Rouge C, et al. Laparoscopic vs open colectomy for sigmoid diverticulitis: a prospective comparative study in the elderly. Surg Endosc 2000;14:1031–1033.
22. Faynsod M, Stamos MJ, Arnell T, et al. A case-control study of laparoscopic versus open sigmoid colectomy for diverticulitis. Am Surg 2000;66: 841–843.
23. Dwivedi A, Chahin F, Agrawal S, et al. Laparoscopic colectomy vs. open colectomy for sigmoid diverticular disease. Dis Colon Rectum 2002;45: 1309–1314.
24. Lawrence DM, Pasquale MD, Wasser TE. Laparoscopic versus open sigmoid colectomy for diverticulitis. Am Surg 2003;69:499–503.

Chapter 11.4

Outcomes After Laparoscopic Colectomy for Crohn's Disease

Jeffrey W. Milsom, Bartholomäus Böhm, and Kiyokazu Nakajima

Crohn's disease (CD) limited to the terminal ileum has become a common indication in the literature for laparoscopic surgical therapy, and laparoscopic methods in the treatment of CD have been described since at least 1993.[1] This chapter will present the current evidence base for the use of laparoscopic techniques in the surgical therapy of Crohn's of the small and large intestine.

Methods

Search of Literature

The literature database MEDLINE was searched for all clinical studies for the years 1991–2004. The MeSh-terms "Crohn's disease," "colectomy," "proctectomy*," "laparoscopy*," and "laparoscopic surgery*" were used for the search and more than 200 publications written in English were found. Laparoscopic, laparoscopic-assisted, and hand-assisted procedures or resections were included. Clinical studies including patients with other diseases or with only laboratory data without any clinical outcome were excluded from further analysis. Studies reported in multiple publications or data given only as abstracts were also excluded.

Outcomes

The studies were carefully analyzed and the following items extracted if given: Morbidity, mortality, the proportion of conversion to a conventional approach, the duration of surgery, time to first flatus, time to resumption of a regular diet, and the length of postoperative hospital stay. All endpoints were looked at in the comparative cohort studies, summarized in an "intent-to-treat" analysis, and compared between laparoscopic and conventional surgery. If long-term results were available, the length of follow-up and recurrence rate were documented.

Data Analysis

The overall quality of the studies would be classified as level of evidence 3–5. Most of the studies we found were very small retrospective or prospective case series which were excluded from this analysis. There is only one randomized controlled trial (RCT) that compare both laparoscopic and open approaches in patients with CD.[2] This RCT and seven comparative cohort studies[3–9] were analyzed (Table 11.4.1).

Table 11.4.1. Method of the comparative cohort studies for CD

Author	Period (months)	n	Rate
Luan et al.[3] In 24 patients for whom a laparoscopic approach was intended. Seven cases were converted. Twenty-three open cases were retrospectively reviewed for comparison.	57	47	0.8
Milsom et al.[2] RCT	52	60	1.2
Duepree et al.[4] Prospective study. Data from two surgical teams.	17	45	2.6
Shore et al.[5] Retrospective study. Elective resections for primary ileocolic disease. The surgeon selected the approach.	60	40	0.7
Bergamaschi et al.[6] Thirty-one laparoscopic resections were compared with a historical group of 53 resections.	108	84	0.8
Benoist et al.[7] Twenty-four consecutive patients who underwent laparoscopic ileocolic resection were matched with 32 patients from a prospective database.	42	56	–
van Allmen et al.[8] Retrospective study from one surgeon performed on teenagers (age 15 ± 3 years)	60	30	0.5
Huilgol et al.[9] A historically open group was compared with a laparoscopic group.	120	40	0.3

The length of the study in months (period) and number of resections (n) was given to calculate the resection rate per month (rate).

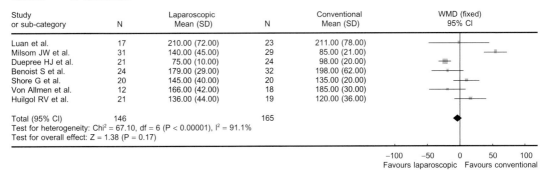

Review: Laparoscopic versus conventional colectomy in Crohn's disease
Comparison: 01 Operative time
Outcome: 01 Operative time

Study or sub-category	N	Laparoscopic Mean (SD)	N	Conventional Mean (SD)
Luan et al.	17	210.00 (72.00)	23	211.00 (78.00)
Milsom JW et al.	31	140.00 (45.00)	29	85.00 (21.00)
Duepree HJ et al.	21	75.00 (10.00)	24	98.00 (20.00)
Benoist S et al.	24	179.00 (29.00)	32	198.00 (62.00)
Shore G et al.	20	145.00 (40.00)	20	135.00 (20.00)
Von Allmen et al.	12	166.00 (42.00)	18	185.00 (30.00)
Huilgol RV et al.	21	136.00 (44.00)	19	120.00 (36.00)
Total (95% CI)	146		165	

Test for heterogeneity: $Chi^2 = 67.10$, df = 6 ($P < 0.00001$), $I^2 = 91.1\%$
Test for overall effect: Z = 1.38 (P = 0.17)

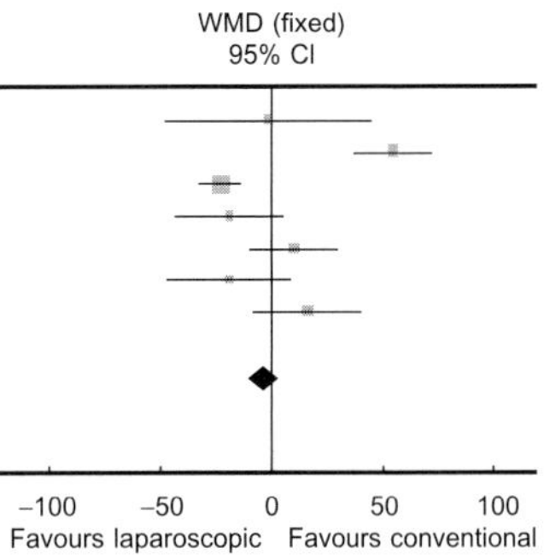

Figure 11.4.1. Operative time [weighted mean difference (WMD) including the 95% confidence interval (CI)] after laparoscopic and conventional surgery for CD.

Results

The indications for elective resection were mainly acute or chronic inflammatory process of the ileocolic region, usually with stenosis and seldom with interenteric fistula or fistula to the bladder. The proportion of conversion was 5%[4] to 41%[3] and depended on the experience as well as the extent of inflammation.

The operative time was not different between groups (Figure 11.4.1; Table 11.4.2). Hospital stay was –2.23 days (–2.94 to –1.53) shorter after laparoscopic surgery (Figure 11.4.2). Morbidity was also not different between groups (Figure 11.4.3). No patient died after laparoscopic or conventional resection.

Table 11.4.2. Comparison of outcomes of comparative cohort studies for CD

Outcome	Studies	Patients	Statistical method	Effect size
Operative time (min)	7	311	WMD (fixed), 95% CI	–4.64 [–11.23, 1.94]
Hospital stay (days)	6	266	WMD (fixed), 95% CI	–2.23 [–2.94, –1.53]
Morbidity	7	318	RR (fixed), 95% CI	0.89 [0.54, 1.48]

WMD, weighted mean difference; CI, confidence interval.

Review: Laparoscopic versus conventional colectomy in Crohn's disease
Comparison: 02 Hospital stay
Outcome: 01 Hospital stay

Study or sub-category	N	Laparoscopic Mean (SD)	N	Conventional Mean (SD)	WMD (fixed) 95% CI
Luan et al.	17	11.00 (2.00)	23	14.00 (2.00)	
Milsom JW et al.	31	5.00 (6.00)	29	6.00 (4.00)	
Benoist S et al.	24	7.70 (3.00)	32	8.00 (2.00)	
Shore G et al.	20	4.25 (1.50)	20	8.25 (4.00)	
Von Allmen et al.	12	5.50 (4.20)	18	11.50 (5.00)	
Huilgol RV et al.	21	6.40 (3.10)	19	8.20 (2.50)	
Total (95% CI)	125		141		

Test for heterogeneity: $Chi^2 = 18.42$, df = 5 (P = 0.002), $I^2 = 72.9\%$
Test for overall effect: Z = 6.21 (P < 0.00001)

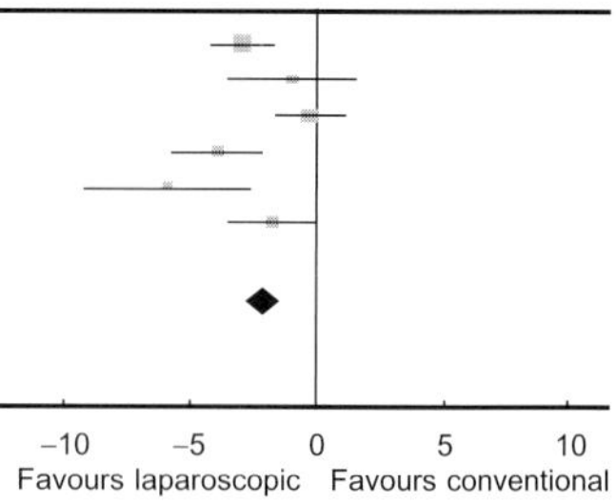

−10 −5 0 5 10
Favours laparoscopic Favours conventional

Figure 11.4.2. Hospital stay [weighted mean difference (WMD) including the 95% confidence interval (CI)] after laparoscopic and conventional surgery for CD.

Discussion

"Pure" laparoscopic treatment of both small and large bowel diseases is uncommonly described in the literature because an incision somewhere on the abdominal wall is needed whether done by a pure method or by an assisted method, and the size of this incision is nearly the same whichever technique is used. Thus, the handling of the thickened Crohn's mesentery and intestine is much easier when an assisted method is used. Whether hand-assisted laparoscopic surgery may facilitate the procedure has to be shown in the future. However, if hand dissection may permit the surgeon to accomplish a procedure in which the only significant incision is placed in the suprapubic area, it may be an advantage.

Review: Laparoscopic versus conventional colectomy in Crohn's disease
Comparison: 03 Morbidity
Outcome: 01 Morbidity

Study or sub-category	Laparoscopic n/N	Conventional n/N	RR (fixed) 95% CI
Luan et al.	3/24	4/23	
Milsom JW et al.	6/31	9/29	
Duepree HJ et al.	3/21	4/24	
Benoist S et al.	5/24	3/32	
Shore G et al.	0/20	1/20	
Von Allmen et al.	1/12	2/18	
Huilgol RV et al.	4/21	3/19	
Total (95% CI)	153	165	

Total events: 22 (Laparoscopic), 28 (Conventional)
Test for heterogeneity: $Chi^2 = 3.10$, df = 6 (P = 0.80), $I^2 = 0\%$
Test for overall effect: Z = 0.44 (P = 0.66)

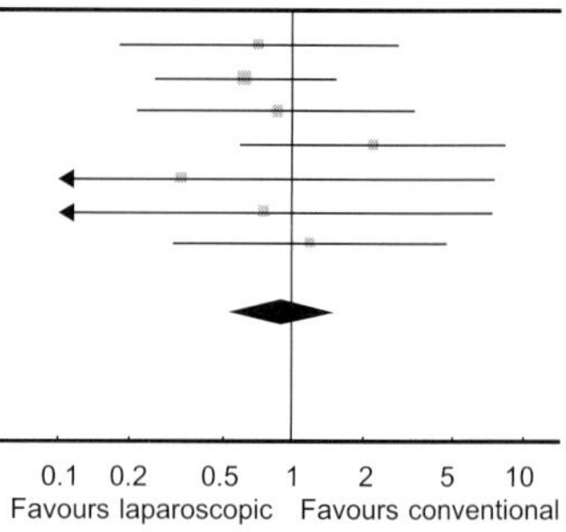

0.1 0.2 0.5 1 2 5 10
Favours laparoscopic Favours conventional

Figure 11.4.3. Morbidity [risk ratio (RR) including the 95% confidence interval (CI)] after laparoscopic and conventional surgery for CD.

Clinical reports have emerged over the past 12 years describing that the treatment of CD using laparoscopic methods, particularly ileocolic resections, are feasible and safe. Most have been uncontrolled, and nonrandomized. There remains only one RCT[2] comparing a laparoscopic-assisted method with open surgery in the treatment of ileocolonic CD. Shorter hospital stay, longer operative time, and less morbidity were described in accordance with the findings of the RCTs for colorectal cancer.

However, the available evidence from the nonrandomized studies do not support a longer operative time or less morbidity. Whether this is attributable to the nonrandomized design of the studies or to the disease cannot be answered yet. Future RCTs have to prove that the benefits seen in laparoscopic colorectal cancer surgery are also available in CD.

Although reliable long-term results after laparoscopic resection for CD are not available, it is assumed that they are not different from the conventional approach because the indication for surgery and the extent of resection are the same.

Conclusion

Laparoscopic surgery for CD is safe and feasible. Based on the current evidence, clinically relevant benefits have not actually been proven at this point in time.

Final Questions for Consideration

1. Is the laparoscopic approach associated with less morbidity?
   No (Recommendation C).
2. Does the laparoscopic approach lead to less mortality?
   No (Recommendation C).
3. What are the short-term advantages to the laparoscopic approach?
   Hospital stay is shorter (Recommendation B).
4. Does the laparoscopic approach increase hospital costs?
   Not known because no RCTs have addressed cost-savings for the hospital or society. (Recommendation D).
5. Are the long-term results in favor of the laparoscopic approach?
   Not known because no studies have addressed the long-term results (Recommendation D).

References

1. Milsom JW, Lavery IC, Böhm B et al. Laparoscopically assisted ileocolectomy in Crohn's disease. Surg Laparosc Endosc 1993;3:77–80.
2. Milsom JW, Hammerhofer KA, Bohm B, et al. Prospective, randomized trial comparing laparoscopic vs. conventional surgery for refractory ileocolic Crohn's disease. Dis Colon Rectum 2001;44:1–8.
3. Luan X, Gross E. Laparoscopic assisted surgery for Crohn's disease: an initial experience and results. J Tongji Med Univ 2000;20:332–335.

4. Duepree HJ, Senagore AJ, Delaney CP, et al. Advantages of laparoscopic resection for ileocecal Crohn's disease. Dis Colon Rectum 2002;45:605–610.
5. Shore G, Gonzalez QH, Bondora A, et al. Laparoscopic vs conventional ileocolectomy for primary Crohn disease. Arch Surg 2003;138:76–79.
6. Bergamaschi R, Pessaux P, Arnaud JP. Comparison of conventional and laparoscopic ileocolic resection for Crohn's disease. Dis Colon Rectum 2003;46:1129–1133.
7. Benoist S, Panis Y, Beaufour A, et al. Laparoscopic ileocecal resection in Crohn's disease: a case-matched comparison with open resection. Surg Endosc 2003;17:814–818.
8. von Allmen D, Markowitz JE, York A, et al. Laparoscopic-assisted bowel resection offers advantages over open surgery for treatment of segmental Crohn's disease in children. J Pediatr Surg 2003;38:963–965.
9. Huilgol RL, Wright CM, Solomon MJ. Laparoscopic versus open ileocolic resection for Crohn's disease. J Laparoendosc Adv Surg Tech A 2004; 14:61–65.

Chapter 11.5

Outcomes After Laparoscopic Total Colectomy or Proctocolectomy

Jeffrey W. Milsom, Bartholomäus Böhm, and Kiyokazu Nakajima

Total colectomy with ileostomy or restorative proctocolectomy is sometimes indicated in patients with ulcerative colitis or familial adenomatosis polyposis (FAP). Both procedures have been described in the literature using laparoscopic approaches. Whether these advanced procedures are feasible, safe, and beneficial compared with an open approach is answered in this chapter.

Methods

Search of Literature

The literature database MEDLINE was searched for all clinical studies for the years 1993–2004. The MeSh-terms "total colectomy," "proctocolectomy," "laparoscopy*," and "laparoscopic surgery*" were used for the search and more than 60 publications written in English were found. Laparoscopic, laparoscopic-assisted, and hand-assisted procedures were included. Individual case reports and small case series (less than 18) were excluded. Clinical studies reported in multiple publications or data given only as abstracts were also excluded from further analysis.

Outcomes

The studies were carefully analyzed and the following items extracted if given: indication for surgery, morbidity, mortality, the proportion of conversion to a conventional approach, the duration of surgery, time to first flatus, time to resumption of a regular diet, and the length of postoperative hospital stay. All endpoints were looked at in the comparative cohort studies, summarized in an "intent-to-treat" analysis, and compared between laparoscopic and conventional surgery. If long-term results were available, the length of follow-up and recurrence rate were documented.

Data Analysis

The overall quality of the studies would be classified as level of evidence 3–5. Most of the studies we found were very small retrospective or prospective case series which were excluded from this analysis. A randomized controlled trial was not found. Six studies[1–6] compared the laparoscopic and open approaches in patients with colitis or FAP (Table 11.5.1). Two studies[7,8] compared the laparoscopic procedure with the hand-assisted laparoscopic surgery procedure.

Table 11.5.1. Method of the comparative cohort studies for total colectomy or proctocolectomy

Author	Period (months)	n	Rate
Marcello et al.[1] Data about 20 laparoscopic procedures were prospectively collected and compared with matched controls in the same period.	72	40	0.6
Brown et al.[3] Retrospective study. Laparoscopic procedures were accomplished 1996–1997 followed by minilaparotomy 1997–1999.	46	25	0.5
Marcello et al.[2] Laparoscopic total colectomy for acute colitis of two institutions were prospectively evaluated and compared with matched controls in the same period.	36	48	1.3
Dunker et al.[4] Retrospective study. Laparoscopic restorative proctocolectomy was compared with matched controls of the same period.	42	35	0.8
Hashimoto et al.[5] Laparoscopic cases were compared with historical controls.	–	25	–
Proctor et al.[10] Laparoscopic cases were compared with historical controls of the same surgeon.	–	18	–

The length of the study in months (period) and number of resections (n) were given to calculate the resection rate per month (rate).

Table 11.5.2. Comparison of outcomes of all comparative studies (n = 5) for total colectomy or proctocolectomy

Outcome	Studies	Patients	Statistical method	Effect size
Operative time (min)	6	187	WMD (random), 95% CI	93.38 [58.25, 128.51]
Hospital stay (days)	6	187	WMD (random), 95% CI	–1.98 [–3.23, –0.73]
Morbidity	6	187	RR (random), 95% CI	0.96 [0.60, 1.52]

WMD, weighted mean difference; CI, 95% confidence interval; RR, risk ratio.

Results

The indications for total colectomy or proctocolectomy were in nearly all cases mucosal ulcerative colitis or FAP. All comparative studies reported no conversions at all.

The laparoscopic approach took more than 90 minutes longer (Table 11.5.2; Figure 11.5.1). The hospital stay was 2 days shorter (Figure 11.5.2). Morbidity was about 25% and not different between groups (Figure 11.5.3).

Dunker et al.[4] did not find any difference in the quality of life after a mean follow-up of 9.5 months between laparoscopic or open proctocolectomy.

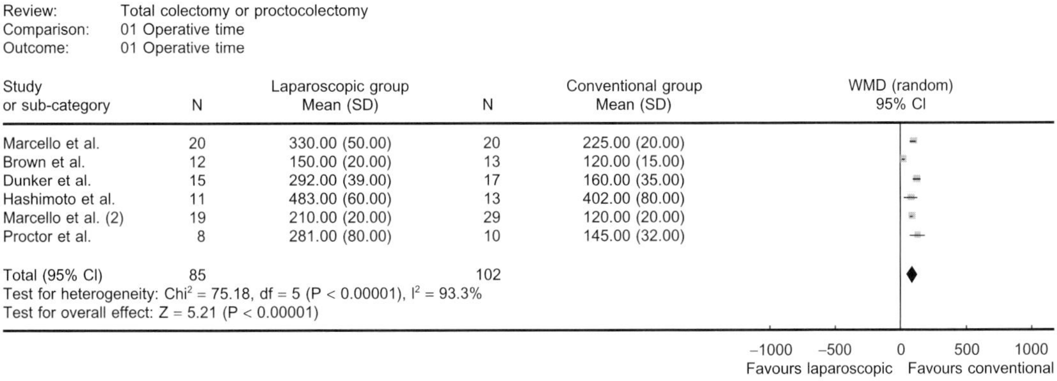

Review: Total colectomy or proctocolectomy
Comparison: 01 Operative time
Outcome: 01 Operative time

Study or sub-category	N	Laparoscopic group Mean (SD)	N	Conventional group Mean (SD)	WMD (random) 95% CI
Marcello et al.	20	330.00 (50.00)	20	225.00 (20.00)	
Brown et al.	12	150.00 (20.00)	13	120.00 (15.00)	
Dunker et al.	15	292.00 (39.00)	17	160.00 (35.00)	
Hashimoto et al.	11	483.00 (60.00)	13	402.00 (80.00)	
Marcello et al. (2)	19	210.00 (20.00)	29	120.00 (20.00)	
Proctor et al.	8	281.00 (80.00)	10	145.00 (32.00)	
Total (95% CI)	85		102		

Test for heterogeneity: $Chi^2 = 75.18$, df = 5 ($P < 0.00001$), $I^2 = 93.3\%$
Test for overall effect: Z = 5.21 ($P < 0.00001$)

–1000 –500 0 500 1000
Favours laparoscopic Favours conventional

Figure 11.5.1. Operative time [weighted mean difference (WMD) including the 95% confidence interval (CI)] after laparoscopic and conventional surgery for total colectomy or proctocolectomy.

Review: Total colectomy or proctocolectomy
Comparison: 02 Hospital stay
Outcome: 01 Hospital stay

Study or sub-category	N	Laparoscopic group Mean (SD)	N	Conventional group Mean (SD)	WMD (random) 95% CI
Marcello et al.	20	7.00 (1.00)	20	8.00 (1.80)	
Brown et al.	12	7.50 (2.00)	13	8.00 (1.30)	
Dunker et al.	15	9.90 (2.40)	17	12.50 (2.70)	
Hashimoto et al.	11	24.00 (4.00)	13	31.00 (5.00)	
Marcello et al. (2)	19	4.00 (1.60)	29	6.00 (3.20)	
Proctor et al.	8	23.00 (16.00)	10	29.00 (8.00)	
Total (95% CI)	85		102		

Test for heterogeneity: Chi² = 14.81, df = 5 (P = 0.01), I² = 66.2%
Test for overall effect: Z = 3.11 (P = 0.002)

–10 –5 0 5 10
Favours laparoscopic Favours conventional

Figure 11.5.2. Hospital stay [weighted mean difference (WMD) including the 95% confidence interval (CI)] after laparoscopic and conventional surgery for total colectomy or proctocolectomy.

Discussion

The available studies prove that a total colectomy and proctocolectomy can be accomplished with a low morbidity, longer operative time, and shorter hospital stay. However, operative time as well as hospital stay varied widely between groups.

Whether hand-assisted laparoscopic surgery may be preferable over the laparoscopic-assisted approach was evaluated in a nonrandomized study by Nakajima et al.[7] and Rivadeneira et al.[8] Both study groups described a similar morbidity and incision length but a shorter operative time.

Even a one-stage laparoscopic restorative proctocolectomy can be safely accomplished. Ky et al.[9] reported a low morbidity on 32 cases.

Review: Total colectomy or proctocolectomy
Comparison: 03 Morbidity
Outcome: 01 Morbidity

Study or sub-category	Laparoscopic group n/N	Conventional group n/N	RR (random) 95% CI
Marcello et al.	4/20	5/20	
Brown et al.	2/12	2/13	
Dunker et al.	2/15	4/17	
Hashimoto et al.	6/11	5/13	
Marcello et al. (2)	3/19	7/29	
Proctor et al.	4/8	5/10	
Total (95% CI)	85	102	

Total events: 21 (Laparoscopic group), 28 (Conventional group)
Test for heterogeneity: Chi² = 1.77, df = 5 (P = 0.88), I² = 0%
Test for overall effect: Z = 0.19 (P = 0.85)

0.1 0.2 0.5 1 2 5 10
Favours laparoscopic Favours conventional

Figure 11.5.3. Morbidity [risk ratio (RR) including the 95% confidence interval (CI)] after laparoscopic and conventional surgery for total colectomy or proctocolectomy.

Conclusion

In conclusion, laparoscopic surgery for total colectomy or proctocolectomy also seems to be safe with good long-term results. Whether or not there are advantages over the open method remains to be proven in larger prospective comparative studies.

Final Questions for Consideration

1. Is the laparoscopic approach associated with less morbidity?
   No (Recommendation C).
2. Does the laparoscopic approach lead to less mortality?
   No (Recommendation C).
3. What are the short-term advantages to the laparoscopic approach?
   Hospital stay is shorter (Recommendation C).
4. Does the laparoscopic approach increase hospital costs?
   Not known because no comparative studies have addressed the costs (Recommendation D).
5. Are the long-term results in favor of the laparoscopic approach?
   Not known because no comparative studies have addressed the long-term results. (Recommendation D)

References

1. Marcello PW, Milsom JW, Wong SK, et al. Laparoscopic restorative proctocolectomy: case-matched comparative study with open restorative proctocolectomy. Dis Colon Rectum 2000;43:604–608.
2. Marcello PW, Milsom JW, Wong SK, et al. Laparoscopic total colectomy for acute colitis: a case-control study. Dis Colon Rectum 2001;44:1441–1445.
3. Brown SR, Eu KW, Seow-Choen F. Consecutive series of laparoscopic-assisted vs. minilaparotomy restorative proctocolectomies. Dis Colon Rectum 2001;44:397–400.
4. Dunker MS, Bemelman WA, Slors JF, et al. Functional outcome, quality of life, body image, and cosmesis in patients after laparoscopic-assisted and conventional restorative proctocolectomy: a comparative study. Dis Colon Rectum 2001;44:1800–1807.
5. Hashimoto A, Funayama Y, Naito H, et al. Laparoscope-assisted versus conventional restorative proctocolectomy with rectal mucosectomy. Surg Today 2001;31:210–214.
6. Proctor ML, Langer JC, Gerstle JT, et al. Is laparoscopic subtotal colectomy better than open subtotal colectomy in children? J Pediatr Surg 2002;37:706–708.
7. Nakajima K, Lee SW, Cocilovo C, et al. Laparoscopic total colectomy: hand-assisted vs standard technique. Surg Endosc 2004;18:582–586.
8. Rivadeneira DE, Marcello PW, Roberts PL, et al. Benefits of hand-assisted laparoscopic restorative proctocolectomy: a comparative study. Dis Colon Rectum 2004;47:1371–1376.
9. Ky AJ, Sonoda T, Milsom JW. One-stage laparoscopic restorative proctocolectomy: an alternative to the conventional approach? Dis Colon Rectum 2002;45:207–210.
10. Proctor ML, Langer JC, Gerstle JT, et al. Is laparoscopic subtotal colectomy better than open subtotal colectomy in children? J Pediatr Surg 2002;37:706–708.

Chapter 11.6

Outcomes After Laparoscopic Treatment for Rectal Prolapse

Jeffrey W. Milsom, Bartholomäus Böhm, and Kiyokazu Nakajima

Rectal prolapse is a rare disease but can usually be cured by surgery. Many abdominal and perineal approaches have been described in the past. Currently, abdominal surgery with some type of rectopexy plus or minus sigmoid resection is the most common abdominal operation to treat rectal prolapse. Because different opinions about the best available procedure are well known and the debate is unsettled, this chapter only discusses whether the laparoscopic approach is beneficial compared with the conventional approach if an abdominal procedure is chosen to treat the prolapse.

Methods

Search of Literature

The literature database MEDLINE was searched for all clinical studies for the years 1993–2004. The MeSh-terms "rectal prolapse," "rectopexy," "laparoscopy*," and "laparoscopic surgery*" were used for the search and more than 100 publications written in English were found. Laparoscopic, laparoscopic-assisted, and hand-assisted procedures were included. Clinical studies including patients with other diseases, studies reported in multiple publications, small case series with less than 18 patients, or data given only as abstracts were excluded from further analysis.

Outcomes

The studies were carefully analyzed and the following items extracted if given: Morbidity, mortality, the proportion of conversion to a conventional approach, the duration of surgery, time to first flatus, time to resumption of a regular diet, and the length of postoperative hospital stay. All endpoints were looked at in the comparative cohort studies, summarized in an "intent-to-treat" analysis, and compared between laparoscopic and conventional surgery. If long-term results were available, the length of follow-up and recurrence rate were documented.

Table 11.6.1. Method of the comparative cohort studies on rectal prolapse

Author	Period (months)	n	Rate
Solomon et al.[1] RCT.	36	39	1.1
Kairaluoma et al.[5] Fifty-six laparoscopic procedures were compared with 56 historical controls which were retrospectively analyzed.	90	56	0.6
Xynos et al.[10] Ten laparoscopic procedures were compared with 8 historical controls. The observational period was not given.	–	18	–
Baker et al.[4] Laparoscopic approach was compared with historical controls.	54	18	0.3

The length of the study in months (period) and number of resections (n) was given to calculate the resection rate per month (rate).

Data Analysis

The overall quality of the studies would be classified as level of evidence 3–5. Most of the studies we found were very small retrospective or prospective case series which were excluded from this analysis. There is only one randomized controlled trial (RCT) that compared both laparoscopic and open approaches in patients with rectal prolapse.[1] A second publication was written on the same trial to evaluate the economic impact.[2] This RCT and three comparative cohort studies[3–5] were analyzed (Table 11.6.1).

Results

The RCT[1] described a longer operative time, shorter hospital stay, and quicker resumption of liquid and normal diet. No conversion was required. The stress response (IL-6, CRP, and catecholamine) was more pronounced after conventional surgery. The morbidity was 3/20 in the laparoscopic group and 9/19 in the conventional group ($P = .03$). The economic analysis showed that the mean hospital costs were £2812 in the laparoscopic group and £3169 in the conventional group. The difference was £357 [95% confidence interval (CI): £164 to £592]. This advantage of the laparoscopic approach is attributed to the longer hospital stay. The costs in the operating room are higher in the laparoscopic group.

Table 11.6.2. Comparison of outcomes of all comparative studies (n = 5) for rectal prolapse

Outcome	Studies	Patients	Statistical method	Effect size
Operative time (min)	4	181	WMD (random), 95% CI	65.54 [46.77, 84.31]
Hospital stay (days)	4	181	WMD (random), 95% CI	−2.00 [−3.91, −0.08]
Morbidity	4	181	RR (random), 95% CI	0.58 [0.30, 1.13]

WMD, weighted mean difference; CI, 95% confidence interval; RR, risk ratio.

The comparative studies and RCTs prove that operative time is about 65 minutes longer (Table 11.6.2; Figure 11.6.1) and hospital stay 2 days shorter (Figure 11.6.2). Morbidity may also be less after laparoscopic surgery (Figure 11.6.3).

Discussion

Whereas the perineal approach (perineal resection or the Delorme procedure) is usually performed in elderly or high-risk patients, the abdominal approach is generally preferred in otherwise healthy patients because of the lower incidence of recurrence.

Different abdominal procedures have been recommended to cure rectal prolapse. Madbouly et al.[6] described good results after laparoscopic Wells procedure (n = 13) and sutured rectopexy with resection (n = 11). The Wells procedure needed less operative time and shorter hospital stay.

The long-term results are overall acceptable. Stevenson et al.[7] reported on no full thickness recurrence after 18 months (n = 26), Kessler et al.[8] on 2/32 recurrence after 33 months, and Bruch et al.[9] on 0/53 recurrences after 30 months.

Review: Rectal prolapse
Comparison: 01 Operative time
Outcome: 01 Operative time

Study or sub-category	N	Laparoscopic group Mean (SD)	N	Conventional group Mean (SD)	WMD (random) 95% CI
Baker et al.	8	177.00 (23.00)	10	87.00 (9.00)	
Xynos et al.	10	130.00 (32.00)	8	80.00 (25.00)	
Solomon et al.	20	153.00 (20.00)	19	102.00 (20.00)	
Kairalouma et al.	53	170.00 (50.00)	53	101.00 (30.00)	
Total (95% CI)	91		90		

Test for heterogeneity: Chi² = 14.68, df = 3 (P = 0.002), I² = 79.6%
Test for overall effect: Z = 6.84 (P < 0.00001)

−100 −50 0 50 100
Favours laparoscopic Favours conventional

Figure 11.6.1. Operative time [weighted mean difference (WMD) including the 95% CI] after laparoscopic and conventional surgery for rectal prolapse.

Review: Rectal prolapse
Comparison: 02 Hospital stay
Outcome: 01 Hospital stay

Study or sub-category	N	Laparoscopic group Mean (SD)	N	Conventional group Mean (SD)	WMD (random) 95% CI
Baker et al.	8	4.00 (0.80)	10	2.90 (0.40)	
Xynos et al.	10	4.70 (1.10)	8	8.30 (1.90)	
Solomon et al.	20	3.90 (0.50)	19	6.60 (2.00)	
Kairalouma et al.	53	5.00 (4.30)	53	7.00 (5.00)	
Total (95% CI)	91		90		

Test for heterogeneity: $Chi^2 = 38.39$, df = 3 ($P < 0.00001$), $I^2 = 92.2\%$
Test for overall effect: Z = 2.05 (P = 0.04)

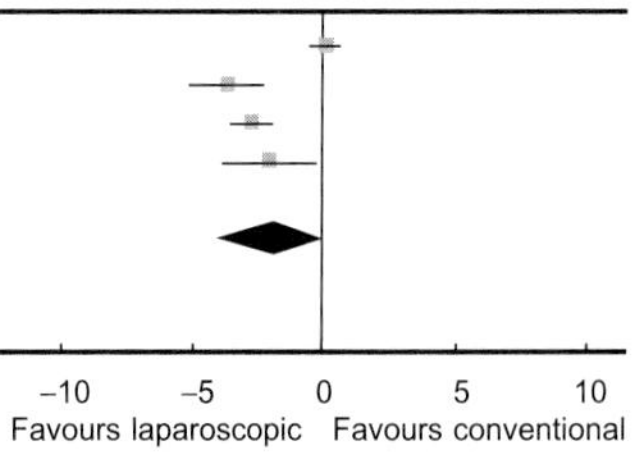

–10 –5 0 5 10
Favours laparoscopic Favours conventional

Figure 11.6.2. Hospital stay [weighted mean difference (WMD) including the 95% CI] after laparoscopic and conventional surgery for rectal prolapse.

Conclusion

In conclusion, laparoscopic surgery for rectal prolapse also seems to be safe with good long-term results. Whether there are advantages over the open method or whether morbidity is really lower has to be proven in further studies.

Final Questions for Consideration

1. Is the laparoscopic approach associated with less morbidity? Likely (Recommendation C).
2. Does the laparoscopic approach lead to less mortality? No (Recommendation C).

Review: Rectal prolapse
Comparison: 03 Morbidity
Outcome: 01 Morbidity

Study or sub-category	Laparoscopic group n/N	Conventional group n/N	RR (random) 95% CI
Baker et al.	1/8	0/10	
Xynos et al.	1/10	3/8	
Solomon et al.	3/20	9/19	
Kairalouma et al.	12/53	16/53	
Total (95% CI)	91	90	

Total events: 17 (Laparoscopic group), 28 (Conventional group)
Test for heterogeneity: $Chi^2 = 3.58$, df = 3 (P = 0.31), $I^2 = 16.1\%$
Test for overall effect: Z = 1.61 (P = 0.11)

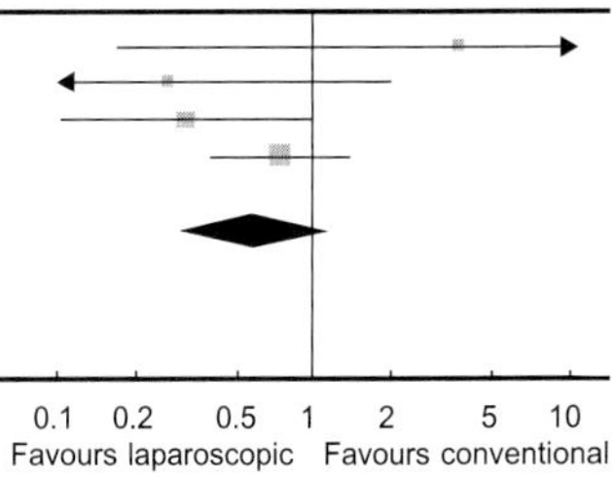

0.1 0.2 0.5 1 2 5 10
Favours laparoscopic Favours conventional

Figure 11.6.3. Morbidity [risk ratio (RR) including the 95% CI] after laparoscopic and conventional surgery for rectal prolapse.

3. What are the short-term advantages to the laparoscopic approach?
   Hospital stay is shorter and morbidity is lower (Recommendation C).
4. Does the laparoscopic approach increase hospital costs?
   No (Recommendation B).
5. Are the long-term results in favor of the laparoscopic approach?
   Not known because no comparative studies have addressed the long-term results (Recommendation D).

References

1. Solomon MJ, Young CJ, Eyers AA, et al. Randomized clinical trial of laparoscopic versus open abdominal rectopexy for rectal prolapse. Br J Surg 2002;89:35–39.
2. Salkeld G, Bagia M, Solomon M. Economic impact of laparoscopic versus open abdominal rectopexy. Br J Surg 2004;91:1188–1191.
3. Xynos E, Chrysos E, Tsiaoussis J, et al. Resection rectopexy for rectal prolapse. The laparoscopic approach. Surg Endosc 1999;13:862–864.
4. Baker R, Senagore AJ, Luchtefeld MA. Laparoscopic-assisted vs. open resection. Rectopexy offers excellent results. Dis Colon Rectum 1995; 38:199–201.
5. Kairaluoma MV, Viljakka MT, Kellokumpu IH. Open vs. laparoscopic surgery for rectal prolapse: a case-controlled study assessing short-term outcome. Dis Colon Rectum 2003;46:353–360.
6. Madbouly KM, Senagore AJ, Delaney CP, et al. Clinically based management of rectal prolapse. Surg Endosc 2003;17:99–103.
7. Stevenson AR, Stitz RW, Lumley JW. Laparoscopic-assisted resection-rectopexy for rectal prolapse: early and medium follow-up. Dis Colon Rectum 1998;41:46–54.
8. Kessler H, Jerby BL, Milsom JW. Successful treatment of rectal prolapse by laparoscopic suture rectopexy. Surg Endosc 1999;13:858–861.
9. Bruch HP, Herold A, Schiedeck T, et al. Laparoscopic surgery for rectal prolapse and outlet obstruction. Dis Colon Rectum 1999;42:1189–1194.
10. Xynos E, Chrysos E, Tsiaoussis J, et al. Resection rectopexy for rectal prolapse. The laparoscopic approach. Surg Endosc 1999;13:862–864.

Chapter 11.7

Outcomes After Laparoscopic Colorectal Cancer Surgery

Wolfgang Schwenk

Four years after the first laparoscopic colectomy was performed, Lacy et al.[1] published the first randomized controlled trial (RCT) comparing the short-term outcomes after laparoscopic and conventional colectomy. Since then, more than 30 publications from RCTs have investigated different aspects of the postoperative course after laparoscopic or conventional colorectal surgery. This chapter presents the results of a thorough search of the literature to identify all RCTs available on this topic up until December 2004. We also performed a metaanalysis and will summarize it here. Please note that nearly all studies done concerned colon cancer and not rectal cancer, a point that will be emphasized during our considerations of this literature.

Methods

Search of Literature

The literature databases MEDLINE, EMBASE, CancerLit, and the Cochrane Central Controlled Trials Register were searched for RCTs for the years 1991–2004. The MeSh-terms "colon*," "colectomy," "proctectomy*," "intestine-large*," "colonic neoplasm," "rectal neoplasm," and "laparosc*" were used for the search and 37 publications found. RCTs that contained only patients with benign disease (i.e., Crohn's disease or rectal prolapse) (n = 2) were excluded from further analysis, as well as publications that gave only laboratory data without any clinical outcome (n = 3). Furthermore, trials using any form of "pseudo-randomization," patients included in multiple publications (n = 8), or data given only as abstracts (n = 3) were also excluded from the analysis. Laparoscopic or laparoscopic-assisted colorectal cancer resections or abdominal wall lift technique were included. "Hand-assisted" laparoscopic procedures were not included in the analysis.

Outcomes

The following short-term outcome measures were analyzed: duration of surgery, estimated intraoperative blood loss, functional data (postoperative pulmonary function, duration of postoperative ileus), postoperative hospital stay, morbidity, and mortality. Subcutaneous wound infection, anastomotic leakage, intraabdominal abscess, ileus, pulmonary, or cardiac complications were analyzed separately.

Whenever available, the following long-term data for long-term outcomes were extracted from the publications: duration of follow-up, tumor recurrence rate (local, metastatic, and total), cancer-related 5-year survival rate, and overall 5-year survival rate.

Data Analysis

All studies that met the selection criteria mentioned above were included in the data analysis. For continuous data, weighted mean differences (WMD) with their corresponding 95% confidence intervals (CIs) were calculated. When no measure of variation was given at all, the study was excluded from the analysis. For dichotomous data, the risk ratio (RR) with their 95% CIs were calculated. Results for dichotomous data were calculated using a random effects model.

Results

Characteristics of Included RCTs

Nineteen RCTs were included in the analysis. The COLOR trial[2] has been published in abstract and was presented at the annual meeting of the European Association of Endoscopic Surgeons in Glasgow Scotland in 2003. Because of the large amount of patients recruited by this trial (>1000), data available from the Glasgow presentation have been included in this analysis. Final data analysis from the COLOR trial is still awaiting publication in printed form. Therefore, slight changes of these data are possible.

The 19 RCTs identified included more than 3500 patients, but 10 trials recruited less than 100 patients. Five RCTs included cancer patients as well as patients with benign indications for surgery. All RCTs included colonic cancer but only seven trials included (mostly upper) rectal cancers. Only six publications gave any information concerning the type of incision used in conventional surgery and these studies all used a midline incision. Details of the postoperative analgesic technique were given in nine publications. In four of these trials, a thoracic epidural analgesia was administered for pain relief, whereas three trials used a systemic opioid patient-controlled analgesia (PCA) regimen, and in two trials opioids were given on demand (Table 11.7.1).

Only six RCTs were considered to be of good methodological quality. Problems with the other RCTs included: Eight publications did not define a main study criterion, only 11 manuscripts mentioned an a priori sample size calculation, and most publications did not give details about the randomization process (i.e., technique and concealment of randomization). Only 11 trials used an "intention-to-treat" approach, analyzing the data of patients converted from laparoscopic to conventional surgery within the laparoscopic group (Table 11.7.1).

Table 11.7.1. Characteristics of RCT comparing laparoscopic and conventional colorectal resection

Author and year	Method	No. of patients	Indications/location	Laparotomy	Analgesia	Outcomes
Ortiz et al.[11] 1996	No SSC; preop. random; no ITT	30	Cancer, benign disease; left/right colon, rectum >2 cm from dl	Not stated	Not stated	MST: duration of ileus; other data: operative time, morbidity
Stage et al.[12] 1997	No SSC; preop. random; no ITT	29	Cancer; colon	Midline or paramedian incision	tPDA-LA/O	MST: not stated; other data: operative time, pain, pulmonary function, morbidity, hospital stay
Hewitt et al.[13] 1998	SSC; random?; no ITT	15	Cancer; left/right colon, rectum >10 cm from dl	Not stated	PCA-O	MST: immunology; other data: operative time, analgetic dose, morbidity, hospital stay
Milsom et al.[14] 1998	SSC; intraop. random; ITT	109	Cancer; left/right colon, no transverse, rectum >12 cm from dl or requiring APR	Midline incision	PCA-O	MST: pulmonary function; other data: operative time, analgetic dose, duration of ileus, morbidity, hospital stay
Leung et al.[15] 2000	SSC; preop. random; ITT	34	Cancer; rectosigmoid >5 cm from dl	Not stated	OD-O	MST: cytokine and C-reactive protein; other data: operative time, pain, analgetic dose, duration of ileus, morbidity, hospital stay
Curet et al.[16] 2000	No SSC; preop. random; no ITT	36	Cancer; left/right colon	Not stated	Not stated	MST: not stated; other data: operative time, morbidity, hospital stay
Tang et al.[17] 2001	SSC; preop. random; no ITT	236	Cancer; left/right colon, no transverse, no TME	Not stated	Not stated	MST: immune and stress response; other data: operative time, morbidity

(Continued)

Table 11.7.1. Characteristics of RCT comparing laparoscopic and conventional colorectal resection (*Continued*)

Author and year	Method	No. of patients	Indications/location	Laparotomy	Analgesia	Outcomes
Lacy et al.[3] 2002	SSC; preop. random; ITT	219	Cancer; left/right colon above 15 cm from dl, no transverse	Not stated	Not stated	MST: cancer-related survival; other data: operative time, duration of ileus, morbidity, hospital stay
Braga et al.[18] 2002	SSC; preop. random; ITT	269	Cancer, benign disease; left/right colon, rectum >4 cm from dl	Not stated	tPDA-LA	MST: morbidity; other data: operative time, duration of ileus, morbidity, hospital stay, recovery of physical function
Liang et al.[19] 2002	No SSC; preop. random; ITT	39	Cancer, polyps; sigmoid colon	Not stated	Not stated	MST: not stated; other data: operative time, duration of ileus, hospital stay, pain, morbidity, disability, inflammatory and immunologic parameter
Schwenk et al.[20] 2002	SSC; intraop. random; ITT	103	Cancer, large polyps; left/right colon, no transverse, rectum >12 cm from dl or requiring APR	Midline	PCA-O	MST: pulmonary function; other data: operative time, duration of ileus, morbidity, hospital stay, fatigue, quality of life
Winslow et al.[10] 2002	No SSC; preop. random; no ITT	83	Cancer; left/right colon, no transverse	Midline	Not stated	MST: wound complications; other data: operative time, morbidity
Danelli et al.[21] 2002	SSC; preop. random; ITT	44	Cancer, benign disease; no location given	Midline	tPDA-LA	MST: perioperative core body temperature; other data: duration of ileus

Weeks et al.[22] 2002	SSC; preop. random; ITT	449	Cancer; left/right colon, no transverse	Not stated	No standard*	MST: quality of life; other data: pain, hospital stay
Hildebrandt et al.[23] 2003	No SSC; preop. random; ITT	42	Cancer, Crohn's disease; left/right colon, no transverse	Midline	Not stated	MST: not stated; other data: operative time, inflammatory and immunologic parameters
Hasegawa et al.[24] 2003	No SSC; preop. random; ITT	50	Cancer; left/right colon, no transverse	Not stated	tPDA-LA/O	MST: not stated; other data: operative time, inflammatory and immunologic response, duration of ileus, morbidity, hospital stay
COLOR[2] 2003	SSC; preop. random; ITT	1005	Cancer; left/right colon, no transverse, rectum >15 cm from dl	Not stated	Not stated	MST: cancer-related survival; other data: operative time, duration of ileus, morbidity, mortality, postoperative hospital stay
COST[5] 2004	SSC; preop. random; ITT	863	Cancer; left/right colon, no transverse	Not stated	No standard*	MST: time to tumor recurrence; other data: overall and cancer-related survival, morbidity, mortality, hospital stay
Leung et al.[4] 2004	SSC, preop. random; ITT	403	Rectosigmoid cancer	Not stated	OD-O	MST: survival; other data: morbidity, mortality, hospital stay

SSC, sample size calculation; random, time of randomization; ITT, "intention-to-treat" analysis; dl, dentate line; tPDA, thoracic epidural analgesia; OD, on demand; O, opioid; LA, local anesthetic; MST, main study criterion.
*Not standardized in a multicenter study.

Review: Short term benefits of laparoscopic colorectal resection (boehmbuch)
Comparison: 02 Operative data
Outcome: 03 Blood loss

Study or sub-category	N	Laparoscopic Mean (SD)	N	Conventional Mean (SD)
Milsom et al.	55	252.00 (222.00)	54	344.00 (626.00)
Curet et al.	18	284.00 (284.00)	18	407.00 (407.00)
Leung et al.	17	103.00 (103.00)	17	141.00 (141.00)
Braga et al.	40	123.00 (107.00)	39	319.00 (307.00)
Braga et al. (2)	136	170.00 (107.00)	133	286.00 (242.00)
Danelli et al.	23	300.00 (300.00)	21	300.00 (300.00)
Lacy et al.	111	105.00 (99.00)	108	193.00 (212.00)
Hasegawa et al.	24	58.00 (0.00)	26	137.00 (0.00)
COLOR study	500	100.00 (100.00)	505	175.00 (175.00)
Leung et al. (2)	203	169.00 (169.00)	200	238.00 (238.00)
Total (95% CI)	1127		1121	

Test for heterogeneity: $\text{Chi}^2 = 10.08$, df = 8 (P = 0.26), $I^2 = 20.7\%$
Test for overall effect: Z = 8.20 (P < 0.00001)

WMD (random) 95% CI

−1000 −500 0 500 1000
Favours laparoscopic Favours conventional

Figure 11.7.1. Blood loss (WMD including the 95% CI) after laparoscopic and conventional surgery for colorectal cancer.

Outcomes

Short-term Outcome

Intraoperative blood loss was estimated in 2248 patients from nine trials. The WMD between the laparoscopic and conventional group was −84 (−104 to −64) cc (Figure 11.7.1). Operative time was 50 (37–64) minutes longer in laparoscopic compared with conventional procedures (Figure 11.7.2).

Postoperative pulmonary function was assessed in three RCTs. Because of the different time intervals in which postoperative pulmonary function was measured and different approaches in visualizing

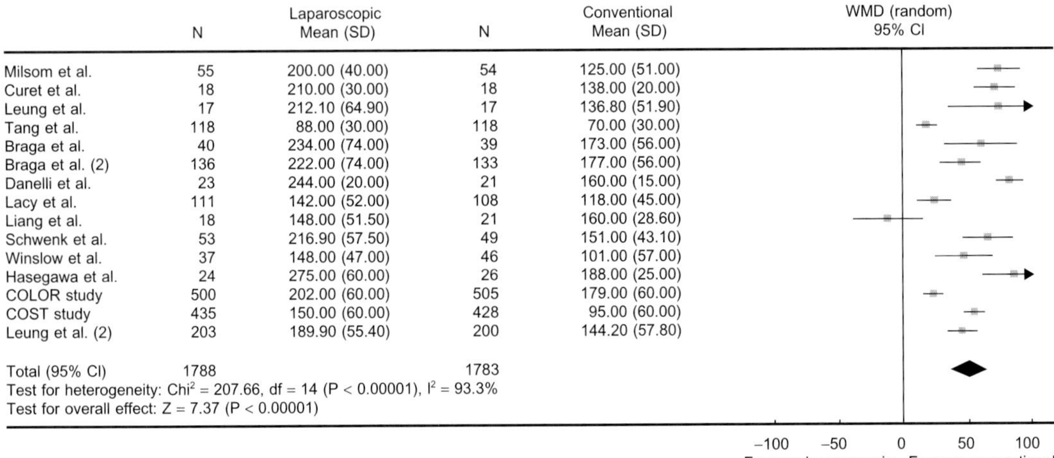

	N	Laparoscopic Mean (SD)	N	Conventional Mean (SD)
Milsom et al.	55	200.00 (40.00)	54	125.00 (51.00)
Curet et al.	18	210.00 (30.00)	18	138.00 (20.00)
Leung et al.	17	212.10 (64.90)	17	136.80 (51.90)
Tang et al.	118	88.00 (30.00)	118	70.00 (30.00)
Braga et al.	40	234.00 (74.00)	39	173.00 (56.00)
Braga et al. (2)	136	222.00 (74.00)	133	177.00 (56.00)
Danelli et al.	23	244.00 (20.00)	21	160.00 (15.00)
Lacy et al.	111	142.00 (52.00)	108	118.00 (45.00)
Liang et al.	18	148.00 (51.50)	21	160.00 (28.60)
Schwenk et al.	53	216.90 (57.50)	49	151.00 (43.10)
Winslow et al.	37	148.00 (47.00)	46	101.00 (57.00)
Hasegawa et al.	24	275.00 (60.00)	26	188.00 (25.00)
COLOR study	500	202.00 (60.00)	505	179.00 (60.00)
COST study	435	150.00 (60.00)	428	95.00 (60.00)
Leung et al. (2)	203	189.90 (55.40)	200	144.20 (57.80)
Total (95% CI)	1788		1783	

Test for heterogeneity: $\text{Chi}^2 = 207.66$, df = 14 (P < 0.00001), $I^2 = 93.3\%$
Test for overall effect: Z = 7.37 (P < 0.00001)

Figure 11.7.2. Operative time (WMD including the 95% CI) after laparoscopic and conventional surgery for colorectal cancer.

Review: Short term benefits of laparoscopic colorectal resection
Comparison: 05 Ileus
Outcome: 02 Duration until bowel movement

Study or sub-category	N	Laparoscopic Mean (SD)	N	Conventional Mean (SD)
Milsom et al.	55	4.80 (4.80)	54	4.80 (4.80)
Leung et al.	17	3.00 (3.00)	17	3.00 (3.00)
Braga et al.	40	5.00 (5.00)	39	6.00 (6.00)
Braga et al. (2)	136	4.70 (0.80)	133	5.70 (1.10)
Danelli et al.	23	3.00 (3.00)	21	4.00 (4.00)
Schwenk et al.	53	2.89 (1.32)	49	3.78 (0.91)
COLOR study	539	2.85 (2.85)	466	3.73 (3.73)
Leung et al. (2)	203	4.00 (4.00)	200	4.60 (4.60)
Total (95% CI)	1066		979	

Test for heterogeneity: $Chi^2 = 2.88$, df = 7 ($P = 0.90$), $I^2 = 0\%$
Test for overall effect: $Z = 10.30$ ($P < 0.00001$)

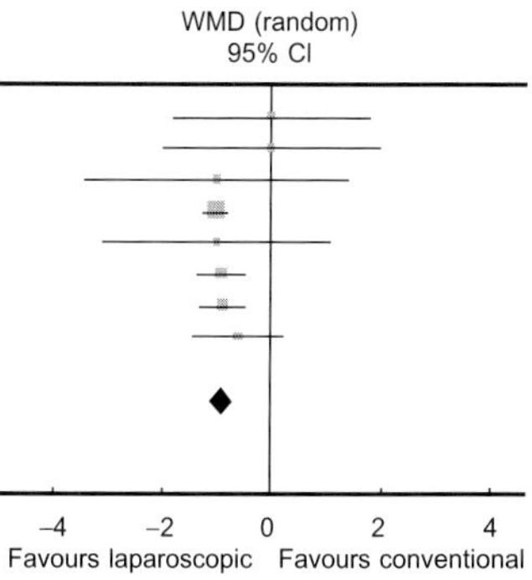

Figure 11.7.3. Time until first bowel movement (WMD including the 95% CI) after laparoscopic and conventional surgery for colorectal cancer.

postoperative recovery of pulmonary function (mean of each measurement vs. patients recovering 80% of preoperative function), different patients' numbers were measured on postoperative days 1–3. On postoperative days 1–3, pulmonary function was less impaired in laparoscopic patients. During this time, the WMDs between both groups ranged from 200 to 560 cc. Recovery of 80% of the preoperative pulmonary function was achieved 8 hours earlier in the laparoscopic group.

Duration of postoperative ileus was measured by time interval from surgery to the first bowel movement in seven RCTs. Gastrointestinal function was restored 0.93 days (0.75–1.1) earlier in patients undergoing laparoscopic surgery compared with conventional patients (Figure 11.7.3).

Patients operated on laparoscopically had a shorter hospital stay of 1.5 days (0.9–2.0) than patients who underwent conventional colorectal cancer resection (Figure 11.7.4).

Review: Short term benefits of laparoscopic colorectal resection
Comparison: 06 Hospital stay
Outcome: 01 Postoperative hospital stay

Study or sub-category	N	Laparoscopic Mean (SD)	N	Conventional Mean (SD)
Milsom et al.	55	6.00 (4.00)	54	7.00 (4.00)
Curet et al.	18	5.20 (1.00)	18	7.30 (2.00)
Braga et al.	40	9.10 (2.90)	39	11.70 (5.10)
Braga et al. (2)	136	10.40 (2.90)	133	12.50 (4.10)
Lacy et al.	111	5.20 (2.10)	108	7.90 (9.30)
Schwenk et al.	53	9.10 (2.90)	49	10.60 (2.04)
Weeks et al.	228	5.60 (0.30)	221	6.40 (0.20)
Leung et al. (2)	203	8.20 (3.20)	200	8.70 (3.70)
Total (95% CI)	844		822	

Test for heterogeneity: $Chi^2 = 25.73$, df = 7 ($P = 0.0006$), $I^2 = 72.8\%$
Test for overall effect: $Z = 5.11$ ($P < 0.00001$)

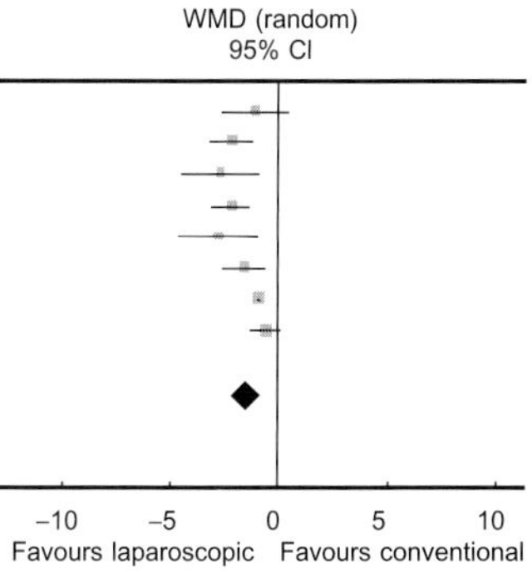

Figure 11.7.4. Hospital stay (WMD including the 95% CI) after laparoscopic and conventional surgery for colorectal cancer.

The relative risk of postoperative morbidity was 0.72 (0.56–0.92) in the laparoscopic group compared with the conventional approach (Figure 11.7.5). The absolute risk reduction (ARR) was 4.4% and therefore the number to avoid one complication (NNT) was 23. There was an ARR of 1.1% for pulmonary morbidity (P = .07) when patients were treated laparoscopically, meaning that 91 patients would have to undergo laparoscopic surgery to prevent one pulmonary complication. No differences were detected for cardiac morbidity. The relative risk of wound infections was 0.65 (0.47–0.90) in the laparoscopic group (Figure 11.7.6) compared with conventional surgery. The ARR was 2.7% and the NNT was 37 patients. There was no difference in the risk of anastomotic leakage, intraabdominal abscess, or reoperation within 30 days after surgery. The relative risk of postoperative ileus was 0.45 (0.26–0.77) compared with open surgery (Figure 11.7.7). The ARR was 3.3% and the NNT was 31. Mortality was overall low, the relative risk in the laparoscopic group was 0.55 (0.26–1.18) and not significantly different between groups (Figure 11.7.8).

Long-term Outcome

Only few of the RCTs gave additional information on the long-term outcome of laparoscopic or conventional colorectal cancer resection.

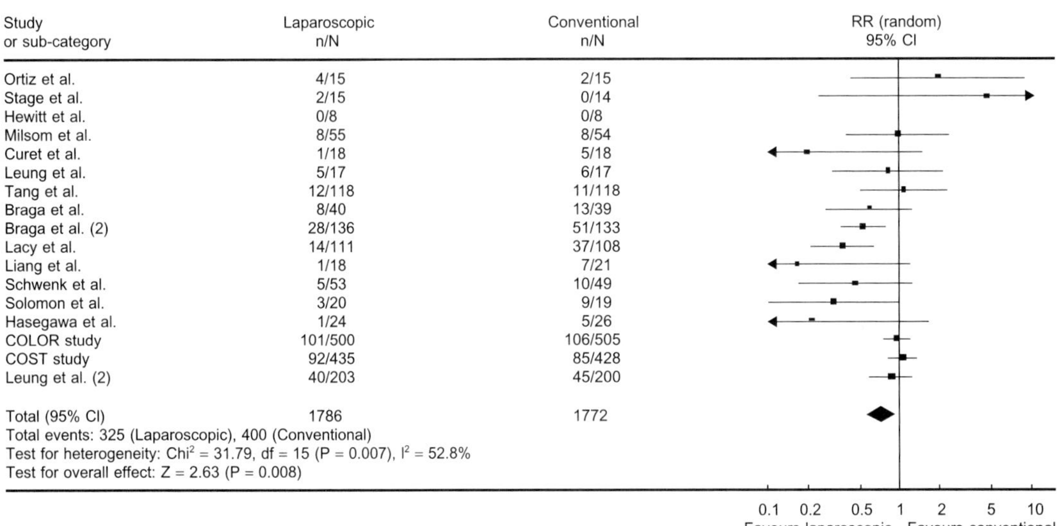

Review: Short term benefits of laparoscopic colorectal resection
Comparison: 08 Morbidity
Outcome: 01 Total
Study or sub-category | Laparoscopic n/N | Conventional n/N | RR (random) 95% CI
Ortiz et al. 4/15 2/15
Stage et al. 2/15 0/14
Hewitt et al. 0/8 0/8
Milsom et al. 8/55 8/54
Curet et al. 1/18 5/18
Leung et al. 5/17 6/17
Tang et al. 12/118 11/118
Braga et al. 8/40 13/39
Braga et al. (2) 28/136 51/133
Lacy et al. 14/111 37/108
Liang et al. 1/18 7/21
Schwenk et al. 5/53 10/49
Solomon et al. 3/20 9/19
Hasegawa et al. 1/24 5/26
COLOR study 101/500 106/505
COST study 92/435 85/428
Leung et al. (2) 40/203 45/200
Total (95% CI) 1786 1772
Total events: 325 (Laparoscopic), 400 (Conventional)
Test for heterogeneity: Chi² = 31.79, df = 15 (P = 0.007), I² = 52.8%
Test for overall effect: Z = 2.63 (P = 0.008)
0.1 0.2 0.5 1 2 5 10
Favours laparoscopic Favours conventional

Figure 11.7.5. Morbidity [(risk ratio (RR) including the 95% CI] after laparoscopic and conventional surgery for colorectal cancer.

Review: Short term benefits of laparoscopic colorectal resection
Comparison: 08 Morbidity
Outcome: 08 Wound infection

Study or sub-category	Laparoscopic n/N	Conventional n/N
Ortiz et al.	2/15	1/15
Curet et al.	1/18	1/18
Leung et al.	0/17	1/17
Tang et al.	3/118	3/118
Braga et al. (2)	8/136	20/133
Lacy et al.	8/111	18/108
Liang et al.	0/18	2/21
Schwenk et al.	1/53	5/49
Winslow et al.	5/37	5/46
Hasegawa et al.	1/24	3/26
COLOR study	18/500	16/505
Leung et al. (2)	9/203	15/200
Total (95% CI)	1250	1256

Total events: 56 (Laparoscopic), 90 (Conventional)
Test for heterogeneity: $Chi^2 = 10.23$, df = 11 (P = 0.51), $I^2 = 0\%$
Test for overall effect: Z = 2.57 (P = 0.01)

RR (random) 95% CI: 0.1 0.2 0.5 1 2 5 10
Favours laparoscopic Favours conventional

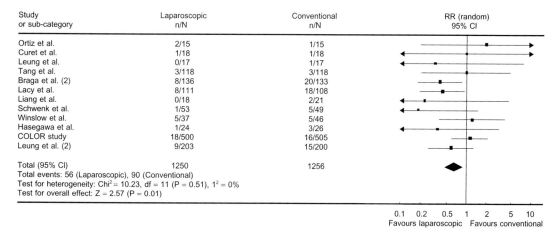

Figure 11.7.6. Wound infections (RR including the 95% CI) after laparoscopic and conventional surgery for colorectal cancer.

Length of follow-up was very short in 4 of 5 RCTs that provided long-term data. Only three trials with an adequate length of follow-up have been published by Lacy et al.,[3] Leung et al.,[4] and the COST Study Group.[5] All other RCTs giving follow-up data lacked a sufficient number of patients as well as an adequate length of follow-up. Therefore, these

Review: Short term benefits of laparoscopic colorectal resection
Comparison: 08 Morbidity
Outcome: 09 Postoperative ileus

Study or sub-category	Laparoscopic n/N	Conventional n/N
Ortiz et al.	1/15	0/15
Curet et al.	0/18	1/18
Braga et al. (2)	3/136	6/133
Lacy et al.	3/111	8/108
Winslow et al.	2/37	14/46
Hasegawa et al.	0/24	2/26
COLOR study	9/500	15/505
Total (95% CI)	841	851

Total events: 18 (Laparoscopic), 46 (Conventional)
Test for heterogeneity: $Chi^2 = 3.99$, df = 6 (P = 0.68), $I^2 = 0\%$
Test for overall effect: Z = 2.92 (P = 0.004)

RR (random) 95% CI: 0.1 0.2 0.5 1 2 5 10
Favours laparoscopic Favours conventional

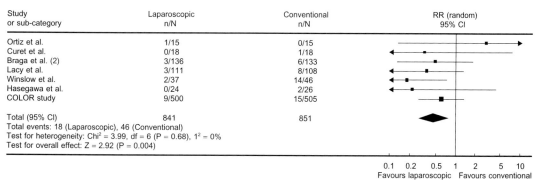

Figure 11.7.7. Postoperative ileus (RR including the 95% CI) after laparoscopic and conventional surgery for colorectal cancer.

Review: Short term benefits of laparoscopic colorectal resection
Comparison: 08 Morbidity
Outcome: 17 Mortality

Study or sub-category	Laparoscopic n/N	Conventional n/N	RR (random) 95% CI
Ortiz et al.	0/15	0/15	
Stage et al.	0/15	0/14	
Hewitt et al.	0/8	0/8	
Milsom et al.	1/55	1/54	
Curet et al.	0/18	0/18	
Leung et al.	0/17	0/17	
Braga et al.	0/40	0/39	
Braga et al. (2)	1/136	0/133	
Lacy et al.	1/111	3/108	
Liang et al.	0/18	0/21	
Schwenk et al.	0/53	1/49	
Hasegawa et al.	0/24	0/26	
COLOR study	6/500	10/505	
Leung et al. (2)	1/203	4/200	
Total (95% CI)	1213	1207	

Total events: 10 (Laparoscopic), 19 (Conventional)
Test for heterogeneity: $Chi^2 = 2.12$, $df = 5$ $(P = 0.83)$, $I^2 = 0\%$
Test for overall effect: $Z = 1.53$ $(P = 0.13)$

0.1 0.2 0.5 1 2 5 10
Favours laparoscopic Favours conventional

Figure 11.7.8. Mortality (RR including the 95% CI) after laparoscopic and conventional surgery for colorectal cancer.

three larger RCTs provided between 64% (locoregional recurrence) and 100% (port site recurrences) of the pooled data.

Rccurrences (Figure 11.7.9) and survival (Figure 11.7.10) were not different between both groups. See Table 11.7.2 for a summary of the outcome statistics.

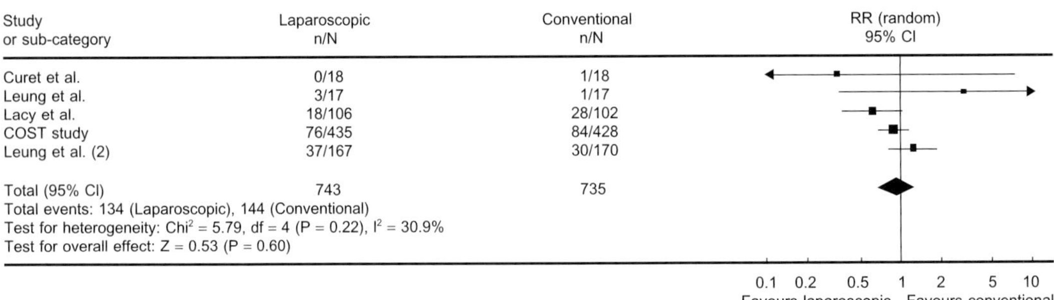

Review: Short term benefits of laparoscopic colorectal resection
Comparison: 10 Follow-up data
Outcome: 02 Recurrences
Study or sub-category
Laparoscopic n/N
Conventional n/N
RR (random) 95% CI
Curet et al. 0/18 1/18
Leung et al. 3/17 1/17
Lacy et al. 18/106 28/102
COST study 76/435 84/428
Leung et al. (2) 37/167 30/170
Total (95% CI) 743 735
Total events: 134 (Laparoscopic), 144 (Conventional)
Test for heterogeneity: Chi² = 5.79, df = 4 (P = 0.22), I² = 30.9%
Test for overall effect: Z = 0.53 (P = 0.60)
0.1 0.2 0.5 1 2 5 10
Favours laparoscopic Favours conventional

Figure 11.7.9. Tumor recurrence (RR including the 95% CI) after laparoscopic and conventional surgery for colorectal cancer.

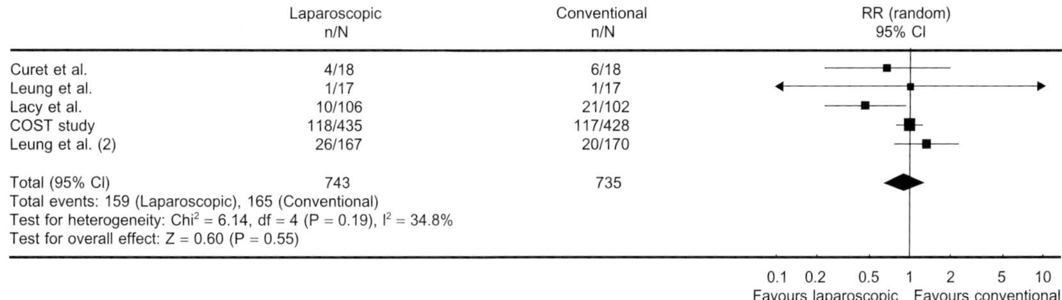

Figure 11.7.10. Long-term survival (RR including the 95% CI) after laparoscopic and conventional surgery for colorectal cancer.

Table 11.7.2. Comparison of outcomes of RCTs for colorectal cancer

Outcome	Studies	Participants	Statistical method	Effect size
Operative time	15	3571	WMD (random), 95% CI	50.34 [36.95, 63.74]
Blood loss	9	2248	WMD (random), 95% CI	−84.14 [−104.24, −64.04]
Bowel movement	8	2045	WMD (random), 95% CI	−0.93 [−1.10, −0.75]
Hospital stay	8	1666	WMD (random), 95% CI	−1.45 [−2.01, −0.90]
Morbidity	16	3558	RR (random), 95% CI	0.72 [0.56, 0.92]
Wound infection	12	2506	RR (random), 95% CI	0.65 [0.47, 0.90]
Postoperative ileus	7	1692	RR (random), 95% CI	0.45 [0.26, 0.77]
Mortality	6	2420	RR (random), 95% CI	0.55 [0.26, 1.18]
Recurrences	5	1478	RR (random), 95% CI	0.92 [0.67, 1.25]
Survival	5	1478	RR (random), 95% CI	0.90 [0.64, 1.27]

Discussion

Within 13 years after the first successful laparoscopic colectomies were reported by Jacobs et al.,[6] more than 30 publications from RCTs comparing laparoscopic and conventional colorectal resection have been published, mainly regarding colon and very sparingly about rectal cancer. When reports with no data on clinical outcome measures, repeated publications from the same trials, ongoing studies, and studies reported only as abstracts were excluded, 19 RCTs with more than 2700 patients were available for analysis.

Despite this huge number of patients included into the metaanalysis, we must recommend cautious interpretation of the data yielded by the identified RCTs. First, many of the RCTs are only small in size and the methodological quality (as far as it was assessable from the publications) was only moderate to poor in about 75% of all RCTs. Simple methodological principles such as the "intention-to-treat" analysis were disregarded in many of the RCTs. Therefore, a meaningful metaanalysis of the data from these trials is problematic. Furthermore, important data on perioperative treatment of the patients were missing in many of the RCTs. Especially the type of incision used for conventional surgery was only given by a minority of authors. All of those who reported the type of laparotomy used the traditional midline or paramedian incision, despite the fact that transverse incisions have been proven to diminish postoperative pain and pulmonary function when compared with midline or paramedian laparotomies. Even more important, the perioperative analgesic technique was not described in 9 of the 17 RCTs and in only 4 studies was a thoracic epidural analgesia used. As a side comment, Kehlet and coworkers have shown in many experimental and clinical trials that perioperative treatment may have a tremendous impact on the postoperative course after abdominal surgery. Effective thoracic epidural analgesia, enforced postoperative mobilization, and early oral feeding (so-called "fast-track" surgery) have an influence on almost all the functional parameters investigated in the 17 RCTs mentioned above. "Fast-track" surgery decreases median postoperative hospital stay to less than 5 days after laparoscopic as well as conventional colorectal resection and may also diminish the incidence of cardiac and pulmonary morbidity.[7–9]

Another important point to consider in this systematic review is the fact that most of the RCTs only included patients with cancers confined to one segment of the colon which was resectable by right hemicolectomy, left hemicolectomy, sigmoid resection, or anterior resection (for tumors >12 cm from the anal verge). Very few patients undergoing low anterior rectal resection or abdominoperineal resection of the rectum were included. Extended colectomies, as required in cancers of the transverse colon, were excluded from all RCTs. Only very few authors reported on how many patients fulfilled the exclusion criteria, why patients were excluded, and none of the trials included a follow-up of excluded patients.

The results of this systematic review of RCTs may be regarded as valid for patients treated with right- or left-sided colonic resection and high anterior rectal resection involving not more than one bowel segment and treated perioperatively in the traditional way with systemic opioid analgesia (either on-demand or PCA), nil-per-mouth for at least 24 hours after surgery, and no enforced mobilization. Considering these prerequisites, short-term significant benefits of laparoscopic compared with conventional colorectal resection were demonstrated for intraoperative blood loss, pulmonary function, duration of postoperative ileus, hospital stay, morbidity, and wound infections. Nevertheless, even advocates of laparoscopic colorectal surgery may be disappointed by the currently proven small extent of the benefits in pulmonary function detected for the laparoscopic group. Although the only disadvantage of laparoscopic surgery, an increased operative time of approximately 50 minutes is not only significant but also (economically) relevant, an ARR for pulmonary complications of 1.1% yielding an NNT of 91 is of questionable clinical relevance.

Because of the reduced size of incisions in laparoscopic colorectal surgery, the reduction of surgical complications, especially wound infections, may have been predicted by some laparoscopic surgeons. But even the reduction of morbidity by 4.4% and of wound infections by 2.7% could be argued to be small advantages for the trade-off of needing to learn an entirely new technique.

Although the incidence of mechanical bowel obstruction caused by intraperitoneal adhesions was not addressed in any of the RCTs so far, Winslow et al.[10] did not detect a difference in the incidence of incisional hernia in their RCT including only 83 patients. Therefore, these non-oncologic long-term results of laparoscopic versus conventional colorectal surgery have to be further investigated in RCTs.

Finally, only three RCTs with adequate sample size provide any data on long-term outcomes. In 2002, Lacy et al.[3] published a lower locoregional tumor recurrence rate ($P = .08$) and an improved cancer-related survival ($P < .05$) after laparoscopic compared with conventional resection. However, the results of this trial have been questioned by several other surgeons because of methodologic problems and clinically relevant differences in postoperative adjuvant therapy of laparoscopic and conventional patients. Furthermore, two RCTs published by Leung et al.[4] (including only rectosigmoid carcinoma) and the COST Study Group[5] did not find any differences in oncologic outcome. Altogether, pooled data from these three trials on tumor recurrences, port site metastasis, or survival were not different among groups. In summary, there is no evidence from RCTs today that long-term oncologic results of laparoscopic colorectal cancer surgery is superior or inferior to those achieved by conventional resection. Stated another way, the long-term oncologic results in RCTs, to this point, show no differences between the laparoscopic and conventional techniques, although longer-term follow-up is needed.

Conclusions

Our systematic review showed significant benefits of the laparoscopic technique: Less blood loss, shorter hospital stay, shorter ileus, less morbidity, and less wound infections. However, perioperative treatment of both groups was traditional in almost all RCTs under investigation. Modern multimodal concepts of perioperative treatment may improve the postoperative course regardless of the type of access to the abdominal cavity used.

Long-term outcomes (e.g., survival, recurrence, and complications such as adhesive obstructions and hernias) after curative laparoscopic or conventional resection of colorectal cancer cannot be assessed with adequate accuracy because results from larger multicenter trials are not yet available. Within the next 3 to 5 years, several multicenter randomized controlled studies from the United Kingdom (CLASSICC trial), Europe (COLOR and LAPKON II trials), and Japan (JCOG trial) will deliver data on long-term outcomes of more than 2000 additional patients.

Final Questions for Consideration

1. Does the laparoscopic approach lead to less morbidity?
   Yes (Recommendation A).
2. Does the laparoscopic approach lead to less mortality?
   It may have a moderate effect because the relative risk of the laparoscopic approach was lower (Recommendation A).
3. Has the laparoscopic approach led to any short-term advantages?
   Under traditional perioperative treatment, the laparoscopic treatment will result in less pain, less analgetic consumption, better pulmonary function, and a shorter duration of postoperative ileus. However, it remains unclear whether this will still hold true when a perioperative multimodal treatment is used (Recommendation A).
4. Does the laparoscopic approach increase hospital costs?
   Until now, no RCTs have addressed cost savings for the hospital or the society, if patients are treated laparoscopically. However, operative time is increased in laparoscopic surgery and this may increase costs caused by the operation itself. The true cost effectiveness of laparoscopic colon surgery has yet to be determined (Recommendation D).
5. Are the long-term results in favor of the laparoscopic approach?
   Oncologic results of laparoscopic and conventional resection of colorectal carcinoma do not seem to be different (Recommendation A).

   It has been hypothesized that the laparoscopic approach may reduce the long-term incidence of hernia, intraperitoneal adhesions, and reoperations for mechanical ileus. However, there are no data from RCTs available yet to support or contradict this hypothesis (Recommendation D).

References

1. Lacy AM, Garcia-Valdecasas JC, Piqué JM, et al. Short-term outcome analysis of a randomized study comparing laparoscopic versus open colectomy for colon cancer. Surg Endosc 1995;9:1101–1105.
2. Hazebroek EJ. COLOR: a randomized clinical trial comparing laparoscopic and open resection for colon cancer. Surg Endosc 2002;16:949–953.
3. Lacy AM, Garcia-Valdecasa JC, Delgado S, et al. Laparoscopy-assisted colectomy versus open colectomy for treatment of non-metastatic colon cancer: a randomised trial. Lancet 2002;359:2224–2229.
4. Leung KL, Kwok SP, Lam SC, et al. Laparoscopic resection of rectosigmoid carcinoma: prospective randomised trial. Lancet 2004;363:1187–1192.
5. The Clinical Outcomes of Surgical Therapy Study Group. A comparison of laparoscopically assisted and open colectomy for colon cancer. N Engl J Med 2004;350:2050–2059.
6. Jacobs M, Verdeja JC, Goldstein HS. Minimally invasive colon resection (laparoscopic colectomy). Surg Laparosc Endosc 1991;1:144–150.
7. Basse L, Hjort JD, Billesbolle P, et al. A clinical pathway to accelerate recovery after colonic resection. Ann Surg 2000;232:51–57.
8. Wilmore DW, Kehlet H. Management of patients in fast track surgery. BMJ 2001;322:473–476.
9. Schwenk W, Raue W, Haase O, et al. ["Fast-track" colonic surgery-first experience with a clinical procedure for accelerating postoperative recovery]. Chirurg 2004;75:508–514.
10. Winslow ER, Fleshman JW, Birnbaum EH, et al. Wound complications of laparoscopic vs open colectomy. Surg Endosc 2002;16:1420–1425.
11. Ortiz H, Armendariz P, Yarnoz C. Early postoperative feeding after elective colorectal surgery is not a benefit unique to laparoscopy-assisted procedures. Int J Colorectal Dis 1996;11:246–249.
12. Stage JG, Schulz S, Moller P, et al. Prospective randomized study of laparoscopic versus open colonic resection for adenocarcinoma. Br J Surg 1997;84:391–396.
13. Hewitt OM, Ip SM, Kwok SPY, et al. Laparoscopic-assisted vs. open surgery for colorectal cancer. Dis Colon Rectum 1998;41:901–909.
14. Milsom JW, Böhm B, Hammerhofer KA, et al. A prospective randomized trial comparing laparoscopic versus conventional techniques in colorectal cancer surgery: a preliminary report. J Am Coll Surg 1998;187:46–57.
15. Leung KL, Lai PB, Ho RL, et al. Systemic cytokine response after laparoscopic-assisted resection of rectosigmoid carcinoma: a prospective randomized trial. Ann Surg 2000;231:506–511.
16. Curet MJ, Putrakul K, Pitcher DE, et al. Laparoscopically assisted colon resection for colon carcinoma. Surg Endosc 2000;14:1062–1066.
17. Tang CL, Eu KW, Tai BC, et al. Randomized clinical trial of the effect of open versus laparoscopically assisted colectomy on systemic immunity in patients with colorectal cancer. Br J Surg 2001;88:801–807.
18. Braga M, Vignali A, Gianotti L, et al. Laparoscopic versus open colorectal surgery: a randomized trial on short-term outcome. Ann Surg 2002;236:759–766.
19. Liang JT, Shieh MJ, Chen CN, et al. Prospective evaluation of laparoscopy-assisted colectomy versus laparotomy with resection for management of complex polyps of the sigmoid colon. World J Surg 2002;26:377–383.
20. Schwenk W, Neudecker J, Böhm B, et al. Kurzfristiger postoperativer Verlauf nach laparoskopischen oder konventionellen Resektionen kolorektaler Tumoren. Minimal Invasive Chirurgie 2002;11:112–118.

21. Danelli G, Berti M, Perotti V, et al. Temperature control and recovery of bowel function after laparoscopic or laparotomic colorectal surgery in patients receiving combined epidural/general anesthesia and postoperative epidural analgesia. Anesth Analg 2002;95:467–471, Table.
22. Weeks JC, Nelson H, Gelber S, et al. Short-term quality-of-life outcomes following laparoscopic-assisted colectomy vs open colectomy for colon cancer. JAMA 2002;287:321–328.
23. Hildebrandt U, Kessler K, Plusczyk T, et al. Comparison of surgical stress between laparoscopic and open colonic resections. Surg Endosc 2003;17: 242–246.
24. Hasegawa H, Kabeshima Y, Watanabe M, et al. Randomized controlled trial of laparoscopic versus open colectomy for advanced colorectal cancer. Surg Endosc 2003;17:636–640.

Chapter 11.8

Dissemination of Tumor Cells During Laparoscopic Surgery

James Yoo

Because the most common indication for a large bowel (colon or rectum) resection in industrialized countries is adenocarcinoma, it is not surprising that the majority of the laparoscopic colorectal procedures in the early 1990s were done for this indication. Great controversy immediately enveloped the use of laparoscopy for colon and rectal cancer because it was a new technique and the phenomenon of port-site metastasis initially seemed to be somehow related to the laparoscopic technique. Early reports of port-site metastases in small case series as high as 21%[1] led to justifiable concerns over the oncologic safety of a laparoscopic approach to colorectal cancer, and many surgeons questioned whether there was a novel risk for tumor cell dissemination during laparoscopy compared with "open" or conventional surgery. Based on these early concerns, over the past decade, many clinical and laboratory studies were performed in search of a realistic incidence and for the etiology of port-site recurrences. Other concerns were whether there was accelerated or unusual tumor growth related to the laparoscopic technique. In this chapter, we will review the results of clinical and laboratory studies, along with currently available long-term data from large prospective randomized trials that have investigated the safety of laparoscopic approaches in the surgical management of colon and rectal cancers.

The Phenomenon of Port-Site Metastasis

Port-site metastasis is defined as cancer recurrence at a trocar insertion site without evidence of recurrence anywhere else, and was first described by Dobronte et al.[2] in 1978 after an ovarian cancer operation. Although the etiology is unclear, the development of recurrent cancer at a previous surgical site is not unique to laparoscopic surgery, but occurs after open surgery as well. Two retrospective reviews of open colectomy for colorectal cancers, with more than 1500 patients in each review, demonstrated a 0.6%–0.68% incidence of incisional tumors, with overall abdominal wall tumors having an incidence of 1%.[3,4]

Table 11.8.1. Incidence of port-site metastasis in randomized trials after laparoscopic (lap) or conventional (open) resection for colorectal cancer

Author	Year	Patients	Lap (%)	Open (%)	Follow-up (years)
COST study[43]	2004	872	0.5	0.2	Median 4.4
Lacy et al.[6]	2002	219	0.9	0	Median 3.7
Milsom et al.[44]	1998	42	0	0	Median 1.5

Multiple studies have now demonstrated that the incidence of port-site metastasis after laparoscopic surgery is much lower than originally reported. A prospective evaluation by the Laparoscopic Bowel Surgery Registry, which was initiated in 1992 by the American Society of Colon and Rectal Surgeons, the American College of Surgeons, and the Society of American Gastrointestinal Endoscopic Surgeons, reported the rate of this complication to be at 1.1%,[5] similar to open results (Table 11.8.1). Recent prospective randomized trials evaluating the outcomes of laparoscopic colectomies for cancer have also reported a very low incidence of port-site metastases.[6]

The Etiology of Port-Site Metastases

Although the etiology of port-site metastases is still unclear, the likely mechanism involves direct tumor cell contact and implantation. Possible contributing factors influencing tumor cell dissemination include:

1) Instrument or trocar/cannula contamination
2) Direct wound implantation (during specimen retrieval)
3) Trocar leakage of gas causing tumor cell implantation (so-called "chimney effect")
4) Trophic effects of the carbon dioxide (CO_2) pneumoperitoneum
5) Tumor cell aerosolization

These mechanisms have been studied in a number of clinical and experimental models.

Instrument or Trocar/Cannula Contamination

Tumor implantation and growth at trocar wound sites may occur as a result of direct contact after instrument or trocar contamination. Many experimental animal studies using a cell suspension model have been used to study this mechanism of port-site metastases. In this model, an inoculum of varying concentrations is injected intraperitoneally, followed by a variety of experimental conditions ranging from the placement and use of trocars, creation of the pneumoperitoneum using insufflation with various gases at varying pressures, and also open laparotomy. Although this experimental model is not likely to correlate with the clinical scenario present in humans, especially because the high concentration of tumor inoculum generally used does not mimic true intraperitoneal tumor concentrations, it has still provided a great deal of insight into possible mechanisms of port-site metastases. Several studies have used this model to demonstrate that trocar contamination is related to the concentration of tumor inoculum present, and that trocar contamination predisposes to tumor cell deposition directly at trocar sites.[7,8] Studies have also demonstrated greater contamination on instruments used by the operating surgeon as opposed to the assistant,[9,10] which is consistent with the finding that increased contamination occurs with increased trocar manipulation.[11]

Direct Wound Implantation/Cannula Leakage of Gas

Tumor shedding at the time of specimen extraction is another proposed mechanism for direct inoculation of wounds.[12] However, metastases have been clinically reported in port sites that had no direct contact with the surgical specimen.[13] Tumor adherence secondary to a cannula leak, presumably from contact of contaminated peritoneal fluid, may also theoretically occur and has been shown experimentally.[14,15] In fact, experimental models have demonstrated that cannula fixation, prevention of gas leaks, and rinsing of instruments, cannula, and wounds with povidone-iodine reduced the incidence of port-site metastases from 63.8% to 13.8%.[16]

Trophic Effects of the CO_2 Gas and Tumor Cell Aerosolization

Interestingly, port-site metastases have also been reported in the absence of obvious tumor manipulation,[17,18] suggesting that other factors come into play, such as the presence of CO_2 pneumoperitoneum or aerosolization of tumor cells. Very little is known about the effect of CO_2 pneumoperitoneum on intraperitoneal tumor growth.[19] Some animal models showed no difference in tumor growth comparing CO_2 laparoscopy, gasless laparoscopy, or midline laparotomy,[10,20–22] whereas others demonstrated greater tumor growth with CO_2 insufflation.[23–25] Intraperitoneal pressures have been shown in some studies to have no effect on tumor growth, whereas increased pressures significantly increased instrument contamination and tumor recurrence in other models.[21,26] Several studies suggest that stable aerosolization of cells after CO_2 insufflation does not occur in numbers that would lead to tumor implantation,[15,27] making this an unlikely mode of tumor cell transport.

Related Clinical and Laboratory Phenomena

There are many clinical reports that tumor cells have deposited at hemorrhoidectomy sites, fissures, and fistulas, suggesting that wound healing sites, which include cannula sites and midline abdominal incisions, may be rich in growth factors that create a favorable environment for tumor cell implantation and growth. Experimental animal models have shown increased tumor deposits at sites of tissue trauma.[14,28] If this mechanism does contribute to tumor growth, the risk of metastases after laparoscopic port placement would likely not be greater than from a larger abdominal incision after open colectomy. Tumor cell dissemination after surgery, whether laparoscopic or open, involves the liberation of viable tumor cells, transportation, and implantation at a new site, followed by growth. This process may occur through either direct contact, as described above, or via hematogenous spread. It is well known that 20%–40% of patients who undergo R0 resections (no detectable gross or microscopic residual disease at the time of surgical therapy) for "curable" colorectal cancer will still go on to develop recurrent disease. Presumably, disseminated disease is present but undetectable at the time of surgery. Minimizing further tumor cell dissemination at the time of surgery was the theory behind the "no-touch isolation" technique initially described by Barnes.[29] This technique argues for early lymphovascular pedicle ligation based on the concept that tumor cell dissemination may result from surgical manipulation. This technique has not gained widespread acceptance because of a lack of evidence demonstrating clear benefit. However, recent data involving the use of reverse transcriptase-polymerase chain reaction (RT-PCR) to detect occult tumor cells in blood and peritoneal fluid suggests that tumor cell dissemination does occur at the time of surgery.[30–35] The impact of laparoscopic techniques on tumor cell dissemination using similar methodologies, as well as the prognostic significance of these findings, has not yet been studied.[36]

The dissemination of viable tumor cells at the time of surgery may occur both hematogenously[37–39] and via direct tumor cell exfoliation into the peritoneal cavity. In a study by Hansen et al.,[38] blood collected from the surgical field in 57 of 61 patients who underwent open oncologic surgery contained tumor cells. Interestingly, peritoneal carcinomatosis and incomplete resection were present in only three cases, and intraperitoneal tumor cells were even identified in nine patients with T1 lesions. In this study, the number of intraperitoneal tumor cells increased with T stage, which supports the finding that advanced-stage cancer may be an independent risk factor for tumor dissemination.

Thus, there is a body of evidence that suggests that tumor cell dissemination after tumor manipulation does occur and may contribute to tumor recurrence that is seen in both open and laparoscopic surgery. In a study by Hayashi et al.,[39] evidence for tumor cell dissemination after tumor manipulation in open colectomies for cancer was evaluated using the mutant-allele-specific amplification method, which is based on the technique of PCR. Tumor cells were identified in the portal vein during resection of colorectal cancer in 8 of the 11 patients (73%) evaluated. Similar studies have demonstrated the new presence of tumor cells in peripheral blood after colorectal cancer resection in patients who had no preoperative evidence of disseminated tumor cells. Again, the clinical significance of these phenomena is unknown as yet.

Comparing the risk of tumor cell dissemination between laparoscopic-assisted and open colectomies, a human study by Bessa et al.[40] examined carcinoembryonic antigen mRNA levels by RT-PCR in the peritoneal fluid, portal and peripheral blood with specimens taken preoperatively, after tumor removal, and 24 hours later. They found that although neoplastic cell mobilization seemed to occur, there was no statistically significant difference between the laparoscopic and open groups. Further studies with larger sample sizes need to be performed, but this preliminary evidence using sophisticated detection systems suggests that the risk of tumor cell dissemination is not inherently different between these surgical approaches.

The Effects of Surgical Technique

These recent data imply that excessive tumor manipulation may increase the risk of tumor cell dissemination at the time of surgery, even though we do not as yet understand the long-term consequences of this. Because the performance of a laparoscopic colectomy is technically demanding, especially early in the learning curve, rough or repeated handling of tissues as this technique is mastered may contribute to increased tumor cell shedding and the risk of wound metastases. This has been demonstrated in several animal models.[41,42] In a mouse solid tumor model, isolated splenic tumors were established and then resected by either laparoscopic or open techniques.[41] The study showed that, because of the initial difficulty in performing the laparoscopic technique, rough handling of the tumor seemed to be associated with an increased incidence of abdominal wound recurrences compared with open resection. The incidence of abdominal recurrences decreased as the laparoscopic resection was performed with less grasping and manipulation, ultimately demonstrating the same incidence seen with open surgical techniques. Similarly, in the study by Hayashi et al.[39] described above, which identified tumor cells in the portal vein during resection of colorectal cancer in 8 of the 11 patients (73%) evaluated, when the no-touch isolation technique was used, only 1 of 7 patients (14%) had tumor cells identified in portal blood, suggesting that surgical technique may reduce hematogenous shedding of tumor cells during colorectal cancer resections. The prognostic significance of these findings is still unclear but warrants further investigation. These findings could be interpreted as follows: resection of colorectal cancer by the laparoscopic (or the open) approach is affected by the skill of the surgeon.

Summary

The current evidence suggests that the incidence of port-site metastases after laparoscopic surgery for colon and rectal cancer does not seem to be different from that seen after open procedures, a concept brought forward both in the previous chapter as well as this one. The levels of clinical evidence are primarily levels 2 and 3, with many animal studies supporting these clinical studies. These data also suggest that tumor cell dissemination after laparoscopic and open procedures may occur by a similar underlying mechanism, and that there are few data to support the early concerns that some type of unique tumor-disseminating mechanism exists for laparoscopic colorectal cancer surgery compared with conventional or open techniques. The pathogenesis behind this phenomenon of tumor dissemination during surgery has been studied in a number of clinical and experimental models, although its etiology still remains uncertain.

Poor surgical technique may be the most significant factor in increasing the risk of early tumor growth in surgical sites, regardless of whether the operation was performed laparoscopically or open. In support of this is the fact that the high port-site metastasis incidence, reported in small clinical series in the early 1990s, has not been seen in clinical series reported by surgeons who have a large experience in performing this type of surgery. Additionally, tumor dissemination at the time of surgery, or early recurrence at the wound after surgery may simply be a function of underlying tumor biology. This behavior is outside the bounds of what the surgeon may accomplish for his/her patient. In the meantime, strict adherence to the basic principles of oncologic surgery is likely to be the most important factor in minimizing this phenomenon.

References

1. Berends FJ, Kazemier G, Bonjer HJ, et al. Subcutaneous metastases after laparoscopic colectomy. Lancet 1994;344:58.
2. Dobronte Z, Wittmann T, Karacsony G. Rapid development of malignant metastases in the abdominal wall after laparoscopy. Endoscopy 1978;10: 127–130.
3. Reilly WT, Nelson H, Schroeder G, et al. Wound recurrence following conventional treatment of colorectal cancer. A rare but perhaps underestimated problem. Dis Colon Rectum 1996;39:200–207.
4. Hughes ES, McDermott FT, Polglase AL, et al. Tumor recurrence in the abdominal wall scar tissue after large-bowel cancer surgery. Dis Colon Rectum 1983;26:571–572.
5. Vukasin P, Ortega AE, Greene FL, et al. Wound recurrence following laparoscopic colon cancer resection. Results of the American Society of Colon and Rectal Surgeons Laparoscopic Registry. Dis Colon Rectum 1996;39: S20–S23.
6. Lacy AM, Garcia-Valdecasa JC, Delgado S, et al. Laparoscopy-assisted colectomy versus open colectomy for treatment of non-metastatic colon cancer: a randomised trial. Lancet 2002;359:2224–2229.
7. Brundell SM, Tucker K, Texler M, et al. Variables in the spread of tumor cells to trocars and port sites during operative laparoscopy. Surg Endosc 2002;16:1413–1419.
8. Hewett PJ, Texler ML, Anderson D, et al. In vivo real-time analysis of intraperitoneal radiolabeled tumor cell movement during laparoscopy. Dis Colon Rectum 1999;42:868–875.
9. Allardyce R, Morreau P, Bagshaw P. Tumor cell distribution following laparoscopic colectomy in a porcine model. Dis Colon Rectum 1996;39: S47–S52.
10. Wilkinson NW, Shapiro AJ, Harvey SB, et al. Port-site recurrence reproduced in the VX-2 rabbit carcinoma model: an in vivo model comparing laparoscopic port sites and open incisions. JSLS 2001;5: 221–226.
11. Allardyce RA, Morreau P, Bagshaw PF. Operative factors affecting tumor cell distribution following laparoscopic colectomy in a porcine model. Dis Colon Rectum 1997;40:939–945.

12. Paolucci V, Schaeff B, Schneider M, et al. Tumor seeding following laparoscopy: international survey. World J Surg 1999;23:989–995.
13. Nduka CC, Monson JR, Menzies-Gow N, et al. Abdominal wall metastases following laparoscopy. Br J Surg 1994;81:648–652.
14. Tseng LN, Berends FJ, Wittich P, et al. Port-site metastases. Impact of local tissue trauma and gas leakage. Surg Endosc 1998;12:1377–1380.
15. Whelan RL, Sellers GJ, Allendorf JD, et al. Trocar site recurrence is unlikely to result from aerosolization of tumor cells. Dis Colon Rectum 1996;39: S7–S13.
16. Schneider C, Jung A, Reymond MA, et al. Efficacy of surgical measures in preventing port-site recurrences in a porcine model. Surg Endosc 2001;15:121–125.
17. Neuhaus S, Hewett P, Disney A. An unusual case of port site seeding. Surg Endosc 2001;15:896.
18. Siriwardena A, Samarji WN. Cutaneous tumor seeding from a previously undiagnosed pancreatic carcinoma after laparoscopic cholecystectomy. Ann R Coll Surg Engl 1993;75:199–200.
19. Pearlstone DB, Feig BW, Mansfield PF. Port site recurrences after laparoscopy for malignant disease. Semin Surg Oncol 1999;16:307–312.
20. Lecuru F, Agostini A, Camatte S, et al. Impact of pneumoperitoneum on tumor growth. Surg Endosc 2002;16:1170–1174.
21. Agostini A, Robin F, Aggerbeck M, et al. Influence of peritoneal factors on port-site metastases in a xenograft ovarian cancer model. BJOG 2001;108: 809–812.
22. Dorrance HR, Oien K, O'Dwyer PJ. Effects of laparoscopy on intraperitoneal tumor growth and distant metastases in an animal model. Surgery 1999;126:35–40.
23. Jones DB, Guo LW, Reinhard MK, et al. Impact of pneumoperitoneum on trocar site implantation of colon cancer in hamster model. Dis Colon Rectum 1995;38:1182–1188.
24. Watson DI, Mathew G, Ellis T, et al. Gasless laparoscopy may reduce the risk of port-site metastases following laparoscopic tumor surgery. Arch Surg 1997;132:166–168.
25. Jacobi CA, Sabat R, Bohm B, et al. Pneumoperitoneum with carbon dioxide stimulates growth of malignant colonic cells. Surgery 1997;121:72–78.
26. Moreira H Jr, Yamaguchi T, Wexner S, et al. Effect of pneumoperitoneal pressure on tumor dissemination and tumor recurrence at port-site and midline incisions. Am Surg 2001;67:369–373.
27. Wittich P, Marquet RL, Kazemier G, et al. Port-site metastases after CO(2) laparoscopy. Is aerosolization of tumor cells a pivotal factor? Surg Endosc 2000;14:189–192.
28. Aoki Y, Shimura H, Li H, et al. A model of port-site metastases of gallbladder cancer: the influence of peritoneal injury and its repair on abdominal wall metastases. Surgery 1999;125:553–559.
29. Barnes JP. Physiologic resection of the right colon. Surg Gynecol Obstet 1952;94:722–726.
30. Sales JP, Wind P, Douard R, et al. Blood dissemination of colonic epithelial cells during no-touch surgery for rectosigmoid cancer. Lancet 1999;354: 392.
31. Chen WS, Chung MY, Liu JH, et al. Impact of circulating free tumor cells in the peripheral blood of colorectal cancer patients during laparoscopic surgery. World J Surg 2004;28(6):552–557.
32. Ito S, Nakanishi H, Hirai T, et al. Quantitative detection of CEA expressing free tumor cells in the peripheral blood of colorectal cancer patients during

surgery with real-time RT-PCR on a LightCycler. Cancer Lett 2002;183: 195–203.
33. Bessa X, Castells A, Lacy AM, et al. Laparoscopic-assisted vs. open colectomy for colorectal cancer: influence on neoplastic cell mobilization. J Gastrointest Surg 2001;5:66–73.
34. Guller U, Zajac P, Schnider A, et al. Disseminated single tumor cells as detected by real-time quantitative polymerase chain reaction represent a prognostic factor in patients undergoing surgery for colorectal cancer. Ann Surg 2002;236:768–775.
35. Yamaguchi K, Takagi Y, Aoki S, et al. Significant detection of circulating cancer cells in the blood by reverse transcriptase-polymerase chain reaction during colorectal cancer resection. Ann Surg 2000;232:58–65.
36. Tsavellas G, Patel H, Allen-Mersh TG. Detection and clinical significance of occult tumour cells in colorectal cancer. Br J Surg 2001;88:1307–1320.
37. Weitz J, Kienle P, Lacroix J, et al. Dissemination of tumor cells in patients undergoing surgery for colorectal cancer. Clin Cancer Res 1998;4:343–348.
38. Hansen E, Wolff N, Knuechel R, et al. Tumor cells in blood shed from the surgical field. Arch Surg 1995;130:387–393.
39. Hayashi N, Egami H, Kai M, et al. No-touch isolation technique reduces intraoperative shedding of tumor cells into the portal vein during resection of colorectal cancer. Surgery 1999;125:369–374.
40. Bessa X, Pinol V, Castellvi-Bel S, et al. Prognostic value of postoperative detection of blood circulating tumor cells in patients with colorectal cancer operated on for cure. Ann Surg 2003;237:368–375.
41. Lee SW, Gleason NR, Bessler M, et al. Port site tumor recurrence rates in a murine model of laparoscopic splenectomy decreased with increased experience. Surg Endosc 2000;14:805–811.
42. Mutter D, Hajri A, Tassetti V, et al. Increased tumor growth and spread after laparoscopy vs laparotomy: influence of tumor manipulation in a rat model. Surg Endosc 1999;13:365–370.
43. The Clinical Outcomes of Surgical Therapy Study Group. A comparison of laparoscopically assisted and open colectomy for colon cancer. N Engl J Med 2004;350:2050–2059.
44. Milsom JW, Böhm B, Hammerhofer KA, et al. A prospective randomized trial comparing laparoscopic versus conventional techniques in colorectal cancer surgery: a preliminary report. J Am Coll Surg 1998;187:46–57.

Chapter 12

Educating the Surgical Team

Kiyokazu Nakajima, Jeffrey W. Milsom, and Bartholomäus Böhm

Laparoscopic colorectal surgery requires advanced laparoscopic surgical skills such as full ambidexterity, the ability to manipulate fragile structures with long instruments under minimal tactile feedback, and the ability to identify surgical anatomy and dissect into proper tissue planes with two-dimensional images. Ideally, these skills are to be acquired in the operating room under adequate supervision of experienced laparoscopic surgeons. However, such a traditional type of teaching may be inefficient in initial phases of laparoscopic training, because novice surgeons are usually unable to mimic the movements of the more experienced surgeon without acquiring basic laparoscopic skills.[1–3] In addition, financial, moral, and ethical constraints have made teaching surgical residents in the operating room more difficult.[4] Therefore, a structured training program outside the operating room has become increasingly important.

Several options exist for teaching laparoscopic skills outside the operating room: e.g., introductory sessions, inanimate (bench) models, virtual reality surgical simulators, animal labs, and cadavers (Table 12.1).[2–5] Training program directors should be aware that each modality has its assets and shortcomings. The final goal is to "transfer" an improvement of skill level on these non-patient-based trainings into an improvement in operative performance. A team approach must also be emphasized, because without a skilled team (surgeon, assistants, and nursing staff), laparoscopic colorectal surgical efforts will founder. Ideally, the paramedical staff should be aggressively involved in introductory sessions and basic hands-on training courses to enhance their ability to troubleshoot problems related to the laparoscopic instruments and equipment.

Introductory Sessions

The introductory sessions initially involve short lectures for trainees to help in understanding basic principles of laparoscopic surgery. Through text, videos, and PC presentations, trainees can develop a perception

Table 12.1. Currently available modalities of "outside OR" laparoscopy training

Lectures
Didactic sessions (videos/textbooks)
Interactive sessions (PC-/web-based)
Live surgery observations (+telementoring)
Box trainers
Mechanical
Organ models
Tissue labs
VR surgical simulators
Animate labs (hands-on)
Cadaveric labs (hands-on)

of the essentials of laparoscopic surgery: e.g., how to prepare video equipment, how to select sites for port placement. In addition, ergonomic principles of laparoscopic surgery (e.g., optimal height of operating table, optimal working angle between two instruments) have to be taught at this phase of training, so that the trainees can start hands-on training after this lecture with maximal efficiency.[6]

With recent technological advances, multimedia interactive computer-based educational programs have become available, and have been reported to be effective to improve residents' subjective knowledge level and comfort level.[7] In addition to CD-ROM and DVD formats, internet-based educational materials (e.g., WebSurg) are also available.[8] Because these programs are basically self-directed and interactive,[7] trainees can learn basics and details of each specific procedure at their own paces, without supervision of senior surgeons. Although computer-based training programs will not totally replace traditional laparoscopic training courses, they will be a valuable adjunct in future laparoscopic training.

Inanimate Models

After the introductory session, the actual laparoscopic training begins using inanimate models (e.g., bench models or training boxes). The inanimate models are totally risk-free, reproducible, readily available, inexpensive, offer unlimited practice, and basically require no intense supervision.[4] The purposes of this training are: 1) To become comfortable working with both hands using laparoscopic instruments; 2) to become familiar with the video and laparoscopic equipment; and 3) to begin learning basic laparoscopic techniques.

The inanimate model is basically a clear (transparent) plastic box that may initially be used with direct visualization (without using a video camera) of instruments and models placed in the box (Figure 12.1).[9] Trainees can experience various types of drills by simply changing the models in the see-through box, and can gradually acclimate themselves to instruments that are limited in their range of motion by the fixation of the cannula. At this phase of training, use of various types of unique instruments (with pistol-grip handles) is strongly encouraged. Techniques, such as cannula insertion, "running" (manipulating) the small bowel, cutting, suturing, dissecting, knot-tying, and applying endoscopic clips/staplers may be practiced under direct vision. To promote efficiency of these practices, many kinds of training "modules" have been proposed from academic centers, and some of them have been validated.[4,9–11] Course tutors have to determine optimal combination of these modules according to trainees' basal (pretraining) skill levels and their demands.

Once the surgeon becomes comfortable performing these techniques under direct vision, the modules are placed in the laparoscopic training box, and the surgeon performs the same tasks under laparoscopic visualization with the video camera (Figure 12.2). This phase of training will require several hours of concentrated effort. The team must be capable of performing accurate and precise work in the inanimate model before graduating to the animal model. While the surgeon focuses on primary skills of surgery, the assistant surgeon should simultaneously practice similar skills on a separate trainer, or hold the video camera for the surgeon. The operating room nurses should use this time to familiarize themselves with equipment, assist the surgeon,

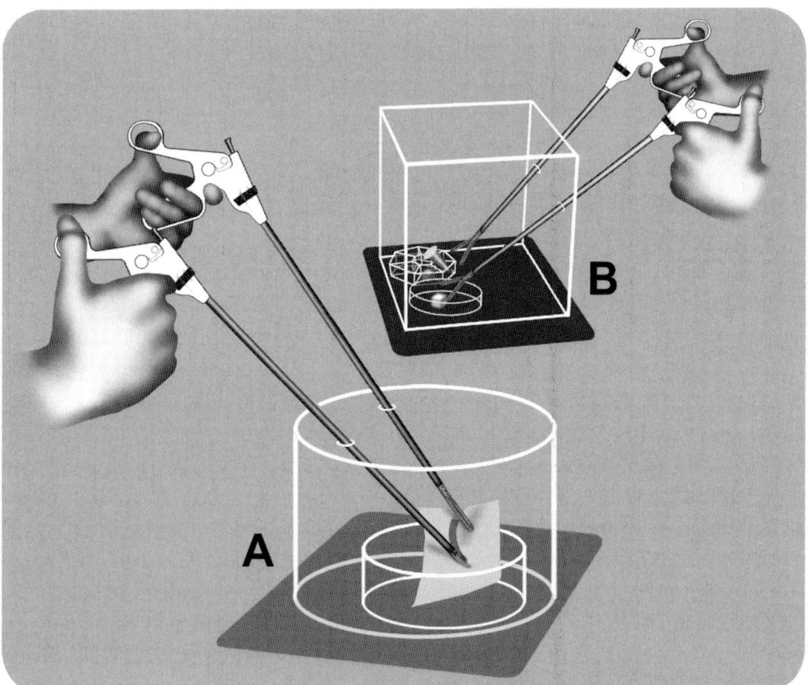

Figure 12.1. "See-through" training boxes for novice surgeons. Training is done under three-dimensional visualization so that trainees can first understand the unique action of delicate and long-handled instruments. **A** Pattern cutting. **B** Peg transfer.

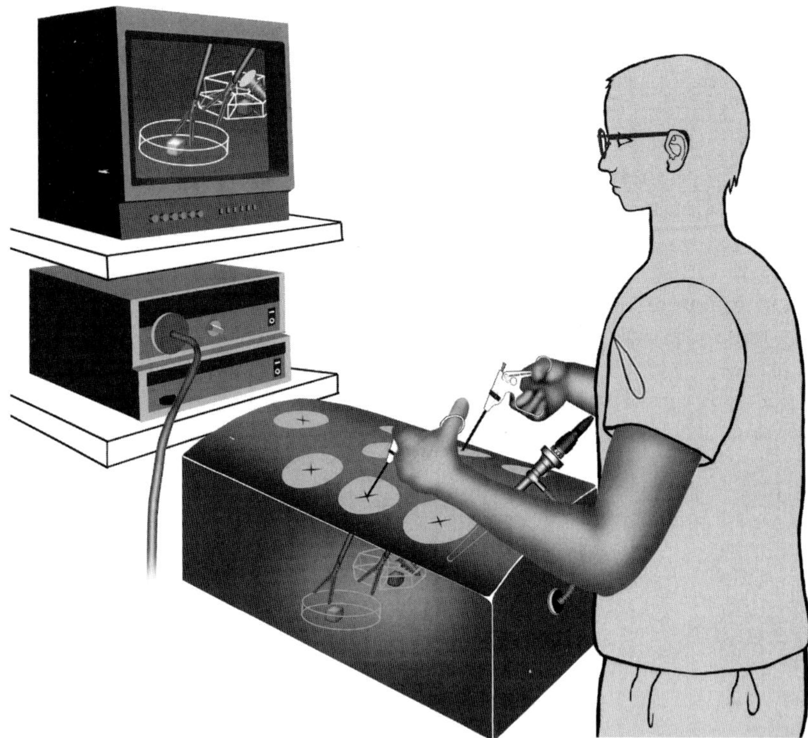

Figure 12.2. "Laparoscopic" training system for basic skill training under two-dimensional visualization. Currently, several systems are commercially available.

and learn the techniques so as to promote maximal efficiency in the operating environment.

Although training programs using inanimate models have become increasingly widespread, there remains one question raised by tutors and trainees: Can such programs provide residents with skills that are transferable to the operating room? Scott et al.[4] randomized 27 junior (2PGY and 3PGY) residents into two groups: A group that received formal inanimate training and a control group. The training group practiced the video-trainer tasks as a group for 30 minutes daily for 10 days, whereas the control group received no formal training. All residents underwent a video-trainer test and validated global assessment of their ability to perform a laparoscopic cholecystectomy based on direct observation by blinded evaluators before and after the rotation. The trained group achieved significantly greater adjusted improvement in video-trainer scores and global assessments, compared with controls. They concluded that laparoscopic training on bench models improves video-eye-hand skills and translates into improved operative performance for junior surgery residents.

Animal Models

Several studies have shown that large-animal models can be successfully used to perform laparoscopic intestinal resections and to develop intraperitoneal anastomotic techniques.[12,13] Although the use of large animals is becoming increasingly difficult because of restrictive legislation, public concern, and economic factors, we still believe that using animal models for training is justified because certain skills cannot currently be acquired in inanimate models: e.g., avoiding tissue injury while grasping tissue with instruments; controlling bleeding vessels with coagulation, ligation, or clips; and accomplishing intestinal anastomoses, especially those performed laparoscopically. These skills, practiced and perfected in animal models, are essential for safety and success in human laparoscopic colorectal surgery.[14]

Virtual Reality Simulators

The term virtual reality (VR) refers to a computer-generated representation of an environment allowing sensory interaction (sound, sight, and touch), thus giving the impression of true realism. Because of the nature of laparoscopy, it will likely benefit from developments in VR technology.[15] In fact, elaborating on the successful paradigm of flight-simulator training for pilots, the potential of VR applications for laparoscopic surgical skills training was proposed almost a decade ago. Recent advances in computer technology, combined with the consensus about the need for training surgeons outside the operating room but equally informative teaching settings, have led to the rapid development of laparoscopic VR simulators. Evidence has been accumulating that such simulators seem to be valid instruments in the acquisition of laparoscopic surgical skills. Moreover, a recent randomized trial has demonstrated that skills obtained through VR simulators can be transferred into the operating room.[5]

Ideal laparoscopic VR simulators must generate three-dimensional images on a two-dimensional monitor that appear to be "natural," allowing a high level of interactivity, stability, and reactivity to the surgeon's actions (Figure 12.3). Organs appearing on the monitor must be anatomically correct, with natural real-time deformation properties and resistance when manipulated, preserving natural traits such as bleeding or leakage when treated abusively.[5] Haptic feedback is optional; however, it will be provided in all types of simulators in the near future. VR surgical simulators are still expensive, but can potentially be a beneficial adjunct to traditional laparoscopic training programs outside the operating room.

One additional but significant advantage of VR surgical simulators is the ability to evaluate trainee's psychomotor skill level objectively.[15] Each trainee's psychomotor skill level can be easily scored and recorded. In case of MIST VR simulators, for example, each trainee's performance for both left and right hands, is objectively scored for time, error rate, and efficiency of movement for each task (Table 12.2). This use of VR

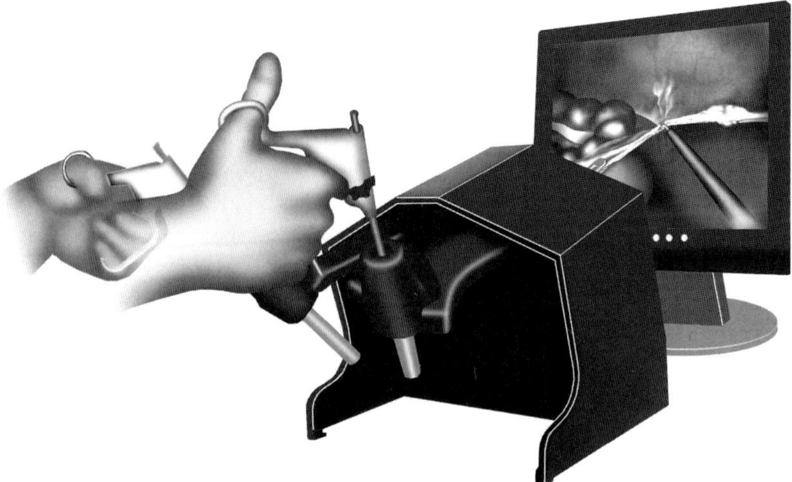

Figure 12.3. "Virtual reality" surgical simulator for advanced laparoscopic training. The risk-free training environment such as this may become a mainstream in future surgical education.

simulators as a metric has been considered to be important, providing trainees with a performance reference point.[1] This may help in setting the benchmark of training, and also help in keeping trainees highly motivated throughout the training program.

Cadavers

Cadavers have been used for centuries to teach human anatomy. In laparoscopic training as well, cadavers offer a high degree of fidelity to the living patient and a nonpressured learning atmosphere.[4] Creation of a pneumoperitoneum is simple and performed exactly as in the operating room. The gas is well maintained, is not absorbed, and does not leak, which leads to a significant reduction in gas utilization.[3] Cadavers do not bleed and hence allow a clear and bloodless vision of the surgical field.

Table 12.2. Summary of performance comparison by MIST VR before and after box training

MIST VR Parameter	Before training	After training
Number of target mispointing	0.9 ± 0.6	1.1 ± 0.4
Movement efficiency		
Dominant hands	6.2 ± 0.6	4.4 ± 1.3*
Nondominant hands	3.5 ± 0.3	3.9 ± 0.6
Time to complete virtual task (seconds)	28.2 ± 10.8	16.7 ± 5.8*

Lower value of movement efficiency means better performance. $^*P < .05$ versus before training.[9]

Although cadaveric laparoscopy training has not been well validated, previous studies have demonstrated that the anatomic landmarks were clearly visible in cadavers. The trainees were satisfied by cadaveric laparoscopy and found it superior to other teaching modalities. The tutors had considered the cadaveric training as satisfactory as well, mainly in terms of operative strategy, surgical anatomy, and the performance of specific procedures.

This modality has few limitations. Fresh cadavers have to be used and are not always readily available, making the logistics of such seminar courses more complicated.[3] Countries and cultures differ in their attitude toward utilization of human cadavers for teaching and research purposes. This may limit the worldwide acceptance of this modality. Cadavers do not bleed and one cannot learn the principles of hemostasis. Cadavers have noncompliant tissue that may be difficult to use for operations. Because of these limitations, we believe that cadaveric laparoscopy should not be an initial training tool. Laparoscopic training should be stepwise. Trainees should use inanimate models for basic skills and then perform large-animal laparoscopy to gain experience with hemostasis, dissection, and performing basic procedures. Cadaveric laparoscopy should be reserved for the advanced trainees, practicing colorectal procedures.

Human Laparoscopic Colorectal Surgery

Once proficiency has been achieved in inanimate trainers and animal/cadaver models, the surgical laparoscopic team may begin to consider human laparoscopic colorectal surgery. Although additional laparoscopic training opportunities after surgical residency (i.e., laparoscopic fellowship) have increased in general, only a few surgical training programs currently have formal training in laparoscopic colorectal surgery. Surgeons who want to start laparoscopic colorectal procedures must act as preceptors for other surgeons or surgical departments. Preceptors should have surgical privileges at the hospital so that he/she may perform at least some of the operative technique if necessary. Although the described large-animal models are valuable, human tissue dissection and anatomy may be quite different, particularly in pathologic states.

Initially, the beginner in laparoscopic colorectal surgery should choose simple, uncomplicated cases (such as diagnostic laparoscopy, biopsy, or loop ileostomy, or colostomy) in thin patients who have not undergone previous abdominal surgery. Next, the surgeon should proceed to limited resections for benign disease with or without intraperitoneal mesenteric dissection or anastomosis. More demanding procedures, such as resection for inflammatory bowel disease (such patients often have a thickened mesentery and inflamed fragile tissue) or oncologic resections, should be performed only if the surgeon is very comfortable with laparoscopic colorectal techniques.

The entire laparoscopic team must be involved in learning from the preceptor, because the skills of the entire team must be developed. This should involve preliminary discussions of every step of the procedure, from setup of the operating room to placement of the last suture, to postoperative care. The procedure should be standardized as much as possible so that all members of the laparoscopic team can predict what the next step in the procedure will be. Standardization will increase safety and efficacy of laparoscopic procedures and minimize frustration.

Establishing Structured Training Program

The long-term success and development of laparoscopic colorectal surgery (and all of advanced laparoscopic surgery, for that matter) rests on incorporating laparoscopic training into current surgical education programs. A well-structured laparoscopic training program will lead to overall improvement of morbidity and mortality rates after laparoscopic colorectal surgery.

References

1. Gallagher AG, Satava RM. Virtual reality as a metric for the assessment of laparoscopic psychomotor skills. Learning curves and reliability measures. Surg Endosc 2002;16:1746–1752.
2. Adrales GL, Park AE, Chu UB, et al. A valid method of laparoscopic simulation training and competence assessment. J Surg Res 2003;114:156–162.
3. Katz R, Hoznek A, Antiphon P, et al. Cadaveric versus porcine models in urological laparoscopic training. Urol Int 2003;71:310–315.
4. Scott DJ, Bergen PC, Rege RV, et al. Laparoscopic training on bench models: better and more cost effective than operating room experience? J Am Coll Surg 2000;191:272–283.
5. Seymour NE, Gallagher AG, Roman SA, et al. Virtual reality training improves operating room performance: results of a randomized, double-blinded study. Ann Surg 2002;236:458–463.
6. Berquer R, Smith WD, Davis S. An ergonomic study of the optimum operating table height for laparoscopic surgery. Surg Endosc 2002;16:416–421.
7. Ramshaw BJ, Young D, Garcha I, et al. The role of multimedia interactive programs in training for laparoscopic procedures. Surg Endosc 2001; 15:21–27.
8. Marescaux J, Soler L, Mutter D, et al. Virtual university applied to telesurgery: from teleeducation to telemanipulation. Stud Health Technol Inform 2000;70:195–201.
9. Nakajima K, Wasa M, Takiguchi S, et al. A modular laparoscopic training program for pediatric surgeons. JSLS 2003;7:33–37.
10. Jones DB, Brewer JD, Soper NJ. The influence of three-dimensional video systems on laparoscopic task performance. Surg Laparosc Endosc 1996;6:191–197.
11. Rosser JC Jr, Rosser LE, Savalgi RS. Objective evaluation of a laparoscopic surgical skill program for residents and senior surgeons. Arch Surg 1998;133:657–661.
12. Fleshman JW, Brunt M, Fry RD, et al. Laparoscopic anterior resection of the rectum using a triple stapled intracorporeal anastomosis in the pig. Surg Laparosc Endosc 1993;3:119–126.

13. Bohm B, Milsom JW, Kitago K, et al. Laparoscopic oncologic total abdominal colectomy with intraperitoneal stapled anastomosis in a canine model. J Laparoendosc Surg 1994;4:23–30.
14. Bohm B, Milsom JW. Animal models as educational tools in laparoscopic colorectal surgery. Surg Endosc 1994;8:707–713.
15. Schijven M, Jakimowicz J. Virtual reality surgical laparoscopic simulators. Surg Endosc 2003;17:1943–1950.

Chapter 13

Future Aspects of Laparoscopic Colorectal Surgery

Jeffrey W. Milsom, Bartholomäus Böhm, and Kiyokazu Nakajima

Ten years ago, the adoption of laparoscopic techniques into commonplace use in the practice of colorectal surgery was uncertain. Today, most surgeons would agree that this field is evolving rapidly, and some would say that minimally invasive surgery is only at its beginning. In this chapter, we will briefly present some of the interesting developments shaping the future development of the field of laparoscopic colorectal surgery.

Surgical Energy

The ability to successfully transect tissues without bleeding has improved dramatically in the past decade. The biggest changes have occurred with the use of ultrasonic tools and of the bipolar electrosurgery devices which permit rapid cutting and coagulation of even large vessels.

Prediction: In the next decade, many further developments in energy devices will occur, permitting faster, safer, and less traumatic division of tissues. These new tools will allow more facile dissection of tissues, and this will extend the range and safety of current laparoscopic methods. Example: A rectal dissection without blood loss, and clean and quick dissection of the correct planes, minimizing also the potential for nerve damage.

Computer-Assisted Instruments, Including Staplers and Endoscopes

Many of the decisions which only humans have made in the past will be made by computers. Current simple examples include the decision as to when the surgical tissue is safe to cut when the LigaSure bipolar instrument is used. A "beep" from the machine tells the surgeon that the impedance of the tissue is at a point that permits safe cutting of the tissue such that it will not bleed. An expansion of such decisions will be applied to stapling tools ("tissue is at the proper thickness to staple and cut") as is seen in the Powermedical stapling tools (New Hope, PA). All of their stapling devices are attached to a computer by a thick sterile cable, enabling feedback between computer and the human tissue. Another example of this type of interface will occur in the use of endoscopic tools in the operating room. Surgeons (and endoscopists) will increasingly rely on computer-acquired information to make decisions and treat patients.

Prediction: Surgical devices used in the human body will increasingly have interfaces with sophisticated monitoring equipment, which should allow for better judgment in the operating room (Is the tissue ischemic or not? Is this a malignant or benign process?), and more precise dissection of tissues. This will mean LESS and LESS invasive surgery, because the surgeon will know much more about the environment in which he/she is working.

Biological Glues and Adhesives

The role of these agents in the treatment of surgical diseases is increasing. Glues such as Tisseel (Baxter Healthcare Corp., Deerfield, IL) and BioGlue (Cryolife, Kennesaw, GA), which are derivatives of fibrin, are in common use in multiple disciplines such as vascular, cardiac, and neurosurgery. There they are used to stop bleeding from pinpoint areas. The companies manufacturing these products are exploring a wide array of clinical applications in the abdomen, and some areas, such as the cut edge of the liver, are ideal applications for an effective hemostatic agent. Cyanoacrylic glues also seem to be acceptable agents in the treatment of certain bleeding areas of the brain. There are countless possibilities for using such agents, especially if they can be inserted through laparoscopic applicators, or endoscopically.

Prediction: Biological glues and adhesives will expand dramatically over the next decade, and have the potential to challenge the suture and staple as a mainstay of tissue apposition. Laparoscopic and endoscopic applications will soon be used to supplement these current methods.

Robotics

There is no field of minimally invasive surgery that is more eagerly anticipated than the use of robotic tools. These tools have been shown to increase the precision of many surgical actions, including the suturing of small vessels. For radical prostatectomy, the current commercially available robot ("Da Vinci"; Intuitive Surgery, Mountain View, CA) seems to afford some advantages compared with open prostatectomy. Again, some of this is attributable to the magnification afforded by the stereoscopic laparoscope, and using the Da Vinci's small graspers equipped with wrists is also helpful in performing the cystourethral anastomosis. The field of laparoscopic colorectal surgery has not yet found applications mainly because of our needs to move through multiple quadrants of the abdomen while performing a single operation, which the current Da Vinci does not readily permit. Also, the use of the small robotic arms within the abdominal cavity does not easily permit retraction of the small and large intestines, a major impediment.

Prediction: Robotics will continue to improve, and the merging of surgical therapy and robotics will result in many applications, although this evolution will occur slowly because of the tremendous amount of technology and expense involved in making this transformation. Capsule endoscopy is a forerunner of such tools which may perform surgical actions, under guidance from a surgeon, or on their own ("seek and destroy missions").

Other Technologies of Importance

Image processing (e.g., miniaturization, three-dimensional, HDTV), changes in the laparoscope function and design, and use of wireless technologies will transform how we procure images in the operating room and use them in the surgical treatment of patients. Photodocumentation is now easy to obtain during any operation, and most are high-quality, digital images. Along with commercial applications, surgery will experience further important improvements in these technologies in the near future. Improvements in these images will accelerate our ability to transmit knowledge and teach new methods of minimally invasive surgery. This will lead to further progress in understanding diseases and progress in the treatment of patients.

Telesurgery

This topic deserves a separate discussion, although it involves many different technologies, techniques, and educational concepts. From the earliest time of using the miniaturized cameras of the laparoscope, the transmittal of these images to remote locations (telesurgery) has been a fundamentally important part of the "laparoscopic revolution" (Figure 13.1). This permitted many individuals to see, witness, and learn about new methods of performing surgery. For the first time, many surgeons could witness an expert throughout a complex operation, potentiating the learning experience of surgery.

The topic of telementoring deserves some mention. The possibility of an expert surgeon to observe, and render advice/teach actively during an operation which is some distance away from this expert, is likely to become an important part of the future of surgery (Figure 13.2). The possibilities of using such expert instruction from a distance means that new ideas and technologies could be quickly disseminated without the need for "on-site" instructions or labs, and it could also form a means of getting rapid operating room teleconsultations in remote areas, if the need arose, from a centralized source of expertise.

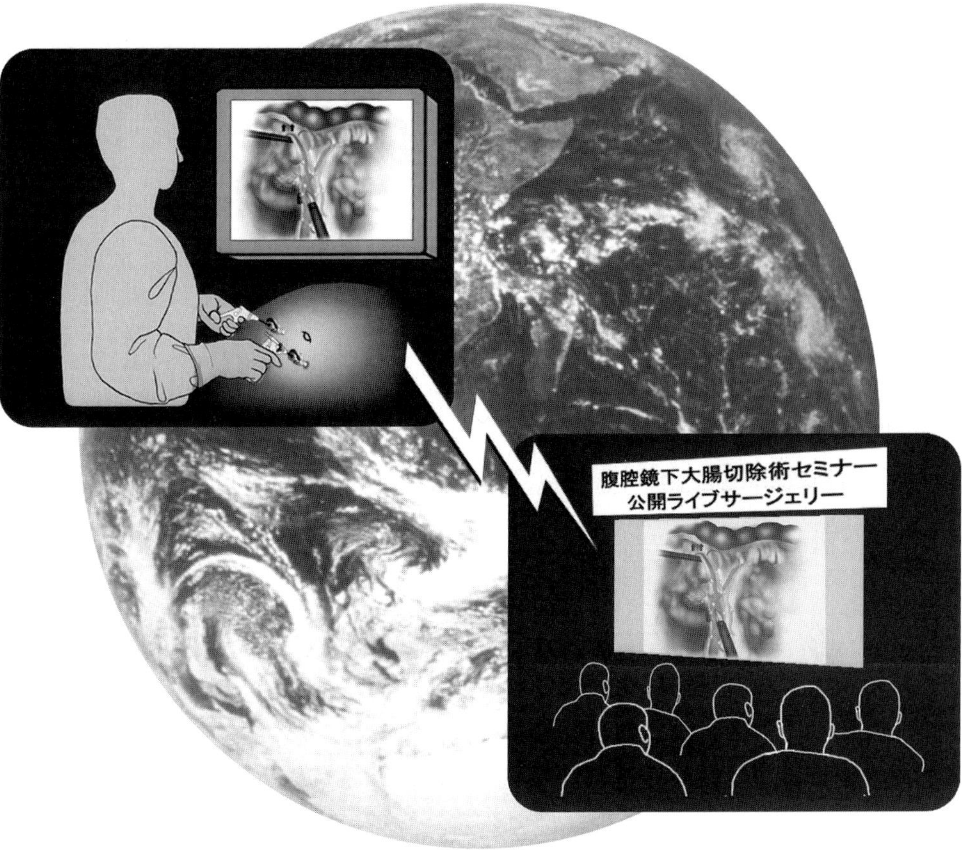

Figure 13.1. Telesurgery, now widely practiced, will expand in the future to permit more widespread dissemination of new ideas and technology.

A further source of expert help will combine telementoring with some of the emerging aspects of robotics, telepresence, and miniaturization of instruments. This means that the expert surgeon will be capable of entering the operating room as a "robotic" surgeon and performing surgical actions, assisting the team there (Figure 13.3). Even our uses of robotics will change, because robots may be expected to enter the body on their own, identify body structures, and make decisions with or without human directions (Figure 13.4). This scenario will challenge both our technological as well as ethical frontiers, and it is one that we must prepare for, because there is no doubt, at least among the editors of this book, that this will occur.

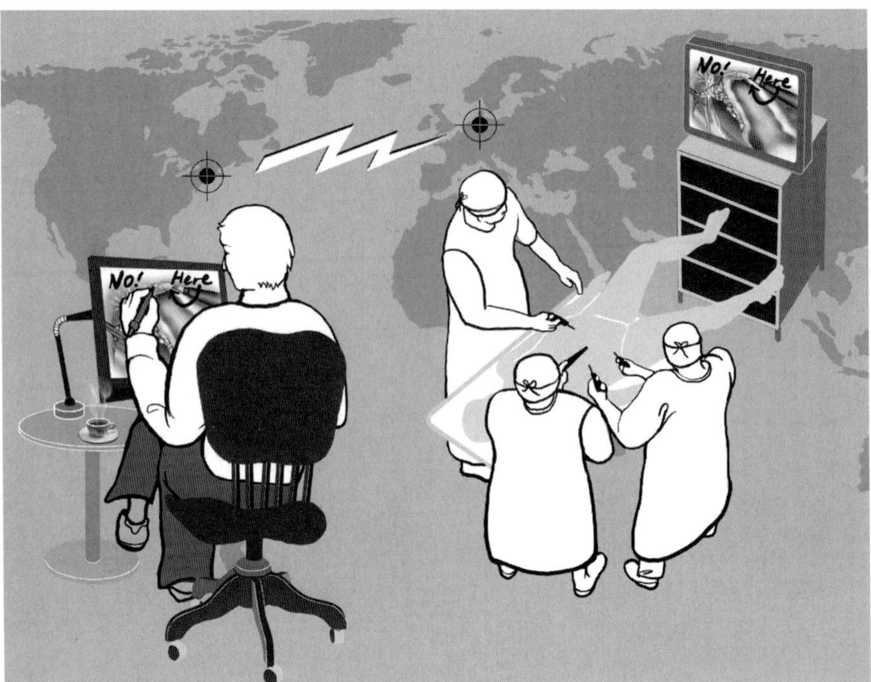

Figure 13.2. Telementoring, which involves direct instruction of a laparoscopic mentor interacting with a surgical team in real time, will expand the use of new methods and technologies.

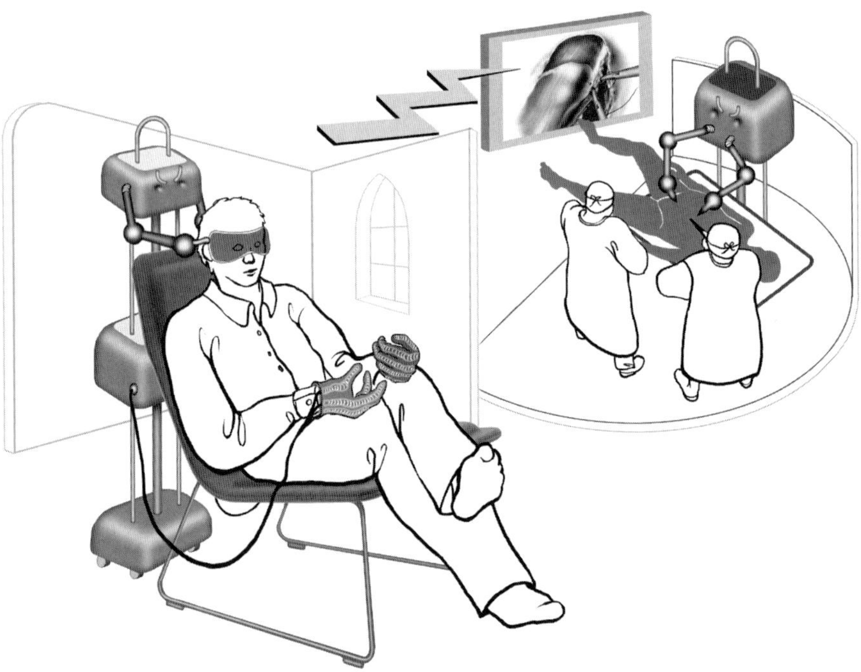

Figure 13.3. Robotic-assisted surgery will permit surgical experts to DIRECTLY perform surgeries in remote locations, with the assistance of a local team.

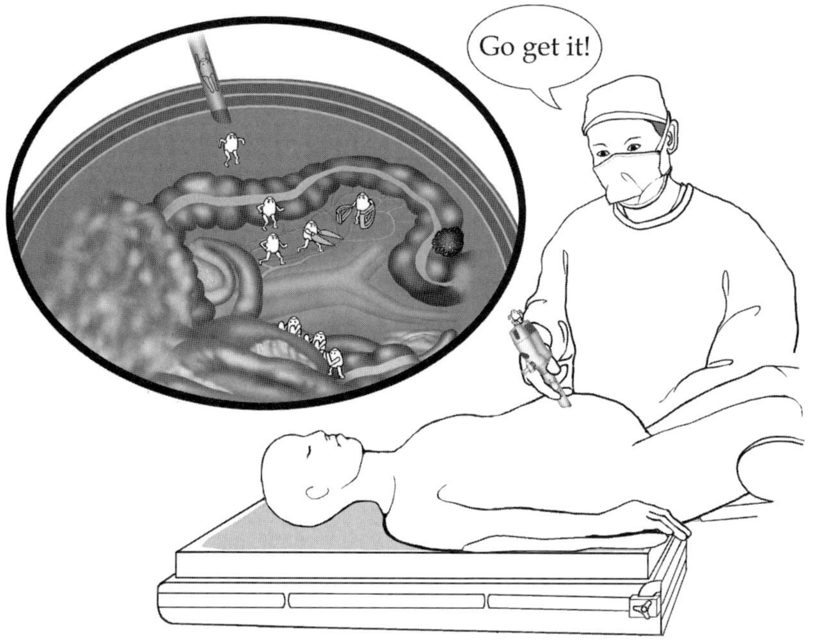

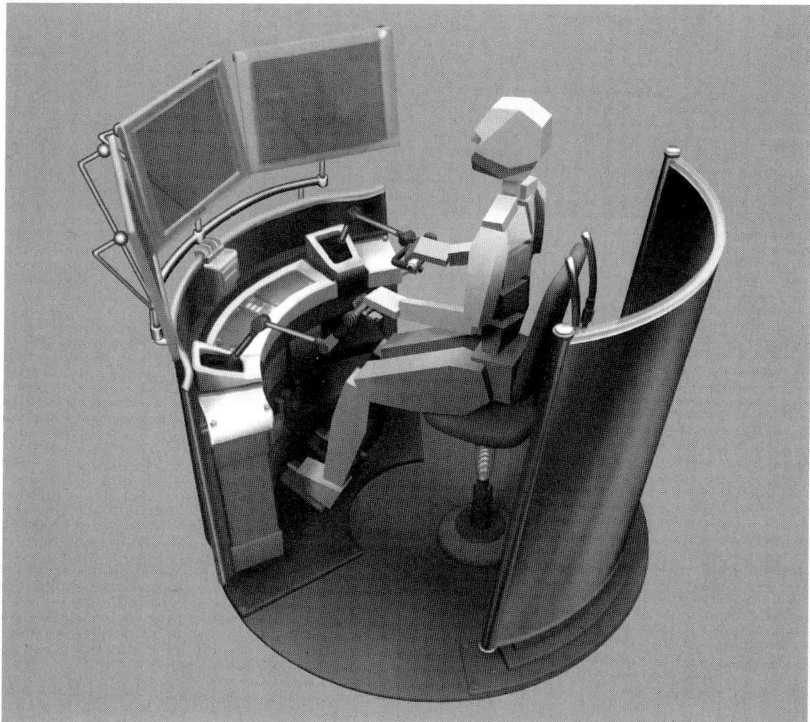

Figure 13.4. A Minute robots themselves, under the guidance of surgical experts, may be expected to actively enter the scene of surgery in the future. **B** Robots may also actively enter the scene of surgery to make complex decisions about cases on their own. This could be particularly important in battlefield situations, where actual surgeons would be directing the robots from a "safe" location.

Conclusions

The field of laparoscopic colorectal surgery is squarely in the middle of the great technological changes that are occurring in surgery. The complexity of laparoscopic colorectal procedures has made it necessary to proceed slowly over the first decade, but now many new tools are emerging that are going to improve on the efficiencies and outcomes of patients requiring laparoscopic treatment of their colorectal diseases.

We have reviewed some of the important changes occurring, albeit briefly, which are now upon us, and have also made some predictions.

The operating room of the future will be a highly complex environment, filled with tools that will change the outcomes of patients in a dramatically positive way. The potential for improvements will depend on the cooperation of surgeons and the surgical industries to continue to innovate and work together.

Index

C

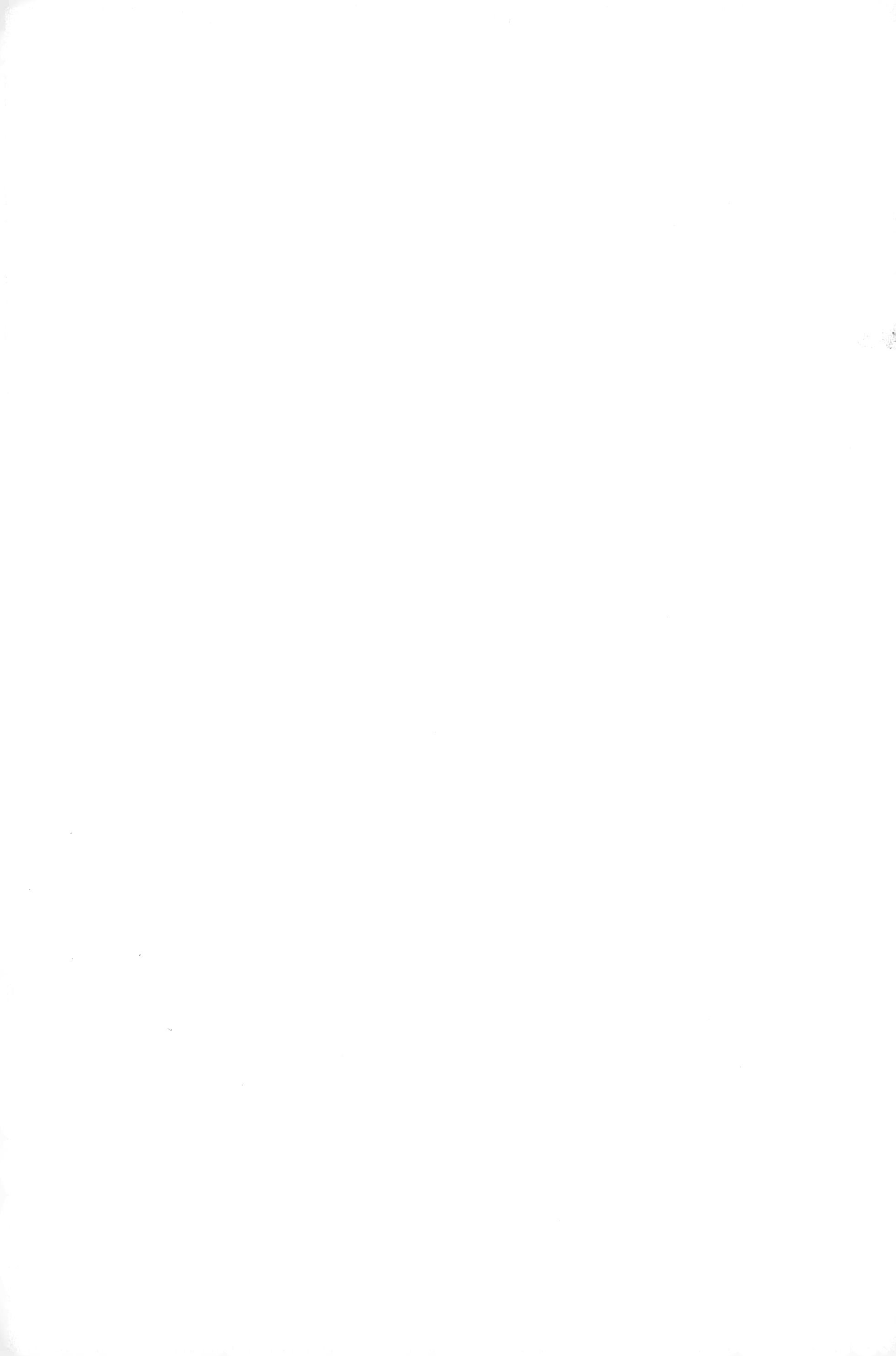